BIOTHERAPEUTIC APPROACHES TO ASTHMA

LUNG BIOLOGY IN HEALTH AND DISEASE

1. Immunologic and Infectious Reactions in the Lung, *edited by C. H. Kirkpatrick and H. Y. Reynolds*
2. The Biochemical Basis of Pulmonary Function, *edited by R. G. Crystal*
3. Bioengineering Aspects of the Lung, *edited by J. B. West*
4. Metabolic Functions of the Lung, *edited by Y. S. Bakhle and J. R. Vane*
5. Respiratory Defense Mechanisms (in two parts), *edited by J. D. Brain, D. F. Proctor, and L. M. Reid*
6. Development of the Lung, *edited by W. A. Hodson*
7. Lung Water and Solute Exchange, *edited by N. C. Staub*
8. Extrapulmonary Manifestations of Respiratory Disease, *edited by E. D. Robin*
9. Chronic Obstructive Pulmonary Disease, *edited by T. L. Petty*
10. Pathogenesis and Therapy of Lung Cancer, *edited by C. C. Harris*
11. Genetic Determinants of Pulmonary Disease, *edited by S. D. Litwin*
12. The Lung in the Transition Between Health and Disease, *edited by P. T. Macklem and S. Permutt*
13. Evolution of Respiratory Processes: A Comparative Approach, *edited by S. C. Wood and C. Lenfant*
14. Pulmonary Vascular Diseases, *edited by K. M. Moser*
15. Physiology and Pharmacology of the Airways, *edited by J. A. Nadel*
16. Diagnostic Techniques in Pulmonary Disease (in two parts), *edited by M. A. Sackner*
17. Regulation of Breathing (in two parts), *edited by T. F. Hornbein*
18. Occupational Lung Diseases: Research Approaches and Methods, *edited by H. Weill and M. Turner-Warwick*
19. Immunopharmacology of the Lung, *edited by H. H. Newball*
20. Sarcoidosis and Other Granulomatous Diseases of the Lung, *edited by B. L. Fanburg*
21. Sleep and Breathing, *edited by N. A. Saunders and C. E. Sullivan*
22. *Pneumocystis carinii* Pneumonia: Pathogenesis, Diagnosis, and Treatment, *edited by L. S. Young*
23. Pulmonary Nuclear Medicine: Techniques in Diagnosis of Lung Disease, *edited by H. L. Atkins*
24. Acute Respiratory Failure, *edited by W. M. Zapol and K. J. Falke*
25. Gas Mixing and Distribution in the Lung, *edited by L. A. Engel and M. Paiva*

26. High-Frequency Ventilation in Intensive Care and During Surgery, *edited by G. Carlon and W. S. Howland*
27. Pulmonary Development: Transition from Intrauterine to Extrauterine Life, *edited by G. H. Nelson*
28. Chronic Obstructive Pulmonary Disease: Second Edition, *edited by T. L. Petty*
29. The Thorax (in two parts), *edited by C. Roussos and P. T. Macklem*
30. The Pleura in Health and Disease, *edited by J. Chrétien, J. Bignon, and A. Hirsch*
31. Drug Therapy for Asthma: Research and Clinical Practice, *edited by J. W. Jenne and S. Murphy*
32. Pulmonary Endothelium in Health and Disease, *edited by U. S. Ryan*
33. The Airways: Neural Control in Health and Disease, *edited by M. A. Kaliner and P. J. Barnes*
34. Pathophysiology and Treatment of Inhalation Injuries, *edited by J. Loke*
35. Respiratory Function of the Upper Airway, *edited by O. P. Mathew and G. Sant'Ambrogio*
36. Chronic Obstructive Pulmonary Disease: A Behavioral Perspective, *edited by A. J. McSweeny and I. Grant*
37. Biology of Lung Cancer: Diagnosis and Treatment, *edited by S. T. Rosen, J. L. Mulshine, F. Cuttitta, and P. G. Abrams*
38. Pulmonary Vascular Physiology and Pathophysiology, *edited by E. K. Weir and J. T. Reeves*
39. Comparative Pulmonary Physiology: Current Concepts, *edited by S. C. Wood*
40. Respiratory Physiology: An Analytical Approach, *edited by H. K. Chang and M. Paiva*
41. Lung Cell Biology, *edited by D. Massaro*
42. Heart–Lung Interactions in Health and Disease, *edited by S. M. Scharf and S. S. Cassidy*
43. Clinical Epidemiology of Chronic Obstructive Pulmonary Disease, *edited by M. J. Hensley and N. A. Saunders*
44. Surgical Pathology of Lung Neoplasms, *edited by A. M. Marchevsky*
45. The Lung in Rheumatic Diseases, *edited by G. W. Cannon and G. A. Zimmerman*
46. Diagnostic Imaging of the Lung, *edited by C. E. Putman*
47. Models of Lung Disease: Microscopy and Structural Methods, *edited by J. Gil*
48. Electron Microscopy of the Lung, *edited by D. E. Schraufnagel*
49. Asthma: Its Pathology and Treatment, *edited by M. A. Kaliner, P. J. Barnes, and C. G. A. Persson*
50. Acute Respiratory Failure: Second Edition, *edited by W. M. Zapol and F. Lemaire*
51. Lung Disease in the Tropics, *edited by O. P. Sharma*
52. Exercise: Pulmonary Physiology and Pathophysiology, *edited by B. J. Whipp and K. Wasserman*
53. Developmental Neurobiology of Breathing, *edited by G. G. Haddad and J. P. Farber*
54. Mediators of Pulmonary Inflammation, *edited by M. A. Bray and W. H. Anderson*
55. The Airway Epithelium, *edited by S. G. Farmer and D. Hay*

56. Physiological Adaptations in Vertebrates: Respiration, Circulation, and Metabolism, *edited by S. C. Wood, R. E. Weber, A. R. Hargens, and R. W. Millard*
57. The Bronchial Circulation, *edited by J. Butler*
58. Lung Cancer Differentiation: Implications for Diagnosis and Treatment, *edited by S. D. Bernal and P. J. Hesketh*
59. Pulmonary Complications of Systemic Disease, *edited by J. F. Murray*
60. Lung Vascular Injury: Molecular and Cellular Response, *edited by A. Johnson and T. J. Ferro*
61. Cytokines of the Lung, *edited by J. Kelley*
62. The Mast Cell in Health and Disease, *edited by M. A. Kaliner and D. D. Metcalfe*
63. Pulmonary Disease in the Elderly Patient, *edited by D. A. Mahler*
64. Cystic Fibrosis, *edited by P. B. Davis*
65. Signal Transduction in Lung Cells, *edited by J. S. Brody, D. M. Center, and V. A. Tkachuk*
66. Tuberculosis: A Comprehensive International Approach, *edited by L. B. Reichman and E. S. Hershfield*
67. Pharmacology of the Respiratory Tract: Experimental and Clinical Research, *edited by K. F. Chung and P. J. Barnes*
68. Prevention of Respiratory Diseases, *edited by A. Hirsch, M. Goldberg, J.-P. Martin, and R. Masse*
69. *Pneumocystis carinii* Pneumonia: Second Edition, *edited by P. D. Walzer*
70. Fluid and Solute Transport in the Airspaces of the Lungs, *edited by R. M. Effros and H. K. Chang*
71. Sleep and Breathing: Second Edition, *edited by N. A. Saunders and C. E. Sullivan*
72. Airway Secretion: Physiological Bases for the Control of Mucous Hypersecretion, *edited by T. Takishima and S. Shimura*
73. Sarcoidosis and Other Granulomatous Disorders, *edited by D. G. James*
74. Epidemiology of Lung Cancer, *edited by J. M. Samet*
75. Pulmonary Embolism, *edited by M. Morpurgo*
76. Sports and Exercise Medicine, *edited by S. C. Wood and R. C. Roach*
77. Endotoxin and the Lungs, *edited by K. L. Brigham*
78. The Mesothelial Cell and Mesothelioma, *edited by M.-C. Jaurand and J. Bignon*
79. Regulation of Breathing: Second Edition, *edited by J. A. Dempsey and A. I. Pack*
80. Pulmonary Fibrosis, *edited by S. Hin. Phan and R. S. Thrall*
81. Long-Term Oxygen Therapy: Scientific Basis and Clinical Application, *edited by W. J. O'Donohue, Jr.*
82. Ventral Brainstem Mechanisms and Control of Respiration and Blood Pressure, *edited by C. O. Trouth, R. M. Millis, H. F. Kiwull-Schöne, and M. E. Schläfke*
83. A History of Breathing Physiology, *edited by D. F. Proctor*
84. Surfactant Therapy for Lung Disease, *edited by B. Robertson and H. W. Taeusch*
85. The Thorax: Second Edition, Revised and Expanded (in three parts), *edited by C. Roussos*

86. Severe Asthma: Pathogenesis and Clinical Management, *edited by S. J. Szefler and D. Y. M. Leung*
87. *Mycobacterium avium*–Complex Infection: Progress in Research and Treatment, *edited by J. A. Korvick and C. A. Benson*
88. Alpha 1–Antitrypsin Deficiency: Biology • Pathogenesis • Clinical Manifestations • Therapy, *edited by R. G. Crystal*
89. Adhesion Molecules and the Lung, *edited by P. A. Ward and J. C. Fantone*
90. Respiratory Sensation, *edited by L. Adams and A. Guz*
91. Pulmonary Rehabilitation, *edited by A. P. Fishman*
92. Acute Respiratory Failure in Chronic Obstructive Pulmonary Disease, *edited by J.-P. Derenne, W. A. Whitelaw, and T. Similowski*
93. Environmental Impact on the Airways: From Injury to Repair, *edited by J. Chrétien and D. Dusser*
94. Inhalation Aerosols: Physical and Biological Basis for Therapy, *edited by A. J. Hickey*
95. Tissue Oxygen Deprivation: From Molecular to Integrated Function, *edited by G. G. Haddad and G. Lister*
96. The Genetics of Asthma, *edited by S. B. Liggett and D. A. Meyers*
97. Inhaled Glucocorticoids in Asthma: Mechanisms and Clinical Actions, *edited by R. P. Schleimer, W. W. Busse, and P. M. O'Byrne*
98. Nitric Oxide and the Lung, *edited by W. M. Zapol and K. D. Bloch*
99. Primary Pulmonary Hypertension, *edited by L. J. Rubin and S. Rich*
100. Lung Growth and Development, *edited by J. A. McDonald*
101. Parasitic Lung Diseases, *edited by A. A. F. Mahmoud*
102. Lung Macrophages and Dendritic Cells in Health and Disease, *edited by M. F. Lipscomb and S. W. Russell*
103. Pulmonary and Cardiac Imaging, *edited by C. Chiles and C. E. Putman*
104. Gene Therapy for Diseases of the Lung, *edited by K. L. Brigham*
105. Oxygen, Gene Expression, and Cellular Function, *edited by L. Biadasz Clerch and D. J. Massaro*
106. Beta$_2$-Agonists in Asthma Treatment, *edited by R. Pauwels and P. M. O'Byrne*
107. Inhalation Delivery of Therapeutic Peptides and Proteins, *edited by A. L. Adjei and P. K. Gupta*
108. Asthma in the Elderly, *edited by R. A. Barbee and J. W. Bloom*
109. Treatment of the Hospitalized Cystic Fibrosis Patient, *edited by D. M. Orenstein and R. C. Stern*
110. Asthma and Immunological Diseases in Pregnancy and Early Infancy, *edited by M. Schatz, R. S. Zeiger, and H. N. Claman*
111. Dyspnea, *edited by D. A. Mahler*
112. Proinflammatory and Antiinflammatory Peptides, *edited by S. I. Said*
113. Self-Management of Asthma, *edited by H. Kotses and A. Harver*
114. Eicosanoids, Aspirin, and Asthma, *edited by A. Szczeklik, R. J. Gryglewski, and J. R. Vane*
115. Fatal Asthma, *edited by A. L. Sheffer*
116. Pulmonary Edema, *edited by M. A. Matthay and D. H. Ingbar*
117. Inflammatory Mechanisms in Asthma, *edited by S. T. Holgate and W. W. Busse*
118. Physiological Basis of Ventilatory Support, *edited by J. J. Marini and A. S. Slutsky*

119. Human Immunodeficiency Virus and the Lung, *edited by M. J. Rosen and J. M. Beck*
120. Five-Lipoxygenase Products in Asthma, *edited by J. M. Drazen, S.-E. Dahlén, and T. H. Lee*
121. Complexity in Structure and Function of the Lung, *edited by M. P. Hlastala and H. T. Robertson*
122. Biology of Lung Cancer, *edited by M. A. Kane and P. A. Bunn, Jr.*
123. Rhinitis: Mechanisms and Management, *edited by R. M. Naclerio, S. R. Durham, and N. Mygind*
124. Lung Tumors: Fundamental Biology and Clinical Management, *edited by C. Brambilla and E. Brambilla*
125. Interleukin-5: From Molecule to Drug Target for Asthma, *edited by C. J. Sanderson*
126. Pediatric Asthma, *edited by S. Murphy and H. W. Kelly*
127. Viral Infections of the Respiratory Tract, *edited by R. Dolin and P. F. Wright*
128. Air Pollutants and the Respiratory Tract, *edited by D. L. Swift and W. M. Foster*
129. Gastroesophageal Reflux Disease and Airway Disease, *edited by M. R. Stein*
130. Exercise-Induced Asthma, *edited by E. R. McFadden, Jr.*
131. LAM and Other Diseases Characterized by Smooth Muscle Proliferation, *edited by J. Moss*
132. The Lung at Depth, *edited by C. E. G. Lundgren and J. N. Miller*
133. Regulation of Sleep and Circadian Rhythms, *edited by F. W. Turek and P. C. Zee*
134. Anticholinergic Agents in the Upper and Lower Airways, *edited by S. L. Spector*
135. Control of Breathing in Health and Disease, *edited by M. D. Altose and Y. Kawakami*
136. Immunotherapy in Asthma, *edited by J. Bousquet and H. Yssel*
137. Chronic Lung Disease in Early Infancy, *edited by R. D. Bland and J. J. Coalson*
138. Asthma's Impact on Society: The Social and Economic Burden, *edited by K. B. Weiss, A. S. Buist, and S. D. Sullivan*
139. New and Exploratory Therapeutic Agents for Asthma, *edited by M. Yeadon and Z. Diamant*
140. Multimodality Treatment of Lung Cancer, *edited by A. T. Skarin*
141. Cytokines in Pulmonary Disease: Infection and Inflammation, *edited by S. Nelson and T. R. Martin*
142. Diagnostic Pulmonary Pathology, *edited by P. T. Cagle*
143. Particle–Lung Interactions, *edited by P. Gehr and J. Heyder*
144. Tuberculosis: A Comprehensive International Approach, Second Edition, Revised and Expanded, *edited by L. B. Reichman and E. S. Hershfield*
145. Combination Therapy for Asthma and Chronic Obstructive Pulmonary Disease, *edited by R. J. Martin and M. Kraft*
146. Sleep Apnea: Implications in Cardiovascular and Cerebrovascular Disease, *edited by T. D. Bradley and J. S. Floras*
147. Sleep and Breathing in Children: A Developmental Approach, *edited by G. M. Loughlin, J. L. Carroll, and C. L. Marcus*

148. Pulmonary and Peripheral Gas Exchange in Health and Disease, *edited by J. Roca, R. Rodriguez-Roisen, and P. D. Wagner*
149. Lung Surfactants: Basic Science and Clinical Applications, *R. H. Notter*
150. Nosocomial Pneumonia, *edited by W. R. Jarvis*
151. Fetal Origins of Cardiovascular and Lung Disease, *edited by David J. P. Barker*
152. Long-Term Mechanical Ventilation, *edited by N. S. Hill*
153. Environmental Asthma, *edited by R. K. Bush*
154. Asthma and Respiratory Infections, *edited by D. P. Skoner*
155. Airway Remodeling, *edited by P. H. Howarth, J. W. Wilson, J. Bousquet, S. Rak, and R. A. Pauwels*
156. Genetic Models in Cardiorespiratory Biology, *edited by G. G. Haddad and T. Xu*
157. Respiratory-Circulatory Interactions in Health and Disease, *edited by S. M. Scharf, M. R. Pinsky, and S. Magder*
158. Ventilator Management Strategies for Critical Care, *edited by N. S. Hill and M. M. Levy*
159. Severe Asthma: Pathogenesis and Clinical Management, Second Edition, Revised and Expanded, *edited by S. J. Szefler and D. Y. M. Leung*
160. Gravity and the Lung: Lessons from Microgravity, *edited by G. K. Prisk, M. Paiva, and J. B. West*
161. High Altitude: An Exploration of Human Adaptation, *edited by T. F. Hornbein and R. B. Schoene*
162. Drug Delivery to the Lung, *edited by H. Bisgaard, C. O'Callaghan, and G. C. Smaldone*
163. Inhaled Steroids in Asthma: Optimizing Effects in the Airways, *edited by R. P. Schleimer, P. M. O'Byrne, S. J. Szefler, and R. Brattsand*
164. IgE and Anti-IgE Therapy in Asthma and Allergic Disease, *edited by R. B. Fick, Jr., and P. M. Jardieu*
165. Clinical Management of Chronic Obstructive Pulmonary Disease, *edited by T. Similowski, W. A. Whitelaw, and J.-P. Derenne*
166. Sleep Apnea: Pathogenesis, Diagnosis, and Treatment, *edited by A. I. Pack*
167. Biotherapeutic Approaches to Asthma, *edited by J. Agosti and A. L. Sheffer*

ADDITIONAL VOLUMES IN PREPARATION

Proteoglycans in Lung Disease, *edited by H. G. Garg, P. J. Roughley, and C. A. Hales*

Gene Therapy in Lung Disease, *edited by S. M. Albelda*

Disease Markers in Exhaled Breath, *edited by N. Marczin, S. Kharitonov, M. Yacoub, and P. J. Barnes*

Chemokines in the Lung, *edited by R. Strieter, S. L. Kunkel, and T. Standiford*

Sleep-Related Breathing Disorders, *edited by D. Carley and M. Radulovacki*

The Immunological Basis of Asthma, *edited by B. N. Lambrecht, H. C. Hoogsteden, and Z. Diamant*

Lung Volume Reduction Surgery for Emphysema, *edited by H. E. Fessler, J. J. Reilly, Jr., and D. J. Sugarbaker*

The opinions expressed in these volumes do not necessarily represent the views of the National Institutes of Health.

BIOTHERAPEUTIC APPROACHES TO ASTHMA

Edited by

Jan M. Agosti

Immunex Corporation
Seattle, Washington, U.S.A.

Albert L. Sheffer

Harvard Medical School and
Brigham and Women's Hospital
Boston, Massachusetts, U.S.A.

MARCEL DEKKER

MARCEL DEKKER, INC. NEW YORK • BASEL

ISBN: 0-8247-0785-0

This book is printed on acid-free paper.

Headquarters
Marcel Dekker, Inc.
270 Madison Avenue, New York, NY 10016
tel: 212-696-9000; fax: 212-685-4540

Eastern Hemisphere Distribution
Marcel Dekker AG
Hutgasse 4, Postfach 812, CH-4001 Basel, Switzerland
tel: 41-61-260-6300; fax: 41-61-260-6333

World Wide Web
http://www.dekker.com

The publisher offers discounts on this book when ordered in bulk quantities. For more information, write to Special Sales/Professional Marketing at the headquarters address above.

Current printing (last digit):
10 9 8 7 6 5 4 3 2 1

PRINTED IN THE UNITED STATES OF AMERICA

INTRODUCTION

Asthma is a very old disease. Medical writings dating from 2000 B.C. include descriptions of symptoms that today are recognizable as asthma. Thus, it is not surprising that these writings also describe many therapeutic approaches. What is surprising is what these approaches constituted then and in the many centuries that followed. For example, the Ebers Papyrus suggested that enemas would improve conditions resembling asthma! In other ancient cultures, plant extracts were used: Ma Huang, the source of "native" ephedrine, was used by the Chinese.

Over the centuries, asthma received considerable attention that led to the development and use of rather astonishing therapies, at least by current standards. Shell powder and spirits, opiates, and strong coffee were in favor at times. Perhaps most striking was the recommendation that a few puffs of tobacco smoke would alleviate asthma attacks.

Eventually anticholinergics, adrenergics, and theophylline became the treatments of choice. However, this armamentarium of new drugs did not significantly change the impact of asthma as a public health problem.

The latter part of the twentieth century saw an extraordinary revolution in medicine, in the understanding of the pathogenesis of disease, and in drug discovery. In the asthma field, the realization that this condition results from an inflammatory process completely modified the therapeutic approach. Anti-inflammatory agents, primarily glucocorticosteroids, coupled with powerful bronchodilators became standard therapy.

These advances did not slow the research, but rather intensified it. Some investigators dissected the inflammatory pathways, while others identified genetic determinations and DNA variants. The findings are leading to new therapeutic opportunities. And that is what this book is about! It explores and analyzes new therapeutic modalities that are emerging or, in some instances, are already being tested and even in use.

The editors, Dr. Jan Agosti and Dr. Albert Sheffer, have assembled a roster of contributors who are pioneers in their fields. Together, editors and authors represent the best of basic and clinical research—just what the patients need.

Often books give a panoramic view of the past and the present; this volume opens a window on the future and illustrates the benefits that asthma patients can expect.

The Lung Biology in Health and Disease series of monographs is privileged to have the opportunity to present this volume to its readership.

Claude Lenfant, M.D.
Bethesda, Maryland

PREFACE

Despite the current multiple therapeutic options for asthma, in the United States more than 5000 patients annually succumb to asthma. A major proportion of these patients with asthma live with chronic limitation of activity, intermittent exacerbations, decreased quality of life, and progressively declining respiratory function. Elucidating the role of inflammation in the pathogenesis of asthma has led to acceptance of corticosteroids as the requisite controller therapy. However, patients remain reluctant to use inhaled corticosteroids because of concern about the adverse side effects of such therapy. Poor compliance with preventive (controller) therapy only emphasizes the need for improved therapeutic options.

Recent discoveries and our enhanced appreciation of the epidemiological, genetic, and immunological mechanisms that contribute to the pathogenesis of asthma now provide insight into newer approaches for the prevention and treatment of asthma. Clinical trials of the newer therapeutic modalities available as a result of DNA and monoclonal antibody technology have provided clarification of the relative roles of the participating various inflammatory pathways. This volume links such scientific appreciation of asthma to the newer effective asthma therapies.

The book is divided into 9 parts, including 15 chapters, which address the current status of asthma therapy with regard to some of the promising new interventions derived from the enhanced appreciation of the various immunobiological mechanisms participating in the genesis of this disorder.

Part One addresses the inhibition of allergen sensitization. Chapter 1 introduces the hygiene hypothesis and the pertubation of IFN-γ. Chapter 2 presents the current epidemiological understanding of the role of aeroallergens and their primary avoidance in asthma causation.

Part Two discusses the role of anti-IgE therapy in asthma (Chapter 3).

Part Three pertains to the role of mast-cell-mediator inhibition in asthma therapy. Chapter 4 addresses the role of immunoreceptor tyrosine-based inhibitory motifs (ITIM) and Chapter 5 the mast-cell-mediated immune responses in the lung, particularly those mediated by proteases and tryptases.

Part Four focuses on targeting the proallergic cytokines. Chapter 6 covers interleukin-4 inhibition and Chapter 7 covers anti-interleukin-5, anti-interleukin-9, and interleukin-10 for the treatment of asthma. Chapters 8 and 9 discuss therapeutic targeting of chemokines and chemokine receptors, as well as interleukin-13, as therapeutic strategies in asthma therapy. Tumor necrosis factor and interleukin-1 asthma inhibitory therapies are reviewed in Chapter 10.

In Part Five, the development and inhibition of the Th2 response is addressed in Chapter 11.

Part Six addresses cell adhesion molecule blocker/modulators in Chapter 12.

Part Seven relates to allergen-specific immunotherapy (Chapter 13).

Part Eight addresses the glucocorticoid effects on mediator modulation/inhibition (Chapter 14).

Finally, Part Nine is devoted to future asthma therapies. Despite the development of many promising modalities to treat asthma, Chapter 15 enumerates some of the limitations to such therapies and the necessity for focusing on the newer formulations of current pharmacological interventions.

This book assembles information regarding drugs that may soon reach human clinical trials. Newer, more specifically targeted pharmacological interventions may present safe and effective therapeutic modalities that may enhance compliance and, hopefully, reduce asthma morbidity and mortality.

Jan M. Agosti
Albert L. Sheffer

CONTRIBUTORS

Jan M. Agosti, M.D. Medical Director, Department of Clinical Research, Immunex Corporation, Seattle, Washington

Peter J. Barnes, D.M., D.Sc., F.R.C.P. Imperial College, National Heart and Lung Institute, London, England

Larry Borish, M.D. Associate Professor, Department of Medicine, University of Virginia Health System, Charlottesville, Virginia

William W. Busse, M.D. Charles E. Reed Professor of Medicine, Department of Medicine, University of Wisconsin, Madison, Wisconsin

C. J. Corrigan Guy's, King's and St. Thomas' School of Medicine, London, England

Francis M. Cuss, M.A., F.R.C.P. Vice President, Biological Research, Schering-Plough Research Institute, Kenilworth, New Jersey

Azzeddine Dakhama, Ph.D. Assistant Professor, Department of Pediatrics, National Jewish Medical and Research Center, Denver, Colorado

S. Balachandra Dass, Ph.D. Clinical Associate, Merck Research Laboratories, Rahway, New Jersey

Bruce Davidson, M.D., Ph.D. Deputy Medical Director, Bayer Pharmaceutical Corporation, West Haven, Connecticut

Laura L. Dziadzio, M.D. Department of Medicine, University of Wisconsin, Madison, Wisconsin

Elizabeth A. Erwin, M.D. Department of Medicine, University of Virginia, Charlottesville, Virginia

Erwin W. Gelfand, M.D. Chairman, Department of Pediatrics, National Jewish Medical and Research Center, and Professor, Department of Pediatrics and Immunology, University of Colorado Health Sciences Center, Denver, Colorado

Howard R. Katz, Ph.D. Associate Professor, Department of Medicine, Harvard Medical School, and Brigham and Women's Hospital, Boston, Massachusetts

A. Barry Kay, F.R.C.P., Ph.D. Allergy and Clinical Immunology, National Heart and Lung Institute, and Faculty of Medicine, Imperial College, London, England

Johan C. Kips, M.D., Ph.D. Professor, Department of Respiratory Disease, Ghent University Hospital, Ghent, Belgium

Mark Larché, Ph.D. Allergy and Clinical Immunology, National Heart and Lung Institute, and Faculty of Medicine, Imperial College, London, England

Tak H. Lee, M.D., Sc.D., F.R.C.P., F.R.C.Path., F.Med.Sci. Professor, Respiratory Medicine and Allergy, Guy's, King's and St. Thomas' School of Medicine, London, England

T. K. Loke Guy's, King's and St. Thomas' School of Medicine, London, England

Fernando D. Martinez, M.D. Swift-McNear Professor of Pediatrics, Arizona Respiratory Center, University of Arizona, Tucson, Arizona

Romain A. Pauwels, M.D., Ph.D. Professor, Department of Respiratory Diseases, Ghent University Hospital, Ghent, Belgium

Thomas A. E. Platts-Mills, M.D., Ph.D. Professor, Department of Internal Medicine, University of Virginia, Charlottesville, Virginia

Theodore F. Reiss, M.D. Executive Director, Clinical Research, Merck Research Laboratories, Rahway, New Jersey

Marc E. Rothenberg, M.D., Ph.D. Associate Professor, Department of Pediatrics, University of Cincinnati College of Medicine and Director, Division of Allergy and Immunology, Department of Pediatrics, Children's Hospital Medical Center, Cincinnati, Ohio

Richard S. Shames, M.D. Protein Design Labs, Inc., Fremont, California

Albert L. Sheffer Clinical Professor of Medicine, Harvard Medical School, Brigham and Women's Hospital, Boston, Massachusetts

John W. Steinke, Ph.D. Assistant Professor, Department of Medicine, University of Virginia Health System, Charlottesville, Virginia

Richard L. Stevens, Ph.D. Associate Professor, Department of Medicine, Brigham and Women's Hospital, Boston, Massachusetts

Marsha Wills-Karp, Ph.D. Division of Immunobiology, Children's Hospital Medical Center, Cincinnati, Ohio

Nives Zimmermann, M.D. Division of Allergy and Immunology, Department of Pediatrics, Children's Hospital Medical Center, Cincinnati, Ohio

CONTENTS

BIOTHERAPEUTIC APPROACHES TO ASTHMA

1

Strategies for the Primary Prevention of Asthma

FERNANDO D. MARTINEZ

Arizona Respiratory Center
University of Arizona
Tucson, Arizona

I. Introduction

Significant advances have occurred during the last decade in our understanding of the pathogenesis of asthma. The appreciation that asthma has a significant inflammatory component and that this component is associated with chronicity of symptoms and bronchial hyperresponsiveness (1) led to crucial improvements in therapeutic strategies to successfully treat the disease. Expert panels in the United States (2) and at an international level (3) proposed consensus guidelines for the treatment of the different expressions of asthma. Although there were slight differences between the different guidelines, they all conveyed a central concept: successful treatment of the disease requires long-term use of anti-inflammatory medication, especially in subjects with persistent symptoms. There is now convincing evidence that this strategy allows most individuals with asthma to lead a normal life.

Although these advances have been associated with great strides in preventing morbidity in both children and adults with asthma, available evidence suggests that none of the currently available therapies appear to modify the natural history of the disease. Subjects with asthma enrolled in long-term trials with inhaled corticosteroids or other anti-inflammatory medicines have clearly shown remarkable improvements in symptomatology, bronchial hyperresponsiveness (BHR), and both invasive and noninvasive assessments of airway inflammation (4–6). However, almost invariably, all these parameters go back to baseline once the medication is discontinued (7). In the case of the results of the recently reported Childhood Asthma Management Programs (5), children with mild-to-moderate asthma who were treated continuously for a period of 4–6 years with inhaled corticosteroids showed significant clinical improvements with very few side effects. However, much as for other clinical trials, discontinuation of therapy even after these prolonged periods of treatment was associated with very rapid return to the levels of bronchial hyperresponsiveness observed at the beginning of the trial.

The results of these studies suggest that although chronic airway inflammation is a crucial characteristic of asthma, adequate control of this inflammatory process does not revert some of the essential mechanisms that are responsible for the long-term expression of the disease.

This understanding of the effectiveness but, at the same time, the limitations of current available therapy for asthma, has focused new attention on studies of the natural history and the genetic, environmental, and immunological factors that determine the initiation of the disease. By definition, any attempt at primary prevention of asthma will entail an intervention at the time of the inception of the disease and before the disease has reached its chronic phase. However, it is now clear from epidemiological studies that asthma is a heterogeneous disease. Individuals who meet the definition of asthma, as proposed in the various guidelines quoted earlier, may have reached their disease status through different disease mechanisms. It has therefore been very difficult to define markers of disease that have sufficient specificity and sensitivity to identify individuals at high risk of chronic asthma. Nevertheless, recent longitudinal studies clearly suggest that in most cases of chronic asthma, symptoms initiate during the first years of life (8). Specifically, over half of all subjects with asthma at any age have reports of asthma-like symptoms before age 3 (9), and over 75% before age 5 (10). Therefore, from the point of view of public health, any strategy for the primary prevention of asthma will require interventions during the preschool years.

II. The Beginnings of Asthma

Several recent studies have addressed the environmental factors that may enhance or prevent the development of asthma. This emphasis is well placed. Assessment of the prevalence of asthma in different countries both in children (11) and in adults (12) has suggested a large variability in the clinical expression of the disease worldwide. Even among populations with the same ethnic background and presumably similar genetic susceptibility, very large differences in asthma prevalence have been reported (13). This has suggested the logical conclusion that a better understanding of the environmental factors that are responsible for these wide variations could offer significant clues as to the factors that determine the inception of the disease. In addition, if environmental factors could be identified that either protect or enhance the development of the disease, then strategies for the primary prevention of asthma could be based on the systematic inclusion or exclusion of these factors from the environment.

III. Role of Exposure to Allergens

The majority of children and adults with chronic asthma symptoms show skin test reactivity against aeroallergens that are prevalent in the geographical areas in which they were born and raised (14,15). Several etiological (16) and experimental (17) studies have shown that exposure to allergens against which the individual has developed IgE antibodies is associated with acute or chronic symptoms of airway obstruction. This strong association between prevalence of asthma and asthma symptoms and allergic sensitization and exposure to aeroallergens suggested the conclusion that such exposure was a causal factor in the development of asthma (18,19). In discussing this issue, it is important to distinguish the potential role of exposure to allergens as a *trigger* of acute asthma symptoms in the individuals who already have asthma from the putative role of allergen exposure as a determinant of the *inception* of the disease.

There is at this time quite convincing evidence from experimental studies that indeed exposure to aeroallergens in susceptible individuals is associated with a well-defined series of responses, both immediate and late-phase, that are associated with bronchial hyperresponsiveness (BHR), drops in pulmonary function, local lung inflammation, and asthma-like symptoms. On the other hand, the evidence that exposure to aeroallergens may be directly involved in the initiation of the process that leads to chronic asthma is at best circumstantial. For example, it has been established that in coastal regions, most children and young adults with asthma are sensitized against an aeroallergen that is prevalent in these regions, *Dermatophagoides pteronyssinus* (the house dust mite). The association is indeed very strong, and a classic study from the United Kingdom suggested that individuals who are more heavily exposed to house dust mites in their homes during the first years of life are more likely to develop earlier symptoms of asthma than those who are less exposed (20). It is thus not surprising that for years the house dust mite was considered a causal agent for asthma and that strategies for the prevention of asthma were proposed that implied avoiding exposure to this allergen during the first years of life (21). This paradigm appeared to be supported that the observation that in many workplaces individuals who are exposed to allergens that are specific to that environment develop significant asthma symptoms and increased bronchial hyperresponsiveness, with significant improvement of these clinical features after exposures are avoided (22). It was thus to be expected that prospective studies in which exposure to house dust mites was systematically measured in the homes of young infants, those with high exposures should develop a higher frequency of both sensitization to house dust mites and asthma symptoms, particularly during the school years when symptoms related to allergic sensitization are more frequent.

A study with this precise design was conducted by Lau et al. (23) in several cities in Germany (MAS Study). These authors painstakingly and systematically measured levels of house dust mites in samples obtained from homes of children who were enrolled at birth. The authors then measured allergic sensitization to house dust mites and asthma symptoms at the age of 7 years in a follow-up study. As expected, individuals who were exposed to higher levels of house dust mites in their homes were more likely to be sensitized to the mites at the end of the follow-up period. Moreover, sensitization to house dust mites was strongly associated with the likelihood of having asthma symptoms at age 7. However, there was no association between exposure to house dust mites and the development of asthma symptoms at the age of 7.

Although these results may appear surprising, several lines of evidence suggest that indeed the relation between exposure to house dust mites or any other specific aeroallergen and the development of asthma is not a simple, straightforward cause-and-effect association. Several years ago, Charpin et al. (24) compared frequency of allergic sensitization to house dust mites and frequency of asthma in two populations in France: one living in a coastal region and one living in an alpine region at high altitude. Because prevalence of house dust mites was extremely low in the alpine region, they expected to observe much lower frequency of sensitization to this allergen in the alpine region than in the coastal region. This was indeed the result obtained, but, interestingly, the frequency of asthma symptoms in individuals of similar ages and gender was not very different between the alpine region and the coastal region in spite of marked differences in levels of exposure to mites. Similarly, the frequency of asthma is very similar in regions of Australia with marked differences in the level of exposure to house dust mites. In coastal regions, where exposure is very high, the prevalence is similar to that observed in inland desert regions where exposure to house dust mites is low. In the latter regions, the most important allergen associated with asthma is *Alternaria* (25). Similarly, we observed that in Tucson, Arizona, where exposure to house dust mites is lower than that observed in coastal regions, the main aeroallergen associated with asthma in school-age children is also *Alternaria*, with house dust mites showing a much lower association with the prevalence of asthma symptoms (26).

The picture becomes even more complex when other locales are studied. For example, in the inner cities of the United States, the most important aeroallergens associated with asthma appear to be those of the common cockroach (27).

Researchers investigating the association between aeroallergens and asthma in the arctic regions of Sweden, on the other hand, have observed that the most prevalent allergens associated with asthma in these regions are those of indoor pets such as cats and dogs (28). However, in these same regions, the majority of children with asthma show no sensitization to any known allergen, although those who are not sensitized to allergens show marked increases in total serum IgE levels.

The above observations outline a complex picture for our understanding of the potential causal role of sensitization of specific aeroallergens and the development of asthma. There is little doubt that individuals who are more likely to develop asthma are also more likely to become sensitized to aeroallergens that are more prevalent in the areas where they are raised. The German MAS study strongly suggests a dose–response relationship between sensitization and exposure to aeroallergens in the general population but not among asthmatics. Therefore, although specific aeroallergens may be the cause of asthma symptoms in individuals who already have the disease, they do not appear to be casual agents in the development of the disease. This conclusion is supported by the observation that most individuals who develop asthma-like symptoms when exposed to workplace allergens either have asthma already or have significant evidence for allergic disease (29). More than exposure to aeroallergens being a causal fact in asthma, the evidence suggests that individuals who are predisposed to asthma are also predisposed to becoming sensitized to those allergens that they encounter at crucial times during the development of their disease.

IV. Farm Life and Asthma: Exposure to Endotoxin

A second set of potential exposures that could shed light on the mechanisms for the initiation of asthma are those associated with a farm environment. Several recent reports suggest that children raised in rural communities and in close proximity to animal farms have much lower rates of allergic sensitization and asthma symptoms than children raised in the same rural communities but away from animal farms (30–33). This observation is a result of carefully performed cross-sectional studies in which several potential confounders and effect modifiers were also taken into account. The suggestion from these studies is that certain exposures associated with animal farms, particularly when these exposures occur during the first months of life, may somehow protect against the development of the form of allergic sensitization that is associated with asthma.

Naturally, many factors are present in the environment of individuals raised in farms that could influence the development of the immune system. However, the observation that living close to animal farms is a protective factor for asthma seems to go in the same direction as those made in urban environments and related to exposure to household pets. Burney and coworkers (34) observed that there was an inverse association between the likelihood of being sensitized to aeroallergens and the presence of pets in the homes. In studies performed in Tucson, Arizona, Remes et al. (35) reported that although there was no association between allergic sensitization and the presence of dogs in the home, there were remarkable differences in the incidence of asthma-like symptoms from dog exposure. Specifically, individuals who were exposed to two or more dogs in the home showed significantly lower incidence rates of asthma-like symptoms than those who were not exposed. Moreover, when exposure to dogs was discontinued at some time during the first 5 years of life, significant increases in incidence rates of asthma occurred during the subsequent years. Platts-Mills and coworkers performed a cross-sectional study of children aged 12–14 years. They observed that those children who were highly exposed to cat allergens were less likely to develop sensitization to cats than those who were less exposed to these same allergens (36). They interpreted their finding as suggesting that a form of immune tolerance occurred for the cat antigens in highly exposed individuals. Because no such tolerance was observed in the case of house dust mites, however, they suggested that a high enough level of exposure was not reached for house dust mites so that tolerance could occur. More recently, Ownby et al. (37) observed that children who were exposed to two or more animals in the home were less likely to develop asthma-like symptoms, bronchial hyperresponsiveness, and sensitization to aeroallergens in general that those who were not so heavily exposed, and this was true for both children exposed to cats and those exposed to dogs. This observation seems to contradict the hypothesis that there is a specific immune tolerance mechanism that is responsible for the lower levels of allergic sensitization and asthma in individuals who are highly exposed to pets. If that were the case, only the risk for sensitization to the specific allergen (in this case, to pet allergen) should be decreased. Moreover, in the Tucson study no effect was observed with respect to sensitization to aeroallergens and the main effect was observed with respect to asthma (38).

These data suggest that both exposure to animal farms and exposure to pets may act through a mechanism that is not specific for any aeroallergen but may be related to a basic developmental pathway of the immune system during early life. Data regarding exposure to endotoxin among children raised in homes close to animal farms provided significant new insight into this potential mechanism. Von Mutius et al. (39) showed that concentration of endotoxin in house dust obtained from homes located close to animal farms was significantly higher than endotoxin concentration in homes from the same rural communities but away from animal farms. They suggested that endotoxin could be the crucial factor explaining the lower prevalence of asthma and asthma-related phenotypes in proximity to animal farms. Endotoxin is a component of the cell wall of gram-negative bacteria that is ubiquitous in nature. It has been shown to be more abundant in homes where pets are kept (40) and thus could be an important marker for the environmental factor or factors that explain the lower risk of asthma and allergic sensitization in children raised in animal farms or close to pets.

More recently, Gereda et al. (41) provided new clues for the understanding of these complex mechanisms. These authors measured levels of endotoxin in house dust in homes of children raised in Denver, Colorado. They observed a strong inverse relation between the level of exposure to endotoxin and the likelihood of becoming sensitized to aeroallergens during the first few years of life. Moreover, individuals who were more highly exposed to endotoxin were also likely to show interferon gamma (IFN-γ) responses by peripheral blood mononuclear cells to nonspecific stimuli. These studies are important because they connect endotoxin exposure to the patterns of development of the immune system in early life. Several authors (42–45) have demonstrated that individuals who are likely to develop early sensitization to local aeroallergens show delayed IFN-γ responses by peripheral blood mononuclear cells during the first year of life. Interestingly, these responses do not appear to be different between individuals who will go on to become sensitized when measured in cord blood or after the third year of life (46). Therefore, there is a specific window during which susceptible individuals (i.e., those with a predisposition for allergies as determined by their family history) show deficits in the development of IFN-γ responses. Because these responses appear to inhibit the synthesis of IgE against aeroallergens in both human studies and experimental animal models, it is reasonable to surmise that deficits in IFN-γ responses during these critical periods may be a causal factor in the development of IgE-mediated responses against local aeroallergens in susceptible individuals.

The work by Gereda and coworkers cited earlier suggests that not only genetic factors may influence the susceptibility to becoming sensitized to aeroallergens. It is possible that exposure to endotoxins may stimulate the development of early IFN-γ responses and therefore, by this mechanism, prevent the development of Th2-mediated IgE responses to local aeroallergens. Experimental studies have shown that, indeed, when exposure to endotoxin occurs together with or shortly before exposure to aeroallergens, IgE-mediated responses to these aeroallergens are repressed (47). Apparently, the biological mechanism for this consists of a direct stimulation of the endotoxin receptor system by endotoxin, and this receptor system, composed of CD14, toll-like receptor 4 (TLR4), lipoprotein-binding protein (LBP), and several other molecules, mediates the production of IL-10, IL-12, and other cytokines by antigen-presenting cells.

V. Gene by Environment Interaction in the Development of Early Allergic Sensitization

If exposure to endotoxin is an important modulator of early allergic sensitization during developmental ''windows'' of susceptibility in early life, it is plausible to surmise that genetic variations in the receptor system for endotoxin could be significant genetic determinants of susceptibility to these environmental exposures. On the basis of this hypothesis, Baldini et al. (48) assessed the association between polymorphisms in the CD14 gene and markers of atopy in children. They screened the promoter region of CD14 for potential polymorphisms and found one such polymorphism at position −159 from the transcription initiation site (CD14/−159). This polymorphism was then genotyped in a group of over 400 children, and the association with circulating levels of soluble CD14 (sCD14), total serum IgE levels, and IFN-γ/IL-4 responses by peripheral blood mononuclear cells (PBMCs) was investigated. CD14/−159 was found to be significantly associated with sCD14, with homozygote carriers of the T allele having 30% higher circulating levels of sCD14 than homozygotes for the C allele. In addition, sCD14 levels were directly related to IFN-γ responses and inversely related to IL-4 responses by PBMC. Finally, carriers of the T allele, especially in homozygote form, were found to have lower serum IgE levels than carriers of the C allele, and this was particularly true for those who were skin test positive, whereas the number of positive skin tests was higher in carriers of the T allele. These findings were recently confirmed, in a Dutch population sample, by Koppelman et al. (49).

Two other groups have tested this same polymorphism in relation to atopic sensitization. In a study performed among the Hutterites, Ober et al. (50) observed that the C allele of CD14/−159 was more frequently transmitted than the T alleles among subjects who were skin test positive to local aeroallergens. They postulated that most likely CD14/−159 was acting as a marker for a different polymorphism occurring in the same chromosomal region that could be responsible for increased likelihood of atopic sensitization. Walley et al. (51) also genotyped CD14/−159 in a population sample from Australia and found that indeed this polymorphism was linked with a high level of significance to atopic sensitization. However, in their study they found no association between CD14/−159 and markers of atopy, again suggesting that this polymorphism may be acting as a marker for a different variant responsible for this signal. Although these findings indicate the complex nature of the association between genetic variants and common diseases such as allergies and asthma, they clearly indicate that perhaps within the same CD14 gene or within the regulatory region of this gene there may be polymorphisms that regulate the expression of allergic disease and asthma. Further studies are currently ongoing to assess the presence of such polymorphisms and their associations with the phenotypes of interest.

Regardless of which polymorphism may be responsible for the linkage and association signals observed in relation to CD14/−159, the results of these studies suggest that genetic variants that may regulate the expression of a gene that codes for a component of the endotoxin receptor system may influence the likelihood of becoming sensitized to local aeroallergens. This provides significant support for the hypothesis that exposure to endotoxin or other factors associated with microbial burden, particularly at times when windows of opportunity are created during the development of the immune system, may modulate the clinical expression of allergic disease and, as a consequence, of the asthma phenotypes.

VI. Mechanisms of Response to Endotoxin

We suggested earlier that one potential mechanism by which endotoxin may influence the likelihood of becoming sensitized to local aeroallergens is an enhanced development of IFN-γ responses at critical times during the development of the immune system. This hypothesis needs to be applied to the complex mechanisms that determine responses to aeroallergens in early life. A detailed analysis of these mechanisms goes beyond the scope of this chapter. However, it appears that the production of IL-12 by antigen-presenting cells at the time of antigen presentation enhances the development of T-helper cells that produce interferon gamma and inhibits the development of T-helper cells that produce IL-4 and IL-13 (52). Because IL-4 and IL-13 are essential signals for the production of IgE by B-cells, it is plausible that endotoxin, by stimulating the production of IL-12 by antigen-presenting cells, may inhibit IgE production.

However, several lines of evidence suggest that the timing of endotoxin exposure may be very important. Studies performed in humans suggest that exposure to endotoxin may *increase* the severity of asthma in individuals who have already developed the disease (53,54). Similarly, in animal models, exposure to endotoxin at a time when B cells have already been committed to the production of IgE seems to enhance IgE-mediated responses (47). Therefore, if this environmental model of asthma prevention will be used as a paradigm for future strategies for the prevention of the disease, timing will be of the essence. More specifically, any exposure used as a surrogate for endotoxin will need to occur very early during the different phases of the development of the immune response against aeroallergens. Observational studies would suggest that this may mean exposures up to the age of 3–5 years.

VII. Role of IL-10 and IgG4 Responses

The mechanisms by which endotoxin (or other microbial products, see below) may influence the development of Th2-like responses may not be limited to the development of IFN-γ production in early life. Recent studies suggest that IL-10, which is produced by, among other cells, antigen-presenting cells, may influence the immunoglobulin responses by Th2-like cells. Elegant in vitro studies have shown that IL-10 has a differential effect on IgG4 versus IgE production by PBMCs (55). IL-10 decreased epsilon transcript and IgE production induced by IL-4 when added during the first 3 days of in vitro culture, suggesting that IL-10 decreases IL-4-induced switching. In contrast, if added later on to B cells that are already IgE switched, IL-10 potentiates IgE production. These results suggest that IL-10 may be a potential mechanism by which exposure to endotoxin may influence IgE production at the time of antigen presentation. However, Jeannin and coworkers also found that, whatever the time of addition, IL-10 increases IL-4-induced γ4 transcript expression and IgG4 production. Therefore, the production of IL-10 at the time of antigen presentation may not inhibit the development of Th2-like cells but may influence the type of immunoglobulin that these cells produce. Therefore, IL-10 may induce a ''Th2-modified'' response (36) and, by this mechanism, may mediate the effects of endotoxin as described earlier. Clearly, these issues require further elucidation.

VIII. Coexposures to Endotoxin and Their Potential Role

In the previous discussion we considered mainly the potential role of endotoxin in determining some of the outcomes observed in individuals exposed to either animal farms or pets. However, it is likely that substances other than endotoxin that are also associated with microbial exposure and for which endotoxin is acting as a marker may influence the development of the immune system in early life. Of particular interest are CpG-containing DNA sequences. For years, it was known that bacterial DNA could activate inflammatory cells but the specific mechanism was unknown. It has now been established that there are subtle structural differences between bacterial and eukaryotic DNA that account for the ability of bacterial DNA to serve as an immune-activating agent. Bacterial DNA contains a high proportion of short sequences with unmethylated CpG dinucleotides. On the other hand, mammalian DNA contains many fewer CpG motifs and the cytosine present in CpG dinucleotides in mammalian DNA is usually methylated. It has been shown that bacterial DNA causes activation of B cells and NK cells and the secretion of Th1-like cytokines (56). As explained earlier, Th1 cytokines such as IFN-γ suppress Th2 responses, and, for this reason, exposure to bacterial DNA could be an important determinant of the effects of bacterial exposure on the development of early allergic sensitization and asthma. In animal models of asthma, CpG-motif oligodeoxynucleotides, when administered together with antigen, prevented airway eosinophilia, Th2 cytokine production, IgE production, and bronchial hyperreactivity (57). Moreover, bacterial DNA acts synergistically with LPS to activate macrophages. In a murine macrophage cell line, bacterial DNA enhanced TNF-α secretion when administered together with substimulatory concentrations of LPS (58). Interestingly, at least in these animal models, it appears that the molecular mechanisms by which CpG enhances production of TNF-α (and presumably other cytokines) are complementary to and different from those by which LPS activates these same macrophages. Specifically, whereas LPS acts at a transcriptional level, CpG motifs seem to act through a post-translational event (58). Moreover, very recent findings suggest that CpG motifs may induce immune responses through a receptor system that is different from that involved in LPS responses. As explained earlier, LPS interacts with the CD14/TLR4 receptor system, whereas CpG motifs interact with TLR9 receptors (59).

The relative roles of DNA CpG motifs and LPS as determinants of the effects of bacterial exposure on the risk of allergies and asthma is at present unknown. This is certainly an important issue, because if ''imitating nature'' prevention strategies are to be developed, the precise biological mechanisms involved need to be well understood (see below).

It is also important to stress here that not only components of gram-negative bacteria may be involved in the preventive influences of bacterial exposure. It is plausible to surmise that individuals who are exposed to high levels of endotoxin may also be exposed to high levels of gram-positive bacteria, mycobacteria, and even viruses. All of these microbes interact with the innate immune system through pattern recognition receptor systems that are not very dissimilar from those involved in responses to LPS and CpG motifs. Gram-positive bacteria, for example, induce dendritic cell activation through the interaction of lipoteichoic acid with TLR2 (60). Peptidoglycans are other major components of the cell wall of gram-positive bacteria, and they have also been shown to interact with TLR2 in activating macrophages (61). Cell walls of mycobacteria contain lipoarabinomannans, which also activate macrophages via TLR (62). Finally, recent observations suggest that viruses may interact with pattern recognition receptors to activate antigen-presenting cells (63).

All these mechanisms may thus be involved in what we have here generically called ''microbial burden.'' Because most of these mechanisms may activate different responses by macrophages and thus may shift specific immune responses in different directions depending on dose, timing, and coexposure with each other and with antigen, much more work needs to be done to better understand the exact immune pathways that are activated by different microbial exposures to determine patterns of maturation of the immune system in early life.

IX. Conclusions

It is now clear that complex interactions occur between allergen antigens, microbial exposures, and genetic background of the individual to determine the type of immune responses to aeroallergens during the first years of life. Because early sensitization to these aeroallergens appears to be a crucial risk factor for the development of asthma (64,65), understanding the molecular mechanisms involved may be crucial for the development of strategies for the primary prevention of asthma. Specifically, our aim should be to identify substances to which individual infants can be exposed that will produce the same preventive effects observed for microbial burden but that will not be associated with the increased risk of acute infectious disease observed in early life in populations heavily exposed to such microbes. In addition, identification of those genetic variations that make subjects more or less susceptible to certain exposures may allow us to target different exposures to different individuals, thus maximizing effect and minimizing potential toxicity.

These approaches offer the best hope to finding therapeutic approaches for the primary prevention of asthma in the next decade.

References

1. Holgate ST, ed. The Role of Inflammatory Processes in Airway Hyperresponsiveness. London: Blackwell Scientific, 1989.
2. National Asthma Education Prevention Program Coordinating Committee. Guidelines for the diagnosis and management of asthma. Bethesda, MD: National Institutes of Health, 1997.
3. Von Mutius E. Presentation of new GINA guidelines for paediatrics. The Global Initiative on Asthma. Clin Exp Allergy 2000; 30(suppl 1):6–10.
4. Haahtela T, Jarvinen M, Kava T, Kiviranta K, Koskinen S, Lehtonen K, Nikander K, Persson T, Selroos O, Sovijarvi A. Effects of reducing or discontinuing inhaled budesonide in patients with mild asthma. N Engl J Med 1994; 331(11):700–705.
5. The Childhood Asthma Management Program Research Group. Long-term effects of budesonide or nedocromil in children with asthma. The Childhood Asthma Management Program Research Group. N Engl J Med 2000; 343(15):1054–1063.
6. Booth H, Richmond I, Ward C, Gardiner PV, Harkawat R, Walters EH. Effect of high dose inhaled fluticasone propionate on airway inflammation in asthma. Am J Respir Crit Care Med 1995; 152(1):45–52.
7. Haahtela T. Early treatment of asthma. Allergy 1999; 54(suppl 49):74–81.
8. Yunginger J, Reed CE, O'Connell EJ, Melton LJ, O'Fallon WM, Silverstein MD. A community-based study of the epidemiology of asthma. Incidence rates, 1964–1983. Am Rev Respir Dis 1992; 146:888–894.
9. Anderson HR, Pottier AC, Strachan DP. Asthma from birth to age 23: Incidence and relation to prior and concurrent atopic disease. Thorax 1992; 47(7):537–542.
10. Barbee RA, Dodge R, Lebowitz ML, Burrows B. The epidemiology of asthma. Chest 1985; 87(1 suppl):21S–25S.
11. The International Study of Asthma and Allergies in Childhood (ISAAC) Steering Committee. Worldwide variation in prevalence of symptoms of asthma, allergic rhinoconjunctivitis, and atopic eczema: ISAAC. Lancet 1998; 351(9111):1225–1232.
12. Janson C, Chinn S, Jarvis D, Burney P. Physician-diagnosed asthma and drug utilization in the European Community Respiratory Health Survey. Eur Respir J 1997; 10(8):1795–1802.

13. Leung R, Ho P. Asthma, allergy, and atopy in three south-east Asian populations. Thorax 1994; 49(12):1205–1210.
14. Burrows B, Martinez FD, Halonen M, Barbee RA, Cline MG. Association of asthma with serum IgE levels and skin-test reactivity to allergens. N Engl J Med 1989; 320(5):271–277.
15. Platts-Mills TA, Rakes G, Heymann PW. The relevance of allergen exposure to the development of asthma in childhood. J Allergy Clin Immunol 2000; 105(2 Pt 2): S503–S508.
16. Rosenstreich DL, Eggleston P, Kattan M, Baker D, Slavin RG, Gergen P, Mitchell H, McNiff-Mortimer K, Lynn H, Ownby D, Malveaux F. The role of cockroach allergy and exposure to cockroach allergen in causing morbidity among inner-city children with asthma. [see comments]. N Engl J Med 1997; 336(19):1356–1363.
17. Platts-Mills TA, Tovey ER, Mitchell EB, Moszoro H, Nock P, Wilkins SR. Reduction of bronchial hyperreactivity during prolonged allergen avoidance. Lancet 1982; 2(8300):675–678.
18. Peat JK, Tovey E, Toelle BG, Haby MM, Gray EJ, Mahmic A, Woolcock AJ. House dust mite allergens. A major risk factor for childhood asthma in Australia. Am J Respir Crit Care Med 1996; 153(1):141–146.
19. Sporik R, Chapman MD, Platts-Mills TA. House dust mite exposure as a cause of asthma. Clin Exp Allergy 1992; 22(10):897–906.
20. Sporik R, Holgate ST, Platts-Mills TA, Cogswell JJ. Exposure to house-dust mite allergen (Der p I) and the development of asthma in childhood. A prospective study. N Engl J Med 1990; 323(8):502–507.
21. Custovic A, Simpson A, Woodcock A. Importance of indoor allergens in the induction of allergy and elicitation of allergic disease. Allergy 1998; 53(48 suppl):115–120.
22. Montanaro A. Prognosis of occupational asthma. Ann Allergy Asthma Immunol 1999; 83(6 Pt 2):593–596.
23. Lau S, Illi S, Sommerfeld C, Niggemann B, Bergmann R, von Mutius E, Wahn U. Early exposure to house-dust mite and cat allergens and development of childhood asthma: A cohort study. Lancet 2000; 356:1392–1397.
24. Charpin D, Birnbaum J, Haddi E, Genard G, Lanteaume A, Toumi M, Faraj F, Van der Brempt X, Vervloet D. Altitude and allergy to house-dust mites. A paradigm of the influence of environmental exposure on allergic sensitization. Am Rev Respir Dis 1991; 143(5 Pt 1):983–986.
25. Peat JK, Tovey E, Mellis CM, Leeder SR, Woolcock AJ. Importance of house dust mite and Alternaria allergens in childhood asthma: An epidemiological study in two climatic regions of Australia. Clin Exp Allergy 1993; 23(10):812–820.
26. Halonen M, Stern DA, Wright AL, Taussig LM, Martinez FD. Alternaria as a major allergen for asthma in children raised in a desert environment. Am J Respir Crit Care Med 1997; 155(4):1356–1361.
27. Kang BC, Johnson J, Veres-Thorner C. Atopic profile of inner-city asthma with a comparative analysis on the cockroach-sensitive and ragweed-sensitive subgroups. J Allergy Clin Immunol 1993; 92(6):802–811.
28. Perzanowski MS, Ronmark E, Nold B, Lundback B, Platts-Mills TA. Relevance of allergens from cats and dogs to asthma in the northernmost province of Sweden:

Schools as a major site of exposure. J Allergy Clin Immunol 1999; 103(6):1018–1024.
29. Mapp C, Boschetto P, Miotto D, De Rosa E, Fabbri LM. Mechanisms of occupational asthma. Ann Allergy Asthma Immunol 1999; 83(6 Pt 2):645–664.
30. Von Ehrenstein OS, Von Mutius E, Illi S, Baumann L, Bohm O, von Kries R. Reduced risk of hay fever and asthma among children of farmers. Clin Exp Allergy 2000; 30(2):187–193.
31. Riedler J, Eder W, Oberfeld G, Schreuer M. Austrian children living on a farm have less hay fever, asthma and allergic sensitization. Clin Exp Allergy 2000; 30(2):194–200.
32. Braun-Fahrlander C, Gassner M, Grize L, Neu U, Sennhauser FH, Varonier HS, Vuille JC, Wuthrich B. Prevalence of hay fever and allergic sensitization in farmer's children and their peers living in the same rural community. SCARPOL team. Swiss Study on Childhood Allergy and Respiratory Symptoms with Respect to Air Pollution. Clin Exp Allergy 1999; 29(1):28–34.
33. Ernst P, Cormier Y. Relative scarcity of asthma and atopy among rural adolescents raised on a farm. Am J Respir Crit Care Med 2000; 161(5):1563–1566.
34. Svanes C, Jarvis D, Chinn S, Burney P. Childhood environment and adult atopy: Results from the European Community Respiratory Health Survey. J Allergy Clin Immunol 1999; 103(3 Pt 1):415–420.
35. Remes ST, Castro-Rodriquez JA, Holberg CJ, Martinez FD, Wright AL. Dog exposure in infancy decreases the subsequent risk of frequent wheeze but not atopy. J Allergy Clin Immunol 2001:In Press.
36. Platts-Mills T, Vaughan J, Squillace S, Woodfolk J, Sporik R. Sensitisation, asthma, and a modified Th2 response in children exposed to cat allergen: A population-based cross-sectional study. Lancet 2001; 357(9258):752–756.
37. Ownby DR, Johnson CC, Peterson EL. Exposure to cats and dogs during the first year of life reduces atopy and improves lung function in boys. Am J Respir Crit Care Med 2001; 163(5):A722.
38. Remes ST, Korppi M, Remes K, Pekkanen J. Prevalence of asthma at school age: A clinical population-based study in eastern Finland. Acta Paediatr 1996; 85(1):59–63.
39. Von Mutius E, Braun-Fahrlander C, Schierl R, Riedler J, Ehlermann S, Maisch S, Waser M, Nowak D. Exposure to endotoxin or other bacterial components might protect against the development of atopy. Clin Exp Allergy 2000; 30(9):1230–1234.
40. Gereda JE, Klinnert MD, Price MR, Leung DY, Liu AH. Metropolitan home living conditions associated with indoor endotoxin levels. J Allergy Clin Immunol 2001; 107(5):790–796.
41. Gereda JE, Leung DYM, Thatayatikon A, Streib JE, Price MR, Klinnert MD, Liu AH. Relation between house-dust endotoxin exposure, type 1 T-cell development, and allergen sensitization in infants at high risk of asthma. Lancet 2000; 355:1680–1683.
42. Prescott SL, Macaubes C, Yabuhara A, Venaille TJ, Holt BJ, Habre W, Loh R, Sly PD, Holt PG. Developing patterns of T cell memory to environmental allergens in the first two years of life. Int Arch Allergy Immunol 1997; 113(1–3):75–79.
43. Martinez FD, Stern DA, Wright AL, Holberg CJ, Taussig LM, Halonen M. Associa-

tion of interleukin-2 and interferon-gamma production by blood mononuclear cells in infancy with parental allergy skin tests and with subsequent development of atopy. J Allergy Clin Immunol 1995; 96(5 Pt 1):652–660.
44. Prescott SL, Macaubas C, Smallacombe T, Holt BJ, Sly PD, Holt PG. Development of allergen-specific T-cell memory in atopic and normal children. Lancet 1999; 353(9148):196–200.
45. Kondo N, Kobayashi Y, Shinoda S, Takenaka R, Teramoto T, Kaneko H, Fukao T, Matsui E, Kasahara K, Yokoyama Y. Reduced interferon gamma production by antigen-stimulated cord blood mononuclear cells is a risk factor of allergic disorders—6-year follow-up study. Clin Exp Allergy 1998; 28(11):1340–1344.
46. Holt PG, Rudin A, Macaubas C, Holt BJ, Rowe J, Loh R, Sly PD. Development of immunologic memory against tetanus toxoid and pertactin antigens from the diphtheria-tetanus-pertussis vaccine in atopic versus nonatopic children. J Allergy Clin Immunol 2000; 105(6 Pt 1):1117–1122.
47. Tulic MK, Wale JL, Holt PG, Sly PD. Modification of the inflammatory response to allergen challenge after exposure to bacterial lipopolysaccharide. Am J Respir Cell Mol Biol 2000; 22(5):604–612.
48. Baldini M, Lohman IC, Halonen M, Erickson RP, Holt P, Martinez FD. A polymorphism in the 5′-flanking region of the CD14 gene is associated with circulating soluble CD14 levels and with total serum IgE. Am J Resp Cell Mol Biol 1999; 20(5): 976–983.
49. Koppelman GH, Reijmerink NE, Colin Stine O, Howard TD, Whittaker PA, Meyers DA, Postma DS, Bleecker ER. Association of a promoter polymorphism of the CD14 gene and atopy. Am J Respir Crit Care Med 2001; 163(4):965–969.
50. Ober C, Tsalenko A, Willadsen S, Newman D, Daniel R, Wu X, Andal J, Hoki D, Schneider D, True K, Schou C, Parry R, Cox N. Genome-wide screen for atopy susceptibility alleles in the Hutterites. Clin Exp Allergy 1999; 29(suppl 4):11–15.
51. Walley AJ, Wiltshire S, Ellis CM, Cookson WO. Linkage and allelic association of chromosome 5 cytokine cluster genetic markers with atopy and asthma associated traits. Genomics 2001; 72(1):15–20.
52. Sieling PA, Modlin RL. Activation of toll-like receptors by microbial lipoproteins. Scand J Infect Dis 2001; 33(2):97–100.
53. Michel O, Kips J, Duchateau J, Vertongen F, Robert L,Collet H, Pauwels R, Sergysels R. Severity of asthma is related to endotoxin in house dust. Am J Respir Crit Care Med 1996; 154(6 Pt 1):1641–1646.
54. Michel O, Nagy AM, Schroeven M, Duchateau J, Neve J, Fondu P, Sergysels R. Dose-response relationship to inhaled endotoxin in normal subjects. Am J Respir Crit Care Med 1997; 156(4 Pt 1):1157–1164.
55. Jeannin P, Lecoanet S, Delneste Y, Gauchat JF, Bonnefoy JY. IgE versus IgG4 production can be differentially regulated by IL-10. J Immunol 1998; 160(7):3555–3561.
56. Wild JS, Sur S. CpG oligonucleotide modulation of allergic inflammation. Allergy 2001; 56(5):365–376.
57. Kline JN, Waldschmidt TJ, Businga TR, Lemish JE, Weinstock JV, Thorne PS, Krieg AM. Modulation of airway inflammation by CpG oligodeoxynucleotides in a murine model of asthma. J Immunol 1998; 160(6):2555–2559.

58. Gao JJ, Xue Q, Papasian CJ, Morrison DC. Bacterial DNA and lipopolysaccharide induce synergistic production of TNF-alpha through a post-transcriptional mechanism. J Immunol 2001; 166(11):6855–6860.
59. Takeshita F, Leifer CA, Gursel I, Ishii KJ, Takeshita S, Gursel M, Klinman DM. Cutting edge: Role of toll-like receptor 9 in CPG DNA-induced activation of human cells. J Immunol 2001; 167(7):3555–3558.
60. Kawowaki N, Ho S, Antonenko S, de Waal Malefyt R, Kastelein RA, Bazen F, Liu YJ. Subsets of human dendritic cell precursors express different toll-like receptors and respond to different microbial antigens. J Exp Med 2001; 194(6):863–870.
61. Schwandner R, Dziarski R, Wesche H, Rothe M, Kirschning CJ. Peptidoglycan- and lipoteichoic acid-induced cell activation is mediated by toll-like receptor 2. J Biol Chem 1999; 274(25):1746–1749.
62. Jones BW, Means TK, Heldwein KA, Keen MA, Hill PJ, Belisle JT, Fenton MJ. Different toll-like receptor agonists induce distinct macrophage responses. J Leukoc Biol 2001; 69(6):1036–1044.
63. Kurt-Jones EA, Popova L, Kwinn L, Haynes LM, Jones LP, Tripp RA, Walsh EE, Freeman MW, Golenbock DT, Anderson LJ, Finberg RW. Pattern recognition receptors TLR4 and CD14 mediate response to respiratory syncytial virus. Nat Immunol 2000; 1(5):398–401.
64. Peat JK, Salome CM, Woolcock AJ. Longitudinal changes in atopy during a 4-year period: Relation to bronchial hyperresponsiveness and respiratory symptoms in a population sample of Australian schoolchildren. J. Allergy Clin Immunol 1990; 85(1 Pt 1):65–74.
65. Halonen M, Stern DA, Lohman C, Wright AL, Brown MA, Martinez FD. Two subphenotypes of childhood asthma that differ in maternal and paternal influences on asthma risk. Am J Respir Crit Care Med 1999; 160(2):564–570.

2

The Role of Aeroallergens

What Is the Case for Primary Avoidance?

ELIZABETH A. ERWIN and THOMAS A. E. PLATTS-MILLS

University of Virginia
Charlottesville, Virginia

I. Introduction

In the mid-1800s when Charles Blackley began to investigate hay fever, there were many theories regarding its causation. The theories at the time included that it was caused by inhalation of benzoic acid or the odor of hay (or other odors); that it was due to the action of ozone, the effects of dust, or the influence of light and heat; and finally that it was caused by inhaling pollen. By experimenting on himself, Blackley was able to exclude all causative mechanisms other than pollen and dust. During his investigations, which included various challenges, not only did he provoke symptoms of allergic rhinitis, but on many occasions he also provoked an attack of asthma. His observations of those who suffered from the disease suggested that it was most predominant in well-educated people. He observed a lack of symptoms among farming classes, which he attributed to poor education and the possibility that they had developed immunity because of their great exposure to pollen. Even at that time he was concerned that hay fever was increasing, which he attributed to increased education and a change in the proportion of people involved in farming activities (1).

Today we are left with many of the same observations and questions. As asthma continues to increase, there are several current theories. One of the hypotheses is that a decline in certain childhood infections or a lack of exposure to infectious agents during the first years of life is related to the rise of asthma. More specifically, environmental endotoxin exposure has been considered to have a possible role in the prevention of atopic disease (2). In spite of interesting observations, it is early to draw any conclusions. Despite clear evidence that ozone and diesel particulates can contribute to inflammation in the respiratory tract, there is only limited evidence that outdoor pollution contributes to either the prevalence of sensitization or the increasing morbidity of asthma (3). Observations that the risk of atopic sensitization is particularly high in industrialized societies and evidence that high socioeconomic status is considered a risk factor have raised issues of Western lifestyle. These lifestyle-related factors include diet, obesity, sedentary entertainment, and the decreased number of people having any contact with farming and rural lifestyle (4). (See Table 1.)

Before discussing the causes of the increasing rate of asthma any further, a factor that must be addressed is the challenge of differentiating between two overlapping conditions, wheezing early in life and persistent asthma. It has long been known that children who wheeze early in life often lose these symptoms later in childhood. Several groups have noted a high incidence of asthma around age 8 as well as a common occurrence of remission (5–7). Ronmark et al. (5) found a 10% remission rate that was associated with negative skin tests. Williams and McNicol (6) found that 11% of all children had wheezed before age 10 but only 30% of those continued to have symptoms. Martinez et al. (7) observed a similar remission rate (60%) in children less than 3 years of age who wheezed with lower respiratory tract illness. The type of viral infection present is the key differentiating feature. In pediatric patients treated in the emergency room, respiratory viruses, most commonly respiratory syncytial virus (RSV), were detected

Table 1 Factors Contributing to the Increased Prevalence of Asthma

Increased exposure
Allergens: Housing modifications and time indoors
Passive tobacco/air pollution
Increased response
Decreased infections
Decreased rural lifestyle
Lifestyle change
Obesity, immobility
Diet
Immunization
Antibiotics

in 82% of wheezing infants. In the same study, 83% of children between the ages of 2 and 16 had evidence of viral infection; however, rhinovirus was the most common pathogen. With increasing age, sensitization increases, and in children aged 2–16 years positive tests for allergic inflammation showed the presence of elevated eosinophil cationic protein (ECP) in nasal wash fluid and increased serum IgE level (8). (See Table 2.)

In patients with persistent asthma, the role of environmental allergens has been extensively studied. A clear association between exposure and sensitization has been observed for several allergens. In addition, a clear association between sensitization and the development of asthma has been documented, such that >70% of patients over 4 years of age with asthma are sensitized. Measurement of quantity of dust mite exposure suggested that there was a critical level of exposure, i.e., 2 μg/g Der p 1/g of dust for sensitization and 10 μg of Der p 1/g also suggested that as a risk for increased symptoms of asthma. Sporik et al. (9) found that the relative risk for active asthma was 4.8 times greater in those exposed to Der p 1 > 10 μg/g dust at age 1 or 2 years, suggesting a causal relationship between exposure to allergens and asthma.

Whereas there is little debate about the causal relationship between exposure to allergens and sensitization and regarding the strength of the association between sensitization and asthma, a direct connection between exposure and asthma is disputed. Recently several investigators argued that the case for allergen exposure as a major primary cause of asthma is based on indirect evidence (10,11). Of course, evidence of a dose–response relationship would provide support for causality, but there are several factors that will obscure that connection. First, if the relationship is not linear, i.e., sigmoidal with a plateau or bell-shaped, it may be that all the houses in areas of high exposure would have sufficient allergen to maintain bronchial hyperreactivity in those who are predisposed. Second, individual differences in the local inflammatory response in the lungs may be only weakly correlated with our measures of sensitization such as skin test results or the titer of specific IgE. A third issue is the interplay of many different irritants such as cold air, exercise, passive smoke, and changes in weather. Fourth

Table 2 Incidence and Natural History of Wheezing in Childhood

Age	≤ 2 years	2–16 years
% Children	30%[a]	5–15%
Risk factors	Small lungs	Increased sensitization
	Passive smoke	Elevated total IgE
	RSV	Rhinovirus

[a] 30–40% persist.

is the relative inaccuracy of measurements of allergen in an environment as a method of predicting the quantity of allergen entering the lungs. Finally, for many patients, multiple allergens contribute to their symptoms (12). (See Fig. 1.)

The continuing high prevalence and severity of asthma has led many groups to investigate the potential for primary and secondary prevention. Primary prevention is designed to decrease sensitization to allergens and the onset of asthma. It has the advantage that it targets a population that is healthy but would be much simpler if at-risk children could be identified. On the other hand, if the measures proposed were simple and carried no risk (e.g., environmental control in the home), then primary prevention might be a reasonable strategy for a population.

There are several issues that affect the design of and evaluation of avoidance studies:

1. Can at-risk children be identified by history, blood tests, or genetics?
2. Do we know what form of immune response creates the risk of asthma,

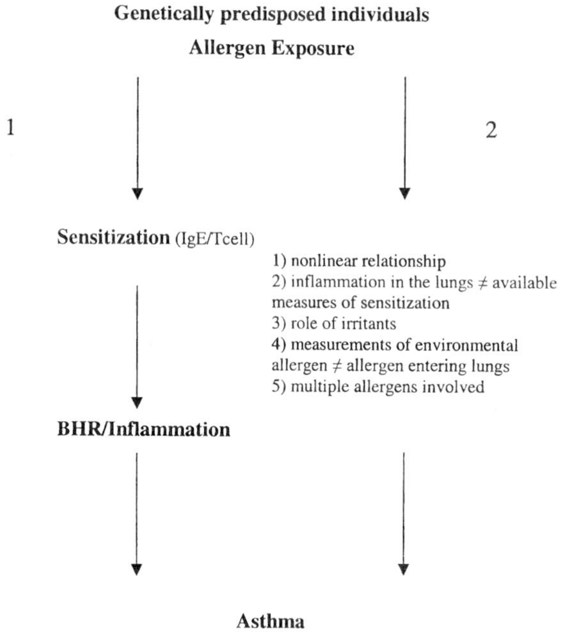

Figure 1 Factors influencing the dose–response relationship between allergen exposure and asthma. (1) The natural response to allergens requires sensitization and inflammation, which may be enough to obscure a dose response. (2) Attempts to define a direct relationship between allergen exposure and asthma are unlikely to succeed because too many factors interfere with the response.

and, equally important, when does the allergen-specific response begin?

3. Avoidance as a strategy implies that the dose response is linear, which may be true for dust mite but not for cat.
4. Are the strategies recommended for primary and secondary avoidance consistently effective at decreasing exposure or disease?

The present chapter addresses most of these issues. However, it is always important to keep in perspective the fact that the causes of the increased severity of asthma are not established. Without correctly identifying the causes of the epidemic, it is unlikely that we will control it.

II. Identification of At-Risk Infants

A. Family History and Genetics

Though familial clustering of asthma has been known for a long time, Mendelian inheritance has not been observed. Of course, multifactorial control is not surprising considering the difficulties of defining asthma and the variation in phenotypes. Many investigators are involved in studies to determine the genetic factors involved and their relevance. The collaborative Study on the Genetics of Asthma is a multicenter study begun with the intention of identifying important genetic loci for asthma by multipoint linkage analysis. Novel asthma susceptibility genes have been identified in three ethnic groups. These genetic differences in the setting of varied environmental exposures may contribute to differences in disease prevalence and severity (13). The alternative approach has been to search for polymorphisms of candidate genes that could influence the disease. One group reported linkage of atopy to chromosome 11q, suggesting a mechanism for enhanced IgE responses (14). Marsh et al. (15) reported evidence for linkage in 5q in the coding region of several cytokines with roles in the Th2 phenotype IL-4, IL-5, and IL-13. Rossenwasser et al. (16) found the IL-4 promoter polymorphism in 40% of their asthmatic subjects, and it was associated with higher total IgE levels. Although multiple sites have been identified as related to asthma, and genetic associations with several specific allergens have been identified, they do not yet provide any guidance about (1) the reasons for the increase, (2) specific approaches to treatment, or (3) how to identify individuals in whom primary prevention would be appropriate.

B. Immunological Markers

Elevated serum IgE is known to be a hallmark of atopic diseases, but it does not cross the placenta. On the other hand, the fetus is capable of synthesizing IgE from 11-weeks gestation (17) so that cord blood IgE (CB-IgE) would appear to be a good candidate for the prediction of atopy in infants. Some investigations have suggested that CB-IgE predicts early sensitization. In 1988, Magnusson showed that about 50% of the newborns who develop atopy before 18 months of age have elevated CB-IgE. In agreement with other investigators, Magnusson found that 30–40% of atopic children had a negative family history, suggesting that a screening program should include all newborns (17). Edenharter et al. (18), in conjunction with the German Multicenter Allergy Study, found a strong positive association between CB-IgE and early sensitization at 12 months; however, the predictive performance of elevated CB-IgE after that age was poor. No association between CB-IgE and recurrent wheezing was found (18). Kaan et al. (19) showed that measurable cord blood IgE was a significant risk factor for urticaria due to food but not for any other outcomes at 12 months of age. In addition, they found that a maternal history of asthma was the most important determinant for high cord blood IgE and that infants born during winter months were at significantly higher risk of having high IgE in cord blood (19).

There are several concerns about using IgE as a predictor for atopy. Although IgE is a marker for allergy, it is also influenced by other factors such as pollution and parasitic infection. High levels of IgE may occasionally be due to contamination by maternal blood. Finally, the levels of IgE being measured are in the range of 0.5 kU/L, which is at the lower limits of our capability of measurement.

III. The Evidence for In Utero Sensitization

The design of approaches to primary prevention depends on knowing when sensitization occurs. If sensitization starts during intrauterine life, which may well be true for foods, intervention measures should be instituted before birth. The selection of a specific cytokine phenotypic response for allergen-specific Th memory cells is believed by some to occur early in life. Initial priming may occur in utero as exogenous antigens that leak across the placenta are presented to the fetal immune system (20). Some research has suggested that the fetal environment is one of Th1 suppression and Th2 immunity. Although there is evidence of changes in cytokine profile in utero and early in life, the relationship of these to specific sensitization is not clear (21).

Recently, the response of fetal or cord blood mononuclear cells (CBMCs) has been investigated as a marker of prenatal sensitization to food or inhalant allergens. Early reports suggested that CBMC proliferative reactions at birth were higher in infants who were born to atopic parents and who developed atopic disease by 1 year of age. This led investigators to consider that antenatal sensitization could increase the probability of the development of early atopic disease. It was not known whether this would be due to higher antenatal allergen exposure or innate differences in immune responsiveness (22). Van Duren-Schmidt et al.

(23) suggested that the susceptibility of the fetal immune system to priming with birch or grass pollen varies during gestation because the majority of positive proliferative responses were obtained when maternal pollen exposure occurred during the first 6 months. Other investigators compared cord blood samples from unborn babies to term newborns to evaluate at what gestational age prenatal priming is predominantly initiated. They found no significant difference between responses in groups of preterm and term infants, again suggesting that the window of occurrence of priming was very early (<20 weeks). However, they also found that a lymphoproliferative response to seasonal allergens was uncommon and the response to dust mite was variable. By contrast, they and others have found consistent cord blood responses to β-lactoglobulin, suggesting that placental passage of foods may be normal (24). The most serious question about the significance of the apparent cord blood responses to dust mite comes from the finding by three groups that the prevalence and magnitude of proliferation is unrelated to maternal exposure (19,25,26).

Initial investigations were interesting, but a critical examination of the data seems appropriate. Many technical factors influence lymphocyte proliferation such as the density of cells or additives to the medium, including serum or antibiotics, which can lead to nonspecific stimulation. In addition, the lower number of $CD4RO^+$ cells in an immature individual makes it less likely that proliferative responses will be consistent from culture to culture. Using Bet v 1 and Phl p 1, the proliferative response can be directly examined, and cord blood responses have not been as impressive. Some caution that although it is clear that allergen exposure plays a role in the development of the allergic response, at the present time there is no convincing evidence that responses in cord blood to dust mite or pollen are related to maternal exposure (26).

In conclusion, these data are still open to interpretation. There are very complex in utero changes that help to protect the fetus. These include a relative shift in cytokine production toward a Th2 profile. In addition, it is possible to demonstrate T-cell proliferative responses to some antigens, particularly mite. However, these responses are unrelated to the exposure of the mother and must reflect some aspect of the development of T-cell repertoire. Technical issues come into question as well. In vitro responses are very variable because of the low number of precursors. Thus evaluation of these responses requires multiple replicates. In addition, some cord blood results have shown very high background, which also confuses interpretation.

IV. Methods of Prevention

A. Asthma Vaccine

Several methods of vaccination for protection against asthma and allergy have been suggested based on the mechanisms of sensitization. Holt, making note of tolerance to food allergens after continued antigen exposure, proposed the development of a similar routine for inhalant allergens. He believed this strategy could be accomplished during early childhood when the immune system was still reacting with competing Th1 and Th2-like responses. He suggested two strategies, one being enteral or intranasal administration of allergen, and the other being parenteral vaccination with a mixture of major inhalant allergens, ideally in combination with an appropriate Th1-selective adjuvant (27). Hsu et al. injected plasmid DNA encoding house dust mite allergen in mice resulting in expression of Der p 5-specific IgG1 and IgG2a antibodies as well as suppression of IgE, histamine, and allergen-induced airway hyperresponsiveness (28). These approaches would be different from desensitization, because they are intended to prevent the emergence of Th2 phenotype.

As previously discussed, one factor associated with the rise in atopy is the decline in rates of infectious diseases in developed countries. Childhood respiratory infections that have been proposed to modify the developing immune system include measles, whooping cough, and tuberculosis. Some of these infections may produce an immune response that could be characterized as Th1. Shirakawa et al. (29) found an inverse association between positive tuberculosis tests (≥10 mm induration) and atopic characteristics including symptoms and IgE levels. As the study was performed in Honshu, Japan, where immunization with BCG is established, it has been suggested that immunization with BCG or tuberculosis infection may have the potential to shift the immune response toward a Th1 phenotype (29). However, in Honshu and also in European countries where BCG is used extensively, the prevalence of allergic diseases and the increase in asthma have been no different from those seen in countries where BCG is not given. Similarly, when Arkwright and David (30) immunized patients who had atopic dermatitis with *Mycobacterium vaccae*, they observed significant improvement in the severity of atopic dermatitis by skin surface area affected, dermatitis scores, and potency of topical steroid ointments used. They emphasize the difference between reduction in atopic disease and absence of disease, the endpoint in other investigations (30).

B. Dietary Avoidance

Because allergy to foods is usually the first manifestation of atopy, attempts to manipulate dietary factors make sense. Initial observations that breastfeeding resulted in less atopic dermatitis date back to the 1930s (31). Recent studies have also shown a protective effect of exclusive breastfeeding (≥4 months) against asthma and atopy. This effect may result from several mechanisms including the exclusion of milk and its potentially allergenic components and the transfer of immunomodulatory components in breast milk (32).

Given that allergens are present in breast milk, it was believed that maternal diet may be important in the development of allergy. Strict maternal avoidance diets during breastfeeding resulted in a reduction in food-related allergic disorders and food-specific IgE sensitization, but the prevalence of allergic rhinitis, inhalant sensitization, and asthma was unaffected (33). Falth-Magnusson et al. (34,35). examined the effects of maternal elimination diet during pregnancy only and found no significant difference in allergic disease between the groups.

Food allergens are almost certainly passed to the infant in utero, and cord blood responses are not unusual. In addition, sensitization to food in the first year of life is common. On the other hand, the normal outcome is progressive tolerance with increased IgG/IgG4 antibody responses and decreases in IgE antibody. Although dietary avoidance in pregnancy and infancy may play a role in controlling eczema in children from highly atopic families, there is very little evidence that these measures are helpful in controlling allergic rhinitis or asthma after the first 2–3 years of life.

C. Environmental Control

Studies of asthmatic patients who are sensitive to house dust mites have demonstrated the success of avoidance measures in the control of asthma. Murray and Ferguson performed a 6-week controlled trial in Vancouver, Canada, with dust mite avoidance measures in the bedroom only. They included vinyl covers for pillows, mattresses, and box springs; biweekly washing of blankets and mattress pads; removal of toys, books, upholstered furniture, and carpets; and daily mopping of the floor. Those who were treated experienced fewer days of wheezing, fewer days of medication use, and fewer drops in peak flows. They also exhibited increased tolerance to inhaled histamine (36). We observed nine asthmatic patients who lived in an allergen-free hospital room. In most patients, symptoms and peak flows were improved and medications were reduced. Approximately one-half showed a major decrease in bronchial hyperreactivity to histamine over 3 months. In controlled trials of avoidance where a decrease in mite allergen was observed, there has been a consistent, significant outcome of decreased bronchial hyperreactivity (37). (See Table 3.)

Recommendations for dust mite avoidance are best described because dust mites have been so well characterized. House dust mites are mites of the family Pyroglyphidae with three predominant species: *Dermatophagoides pteronyssinus*, *D. farinae*, and *Euroglyphus maynei*. Other mites that can occur in houses include several species termed storage mites. Purification of proteins and analysis of their allergenic activity resulted in the definition of group I, group II, and now many other allergens and the development of assays. The bedroom is the most important room in the house for pyroglyphid mites, but mites can also be found in carpets, upholstered furniture, soft toys, and clothing (38).

Table 3 Decrease in Bronchial Hyperreactivity: Evidence from Six Controlled Trials

Reference	Time	*N*	Intervention	Decrease in mite allergen	Primary outcome
36	1 yr	10/10	Physical barriers	++	BHR
59	1 yr	22/20	Physical barriers	++	PEFR/BHR
60	1 yr	8/16	Physical barriers, acaricide	++	BHR
61	6 mo	24/25	Physical barriers, acaricide, washing, vacuuming	+	PEFR/BHR
40	6 mo	15/15	Physical barriers, air cleaner	++	BHR
62	6–12 mo	7/8	Hot air, ventilation, steam cleaning	++	BHR

++ = ≥70% reduction for >6 months.

With that in mind, recommendations for avoidance are as follows. The first step is to obtain a dust mite-impermeable mattress and pillow covering. If possible, removal of allergen sources, from old mattresses to carpets, can be helpful. In order to maintain low levels, smooth floor coverings, low levels of indoor humidity, and increased air ventilation are required (38). Because mites can also be present on clothing, it is also important to consider the best laundry procedures to reduce mite populations and allergen. McDonald and Tovey found that at 50°C half the mites were killed but at 55°C all mites were killed. At lower temperatures the concentrations of Der p 1 but not the number of mites were reduced by washing. In contrast, dry cleaning seemed to kill all mites but did not reduce the Der p 1 concentration. The current consensus is that washing every 2 weeks is acceptable (39). It is difficult to demonstrate effectiveness of air cleaners for dust mites because the levels of airborne house dust mite allergen in the absence of disturbance are generally below the limits of detection. As a result, there have been few data demonstrating a relationship between airborne measurements and sensitization or symptoms, but van der Heide et al. (40) showed improvement in airway hyperresponsiveness in patients who used active air cleaners in addition to allergen-impermeable mattress covers.

V. Controlled Trials of Primary Avoidance

The effectiveness of aeroallergen avoidance measures in the primary prevention of asthma has been investigated in only a few prospective, randomized, controlled studies. The first attempt was undertaken by Helken et al. in Denmark in 1988. They selected "high-risk" infants by biparental history of atopy or severe single atopic disposition combined with CB-IgE $\geq$ 0.5 kU/L. To these patients they recommended an allergy prevention program that included either breastfeeding (with an unrestricted maternal diet) or casein hydrolysate formula or ultrafiltrated whey hydrolysate for the first 6 months. In addition, it was recommended that solid foods not be introduced until 6 months of age. Further, avoidance of daily passive tobacco smoke, daily contact with furred pets, damp housing, carpeted floor, and dust-collecting materials in the child's room was recommended. These patients were compared to high-risk infants born 3 years earlier at a time when no such recommendations were made and to a group of infants not considered to be at risk. When the data were examined, at 18 months significantly fewer high-risk patients in the prevention group had atopic symptoms including recurrent wheezing, atopic dermatitis, vomiting/diarrhea, and colic. However, it was noted that compliance was poor, and when the groups were stratified according to environmental differences, the prevalence of atopic symptoms did not change (41).

In 1992, Arshad et al. in the United Kingdom published a prospective, prenatally randomized, controlled study using the same inclusion criteria. In contrast, in their prophylactic group, they recommended a strict maternal avoidance diet for those who were breastfeeding. They also included dust mite impermeable mattress covers, applied acaricide at 3-month intervals, and monitored compliance with home visits that included dust sampling. The infants were assessed for allergy at 1 year of age. Measures to reduce concentrations of Der p 1 were successful. After adjustments for confounding variables, the control group was at significantly greater risk for asthma, atopic dermatitis, and positive skin prick tests. The effect of food and house dust mite avoidance could not be separated (42). When the patients were followed at ages 2 and 4 they continued to show substantially less atopic disease (43,44).

Chan-Yeung et al. looked at the value of intervention in high-risk infants with a first-degree relative with asthma or two first-degree relatives with a history of allergy. The intervention program included breastfeeding with dietary avoidance or hydrolysate as well as dust mite control measures such as impermeable mattress covers, hot water washes of bedding, and application of benzyl benzoate powder or foam. Pet avoidance measures based on knowledge at the time consisted of removal of pets from the home, restriction to outside, or at least exclusion from the bedroom. Parents were also counseled on smoking cessation. Measured mite allergen levels were reduced in the intervention group and infants in the intervention group were breastfed longer with later introduction of solid foods. There was no difference in the prevalence of smoking or pet ownership. Risk for asthma was reduced by 34% in the intervention group. Risk for noninfectious rhinitis was also lower in the intervention group (45).

VI. Other Relevant Allergens

A. Cockroach

Cockroach allergy has been considered an important cause of asthma for years. Furthermore, sensitization to cockroach allergens is strongly associated with asthma in patients presenting to the emergency room (46). Estimates of the prevalence of cockroach allergy among asthmatic individuals range from 17% to 41% (47). Findings of the National Cooperative Inner City Asthma Study suggested that exposure to Bla g 1 levels >8 U/g in children's bedrooms was strongly associated with hospital admissions for asthma. A significant proportion of children (32%) were sensitized at exposure levels of 1–2 U/g, with the proportion of children with a positive skin test response increasing as the amount of Bla g 1 exposure increased and reaching a plateau at 4 U/g. Exposure levels in the bedroom were found to be most important (48). Similarly, in a population-based study of school-age children we found a clear dose–response relationship to cockroach allergen and sensitization. At this point, it appears that there is a dose–response relationship between exposure to cockroach allergen and sensitization (49). In contrast to the case of dust mites, however, early exposure to cockroaches was associated with recurrent wheezing independent of specific IgE antibody responses. Unfortunately, environmental control is not straightforward. Cockroach allergens persist in the indoor environment even after the cockroach population has been reduced, and sustained removal of cockroaches is difficult to achieve. In a recent attempt to reduce cockroach allergen exposure in Atlanta, there was no difference between placebo and treatment groups (50). It is believed that cockroach extermination needs to be done in all rooms and should be combined with thorough cleaning measures; however, an effective controlled trial has yet to be performed (47).

B. The Cat Paradox

In areas where dust mite is not a major allergen such as those with a cold climate, or high altitude giving rise to low humidity, asthma is still increasing. In such places, a significant association with asthma and sensitization to animal dander has been found (odds ratio of 4.2 by one report) (51). Exposure to cat allergens that have become airborne is thought to be much greater than for mite or cockroach allergens. In contrast to dust mite exposure, however, a simple dose–response relationship between exposure and sensitization has not been confirmed. Though Wahn et al. (52) noted a linear dose–response link between cat exposure and sensitization, in several studies the presence of a cat at home has not been identified as a risk factor for asthma or sensitization (53). Most houses with a cat have >8 μg Fel d 1 per gram of dust. In our recent study, we found a very wide range of cat exposure, 0.69–3840 μg/g dust. In that study, the maximum prevalence of sensitization to cat occurred with moderate exposure. By contrast, the number of children with IgG antibody to Fel d 1 was increased among those with the highest exposures. In this exposure group, there were 31 children who had IgG antibody *without* sensitization. Further analysis of their IgG antibodies showed that the amount of IgG4 was on average 20% of the total amount of IgG, very similar to allergic subjects. The primary cytokine that induces IgG4 production is IL-4; thus an antibody response such as this should be regarded as similar to a Th2 response, perhaps a ''modified Th2 response'' (51). (See Table 4.)

The now clear evidence that high exposure to cat allergens is associated with a decreased prevalence of sensitization and asthma raises many questions about the nature of the immune response to allergens as well as practical issues about avoidance. Given the very high levels of exposure to airborne cat allergen, it may not be surprising that many children have exhibited a response. However, the response observed does not have the features of a Th1 response. It includes a high proportion of IgG4, none of the children have delayed hypersensitivity skin tests, and the T-cell responses appear similar to those of allergic individuals. Thus the response may be best seen as a different form of Th2 response. However, many questions remain:

1. Is this IgG/IgG4 response responsible for the decreased prevalence, i.e., is it those children who would have become allergic with moderate exposure who develop IgG without IgE with high exposure?
2. Does this response depend on continued exposure, and if so what happens to individuals who have a dramatic decrease in exposure? To follow up this question, how long would a change in response take?
3. If high exposure to cat allergens can induce a response that is in effect a form of tolerance, why doesn't natural exposure to other allergens have the same effect? Although the answer is not clear, the possibilities include that (1) the quantity of cat allergen inhaled is in reality 100 times higher than that of mite allergen or (2) the enzymatic activity of dust mite (and cockroach) allergens both contributes to their allergenicity and prevents the generation of this form of tolerance.

Regardless, the results strongly suggest that having a cat in the home is associated with less risk of sensitization than moderate exposure. Thus recommending that patients not have a cat in the house may not be sensible advice to prevent sensitization and may well have affected the results of some studies on primary avoidance.

C. Alternaria

Although a consistent association between sensitization to indoor allergens and asthma has been observed, most studies suggested that sensitization to outdoor

Table 4 Characteristics of Purified Allergens: Relationship of Inhaled Dose to Evidence of "Tolerance"

Source	Allergen (mass)	Inhaled daily	Function	Evidence of high-dose tolerance	
				Epi[a]	Serol[b]
Dust mite (feces)	*D. pteronyssinus*	ng	Cysteine protease	No	No
	Der p 1 (25 kDa)		(Epididymal protein)[c]		
	Der p 2 (13 kDa)				
Cats (dander)	*Felis domesticus*	μg	(Uteroglobin)[c]	Yes	Yes
	Fel d 1 (36 kDa)	μg	Albumin	?	?
	Cat albumin				
Dogs (dander)	*Canis familiarus*	μg	Lipocalins	Yes	Yes
	Can f 1 (21 kDa)	μg	Lipocalins		
	Can f 2 (27 kDa)				
Rats (urine)	*Rattus norwegicus*	μg	(Pheromone binding protein)[c]	Yes[d]	Yes
	Rat n 1 (19 kDa)				
Cockroach (saliva)	*Blatella germanica*	ng	Aspartic protease	No	?
	Bla g 2 (36 kDa)	ng	Calycin	No	?
	Bla g 4 (21 kDa)	ng	Glutathione-S-transferase	No	?
	Bla g 5 (23 kDa)				
Fungi (spores, hyphae)	*Alternaria alternata*	?	Not known	No	?
	Alt a 1 (28 kDa)				

[a] Epidemiological.
[b] Serological.
[c] Sequence homology, functional importance not known.
[d] Observed among laboratory animal handlers.

allergens is primarily associated with allergic rhinitis (54). In spite of this, sensitization to *Alternaria*, typically thought of as an outdoor allergen, has been shown as an independent risk factor for asthma, and *Alternaria* has been the major asthma-associated allergen in desert regions of the United States and Australia (55,56). Several issues have made it difficult to determine its role. Only recently was an assay for measuring the major *Alternaria* antigen Alt a 1 developed (57). Application of the assay showed promising results with specificity and sensitivity down to 0.2 ng/mL Alt a 1. When used to assess environmental exposure, however, Alt a 1 was detected in only 6 of 1531 dust samples, suggesting that high levels of environmental fungal exposure were not present. Unfortunately, data measuring spore levels indoors are not available for comparison (58).

VII. Conclusion

The very strong association between sensitization to indoor allergens and asthma has focused attention on this relationship. Furthermore, many of the arguments about the reasons for the increase in allergic disease relate to this relationship. Thus it has been argued (1) that increased disease relates to increased exposure to indoor allergens or (2) that there has been a shift in immune responsiveness such that a larger proportion of the population is becoming allergic. The findings can be summarized as follows.

1. We believe that sensitization as judged by serum IgE antibodies or positive skin tests is dependent on exposure. Thus, in areas of the world where dust mites are absent, e.g., New Mexico or northern Sweden, very few children become sensitized or have any other evidence of an immune response. For dust mite and cockroach, the relationship between exposure and sensitization appears to be linear, strongly implying that decreased exposure in childhood would decrease the prevalence of sensitization. For cat allergen, it now appears certain that very high exposure can induce an immune response that includes IgG/IgG-4 antibodies and that should be regarded as a form of immunological tolerance. Thus for cat allergens, high exposure should prevent sensitization.
2. The association between sensitization and asthma is not only very strong but has been seen in many different environments related to many different allergens, i.e., mite, cockroach, cat, dog, and *Alternaria*. The strength of the association is such that in many environments sensitization dominates the relationship between exposure and asthma. If sensitization defines the relationship between allergens and disease,

then we do not expect to observe a relationship between current allergen exposure and asthma on a population basis.

3. Avoidance of indoor allergens is an important part of the management of allergic disease and has been shown to be effective in the treatment of asthma in dust mite-allergic asthma. For other allergens there are still extensive problems with the regimes recommended for avoidance. In particular, there is evidence that a large part of the problem for cat-allergic patients relates to allergen exposure in public places such as school or in homes without a cat. Primary avoidance studies have shown benefit, and several are ongoing. However, it appears that the results may be confounded by the effects of passive exposure to cat allergen. Interestingly, effective mite avoidance measures may play an indirect role in decreasing exposure to passively transferred cat allergen.
4. Although we have focused on allergen exposure, there is clearly potential for intervention to change immune responses. Our conclusion is that the response to mite allergen as judged by IgG antibodies is unusual before 2 years of age. In parallel with this, we consider that there is little or no evidence to suggest that nonallergic individuals mount a Th1 response to mite allergens. Furthermore, our evidence about the response to cat allergen suggests that increasing exposure to inhaled allergens will lead to an altered or modified Th2 response. We consider this form of "tolerance" the correct target for intervention either prior to or after sensitization.
5. Asthma is a complex disease during which changes in the lungs may be influenced by (1) genetics, (2) allergen sensitization, (3) allergen exposure, (4) the inflammatory response, and (5) multiple additional "enhancers" such as ozone, diesel particulates, and rhinovirus. However, it is not clear that any of these can adequately explain the increase in asthma over the last 30 years of the twentieth century. Thus it remains possible that some other aspect of Western lifestyle has decreased the threshold for wheezing or removed some protective effect for the lungs. It is clear that allergen exposure, the immune response to allergen, and the inflammatory response provide important targets both pharmacological and allergen-specific. However, the true causes of the increase in asthma have not been defined, and it is essential to consider all aspects of Western lifestyle that could influence the immunology, immunopathology, and physiology of the lungs. In particular, these issues are enormously important for children living in poverty in American cities where some but not all of the changes of Western society have been very marked.

References

1. Taylor G, Walker J. Charles Harrison Blackley. Clin Allergy 1973; 3:103–108.
2. Wahn U, von Mutius E. Childhood risk factors for atopy and the importance of early intervention. J Allergy Clin Immunol 2001; 107:567–574.
3. Waldron G, Pottle B, Dod J. Asthma and the motorways: One district's experience. J Public Health Med 1995; 17:85–89.
4. Bergman RL, Edenharter G, Bergmann KE, Lau S, Wahn U. Socioeconomic status is a risk factor for allergy in parents but not in their children. Clin Exp Allergy 2000; 30:1740–1745.
5. Ronmark E, Jonsson E, Platts-Mills TAE, Lundback B. Incidence and remission of asthma in schoolchildren: Report from the obstructive lung disease in northern Sweden studies (abstr). Pediatrics 2001; 107:578.
6. Williams H, McNicol KN. Prevalence, natural history, and relationship of wheezy bronchitis and asthma in children. An epidemiological study. Br Med J 1969; 4: 321–325.
7. Martinez FD, Wright AL, Taussig LM, Holburg CJ, Halonen M, Morgan WJ. Asthma and wheezing in the first six years of life. N Engl J Med 1995; 332:133–138.
8. Rakes GP, Arruda E, Ingram JM, Hoover GE, Zambrano JC, Hayden FG, Platts-Mills TAE, Heymann PW. Rhinovirus and respiratory syncytial virus in wheezing children requiring emergency care. IgE and eosinophil analyses. Am J Respir Crit Care Med 1999; 159:785–790.
9. Sporik RB, Holgate ST, Platts-Mills TAE, Cogswell J. Exposure to house dust mite allergen (Der p I) and the development of asthma in childhood: A prospective study. N Engl J Med 1990; 323:502–507.
10. Pearce N, Douwes J, Beasley R. Is allergen exposure the major primary cause of asthma? Thorax 2000; 55:424–431.
11. Lau S, Illi S, Sommerfeld C, Niggemann B, Bergmann R, von Mutius E, Wahn U, and the MAS group. Early exposure to house-dust mite and cat allergens and development of childhood asthma: A cohort study. Lancet 2000; 356:1392–1397.
12. Platts-Mills TAE, Sporik RB, Wheatley LM, Heymann PW. Is there a dose response relationship between exposure to indoor allergens and symptoms of asthma? J Allergy Clin Immunol 1995; 96:435–440.
13. Collaborative Study of the Genetics of Asthma. A genome-wide search for asthma susceptibility loci in ethnically diverse populations. Nat Genet 1997; 15:389–397.
14. Cookson WOCM, Sharp PA, Faux JA, Hopkin JM. Linkage between immunoglobulin E responses underlying asthma and rhinitis and chromosome 11q. Lancet 1989; 1:1292–1295.
15. Marsh DG, Neely JD, Breazeale DR, Ghosh B, Friedhoff LR, Ehrlich-Kautzky E, Schou C, Krishnaswamy G, Beaty TH. Linkage analysis of IL-4 and other chromosome 5q31.1 markers and total serum immunoglobulin E concentrations. Science 1994; 264:1152–1156.
16. Rossenwasser LJ, Klemm DJ, Dresback JK, Inamura H, Mascali JJ, Klinnert M, Borish L. Promoter polymorphisms in the chromosome 5 gene cluster in asthma and atopy. Clin Exp Allergy 1995; 25:74–78.

17. Magnusson CGM. Cord serum IgE in relation to family history and as predictor of atopic disease in early infancy. Allergy 1988; 43:241–251.
18. Edenharter G, Bergmann RL, Bergmann KE, Wahn V, Foster J, Zepp F, Sahn U. Cord blood-IgE as a risk factor and predictor for atopic diseases. Clin Exp Allergy 1998; 28:671–678.
19. Kaan A, Dimich-Ward H, Manfreda J, Becker A, Watson W, Ferguson A, Chan H, Chan-Yeung M. Cord blood IgE: Its determinants and prediction of development of asthma and other allergic disorders at 12 months. Ann Allergy, Asthma Immunol 2000; 84:37–42.
20. Prescott SL, Macaubas C, Holt BJ, Smallacombe TB, Loh R, Sly PD, Holt PG. Transplacental priming of the human immune system to environmental allergens: Universal skewing of initial T cell responses toward the T_H2 cytokine profile. J Immunol 1998; 160:4730–4737.
21. Wegmann TG, Lin H, Guilbert L, Mosmann TR. Bidirectional cytokine interactions in the maternal–fetal relationship: Is successful pregnancy a T_H2 phenomenon? Immunol Today 1993; 14:353–356.
22. Miles EA, Warner JA, Jones AC, Colwell BM, Bryant TN, Warner JO. Peripheral blood mononuclear cell proliferative responses in the first year of life in babies born to allergic parents. Clin Exp Allergy 1996; 26:780–788.
23. Van Duren-Schmidt K, Pichler J, Ebner C, Bartmann P, Forster E, Urbanek R, Szepfalusi Z. Prenatal allergen contact with aeroallergens. Pediatr Res 1997; 41:128–131.
24. Szepfalusi Z, Pichler J, Elsasser S, van Duren K, Ebner C, Bernaschek G, Urbanek R. Transplacental priming of the human immune system with environmental allergens can occur early in gestation. J Allergy Clin Immunol 2000; 106:530–536.
25. Smillie FI, Elderfield AJ, Cain G, Patel FY, Tavernier G, Brutsche M, Simpson B, Simpson A, Custovic A, Woodcock AA. Cord blood lymphoproliferative responses in neonates with defined atopic risk and maternal indoor allergen exposure [abstr]. J Allergy Clin Immunol 1999; 103:S109.
26. Platts-Mills TAE, Woodfolk JA. Cord blood proliferative responses to inhaled allergens: Is there a phenomenon? J Allergy Clin Immunol 2000; 106:441–443.
27. Holt PG. A potential vaccine strategy for asthma and allied atopic diseases during early childhood. Lancet 1994; 344:456–458.
28. Hsu CH, Chu KY, Tao MH, Lai YL, Wu HD, Huang SK, Hsieh KH. Immunoprophylaxis of allergen-induced immunoglobulin E synthesis and airway hyperresponsiveness in vivo by genetic immunization. Nat Med 1996; 2:540–544.
29. Shirakawa T, Enomoto T, Shimazu S, Hopkin J. The inverse association between tuberculin responses and atopic disorder. Science 1997; 275:77–79.
30. Arkwright PD, David TJ. Intradermal administration of a killed Mycobacterium vaccae suspension (SRL 172) is associated with improvement in atopic dermatitis in children with moderate-to-severe disease. J Allergy Clin Immunol 2001; 107:531–534.
31. Grulee CG, Sanford HN. The influence of breast and artificial feeding on infantile eczema. J Pediatr 1936; 9:223–225.
32. Oddy WH, Holt PG, Sly PD, Read AW, Landau LI, Stanley FJ, Kendrall GE, Burton PR. Association between breastfeeding and asthma in 6 year old children: Findings of a prospective birth cohort study. Br Med J 1999; 319:815–819.

33. Zeiger RL, Heller S, Mellon MH, Forsythe AB, O'Connor RD, Hamburger RN, Schatz M. Effect of combined maternal and infant food allergen avoidance on development of atopy in early infancy: A randomized study. J Allergy Clin Immunol 1989; 84:72–89.
34. Falth-Magnusson K, Kjellman N-IM. Development of atopic disease in babies whose mothers were receiving exclusion diet during pregnancy: A randomized study. J Allergy Clin Immunol 1987; 80:868–875.
35. Falth-Magnusson K, Kjellman N-IM. Allergy prevention by maternal elimination diet during late pregnancy: A 5-year follow-up of a randomized study. J Allergy Clin Immunol 1992; 89:709–713.
36. Murray AB, Ferguson AC. Dust-free bedrooms in the treatment of asthmatic children with house dust or dust mite allergy: A controlled trial. Pediatrics 1983;71:418–422.
37. Platts-Mills TAE, Mitchell EB, Nock P, Tovey ER, Mosororo H, Wilkins SR. Reduction of bronchial hyperreactivity during prolonged allergen avoidance. Lancet 1982; ii:675–678.
38. Platts-Mills TAE, Thomas WR, Aalberse RC, Vervloet D. Chapman MD. Dust mite allergens and asthma: Report of a second international workshop. J Allergy Clin Immunol 1992; 89:1046–1060.
39. McDonald L, Tovey E. The role of water temperature and laundry procedures in reducing house dust mite populations and allergen content of bedding. J Allergy Clin Immunol 1992; 90:599–608.
40. Van der Heide S, Kauffman HF, Dubois AEJ, deMonchy JGR. Allergen reduction measures in houses of allergic asthmatic patients: Effects of air cleaners and allergen-impermeable mattress covers. Eur Respir J 1997; 10:1217–1223.
41. Halken S, Host A, Hansen LG, Osterballe O. Effect of an allergy prevention programme on incidence of atopic symptoms in infancy. A prospective study of 159 ''high risk'' infants. Allergy 1992; 47:545–553.
42. Arshad SH, Matthews S, Gant C, Hide DW. Effect of allergen avoidance on development of allergic disorders in infancy. Lancet 1992; 339:1493–1497.
43. Hide DW, Matthews S, Matthews L, Stevens M, Ridout S, Twiselton R, Gant C, Arshad SH. Effect of allergen avoidance in infancy on allergic manifestations at age of two years. J Allergy Clin Immunol 1994; 93:842–846.
44. Hide DW, Matthews S, Tariq S, Arshad SH. Allergen avoidance in infancy and allergen at 4 years of age. Allergy 1996; 51:89–93.
45. Chan-Yeung M, Manfreda J, Dimich-Ward H, Ferguson A, Watson W, Becker A. A randomized controlled study on the effectiveness of a multifaceted intervention program in the primary prevention of asthma in high-risk infants. Arch Pediatr Adolesc Med 2000; 154:657–663.
46. Gelber LE, Seltzer LH, Bouzoukis JK, Pollart SM, Chapman MD, Platts-Mills TAE. Sensitization and exposure to indoor allergens as risk factors for asthma among patients presenting to hospital. Am Rev Resp Dis 1993; 147:573–578.
47. Arruda LK, Vailes LD, Ferriani VPL, Santos ABR, Pomes A, Chapman MD. Cockroach allergens and asthma. J Allergy Clin Immunol 2001; 107:419–428.
48. Eggleston PA, Rosenstreich D, Lynn H, Gergen P, Baker D, Kattan M, Mortimer KM, Mitchell H, Ownby D, Slavin R, Malveaux F. Relationship of indoor allergen

exposure to skin test sensitivity in inner-city children with asthma. J Allergy Clin Immunol 1998; 102:563–570.
49. Sporik R, Squillace SP, Ingram JM, Rakes G, Honsinger RW, Platts-Mills TAE. Mite, cat, and cockroach exposure, allergen sensitization, and asthma in children: A case-control study of three schools. Thorax 1999; 54:675–680.
50. Carter MC, Perzanowski MS, Raymond A, Platts-Mills TAE. Home intervention in the treatment of asthma among inner-city children. J Allergy Clin Immunol 2001; 108:732–737.
51. Platts-Mills TAE, Vaughan J, Squillace S, Woodfolk J, Sporik R. Sensitisation, asthma, and a modified T_H2 response in children exposed to cat allergen: A population-based cross-sectional study. Lancet 2001; 357:752–756.
52. Wahn V, Lau S, Bergmann R, Kulig M, Forster J, Bergmann K. Indoor allergen exposure is a risk factor for exposure during the first three years of life. J Allergy Clin Immunol 1997; 99:763–769.
53. Perzanowski M, Ronmark E, Nold B, Lundback B, Platts-Mills TAE. Relevance of allergens from cats and dogs to asthma in the northernmost province of Sweden: Schools as a major site of exposure. J Allergy Clin Immunol 1999; 103:1018–1024.
54. Sporik R, Ingram JM, Price W, Sussman JH, Honsinger RW, Platts-Mills TAE. Association of asthma with serum IgE and skin test reactivity to allergens among children living at high altitude. Tickling the dragon's breath. Am J Resp Crit Care Med 1995; 151:1388–1392.
55. Halonen M, Stern DA, Wright AL, Tallssig LM, Martinez FD. Alternaria as a major allergen for asthma in children raised in a desert environment. Am J Resp Crit Care Med 1997; 155:1356–1361.
56. Perzanowski MS, Sporik R, Squillace SP, Gelber LE, Call R, Carter M, Platts-Mills TAE. Association of sensitization to Alternaria allergens with asthma among school age children. J Allergy Clin Immunol 1998; 101:626–632.
57. Aden E, Weber B, Bossert J, Wahl R, Teppke M, Frank E, Wahl R, Fiebig H, Cromwell O. Standardization of Alternaria alternata: Extraction and quantification of Alt a 1 by using an mAb-based binding assay. J Allergy Clin Immunol 1999; 103:128–135.
58. Vailes L, Sridhara S, Cromwell O, Weber B, Breitenbach M, Chapman M. Quantitation of the major fungal allergens, Alt a 1 and Asp f 1, in commercial allergenic products. J Allergy Clin Immunol 2001; 107:641–646.
59. Walshaw MJ, Evans CC. The effect of seasonal and domestic factors on the distribution of *Euroglyphus maynei* in the homes of *Dermatophagoides pteronyssinus* allergic patients. Clin Allergy 1987; 17:7–14.
60. Ehnert B, Lau-Schadendorf S, Weber A, Buettner P, Schou C, Wahn U. Reducing domestic exposure to dust mite allergen reduces bronchial hyperreactivity in sensitive children with asthma. J Allergy Clin Immunol 1992; 90:135–138.
61. Carswell F, Birmingham K, Oliver J, Crewes A, Weeks J. The respiratory effects of reduction of mite allergen in the bedrooms of asthmatic children—a double-blind controlled trial. Clin Exp Allergy 1996; 26:386–396.
62. Htut T, Higenbottam TW, Gill GW, Darwin R, Anderson PB, Syed N. Eradication of house dust mite from homes of atopic asthmatic subjects: a double-blind trial. J Allergy Clin Immunol 2001; 107:55–60.

3

Anti-IgE and the Treatment of Asthma and Allergic Disease

LAURA L. DZIADZIO and WILLIAM W. BUSSE

University of Wisconsin
Madison, Wisconsin

I. Introduction

Airway hyperresponsiveness and reversible airflow obstruction are characteristic features of asthma that may be mediated, in part, by allergic or nonallergic factors. In allergic patients with asthma, IgE plays a major role in the development and regulation of wheezing and the asthmatic response. Furthermore, serum IgE levels have been correlated with airway hyperresponsiveness both in adults (1,2) and in children (3), and cell-bound IgE is a pivotal signal to mast cell activation. Thus, an antibody to IgE should offer another potential target of therapy for both allergic asthma and rhinitis.

The development of this unique antibody to IgE required the humanization of a mouse monoclonal antibody that binds only to IgE and blocks IgE attachment to mast cells, thereby inhibiting mediator release. Given this property, the antibody, rhuMAb-E25, may ultimately play an important role in the treatment of allergic diseases.

II. IgE Structure, Receptor, and Role in Allergic Disease

The immunoglobulin E isotype participates in both allergic disease and parasitic infections. IgE antibody contains an ε heavy chain and circulates as a bivalent antibody. Functionally, IgE mediates mast cell and basophil activation by binding to the ε chain of Fc receptors regulating the synthesis and release of a variety of proinflammatory mediators and cytokines (4,5) that ultimately lead to the immediate hypersensitivity reaction and eventual inflammatory response.

The pathogenesis of IgE-mediated hypersensitivity follows a typical sequence of events. In atopic patients, allergen exposure stimulates a subpopulation of $CD4^+$ cells (i.e., Th2-like) to release cytokines, including IL-4 and IL-13, as well as other contact-mediated signals to promote B-cell differentiation and production of antibody. IgE circulates and then binds to the high affinity Fc receptors specific for the ε heavy chain on mast cells and basophils. Following this process of sensitization, the subsequent reexposure to antigen binds to IgE Fab fragments, which then causes cross-linking of other cell-surface IgE antibody to signal release of preformed mediators and synthesis of other mediators. The released mediators act upon a variety of target organs, i.e., blood vessels, airway smooth muscle, and circulating cells, to stimulate the acute allergic response, resulting in acute rhinitis, asthma, urticaria, or anaphylaxis.

High affinity Fc receptors for ε heavy chains (FcεRI) are constitutively expressed on mast cells and basophils. The dissociation constant of the FcεRI for IgE is much stronger than that of any other Fc receptor for its ligand. Each FcεRI is composed of three separate transmembrane subunits, one α chain that binds ligand, and three chains involved in signaling (one β chain and two identical γ chains dimerized with disulfide links) (Fig. 1). The binding site for IgE to the FcεRI is at the amino terminus of the α chain and contains two Ig-like domains. The β and γ chains are involved in signal transduction. The β chain crosses the membrane four times and contains one immunoreceptor tyrosine-based activation motif (ITAM) at the carboxy terminus. Each γ chain also contains one ITAM. The γ chain of the FcεRI is a common subunit found in the FcγRI, FcγRIIIA, and FcαR. Tyrosine phosphorylation of the ITAMs is the driving force behind the signaling functions of the FcεRI. IgE upregulates FcεRI expression on mast cells and basophils to amplify IgE-mediated effector functions in parasitic infections and allergic disease.

The low affinity IgE receptor FcεRII is related to C-type mammalian lectins. There are two different isoforms of FcεRII: FcεRIIA, which is B-cell-specific, and FcεRIIB (CD23), which is induced by IL-4 on B cells, monocytes, and eosinophils. The low-affinity receptor for IgE has been implicated in the development of allergy (6,7) because IgE–antigen complexes may interact with the FcεRII on B cells to facilitate antigen presentation to T cells (8), induce lung eosinophilia, and increase cytokine production from Th2 cells (9).

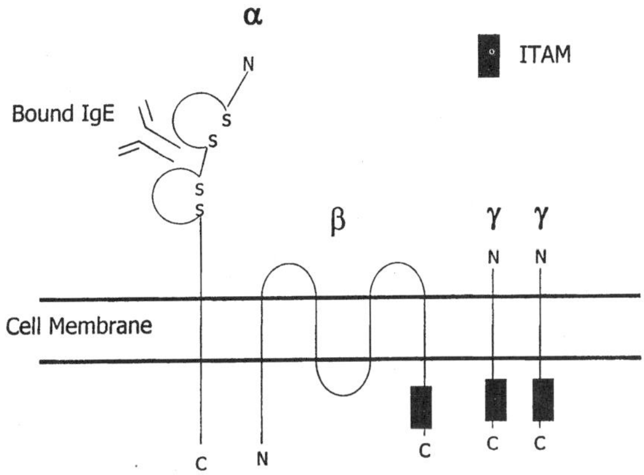

Figure 1 IgE binds Ig-like domains of the α chain of the IgE receptor, whereas the β and γ chains are involved with signal transduction.

Serum IgE levels are variable, affected by age, genetic predisposition, and ethnicity. IgE levels are increased in atopic individuals in response to allergen exposure and may increase two- to fourfold with seasonal pollination (10–12), with peak values 4–6 weeks later. Elevated total serum IgE levels have been shown in children with increased airway hyperresponsiveness, regardless of underlying allergic disease or asthma (3).

III. Development of an Anti-IgE Molecule

Immunoglobulin E has a central role in initiating immediate-type hypersensitivity reactions. The ability to block its receptors and hence IgE activation could be therapeutically effective. The development of a monoclonal antibody to IgE, however, required that a number of properties be considered: (1) a nonanaphylactogenic antibody, by the avoidance of IgE cross-linking and activation of the IgE receptor; (2) the development of a nonimmunogenic antibody; and (3) an absence of iatrogenic immune complex formation.

Two approaches were followed to generate a nonanaphylactogenic antibody to human IgE. First, the structuring of a monoclonal antibody (mAb) that has specificity for the region of membrane IgE exposed on switched B cells was developed (26). Another approach used homology-scanning mutagenesis to generate a murine antibody, MAE-11, that identified the same key amino acids in the C3 domain of IgE as did the α chain of the FcεRI (27). Antibodies selected for FcεRI can also inhibit binding to CD23 (FcεRIIB), because the binding site of IgE for CD23 is in the same region that binds FcεRI (28).

Dimerization of FcεRI is achieved through the binding of antibodies to the Fab of mast cell–bound IgE resulting in anaphylaxis. The development of another antibody that binds FcεRI but does not cause degranulation of IgE-sensitized cells was the goal in the development of anti-IgE as a treatment modality for allergic asthma and rhinitis.

Cross-linking of the FcεRI on mast cells by the anti-IgE molecule could cause degranulation and lead to anaphylaxis. Consequently, a murine monoclonal antibody was developed against the Cε3 domain of the human IgE molecule (29), which is highly specific in its ability to block binding of IgE to receptors. Although this molecule blocked IgE binding to mast cells and did not cross-link receptors, the nonhuman nature of this antibody induced immune responses in human subjects (30).

This response required humanization of the murine monoclonal IgE by the grafting of the antigen-binding loop of the mouse antihuman IgE antibody (MaE11) onto the human IgG1. This modification resulted in a recombinant humanized monoclonal anti-IgE antibody, rhuMAb-E25 (31) (Fig. 2). Ultimately, this molecule contains 95% homology with the human sequence but, due to the specificity of the murine antigen-binding loop, binds IgE at a constant similar to that of the original MaE11.

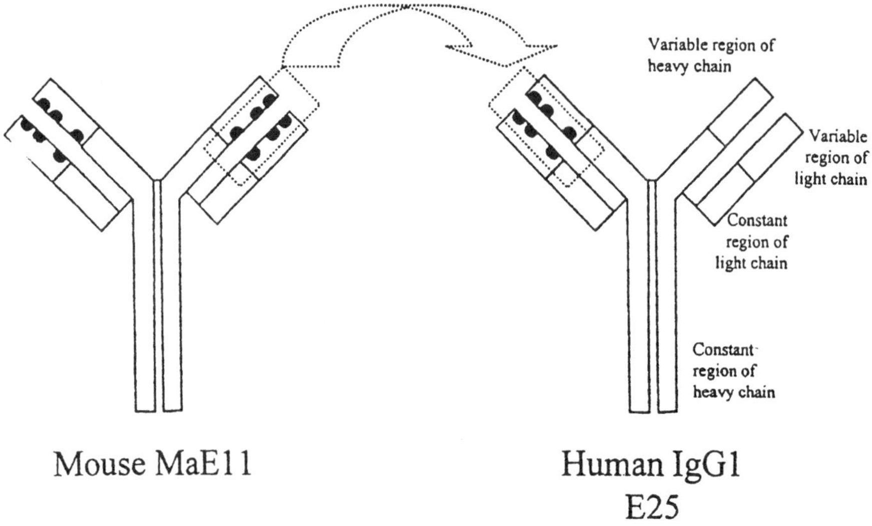

Figure 2 Mouse monoclonal anti-IgE was humanized by exchanging most of the molecule with human IgG1 in order to reduce the risk of immune response to foreign protein. (From Ref. 50.)

Important safety concerns were addressed in the development of rhuMAb-25. The risk for an anaphylactic reaction is reduced because this anti-IgE does not associate with IgE antibodies bound to the FcεI receptor. In addition, concerns regarding immune complex deposition were addressed. Complexes of tetramers and hexamers (two to three molecules of rhuMAb-E25 and two to three molecules of IgE) of rhuMAb-E25 are ultimately formed. The largest of these complexes is approximately 1×10^6 Da, which is too small to fix complement (32) in cynomolgus monkeys at 1 and 96 h after anti-IgE administration and thus do not provoke an immune complex reaction.

One surprising aspect in the development of an anti-IgE molecule involved parasite immunity. Because IgE is thought to be important in the immune response against parasitic infections, there was initial concern that this function of IgE would be attenuated with anti-IgE treatment. Remarkably, in anti-IgE-treated mice that were infected with *Nippostrongylus brasiliensis* (33) or *Schistosoma mansoni* (34) there was normal parasite elimination, a decreased number of eggs, and a diminished number of worms. These changes paralleled the fall in serum IgE. No data are currently available on the effects of anti-IgE in human parasitic infections.

IV. Animal Models Evaluating Anti-IgE

To study further the effects of anti-IgE, murine models were evaluated. A nonanaphylactogenic anti-IgE (mAb1-5) was generated that specifically bound IgE. However, this antibody did not recognize IgE-sensitized murine basophils. At a variety of concentrations, mAb1-5 did not induce histamine release from IgE-sensitized cells (35). Furthermore, systemic administration of mAb1-5 to rats partially inhibited the skin wheal and flare response on day 3 of treatment, with complete inhibition by the fourth day following administration. Eosinophilic recruitment to ovalbumin inhalation was also suppressed up to 90% in mice that were pretreated with anti-IgE. Unlike the skin effects, decreased eosinophilic infiltration to the lung was seen when mice were treated shortly before challenge. The effect on eosinophil infiltration was thought to be due to an interaction between the low affinity CD23 and anti-IgE. Eosinophilic infiltration is considered a feature of allergic asthma, and anti-IgE treatment inhibits lung eosinophilic recruitment to antigen (36). Anti-IgE inhibits eosinophilic inflammation by a CD23 mechanism. It has been shown that in CD23-deficient mice and in mice treated with anti-CD23, mAb1-5 does not affect lung eosinophilia (36). In the same study, administration of anti-IgE after antigen challenge inhibited IL-4 and IL-5 generation from lung T cells.

Antigen-induced bronchoconstriction was also decreased in rats that had been pretreated with mAb1-5. Mice immunized with ovalbumin and then treated with Mab1-5 underwent intravenous and antigen inhalation challenge but had significantly decreased bronchoconstriction and pulmonary hyperreactivity in response to antigen challenge (35). In vitro treatment of monkey bronchi with a nonanaphylactogenic anti-IgE antibody also inhibited the response to antigen (37). From these animal studies, it was apparent than anti-IgE monoclonal antibody treatment could reduce important features of immediate allergic reaction. The next step was trials in human subjects.

V. Human Treatment with Monoclonal Anti-IgE

Phase 1 studies were conducted with single and multiple doses of rhuMAb-E25 to determine whether the antibody was well tolerated and could result in a dose-related decrease in serum-free IgE (38). Free IgE decreased within 5 min of intravenous administration of drug and within 24 h after subcutaneous dosing (39). Total IgE levels (free IgE plus IgE bound to anti-IgE), however, were shown to increase, indicating a slow clearance of the anti-IgE–IgE complexes.

In addition to reducing the amount of free IgE to 1% of pretreatment levels in 15 patients with allergic rhinitis, rhuMAb-E25 decreased the expression of IgE and FcεRI on basophils (40). Over the course of 90 days, subjects received two doses of rhuMAb-E25 (0.015 and 0.03 mg kg^{-1} IU^{-1} mL^{-1}) every 2 weeks. During this treatment period, basophil surface-bound IgE decreased from an average of 240,000 to 2200 molecules per cell. After treatment, total FcεRI density was also reduced from an average of 240,000 receptors per cell to 8300 receptors per basophil. In contrast, unoccupied FcεRI on basophils increased during the treatment from an average of 2700 receptors per basophil to 7100 receptors per basophil ($p = 0.003$). These changes were dependent on regular treatment with rhuMAb-E25 and consistent with a decrease in free IgE, because fewer free molecules would result in more unbound receptor. Within 8 weeks of stopping the 46-week treatment with antibody, FcεRI density returned to 80% of baseline values. In vitro histamine release also returned to normal (41). Within the same time period, free IgE levels had increased to only 16% of pretreatment levels.

Casale et al. (42) studied rhuMAb-E25 treatment of 181 patients with ragweed seasonal allergic rhinitis. Subjects received rhuMAb-E25 treatment weekly [at doses of 0.15 mg/kg intravenously (IV) or subcutaneously (SQ), 0.5 mg/kg IV, or placebo] for 2 weeks, then every 2 weeks. Pharmacokinetic studies revealed a half-life of 20 days for all doses, whether delivered by the intravenous or subcutaneous route. The higher dose of rhuMAb-E25 resulted in lower free IgE levels (30% of baseline) compared to values in patients who received the lower dose (60% of baseline). Only 11 patients (of 181 total subjects) had complete suppression of free IgE. Both total IgE and ragweed-specific IgE were increased in patients who received rhuMAb-E25.

Patients who received rhuMAb-E25 had slightly lower symptom scores compared to placebo during ragweed pollination. These differences were not statistically significant, however, and neither were the use of rescue medication or quality of life scores. Treatment with rhuMAb-E25 was safe, and IV and SQ administration resulted in similar rhuMAb-E25 and free IgE levels. Serum free IgE levels in most of the treated subjects were not decreased to undetectable levels. This lack of effect on IgE may explain the failure of rhuMAb-E25 to modify symptoms of allergic rhinitis.

Treatment with rhuMAb-E25 was also evaluated in subjects with allergic rhinitis to birch pollen (43). In this study, 250 patients received rhuMAb-E25 at a dose that was based on individual serum IgE levels (e.g., levels of <150 IU/mL received 300 mg of anti-IgE or placebo at baseline and at week 4, and levels of >150 IU/mL received 300 mg of anti-IgE or placebo at baseline and at weeks 3 and 6). In 69% of the subjects, free IgE levels 3 or 4 weeks after initiation of treatment were less than 25 ng/mL; they were above 50 ng/mL in only 1.8% of subjects. Symptomatically, rhuMAb-E25-treated subjects had a significant improvement in rhinitis symptoms. There was significant increase in the placebo-treated group's nasal symptom severity during birch season from 0.78 at baseline to 0.98, using a scale of 0 (no symptoms) to 4 (maximal symptoms). In the treated group, there was no change from the baseline severity score of 0.7 during the pollen season. Most notably, efficacy variables were linked to total serum-free IgE concentrations.

Patients with the lowest free IgE had the lowest (1) symptom scores, (2) need for rescue antihistamine use, and (3) proportion of days requiring supplementary medications. Although differences in symptoms between placebo and treatment group were small, they were statistically significant. Moreover, treatment completely resolved symptoms in 21% of patients who received the antibody and in only 2% of those with placebo treatment. Dosing, which was based on total IgE level at initiation of treatment, may also have led to improved outcomes.

VI. Effects of rhuMAb-E25 on Pulmonary Response to Inhaled Antigen

The effects of rhuMAb-E25 were evaluated on the early and late pulmonary response to inhaled allergen (44,45). In a randomized, double-blind, parallel group study, Boulet et al. (44) identified 20 patients with mild allergic asthma who had demonstrated both immediate and late-phase responses to inhaled antigen. The subjects then received an initial dose of rhuMAb-E25 at 2mg/kg IV, followed by dosing of 1 mg/kg rhuMAb-E25 or placebo at weeks 1, 2, 4, 6, 8, and 10. One patient who received the active study drug developed an urticarial rash and was withdrawn from the study. Free IgE levels decreased significantly in the treated group, with mean levels falling from 287 to 30 ng/mL, and to below detection in 7 of 10 patients (Fig. 3). Respiratory symptoms, bronchodilator need, peak flow, and FEV_1 were unchanged in both groups, probably reflecting the mild nature of asthma in these subjects. When given a dose of allergen sufficient to cause an immediate 15% reduction in FEV_1 (median PC_{15}), the dose of antigen required to cause this fall in FEV_1, the treated group increased by 2.3, 2.2, and 2.7 doubling-doses at days 27, 55, and 77 of treatment, respectively. There were no changes in PC_{15} values in the placebo-treated group. Small but significant improvements were also noted in the non-antigen-induced methacholine PC_{20} in the group receiving rhuMAb-E25. The treatment group had an increased mean

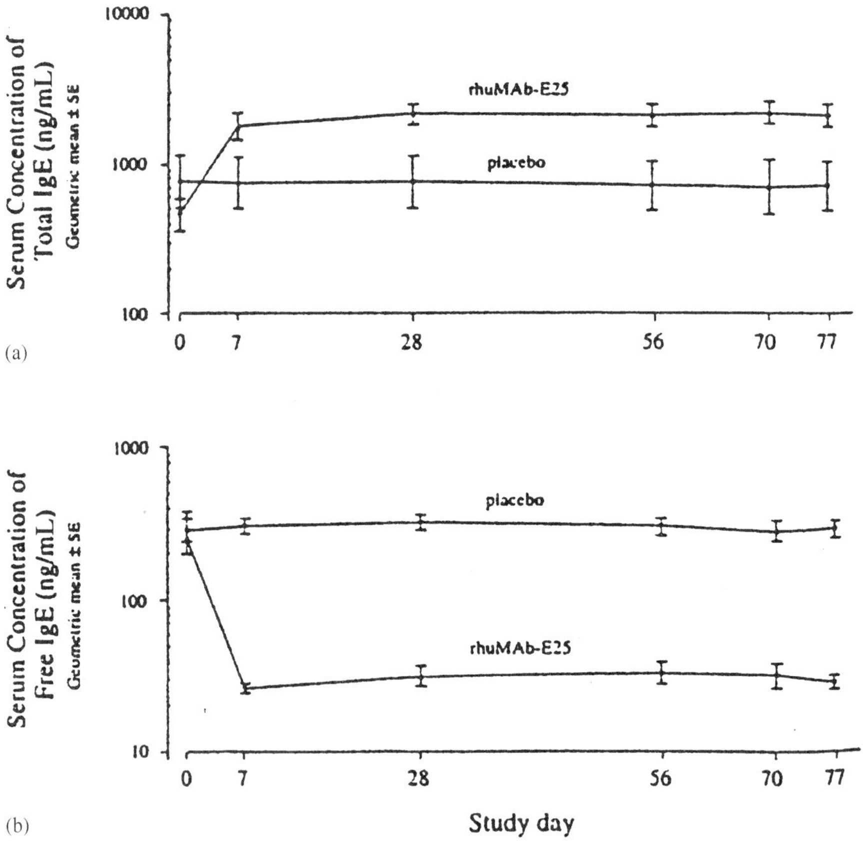

Figure 3 (a) Total serum IgE is elevated in patients treated with rhuMAb-E25, but (b) free-serum IgE is significantly decreased. (From Ref. 44.)

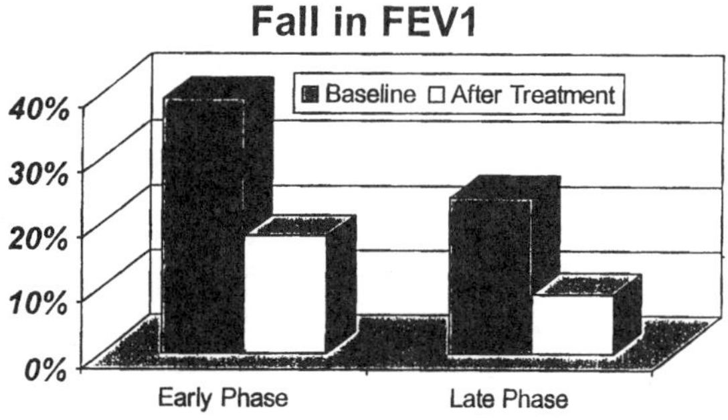

Figure 4 FEV_1 decreased significantly after rhuMAb-25 treatment in early and late phase. (From Ref. 45.)

PC_{20} from 0.73 mg/mL at baseline to 1.34 mg/mL at day 76 (a change of 0.9 doubling dose), which was not seen in the placebo group.

Fahy et al. (45) evaluated the effects of rhuMAb-E25 on the early- and late-phase responses to inhaled antigen in 19 patients with asthma in a parallel-group, randomized, double-blind, placebo-controlled study. The patients receiving rhuMAb-E25 received weekly infusions of 0.5 mg/kg for 9 weeks and had a 90% fall in serum-free IgE. Under these conditions, the early-phase reactions to inhaled antigen were attenuated in patients receiving rhuMAb-E25. The immediate fall in FEV_1 decreased from 39% at pretreatment to 18% after treatment (Fig. 4). Placebo had no effect on this response. The late-phase response was also decreased in patients receiving active therapy. The maximal late-phase fall in FEV_1 in the group receiving rhuMAb-E25 was 24% at baseline and only 9% after treatment. Placebo did not modify the late-phase response to antigen. Although patients treated with rhuMAb-E25 also had less sputum eosinophilia following inhaled antigen, this change was not significant compared with the placebo group.

Symptoms, in contrast, were unaffected by treatment with rhuMAb-E25. For example, values for FEV_1, morning and evening peak expiratory flow, asthma symptoms, and β_2-agonist use did not change significantly in either group during or immediately after treatment. These studies suggest a role for IgE in both early and late allergic response.

VII. rhuMAb-E25 Effects on Clinical Asthma

To assess further the effects of rhuMAb-E25 on patients with active clinical asthma, Milgrom et al. (46) identified 317 patients with moderate-to-severe allergic asthma who required inhaled or oral corticosteroid treatment. The subjects were randomized to receive intravenous rhuMAb-E25 (5.8 μg kg^{-1} ng^{-1} of IgE/mL or 2.4 μg kg^{-1} ng^{-1} of IgE/mL, or placebo) every 2 weeks for 20 weeks. During the first 12 weeks of study the patients were maintained on their usual medications. For the last 8 weeks, corticosteroid doses were tapered, with the objective of either discontinuing this medication or treating with the lowest possible dose. Initially there were no significant differences among the groups, with median doses of inhaled corticosteroid being 800 μg/day, oral corticosteroid doses of 10 mg/day, and mean β-agonist use of 8–9 puffs/day in all groups. The most notable findings in this study involved a reduction in oral and inhaled corticosteroids in all groups. There was a significant ($p = 0.04$) difference in the percentage of patients who experienced a ≥50% decrease in oral corticosteroid dosing in the active treatment phase (78% in the high dose group vs. 33% in the placebo group) (Fig. 5). For patients receiving study drug, regardless of dose, there were more patients who had ≥50% decrease in their oral and inhaled corticosteroid dose than those receiving the placebo, but these differences were not significant. Comparing patients who completely discontinued oral and inhaled corticosteroids, more patients who received rhuMAb-E25 were able to stop steroids than those who received placebo, but again the differences were not significant (oral corticosteroids: 17% discontinued in placebo group, 43% discontinued in low-dose group, and 33% discontinued in high-dose group; inhaled corticosteroids: 12% discontinued in placebo group, 23% discontinued in low-dose group, and 18% discontinued in high-dose group). The most striking finding in this study was that rhuMAb-E25 appeared to act as a corticosteroid-sparing agent, particularly in those subjects with severe asthma, as indicated by a need for daily systemic corticosteroid therapy. In addition, small but statistically significant improvements in quality of life, peak expiratory flow, and symptom scores were noted in those with active treatment.

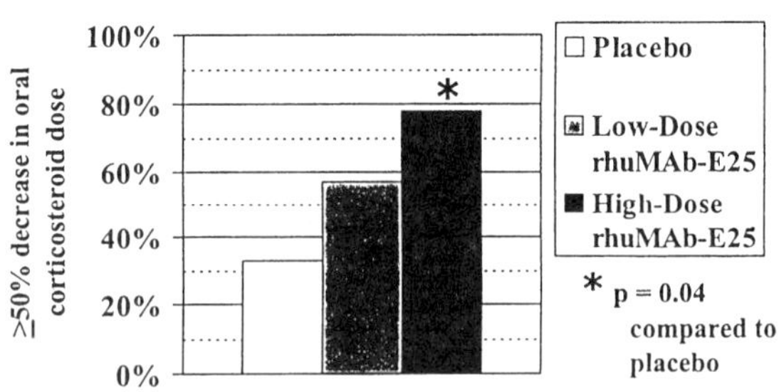

Figure 5 There was a reduction in oral corticosteroid dosing in subjects receiving high-dose rhuMAb-E25 compared with placebo ($p = 0.04$). (From Ref. 46.)

Other markers of disease activity were also evaluated by Milgrom et al. (46). Symptom scores improved in the groups receiving rhuMAb-E25 as well as in the placebo group. There was, however, a significant difference between the active treatment and placebo group symptom score at week 12. Similar improvements in quality of life scores were noted. There was a significant improvement in peak expiratory flow values in the high-dose group (30.7 L/m in the high-dose group, 18.6 L/m in the low-dose group, and 11.3 L/m in the placebo group). Free IgE levels dropped precipitously in the groups receiving rhuMAb-E25 (from 1000 ng/mL to 7.3 ng/mL in the high-dose group and from 1060 ng/mL to 13.9 ng/mL in the low-dose group) within 1 h after the initial dose. Though there was no significant change in FEV_1 among the three groups, the improved PEFR and decreased corticosteroid requirements indicate clinical effect.

To study further the effects of rhuMAb-E25 on patients with moderate to severe asthma (47), a double-blind, placebo-controlled trial was performed with 525 patients who required daily treatment with inhaled corticosteroids. Subjects were randomized to receive placebo or rhuMAb-E25 (150 or 375 mg SQ every 2 or 4 weeks, depending on baseline IgE levels and body weight). Doses of inhaled corticosteroid remained constant over the first 16 weeks of treatment and were then tapered during the last 12 weeks of treatment. Significantly fewer asthma exacerbations occurred in subjects in the active treatment phases of the study than in those receiving placebo. During the corticosteroid reduction phase, patients receiving the active study drug had a median decrease in inhaled corticosteroid dose of 75%, compared with 50% in patients receiving placebo ($p < 0.001$). The percentage of patients who were able to completely discontinue inhaled corticosteroids was also significantly higher in subjects receiving rhuMAb-E25 than in those given placebo (39.6% vs. 19.1%, $p < 0.001$). Rescue albuterol use, asthma symptom scores, and respiratory function were also improved in patients receiving rhuMAb-E25.

The routes of rhuMAb-E25 administration that have been primarily examined have been intravenous and subcutaneous. It appears that both IV and SQ administration effectively achieve appropriate levels of rhuMAb-E25 in serum as well as causing a similar decrease in free IgE. Subcutaneous dosing of drug is of greater ease and less expensive than intravenous dosing. An aerosolized version of rhuMAb-E25 was studied in relationship to alteration of early-phase response to inhaled allergen (48) and serum IgE and rhuMAb-E25 levels. Subjects with mild allergic asthma were enrolled in a randomized, double-blind study in which subjects received placebo or one of two aerosolized rhuMAb-E25 doses (1 mg or 10 mg) on a daily basis for 8 weeks. Although there were detectable serum levels of rhuMAb-E25 in all 10 patients receiving the drug at 10 mg nebulized/day at day 14, by 8 weeks only six of 10 patients still had detectable levels. In the group receiving a nebulized dose of 1 mg/day, four of 12 patients had detectable levels in this series. There was no difference in serum IgE levels, FEV_1, or FEV_1 after antigen challenge (early and late phase). Therefore, nebulized rhuMAb-E25 does not appear to be as effective as either the IV or SQ route of administration.

VIII. Conclusions

Treatment of patients with allergic rhinitis and asthma with rhuMAb-E25, a recombinant, humanized, monoclonal antibody that binds IgE, has been shown to decrease serum-free IgE levels by more than 95% and often to undetectable levels. rhuMAb-E25 is the first monoclonal antibody treatment in allergic disease. It appears safe, with only mild side effects, such as self-limited urticaria, noted in a very small proportion of treated subjects. There have been no reports of anaphylaxis or immune complex disease associated with rhuMAb-E25.

Its clinical effects on allergic rhinitis have been small but in some settings statistically significant. Because the drug is likely to be expensive, alternative therapies involving allergic rhinitis and rhuMAb-E25 may be postulated. In patients with allergic disease requiring immunotherapy who have problems with allergic reactions to this mode of therapy, rhuMAb-E25 may act as a bridging form of treatment. It could potentially be useful in conjunction with standard immunotherapy to diminish its untoward effects, as therapeutic goals of immunotherapy are met.

As studied, rhuMAb-E25 in allergic asthma may also be adjuvant therapy. Its role in the reduction of inhaled and oral corticosteroids in patients with moderate to severe disease may be the most useful and cost-effective use of rhuMAb-E25.

Other monoclonal antibodies, such as anti-CD23, which binds with high affinity to CD23, a membrane protein expressed constitutively at low levels on

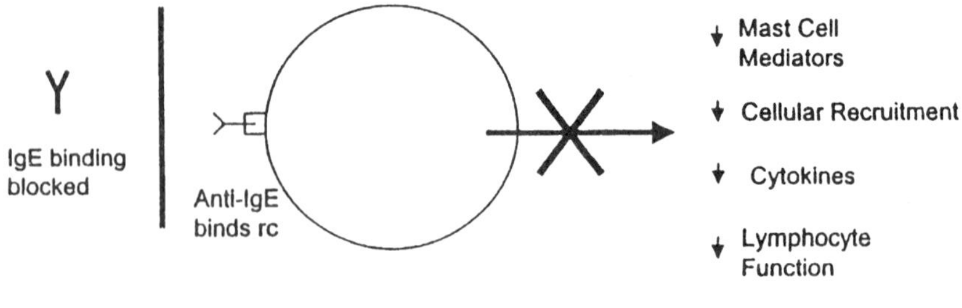

Figure 6 Anti-IgE binding, in addition to blocking IgE, may have anti-inflammatory effects secondary to decreased mast-cell-mediator release, cell recruitment, cytokine generation, and lymphocyte function.

B lymphocytes, as well as on other cell types after incubation with IL-4, may ultimately have a therapeutic role. Phase I studies have shown diminution in IgE levels after treatment with this antibody in patients with allergic asthma (49).

Because as most of the beneficial effects of rhuMAb-E25 have been seen in patients with moderate-to-severe asthma, anti-IgE appears to reduce inflammation and not just block IgE binding. Blocking IgE binding may have other effects on the inflammatory pathways and thus cause the observed changes in the inflammatory response in asthma. As a consequence, prevention of IgE binding may result in not only decreased mast-cell-mediator release but also reduced cellular recruitment, decreased inflammatory cytokine release, and impaired lymphocyte function (Fig. 6). Ultimately, these effects may result in a decrease in inflammation suspected to occur in asthmatic patients treated with rhuMAb-E25.

References

1. Sunyer J, Anto JM, Sabria J, Roca J, Morell F, Rodriguez-Roisin, Rodrigo MJ. Relationship between serum IgE and airway responsiveness in adults with asthma. J Allergy Clin Immunol 1995; 96:699–706.
2. Burrows B, Martinez FD, Halonen M, Barbee RA, Cline MG. Association of asthma with serum IgE levels and skin-test reactivity to allergens. N Engl J Med 1989; 320: 271–277.
3. Sears MR, Burrows B, Flannery EM, Herbison GP, Hewitt CJ, Holdaway MD. Relation between airway responsiveness and serum IgE in children with asthma and in apparently normal children. N Engl J Med 1991; 325:1067–1071.
4. Kinet JP. The high-affinity receptor for immunoglobulin E. Curr Opin Immunol 1990; 2:499–505.
5. Metzget H, Alcaraz G, Hohman R, Kinet JP, Pribluda V, Quarto R. The receptor with high affinity for immunoglobulin E (Review). Annu Rev Immunol 1996; 4: 419–470.
6. Delespesse G, Sarfati H, Hofstetter H. Human IgE-binding factors. Immunol Today 1989; 10:159–164.
7. Delespesse G, Suter U, Mossalyayi, Bettler B, Sarfati M, Hofstetter H, Kilchherr E, Debre P, Dalloul A. Expression, structure, and function of the CD23 antigen. Adv Immunol 1991; 49:149–191.
8. Pirron U, Schlunk T, Prinz JC, Rieber EP. IgE-dependent antigen focusing by human B lymphocytes is mediated by the low-affinity receptor for IgE. Eur J Immunol 1990; 20:1547–1551.
9. Coyle AJ, Wagner K, Bertrand C, Tsuyuki S, Bews J, Heusser C. Central role of immunoglobulin E in the induction of lung eosinophil infiltration and T helper 2 cell cytokine production: Inhibition by a non-anaphylactogenic anti-IgE antibody. J Exp Med 1996; 183:1303–1310.
10. Orgel HA, Lenoir MA, Bazaral M. Serum IgG, IgA, IgM and IgE levels and allergy in Filipino children in the United States. J Allergy Clin Immunol 1974; 53:213–222.

11. Berg T, Johansson SGO. IgE concentrations in children with atopic diseases: A clinical study. Int Arch Allergy Immunol 1969; 36:219–232.
12. Yunginger JW, Gleich GJ. Seasonal changes in serum and nasal IgE concentrations. J Allergy Clin Immunol 1973; 51:174–186.
13. Backer V, Ulrik CS, Wendelboe D, Bach-Mortenson N, Hansen KK, Laursen EM, Dirksen A. Distribution of serum IgE in children and adolescents aged 7 to 16 years in Copenhagen, in relation to factors of importance. Allergy 1992; 47:484–489.
14. Welliver RC, Wong DT, Sun M, Middleton E Jr, Vaughan RS, Ogra PL. The development of respiratory syncytial virus-specific IgE and the release of histamine in the nasopharyngeal secretions after infection. N Engl J Med 1981; 305:841–846.
15. Bahna SL, Horwitz CA, Fiala M, Heiner DC. IgE response in heterophile-positive infectious mononucleosis. J Allergy Clin Immunol 1978; 62:167–173.
16. Skoner DP, Doyle WJ, Tanner EP, Kiss J, Fireman P. Effect of rhinovirus 39 (RV-39) infection on immune and inflammatory parameters in allergic and non-allergic subjects. Clin Exp Allergy 1995; 25:561–567.
17. Wright DN, Nelson RP Jr, Ledford DK, Fernandez-Caldas E, Trudeau WL, Lockey RF. Serum IgE and human immunodeficiency virus (HIV) infection. J Allergy Clin Immunol 1990; 86:445–452.
18. Kaplan LD, Wofsy CB, Volberdring PA. Treatment of patients with acquired immunodeficiency syndrome and associated manifestations. JAMA 1987; 257:1367–1374.
19. Sample S, Chernoff DN, Lenahan GA, Serwonska MH, Rangi S, Sherman JW, Sooy CD, Hollander H, Goetzl EJ. Elevated serum concentrations of IgE antibodies to environmental antigens in HIV-seropositive male homosexuals. J Allergy Clin Immunol 1990; 86:876–880.
20. Miguez-Burbano MJ, Shor-Posner G, Fletchern MA, Lu Y, Moreno JN, Carcarmo C, Page B, Quesada J, Sauberlich H, Baum MK. Immunoglobulin E levels in relationship to HIV-1 disease, route of infection and vitamin E status. Allergy 1995; 50:157–161.
21. Israel-Biet D, Labrousse F, Tourani J, Sors H, Andrieu JM, Even P. Elevation of IgE in HIV-infected subjects: A marker of poor prognosis. J Allergy Clin Immunol 1992; 89:68–75.
22. Lynch NR, Hagel I, Perez M, DiPrisco MC, Lopez R, Alvarez N. Effect of antihelminthic treatment on the allergic reactivity of children in a tropical slum. J Allergy Clin Immunol 1993; 92:404–411.
23. Grove DI, Burston TO, Forbes IJ. Fall in IgE levels after treatment for hookworm. Clin Exp Immunol 1974; 18:565–569.
24. Nielsen BW, Lind P, Hansen B, Reimert CM, Nansen P, Schiotz PO. Immune responses to nematode exoantigens: Sensitizing antibodies and basophil histamine release. Allergy 1994; 49:427–435.
25. Yamaoka KA, Capron M, Bout D, Inuo G, Fujita K. Purified excretory-secretory component of filarial parasite enhances FCεRII/CD23 expression on human splenic B and T cells and IgE synthesis while potentiating T-helper type 2-related cytokine generation from T cells. Immunology 1994; 81:507–512.
26. Peng C, Davis FM, Sun LK, Liou RS, Kim YW, Chang TW. A new isoform of human membrane-bound IgE. J Immunol 1992; 148:129–136.

27. Presta L, Shields R, O'Connell, Lahr S, Porter J, Gorman C, Jardieu P. The binding site on human immunoglobulin E for its high affinity receptor. J Biol Chem 1994; 269:26368–26373.
28. Sutton BJ, Gould HJ. The human IgE network. Nature 1993; 5:493–508.
29. Chang TW, Davis FM, Sun NC, Sun CR, MacGlashan DW Jr, Hamilton RG. Monoclonal antibodies specific for human IgE-producing B-cells, a potential therapeutic for IgE-mediated allergic diseases. Biotechnology 1990; 8:122–126.
30. Shawler DL, Bartholomew RM, Smith LM, Dillman RO. Human immune response to multiple injections of murine monoclonal IgG. J Immunol 1985; 135:1530–1535.
31. Presta LG, Lahr SJ, Shields RL, Porter JP, Gorman CM, Fendly BM, Jardieu PM. Humanization of an antibody directed against IgE. J Immunol 1993; 151:2623–2632.
32. Fox JA, Hotaling TE, Struble C, Ruppel J, Bates DJ, Schoenhoff MB. Tissue distribution and complex formation with IgE of an anti-IgE antibody after intravenous administration in cynomolgus monkeys. J Pharmacol Exp Ther 1996; 279:1000–1008.
33. Marshall JS, Wells PD, Bell EB. Accelerated elimination of *N. brasiliensis* from the small intestine after auto-anti-IgE induction. Immunology 1987; 60:303–308.
34. Amiri P, Haak-Frendscho M, Robbins K, McKerrow JH, Stewart T, Jardier P. Anti-immunoglobulin E treatment decreases worm burden and egg production in *Schistosoma mansoni*-infected normal and interferon knockout mice. J Exp Med 1994; 180: 971–980.
35. Heusser CH, Wagner K, Bowles JPA, Coyle A, Einsle K, Kips J, Eum S-K, Lefort J, Vargaftig BB. Demonstration of the therapeutic potential of non-anaphylactogenic anti-IgE antibodies in murine models of skin reaction, lung function and inflammation. Int Arch Allergy Immunol 1997; 113:231–235.
36. Coyle AJ, Wagner K, Bertrand C, Tsuyuki S, Bews J, Heusser CH. Central role of IgE in the induction of lung eosinophil infiltration and Th2 cell cytokine production: Inhibition by a non-anaphylactogenic anti-IgE antibody. J Exp Med 1996; 183: 1303–1310.
37. Saban R, Haak-Frenscho M, Zine M, Ridgway J, Gorman C, Presta LG, Bjorling D, Saban M, Jardieu P. Human FcεRI-IgG and humanized anti-IgE monoclonal antibody MAE11 block passive sensitization of human and rhesus monkey lung. J Allergy Clin Immunol 1994; 94:836–843.
38. Corne J, Djukanovic R, Thomas L, Warner J, Botta L, Grandordy B, Gygax D, Heusser C, Patalano F, Richardson W, Kilcherr E, Staehelin T, Davis F, Gordon W, Sun L, Liou R, Chang T, Holgate S. The effect of intravenous administration of a chimaeric anti-IgE antibody on serum IgE levels in atopic subjects: Efficacy, safety and pharmacokinetics. J Clin Invest 1997; 99:879–887.
39. Froehlich J, Schoenhoff M, Jardieu P, Ruppel J, Fei D, Buckley P, Bush R. Multiple doses of a recombinant humanized monoclonal anti IgE antibody are safely tolerated and decrease free serum IgE to undetectable levels [abstr]. J Allergy Clin Immunol 1995; 95:356.
40. MacGlashan DW, Bochner BS, Adelman DC, Jardieu PM, Togias A, McKenzie-White J, Sterbinsky SA, Hamilton RG, Lichtenstien LM. Down-regulation of FcεRI expression on human basophils during in vivo treatment of atopic patients with anti-IgE antibody. J Immunol 1997; 158:1438–1445.

41. Saini SS, MacGlashan DW Jr, Sterbinsky SA, Togias A, Adelman DC, Lichtenstien LM, Bochner BS. Down-regulation of human basophil IgE and FCεRIα surface densities and mediator release by anti-IgE-infusions is reversible in vitro and in vivo. J Immunol 1999; 162:5624–5630.
42. Casale TB, Bernstein IL, Busse WW, LaForce CF, Tinkelman DG, Stoltz RR, Dockhorn RJ, Reimann J, Su JQ, Fick RB, Adelman DC. Use of an anti-IgE humanized monoclonal antibody in ragweed-induced allergic rhinitis. J Allergy Clin Immunol 1997; 100:110–121.
43. Adelroth E, Rak KS, Haahtela T, Aasand G, Rosenhall L, Zetterstrom O, Byrne A, Champain K, Thirlwell J, Cioppa GD, Sandstrom T. Recombinant humanized mAB-E25, and anti-IgE mAB, in birch pollen-induced seasonal allergic rhinitis. J Allergy Clin Immunol 2000; 106:253–259.
44. Boulet J, Chapman KR, Cote J, Kalra S, Bhagat R, Swystun VA, Laviolette M, Cleland LD, Deschesnes F, Su JQ, DeVault A, Fick RB Jr, Cockcroft DW. Inhibitory effects of an anti-IgE antibody E25 on allergen-induced early asthmatic response. Am J Respir Crit Care Med 1997; 155:1835–1840.
45. Fahy JV, Fleming E, Wong HH, Liu JT, Su JQ, Reimann J, Fick RB Jr, Boushey HA. The effect of an anti-IgE monoclonal antibody on the early- and late-phase responses to allergen inhalation in asthmatic subjects. Am J Respir Crit Care Med 1997; 155:1828–1834.
46. Milgrom H, Fick RB Jr, Su JQ, Reimann JD, Bush RK, Watrous ML, Metzger WJ. Treatment of allergic asthma with monoclonal anti-IgE antibody. N Engl J Med 1999; 341:1966–1973.
47. Busse W, Corren J, Lanier BQ, McAlary M, Fowler-Taylor A, Rohane P, Gupta N. Omalizumab, anti-IgE recombinant humanized monoclonal antibody, for treatment of allergic asthma. J Allergy Clin Immunol (in press).
48. Fahy JV, Cockcroft DW, Boulet L, Wong HH, Deschesnes F, Davis EE, Ruppel J, Su JQ, Adelman DC. Effect of aerosolized anti-IgE (E25) on airway responses to inhaled allergen in asthmatic subjects. Am J Respir Crit Care Med 1999; 160:1023–1027.
49. Busse WW, Rosenwasser LJ, Lizambri RG, Olejnik RA, Totoritis MC. Results of a phase I, single-dose, dose-escalating trial of a primatized[R] anti-CD23 monoclonal antibody (IDEC-152) in patients with allergic asthma (abstr). J Allergy Clin Immunol 2001; 107(2):S106.

4

Counterregulation of Cell Activation by the Immunoreceptor Tyrosine-Based Inhibitory Motif

HOWARD R. KATZ

Harvard Medical School
and Brigham and Women's Hospital
Boston, Massachusetts

I. Introduction

The activation of immune system cells involved in inflammatory diseases such as asthma was for many years thought to be regulated almost exclusively by activating stimuli such as antigen + specific antibody, adhesion molecule ligands, and cytokines. Over the last few years, it has become apparent that most cells of the hematopoietic system express cell-surface receptors that inhibit activation responses in vitro through a shared cytoplasmic amino acid sequence, termed the immunoreceptor tyrosine-based inhibitory motif (ITIM). ITIM-bearing receptors belong to two superfamilies that are defined by their extracellular domain sequences, namely, the immunoglobulin (Ig) and C-type lectin superfamilies. The mechanisms by which the inhibitory receptors suppress activation responses, the identification of their ligands, and the effects of receptor deficiency in animal models are currently the subjects of considerable investigation, as is the search for additional ITIM-bearing receptors. The animal studies have revealed that many types of inflammation are counterregulated in vivo by inhibitory receptors. Hence, these receptors represent potential therapeutic targets for suppressing chronic inflammation in diseases such as asthma.

This chapter focuses on the biology of ITIM-bearing receptors that either have been shown to be relevant to inflammatory diseases in vivo or are likely to be, based on the types of cells that express them. It is important to note that for each ITIM receptor there is a receptor with a highly homologous extracellular domain but that lacks ITIMs and instead is an activating receptor. Thus, the number of identified activating receptors has grown in parallel with the number of inhibitors, revealing an intricate balancing system in cells that contribute to inflammation.

II. FcγRIIB

The ITIM was first identified in the type IIB Fc-IgG receptor (FcγRIIB) expressed on B cells. These cells are activated when the B-cell antigen receptor (BCR) is cross-linked with $F(ab')_2$ fragments of anti-Ig but not with intact antibody (1–4). However, intact anti-Ig elicits activation if cells are preincubated with anti-FcγRIIB (2,5). These findings implied that intact anti-Ig fails to activate B cells because it coligates the BCR and FcγRIIB with its Fab and Fc regions, respectively. FcγRIIB was therefore implicated as an inhibitory receptor, and mutagenesis studies revealed that a 13-amino acid region of the cytoplasmic domain of FcγRIIB is both necessary and sufficient for inhibiting BCR-induced B-cell activation (5). A tyrosine in the sequence is phosphorylated when FcγRIIB inhibits cell activation, and mutation of the tyrosine to phenylalanine prevents the inhibition. This tyrosine is the core of the ITIM, which has a consensus amino acid sequence of S/I/VXYXXL/V, where X is essentially any amino acid.

The inhibitory effect of FcγRIIB is not limited to B cells, because mouse mast cells and human basophils express the receptor (6–8). Coligation of FcγRIIB with FcεRI inhibits the immediate release of preformed secretory granule mediators and the subsequent generation of cytokines (8–10). As with B cells, inhibition is dependent on coligation of the two receptors to each other and on the presence of the FcγRIIB ITIM (10). Furthermore, coligation of FcγRIIB with the respective activating receptors results in recruitment of a cytosolic inositol phosphatase to the phosphorylated ITIM of FcγRIIB at the plasma membrane (11,12). This src homology 2 domain-containing inositol 5-phosphatase (SHIP) decreases the local levels of phosphatidylinositol-1,3,5-trisphosphate (PIP3), a phospholipid that is important for recruitment and activation of enzymes that ultimately increase intracellular calcium levels, which is necessary for cell activation via the BCR and FcεRI (13–15). The importance of FcγRIIB in the regulation of humoral immunity and inflammation has been demonstrated with mice that have a targeted disruption of the gene that encodes FcγRIIB. $FcγRIIB^-$ mice produce higher Ig levels than normal mice in response to immunization (16). This may occur because $antigen^+$ antibody complexes cannot coligate the BCR with FcγRIIB, an interaction that would suppress B-cell activation. FcγRIIB-deficient mice also exhibit greater susceptibility to pathological effects in certain models of immune complex diseases and antibody-dependent autoimmune diseases. These include the Arthus reaction (17), immune complex alveolitis (18), anti-basement membrane-mediated glomerulonephritis (19), Goodpasture's syndrome (20), and collagen-induced arthritis (21). In addition, FcγRIIB is an important effector for the protection provided by intravenous gamma globulin against antibody-induced thrombocytopenia (22). The mitigating effects of FcγRIIB in these models likely reflect the IgG-mediated coligation of FcγRIIB with FcγRIII, an activating FcγR, on cells such as macrophages. On the other hand, FcγRIIB inhibits FcγRIII$^+$ antibody-mediated cytotoxicity to tumor cells in vivo (23). Naive FcγRIIB-deficient mice are also more prone to developing autoantibodies and autoimmune glomerulonephritis (24), demonstrating the importance of FcγRIIB in maintaining immune homeostasis.

FcγRIIB also downregulates immediate hypersensitivity reactions. FcγRIIB-deficient mice exhibit more vascular permeability in IgG-dependent passive cutaneous anaphylaxis (PCA) than normal animals (16). In addition, FcγRIIB$^-$ mice undergo more hypothermia and death during IgG- and IgE-dependent passive systemic anaphylaxis (25). The effect of FcγRIIB deficiency on IgE-dependent responses is presumably due to the ability of antigen-complexed IgE to bind not only FcεRI but also FcγRIIB on mouse mast cells (26). IgE-dependent PCA (27) and IgE- and IgG-dependent passive systemic anaphylaxis are mast cell–dependent (28). Hence, the findings demonstrate an important role for FcγRIIB on mast cells in downregulating immediate hypersensitivity reactions resulting from anaphylactic mast cell degranulation.

III. The gp49 Family

The mouse gp49 family was originally defined by mAb B23.1, which detected an epitope expressed on the surface of mast cells and macrophages (29–32). Subsequent studies revealed that mAb B23.1 also binds to spleen-derived natural killer (NK) cells expanded in vitro with IL-2 (33,34) or obtained directly from mice undergoing a viral infection (35). The mAb B23.1 epitope is expressed on a 49 kDa glycoprotein (32). cDNA cloning, based on the determined amino-terminal sequence of the immunoreactive 49 kDa protein, revealed a family of highly homologous gp49 molecules belonging to the Ig superfamily, termed gp49A (36), gp49B1, and gp49B2 (37), each of which has two Ig-like domains (Fig. 1). gp49A is encoded by the gp49A gene (38), whereas gp49B1 and gp49B2 are the products of alternate mRNA splicing of the gp49B gene (37). The two 5.6 kb genes are ~94% identical (37,38) and are located ~4.5 kb apart on chromosome 10 (39). gp49A and gp49B1 are transmembrane proteins and are ex-

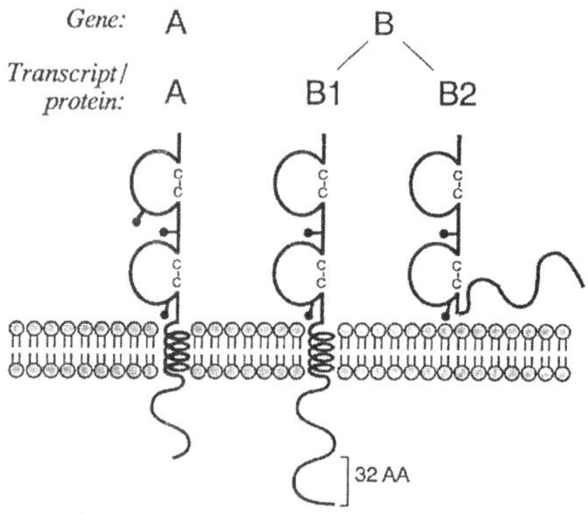

Figure 1 Members of the mouse gp49 family. The 32 amino acid extension in the cytoplasmic domain of gp49B1 that contains the two ITIMs is indicated. AA, amino acids.

pressed in tandem on mast cells (38,40). The gp49B2 transcript lacks exon 6 of the gp49B gene and therefore is predicted to lack a transmembrane domain. If gp49B2 transcripts are translated, gp49B2 would likely be a soluble protein and if secreted could act as a decoy for ligand. Alternatively, nontranslated gp49B2 transcripts may decrease the production of gp49B1 transcripts, which could reduce expression of the transmembrane form.

Of the two transmembrane members of the gp49 family, only gp49B1 has ITIMs. This difference is the result of two fewer nucleotides in exon 8 of the gp49B gene, which extends the carboxyl terminus of gp49B1 by 32 amino acids. Within this extension are two ITIMs (40). Antibody-mediated coligation of gp49B1 with FcεRI on BMMC inhibits the release of secretory granule mediators and leukotriene LTC_4 (40). gp49B1 is also a functional inhibitor in other cell types because expression of a chimeric molecule bearing the cytoplasmic domain of gp49B1 in an NK cell line inhibits NK cell–mediated cytotoxicity (33). In addition, IgG-mediated release of TNF-α from macrophages is inhibited by gp49B1 (41).

As is the case with FcγRIIB, the ITIM tyrosines of gp49B1 are essential for inhibition of cell activation. Mutation of either ITIM tyrosine to phenylalanine partially attenuates the ability of gp49B1 to inhibit FcεRI-directed exocytosis in mast cells, whereas the alteration of both tyrosines abolishes suppression (42). Stimulation of tyrosine phosphorylation in BMMC with sodium pervanadate elicits the phosphorylation of gp49B1 as well as association of the src homology 2 domain-containing tyrosine phosphatases SHP-1 and SHP-2, but not SHIP, with gp49B1 (42). Pervanadate also induces the association of SHP-1 with gp49B1 in NK cells, and the carboxyl SH2 domain of SHP-1 is required for the interaction

(43). In contrast with the effects of pervanadate, only SHP-1 associates with gp49B1 during attenuation of FcεRI-induced mast cell activation (42). The ability of gp49B1 to suppress FcεRI-directed activation is reduced in BMMC generated from mice with an SHP-1 deficiency, thereby demonstrating a requirement for functional SHP-1. In normal BMMC, gp49B1 inhibits FcεRI-induced calcium mobilization, which is required for mast cell exocytosis and LTC_4 generation. Hence, the rapid, FcεRI-induced release of two classes of proinflammatory mediators from mast cells is inhibited by gp49B1 in an ITIM-, SHP-1-, and calcium-dependent manner.

In contrast with FcγRIIB, which binds IgG, and the KIRs, LIR-1, and LIR-2, which bind MHC class I antigens (see below), gp49B1 binds to an integrin, namely, αv3 (44). This interaction inhibits mast cell activation by IgE^{+} antigen, indicating that the binding of a potentially physiological ligand to gp49B1 provides negative signaling to aggregated FcεRI. A notable feature of the interaction is that neither gp49B1 nor αvβ3 generates diversity by recombination or a high mutation rate, as is the case for IgG and MHC class I antigens, respectively. Hence, the inhibition of IgE-dependent mast cell activation by the interaction of gp49B1 with the widely expressed αvβ3 integrin represents a novel example of an innate counterregulatory mechanism for an acquired activation response.

IV. Paired Ig-Like Receptors (PIRs)

The mouse PIR family consists of a single ITIM-bearing receptor, PIR-B, and approximately 7 highly homologous activating receptors, collectively referred to as PIR-A. Like gp49B1, the PIRs are expressed on mast cells, macrophages, and certain NK cells (45–47). However, PIRs have also been detected on B cells, granulocytes, and dendritic cells (45–47). A single gene encodes PIR-B (48,49), which has six Ig-like domains and four potential ITIMs (Fig. 2), although the two membrane-distal motifs appear to be the most important for inhibitory function (50). Coligation of FcεRI in RBL-2H3 cells, or the B-cell receptor in B-cell lines, with transfected, chimeric molecules containing the cytoplasmic domain of PIR-B results in tyrosine phosphorylation of the PIR-B cytoplasmic domain, association of SHP-1 and SHP-2, inhibition of early and late calcium fluxes, and suppression of exocytosis (in RBL-2H3) (50–52). Hence, the mechanisms by which PIR-B and gp49B1 inhibit FcεRI-induced cell activation share a number of common steps. Studies in transfected B cell lines indicate that the src family tyrosine kinase lyn phosphorylates the PIR-B cytoplasmic domain (53). In addition, coligation of the BCR to chimeric PIR-B inhibits BCR-induced phosphorylation and activation of the tyrosine kinases syk and btk as well as phosphorylation of phospholipase C (PLC)-γ2 (54), which likely accounts for the ability of PIR-B to inhibit early and subsequent calcium mobilization.

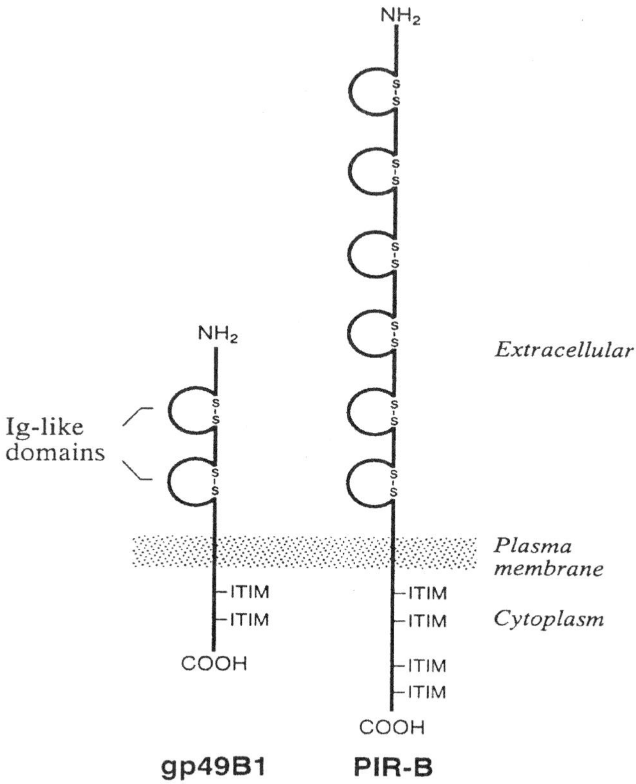

Figure 2 Comparison of the structures of mouse gp49B1 and PIR-B.

A ligand for PIR-B has not been identified. However, PIR-B is constitutively phosphorylated in splenocytes, the level of which is reduced in cells from MHC class I–deficient animals (53). Assuming that the observed phosphorylation results from the interaction of PIR-B with a ligand in the spleen, the data suggest that PIR-B may interact with a class I molecule, similarly to the LIRs and KIRs.

V. KIRs and LIRs/ILTs

In addition to FcγRIIB, human cells express other ITIM receptors whose extracellular domains are more homologous with gp49B1 and PIR-B than with FcγRIIB. The human killer cell Ig-like receptors (KIRs) are expressed primarily on NK cells and certain T-cell populations (55,56). Like gp49B1 and PIR-B, KIRs recruit SHP-1 to their ITIMs as the proximal step in inhibiting cell activation (55,57). KIRs recognize MHC class I molecules (58,59), and essentially all NK cells

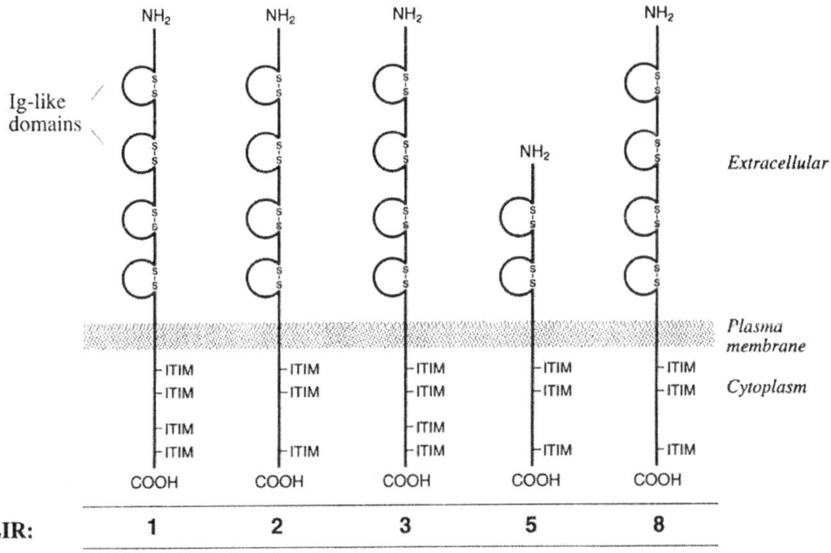

Figure 3 Inhibitory members of the human LIR family.

in an individual express ITIM-bearing KIRs that recognize autologous class I molecules. In this manner, the inhibitory KIRs constitutively prevent NK cells from lysing autologous cells. However, virally infected or transformed cells often express lower amounts of MHC class I molecules than normal cells, which decreases inhibitory KIR ligation so as to foster cytotoxicity when NK cell activating receptors are engaged.

The leukocyte Ig-like receptors (LIRs; also referred to as immunoglobulin-like transcripts and leukocyte-associated immunoglobulin-like receptors) are encoded by a gene complex on human chromosome 19q13.4 near the locus of KIR genes. LIRs are expressed by B cells, mononuclear phagocytes, myeloid cells, mast cells, basophils, eosinophils, and certain NK cells (60–68). ITIM-bearing LIRs (Fig. 3) associate with SHP-1 (63) and hence are likely to provide negative signals similarly to gp49B1, PIRs, and KIRs. LIR-1 and LIR-2 bind MHC class I molecules and a virally encoded class I homolog, UL18 (61,69), whereas the ligands for the other members of the LIR family are unknown.

VI. Mast Cell Function–Associated Antigen

Mast cell function–associated antigen (MAFA) was initially defined by a mAb that bound to rat peritoneal mast cells, the rat basophilic leukemia (RBL) cell line [a mucosal mast cell–like line (70)], and human basophils (71,72). The addition of anti-MAFA to mast cells inhibits IgE^+ antigen-induced signal transduction events that lead to release of immediate mediators and cytokines (71,73). MAFA is a type II transmembrane protein with a C-type (calcium-dependent) lectin domain in its extracellular region that binds mannose and an ITIM motif (SIYSTL) in its cytoplasmic domain that binds SHP-1 in vitro (74–76). Rat MAFA is encoded by a single gene (77).

In mice, a MAFA homolog [mMAFA, also known as ''killer cell lectin-like receptor (KLR) G1''] with 80% amino acid sequence identity to rat MAFA is expressed by splenic NK cells cultured in IL-2 and on $CD8^+$ T cells obtained from virally infected mice (78,79). Surprisingly, mMAFA is not expressed on peritoneal mast cells or BMMC (78,79). mMAFA expression on NK cells is reduced in MHC class I–deficient mice, although this does not occur through a direct interaction of mMAFA with class I antigens (80). mMAFA is encoded by a single gene located on chromosome 6, where the NK cell receptor complex encodes other lectin-like NK cell receptors such as the Ly49 family (79,81).

The human MAFA homolog (hMAFA, also referred to as KLRF1) is expressed not only on basophils and human lung mast cells but also by NK cells and monocytes (82,83). Analysis of the function of hMAFA awaits the development of appropriate reagents but will likely reveal inhibitory functions analogous to those of rMAFA and other ITIM-bearing receptors. The gene that encodes hMAFA is situated in the natural killer cell gene complex located at chromosome 12p12–13 (82), which also encodes the human inhibitory C-type lectin receptors (CD94/NKG2 family).

VII. Conclusions and Implications

It is clear from the studies reviewed in this chapter that cells involved in both the afferent and efferent phases of immune and inflammatory responses express ITIM-bearing receptors. In particular, the expression of inhibitory receptors by human mast cells, basophils, and eosinophils makes it highly probable that activation responses that elicit release of proinflammatory mediators are under reduced negative regulation in chronic inflammatory diseases such as asthma. It also seems clear that at least some of the inhibitory receptors constitutively suppress cellular activation, because ligands such as MHC class I antigens and integrin $\alpha v\beta 3$ are widely expressed under normal conditions. On the other hand, the avidity of integrins frequently increases in response to cell activation (84), raising the possibility that the inhibitory influence of gp49B1 may increase in a milieu rich in activated cells. Moreover, inhibition of cell activation by FcγRIIB is the result of production of antigen-specific IgG through the adaptive immune response and is clearly an example of activation-induced negative feedback through an ITIM-bearing receptor.

Enhancing the function of ITIM-bearing receptors represents a new potential therapeutic approach to the management of allergic inflammation. However, there are still many aspects of the basic human biology of these receptors that need to be resolved. It is not yet clear whether there are individuals with deficiencies in the expression of functional human inhibitory receptors and, accordingly, whether they are more susceptible to inflammatory diseases. If so, the possible beneficial effects of enhancing the expression and function of human inhibitory receptors will be more evident. The ligands for all of the LIRs need to be identified to reveal which LIRs may provide constitutive and/or induced counterregulation of activation and where in the body the interactions take place. A major issue regarding FcγRIIB as a therapeutic target concerns the receptor's diverse effects on antibody homeostasis, response to tumor cells, and beneficial versus pathological inflammation. Indeed, apart from its role as an inhibitor of activating receptors, cross-linking of FcγRIIB molecules elicits apoptosis in B cells (85) and eosinophils (86). Hence, it seems likely that stimulating FcγRIIB expression and/or function in specific cells at limited locations will be a critical component in using the inhibitory power of this receptor as an intervention. Although there is much more to learn about ITIM-bearing receptors, the new appreciation of widespread negative regulation in cells of the immune system is opening entirely new possibilities for counterregulating allergic inflammation.

References

1. Bijsterbosch MK, Klaus GG. Crosslinking of surface immunoglobulin and Fc receptors on B lymphocytes inhibits stimulation of inositol phospholipid breakdown via the antigen receptors. J Exp Med 1985; 162:1825–1836.
2. Cambier JC, Ransom JT. Molecular mechanisms of transmembrane signaling in B lymphocytes. Annu Rev Immunol 1987; 5:175–199.
3. Wilson HA, Greenblatt D, Taylor CW, Putney JW, Tsien RY, Finkelman FD, Chused TM. The B lymphocyte calcium response to anti-Ig is diminished by membrane immunoglobulin cross-linkage to the Fcγ receptor. J Immunol 1987; 138: 1712–1718.
4. Amigorena S, Bonnerot C, Drake JR, Choquet D, Hunziker W, Guillet J-G, Webster P, Sautes C, Mellman I, Fridman WH. Cytoplasmic domain heterogeneity and functions of IgG Fc receptors in B lymphocytes. Science 1992; 256:1808–1812.
5. Muta T, Kurosaki T, Misulovin Z, Sanchez M, Nussenzweig MC, Ravetch JV. A 13-amino-acid motif in the cytoplasmic domain of FcγRIIB modulates B-cell receptor signalling. Nature 1994; 368:70–73.
6. Benhamou M, Bonnerot C, Fridman WH, Daëron M. Molecular heterogeneity of murine mast cell Fcγ receptors. J Immunol 1990; 144:3071–3077.
7. Katz HR, Arm JP, Benson AC, Austen KF. Maturation-related changes in the expression of FcγRII and FcγRIII on mouse mast cells derived in vitro and in vivo. J Immunol 1990; 145:3412–3417.

8. Kepley CL, Cambier JC, Morel PA, Lujan D, Ortega E, Wilson BS, Oliver JM. Negative regulation of FcεRI signaling by FcγRII costimulation in human blood basophils. Allergy Clin Immunol 2000; 106:337–348.
9. Daëron M, Malbec O, Latour S, Arock M, Fridman WH. Regulation of high-affinity IgE receptor-mediated mast cell activation by murine low-affinity IgG receptors. J Clin Invest 1995; 95:577–585.
10. Daëron M, Latour S, Malbec O, Espinosa E, Pina P, Pasmans S, Fridman WH. The same tyrosine-based inhibition motif, in the intracytoplasmic domain of FcγRIIb, regulates negatively BCR-, TCR-, and FcR-dependent cell activation. Immunity 1995; 3:635–646.
11. Ono M, Bolland S, Tempst P, Ravetch JV. Role of the inositol phosphatase SHIP in negative regulation of the immune system by the receptor FcγRIIb. Nature 1996; 383:263–266.
12. Ono M, Okada H, Bolland S, Yanagi S, Kurosaki T, Ravetch JV. Deletion of SHIP or SHP-1 reveals two distinct pathways for inhibitory signaling. Cell 1997; 90:293–301.
13. Fluckiger AC, Li Z, Kato RM, Wahl MI, Ochs HD, Longnecker R, Kinet JP, Witte ON, Scharenberg AM, Rawlings DJ. Btk/Tec kinases regulate sustained increases in intracellular Ca^{2+} following B-cell receptor activation. EMBO J 1998; 17:1973–1985.
14. Scharenberg AM, El-Hillal O, Fruman DA, Beitz LO, Li Z, Lin S, Gout I, Cantley LC, Rawlings DJ, Kinet JP. Phosphatidylinositol-3,4,5-trisphosphate (Ptdins-3,4,5-P_3)/Tec kinase-dependent calcium signaling pathway: A target for SHIP-mediated inhibitory signals. EMBO J 1998; 17:1961–1972.
15. Bolland S, Pearse RN, Kurosaki T, Ravetch JV. SHIP modulates immune receptor responses by regulating membrane association of Btk. Immunity 1998; 8:509–516.
16. Takai T, Ono M, Hikida M, Ohmori H, Ravetch JV. Augmented humoral and anaphylactic responses in FcγRII-deficient mice. Nature 1996; 379:346–349.
17. Schiller C, Janssen-Graalfs I, Baumann U, Schwerter-Strumpf K, Izui S, Takai T, Schmidt RE, Gessner JE. Mouse FcγRII is a negative regulator of FcγRIII in IgG immune complex-triggered inflammation but not in autoantibody-induced hemolysis. Eur J Immunol 2000; 30:481–490.
18. Clynes R, Maizes JS, Guinamard R, Ono M, Takai T, Ravetch JV. Modulation of immune complex-induced inflammation in vivo by the coordinate expression of activation and inhibitory Fc receptors. J Exp Med 1999; 189:179–185.
19. Suzuki Y, Shirato I, Okumura K, Ravetch JV, Takai T, Tomino Y, Ra C. Distinct contribution of Fc receptors and angiotensin II-dependent pathways in anti-GBM glomerulonephritis. Kidney Int 1998; 54:1166–1174.
20. Nakamura A, Yuasa T, Ujike A, Ono M, Nukiwa T, Ravetch JV, Takai T. Fcγ receptor IIB-deficient mice develop Goodpasture's syndrome upon immunization with type IV collagen: A novel murine model for autoimmune glomerular basement membrane disease. J Exp Med 2000; 191:899–905.
21. Yuasa T, Kubo S, Yoshino T, Ujike A, Matsumura K, Ono M, Ravetch JV, Takai T. Deletion of Fcγ receptor IIB renders $H\text{-}2^b$ mice susceptible to collagen-induced arthritis. J Exp Med 1999; 189:187–194.

22. Samuelsson A, Towers TL, Ravetch JV. Anti-inflammatory activity of IVIG mediated through the inhibitory Fc receptor. Science 2001; 291:484–486.
23. Clynes RA, Towers TL, Presta LG, Ravetch JV. Inhibitory Fc receptors modulate in vivo cytoxicity against tumor targets. Nat Med 2000; 6:443–446.
24. Bolland S, Ravetch JV. Spontaneous autoimmune disease in FcγRIIB-deficient mice results from strain-specific epistasis. Immunity 2000; 13:277–285.
25. Ujike A, Ishikawa Y, Ono M, Yuasa T, Yoshino T, Fukumoto M, Ravetch JV, Takai T. Modulation of immunoglobulin (Ig)E-mediated systemic anaphylaxis by low-affinity Fc receptors for IgG. J Exp Med 1999; 189:1573–1579.
26. Takizawa F, Adamczewski M, Kinet J-P. Identification of the low affinity receptor for immunoglobulin E on mouse mast cells and macrophages as FcγRII and FcγRIII. J Exp Med 1992; 176:469–476.
27. Wershil BK, Mekori YA, Murakami T, Galli SJ. ^{125}I-fibrin deposition in IgE-dependent immediate hypersensitivity reactions in mouse skin. Demonstration of the role of mast cells using genetically mast cell-deficient mice locally reconstituted with cultured mast cells. J Immunol 1987; 139:2605–2614.
28. Miyajima I, Dombrowicz D, Martin TR, Ravetch JV, Kinet JP, Galli SJ. Systemic anaphylaxis in the mouse can be mediated largely through IgG1 and FcγRIII. Assessment of the cardiopulmonary changes, mast cell degranulation, and death associated with active or IgE- or IgG1-dependent passive anaphylaxis. J Clin Invest 1997; 99: 901–914.
29. LeBlanc PA, Russell SW, Chang S-MT. Mouse mononuclear phagocyte heterogeneity detected by monoclonal antibodies. J Reticuloendothelial Soc 1982; 32:219–231.
30. LeBlanc PA, Biron CA. Mononuclear phagocyte maturation: A cytotoxic monoclonal antibody reactive with postmonoblast stages. Cell Immunol 1984; 83:242–254.
31. Katz HR, LeBlanc PA, Russell SW. Two classes of mouse mast cells delineated by monoclonal antibodies. Proc Natl Acad Sci USA 1983; 80:5916–5918.
32. Katz HR, Benson AC, Austen KF. Activation- and phorbol ester-stimulated phosphorylation of a plasma membrane glycoprotein antigen expressed on mouse IL-3-dependent mast cells and serosal mast cells. J Immunol 1989; 142:919–926.
33. Rojo S, Burshtyn DN, Long EO, Wagtmann N. Type I transmembrane receptor with inhibitory function in mouse mast cells and NK cells. J Immunol 1997; 158:9–12.
34. Wang LL, Mehta IK, LeBlanc PA, Yokoyama WM. Mouse natural killer cells express gp49B1, a structural homolog of human killer inhibitory receptors. J Immunol 1997; 158:13–17.
35. Wang LL, Chu DT, Dokun AO, Yokoyama WM. Inducible expression of the gp49B inhibitory receptor on NK cells. J Immunol 2000; 164:5215–5220.
36. Arm JP, Gurish MF, Reynolds DS, Scott HC, Gartner CS, Austen KF, Katz HR. Molecular cloning of gp49, a cell surface antigen that is preferentially expressed by mouse mast cell progenitors and is a new member of the immunoglobulin superfamily. J Biol Chem 1991; 266:15966–15973.
37. Castells MC, Wu X, Arm JP, Austen KF, Katz HR. Cloning of the gp49B gene of the immunoglobulin superfamily and demonstration that one of its two products is an early-expressed mast cell surface protein originally described as gp49. J Biol Chem 1994; 269:8393–8401.

38. McCormick MJ, Castells MC, Austen KF, Katz HR. The gp49A gene has extensive sequence conservation with the gp49B gene and provides gp49A protein, a unique member of a large family of activating and inhibitory receptors of the immunoglobulin superfamily. Immunogenetics 1999; 50:286–294.
39. Kuroiwa A, Yamashita Y, Inui M, Yuasa T, Ono M, Nagabukuro A, Matsuda Y, Takai T. Association of tyrosine phosphatases SHP-1 and SHP-2, inositol 5-phosphatase SHIP with gp49B1, and chromosomal assignment of the gene. J Biol Chem 1998; 273:1070–1074.
40. Katz HR, Vivier E, Castells MC, McCormick MJ, Chambers JM, Austen KF. Mouse mast cell gp49B1 contains two immunoreceptor tyrosine-based inhibition motifs and suppresses mast cell activation when coligated with the high-affinity Fc receptor for IgE. Proc Natl Acad Sci USA 1996; 93:10809–10814.
41. Matsumoto Y, Wang LL, Yokoyama WM, Aso T. Uterine macrophages express the gp49B inhibitory receptor in midgestation. J Immunol 2001; 166:781–786.
42. Lu-Kuo JM, Joyal DM, Austen KF, Katz HR. gp49B1 inhibits IgE-initiated mast cell activation through both immunoreceptor tyrosine-based inhibitory motifs, recruitment of the src homology 2 domain-containing phosphatase-1, and suppression of early and late calcium mobilization. J Biol Chem 1999; 274:5791–5796.
43. Wang LL, Blasioli J, Plas DR, Thomas ML, Yokoyama WM. Specificity of the SH2 domains of SHP-1 in the interaction with the immunoreceptor tyrosine-based inhibitory motif-bearing receptor gp49B. J Immunol 1999; 162:1318–1323.
44. Castells MC, Klickstein LB, Hassani K, Cumplido JA, Lacouture ME, Austen KF, Katz HR. gp49B1-αvβ3 interaction inhibits antigen-induced mast cell activation. Nature Immunol 2001; 2:436–442.
45. Hayami K, Fukuta D, Nishikawa Y, Yamashita Y, Inui M, Ohyama Y, Hikida M, Ohmori H, Takai T. Molecular cloning of novel murine cell-surface glycoprotein homologous to killer cell inhibitory receptors. J Biol Chem 1997; 272:7320–7337.
46. Kubagawa H, Burrows PD, Cooper MD. A novel pair of immunoglobulin-like receptors expressed by B cells and myeloid cells. Proc Natl Acad Sci USA 1997; 94: 5261–5266.
47. Kubagawa H, Chen CC, Ho LH, Shimada TS, Gartland L, Mashburn C, Uehara T, Ravetch JV, Cooper MD. Biochemical nature and cellular distribution of the paired immunoglobulin-like receptors, PIR-A and PIR-B. J Exp Med 1999; 189:309–318.
48. Yamashita Y, Fukuta D, Tsuji A, Nagabukuro A, Matsuda Y, Nishikawa Y, Ohyama Y, Ohmori H, Ono M, Takai T. Genomic structures and chromosomal location of p91, a novel murine regulatory receptor family. J Biochem 1998; 123:358–368.
49. Alley TL, Cooper MD, Chen M, Kubagawa H. Genomic structure of PIR-B, the inhibitory member of the paired immunoglobulin-like receptor genes in mice. Tissue Antigens 1998; 51:224–231.
50. Blery M, Kubagawa H, Chen C-C, Vely F, Cooper MD, Vivier E. The paired Ig-like receptor PIR-B is an inhibitory receptor that recruits the protein-tyrosine phosphatase SHP-1. Proc Natl Acad Sci USA 1998; 95:2446–2451.
51. Maeda A, Kurosaki M, Ono M, Takai T, Kurosaki T. Requirement of SH2-containing protein tyrosine phosphatases SHP-1 and SHP-2 for paired immunoglobulin-like receptor B (PIR-B)-mediated inhibitory signal. J Exp Med 1998; 187:1355–1360.

52. Yamashita Y, Ono M, Takai T. Inhibitory and stimulatory functions of paired Ig-like receptor (PIR) family in RBL-2H3 cells. J Immunol 1998; 161:4042–4047.
53. Ho LH, Uehara T, Chen CC, Kubagawa H, Cooper MD. Constitutive tyrosine phosphorylation of the inhibitory paired Ig-like receptor PIR-B. Proc Natl Acad Sci USA 1999; 96:15086–15090.
54. Maeda A, Scharenberg AM, Tsukada S, Bolen JB, Kinet JP, Kurosaki T. Paired immunoglobulin-like receptor B (PIR-B) inhibits BCR- induced activation of syk and btk by SHP-1. Oncogene 1999; 18:2291–2297.
55. Burshtyn DN, Scharenberg AM, Wagtmann N, Rajagopalan S, Berrada K, Yi T, Kinet JP, Long EO. Recruitment of tyrosine phosphatase HCP by the killer cell inhibitory receptor. Immunity 1996; 4:77–85.
56. Olcese L, Lang P, Vely F, Cambiaggi A, Marguet D, Blery M, Hippen KL, Biassoni R, Moretta A, Moretta L, Cambier JC, Vivier E. Human and mouse killer-cell inhibitory receptors recruit PTP1C and PTP1D protein tyrosine phosphatases. J Immunol 1996; 156:4531–4534.
57. Binstadt BA, Brumbaugh KM, Dick CJ, Scharenberg AM, Williams BL, Colonna M, Lanier LL, Kinet J-P, Abraham RT, Leibson PJ. Sequential involvement of Lck and SHP-1 with MHC-recognizing receptors on NK cells inhibits FcR-initiated tyrosine kinase activation. Immunity 1996; 5:629–638.
58. Moretta A, Sivori S, Vitale M, Pende D, Morelli L, Augugliaro R, Bottino C, Moretta L. Existence of both inhibitory (p58) and activatory (p50) receptors for HLA-C molecules in human natural killer cells. J Exp Med 1995; 182:875–884.
59. Colonna M, Samaridis J. Cloning of immunoglobulin-superfamily members associated with HLA-C and HLA-B recognition by human natural killer cells. Science 1995; 268:405–408.
60. Arm JP, Nwankwo C, Austen KF. Molecular identification of a novel family of human immunoglobulin superfamily members that possess immunoreceptor tyrosine-based inhibition motifs and homology to the mouse gp49B1 inhibitory receptor. J Immunol 1997; 159:2342–2349.
61. Borges L, Hsu M-L, Fanger N, Kubin M, Cosman D. A family of human lymphoid and myeloid Ig-like receptors, some of which bind to MHC class I molecules. J Immunol 1997; 159:5192–5196.
62. Cella M, Dohring C, Samaridis J, Dessing M, Brockhaus M, Lanzavecchia A, Colonna M. A novel inhibitory receptor (ILT3) expressed on monocytes, macrophages, and dendritic cells involved in antigen processing. J Exp Med 1997; 185:1743–1751.
63. Colonna M, Navarro F, Bellon T, Llano M, Garcia P, Samaridis J, Angman L, Cella M, Lopez-Botet M. A common inhibitory receptor for major histocompatibility complex class I molecules on human lymphoid and myelomonocytic cells. J Exp Med 1997; 186:1809–1818.
64. Cosman D, Fanger N, Borges L, Kubin M, Chin W, Peterson L, Hsu ML. A novel immunoglobulin superfamily receptor for cellular and viral MHC class I molecules. Immunity 1997; 7:273–282.
65. Meyaard L, Adema GJ, Chang C, Woollatt E, Sutherland GR, Lanier LL, Phillips JH. LAIR-1, a novel inhibitory receptor expressed on human mononuclear leukocytes. Immunity 1997; 7:283–290.
66. Samaridis J, Colonna M. Cloning of novel immunoglobulin superfamily receptors

expressed on human myeloid and lymphoid cells: Structural evidence for new stimulatory and inhibitory pathways. Eur J Immunol 1997; 27:660–665.
67. Colonna M, Samaridis J, Cella M, Angman L, Allen RL, O'Callaghan CA, Dunbar R, Ogg GS, Cerundolo V, Rolink A. Human myelomonocytic cells express an inhibitory receptor for classical and nonclassical MHC class I molecules. J Immunol 1998; 160:3096–3100.
68. Tedla NT, Tassinari P, Austen KF, Borges L, Cosman D, Arm JP. Leukocyte immunoglobulin-like receptors expressed in eosinophils and basophils. FASEB J 2001; 15:A701 (abstr).
69. Navarro F, Llano M, Bellon T, Colonna M, Geraghty DE, Lopez-Botet M. The ILT2 (LIR1) and CD94/NKG2A NK cell receptors respectively recognize HLA-G1 and HLA-E molecules co-expressed on target cells. Eur J Immunol 1999; 29:277–283.
70. Seldin DC, Adelman S, Austen KF, Stevens RL, Hein A, Caulfield JP, Woodbury RG. Homology of the rat basophilic leukemia cell and the rat mucosal mast cell. Proc Natl Acad Sci USA 1985; 82:3871–3875.
71. Ortega E, Schneider H, Pecht I. Possible interactions between the Fcϵ receptor and a novel mast cell function-associated antigen. Int Immunol 1991; 3:333–342.
72. Geller-Bernstein C, Berrebi A, Bassous GL, Ortega E, Licht A, Pecht I. Antibodies specific to membrane components of rat mast cells are cross-reacting with human basophils. Int Arch Allergy Immunol 1994; 105:269–273.
73. Guthmann MD, Tal M, Pecht I. A new member of the C-type lectin family is a modulator of the mast cell secretory response. Int Arch Allergy Immunol 1995; 107: 82–86.
74. Guthmann MD, Tal M, Pecht I. A secretion inhibitory signal transduction molecule on mast cells is another C-type lectin. Proc Natl Acad Sci USA 1995; 92:9397–9401.
75. Binsack R, Pecht I. The mast cell function-associated antigen exhibits saccharide binding capacity. Eur J Immunol 1997; 27:2557–2561.
76. Philosof-Oppenheimer R, Hampe CS, Schlessinger K, Fridkin M, Pecht I. An immunoreceptor tyrosine-based inhibitory motif, with serine at site Y-2, binds SH2-domain-containing phosphatases. Eur J Biochem 2000; 267:703–711.
77. Bocek PJ, Guthmann MD, Pecht I. Analysis of the genes encoding the mast cell function-associated antigen and its alternatively spliced transcripts. J Immunol 1997; 158:3235–3243.
78. Hanke T, Corral L, Vance RE, Raulet DH. 2F1 antigen, the mouse homolog of the rat "mast cell function-associated antigen," is a lectin-like type II transmembrane receptor expressed by natural killer cells. Eur J Immunol 1998; 28:4409–4417.
79. Blaser C, Kaufmann M, Pircher H. Virus-activated CD8 T cells and lymphokine-activated NK cells express the mast cell function-associated antigen, an inhibitory C-type lectin. J Immunol 1998; 161:6451–6454.
80. Corral L, Hanke T, Vance RE, Cado D, Raulet DH. NK cell expression of the killer cell lectin-like receptor G1 (KLRG1), the mouse homolog of MAFA, is modulated by MHC class I molecules. Eur J Immunol 2000; 30:920–930.
81. Voehringer D, Kaufmann M, Pircher H. Genomic structure, alternative splicing, and physical mapping of the killer cell lectin-like receptor G1 gene (KLRG1), the mouse homologue of MAFA. Immunogenetics 2001; 52:206–211.

82. Butcher S, Arney KL, Cook GP. MAFA-1, an ITIM-containing receptor encoded by the human NK cell gene complex and expressed by basophils and NK cells. Eur J Immunol 1998; 28:3755–3762.
83. Lamers MB, Lamont AG, Williams DH. Human MAFA has alternatively spliced variants. Biochim Biophys Acta 1998; 1399:209–212.
84. Van Kooyk Y, Figdor CG. Avidity regulation of integrins: The driving force in leukocyte adhesion. Curr Opin Cell Biol 2000; 12:542–547.
85. Pearse RN, Kawabe T, Bolland S, Guinamard R, Kurosaki T, Ravetch JV. SHIP recruitment attenuates FcγRIIb-induced B cell apoptosis. Immunity 1999; 10:753–760.
86. De Andres B, Mueller AL, Blum A, Weinstock J, Verbeek S, Sandor M, Lynch RG. FcγRII (CD32) is linked to apoptotic pathways in murine granulocyte precursors and mature eosinophils. Blood 1997; 90:1267–1274.

5

Protease-Activated Receptors, Tryptases, and Mast-Cell-Mediated Immune Responses in the Lung

RICHARD L. STEVENS

Brigham and Women's Hospital
Boston, Massachusetts

I. Introduction

Mast cells (MCs) are present in the upper and lower airways. These immune cells express high affinity IgE and complement (C3a and C5a) receptors on their surfaces, and it is widely appreciated that MCs release a diverse array of biologically active molecules (including cytokines, chemokines, leukotrienes, prostaglandins, amines, proteoglycans, and proteases) when activated via either family of receptors. Less widely appreciated is the fact that all MCs that have been examined to date also express functional protease-activated receptor (PAR)1 and PAR2 on their surfaces. The four known members of this family of G protein–coupled receptors possess an exposed amino terminal peptide that when cleaved by thrombin, cathepsin G, or a tryptic-like serine protease at a specific site results in cellular activation. The first aspect of this review focuses on recent advances in the PAR field in the context of the proposed roles of these receptors in the lung and in MC-mediated immune responses.

Mast cells express a large number of neutral proteases, and at least one of these proteases activates cells via a PAR. Tryptases are major constituents of the secretory granules of the MCs residing in the tissues of every species. Tryptases are packaged in the secretory granules ionically bound to serglycin proteoglycans that have either heparin or chondroitin sulfate E chains. One of the biological consequences of cellular activation of an MC is exocytosis of tryptase–proteoglycan macromolecular complexes. Human and mouse MCs express multiple tryptases, and it is now apparent that the individual tryptases evolved to carry out very different functions. The second aspect of this review focuses on the functions of some of these tryptases in MC-mediated immune responses in the lung and other organs.

II. Protease-Activated Receptors

A. Identification and Cloning of Protease-Activated Receptors and Disruption of Their Genes in Mice

Alpha-thrombin activates platelets (1), endothelial cells, epithelial cells, vascular smooth muscle cells, fibroblasts, neurons, and other cell types, but only if this multifunctional, procoagulation serine protease is enzymatically active. These seminal observations eventually led to the cloning of the first thrombin receptor by Coughlin and coworkers in 1991 (2). Four members of this family of protease-responsive receptors in mice and humans have now been identified. Because platelets express all but one member, the initially cloned thrombin receptor (also known as F2R and coagulation factor II receptor) is now designated as PAR1.

PAR2 (also known as F2RL1, coagulation factor II receptor-like 1, and G protein–coupled receptor-11) was cloned by low stringency screening of a mouse genomic DNA library for G protein–coupled receptors (3,4). The isolated mouse PAR2 gene was then used by Nystedt and coworkers to clone its human ortholog (5). The exon/intron organizations of the PAR1 and PAR2 genes are similar, and these genes reside within 100 kb of one another on human chromosome 5q13 and the syntenic region of mouse chromosome 13D2 (6).

Mapping and sequence analysis of a yeast artificial chromosome known to contain the human PAR1 and PAR2 genes resulted in the identification of the physically linked human gene that encodes PAR3 (also known as F2RL2 and coagulation factor II receptor-like 2). PAR3 is only 27% and 28% identical to PAR1 and PAR2, respectively. Nevertheless, the PAR3 gene, like the PAR1 and PAR2 genes, consists of two exons. Human PAR4 (also known as F2RL3 and coagulation factor II receptor-like 3) was cloned by Xu et al. (7) by screening an expressed sequence tag database with the nucleotide sequences that encode PAR1, PAR2, and PAR3. Unlike the other three members of its family, the human PAR4 gene resides on chromosome 19q12. Because the mouse PAR4 gene resides at chromosome 8B3.3 (8) rather than chromosome 13, it also is not physically linked to the other three PAR genes in the mouse genome.

A PAR has been cloned from *Xenopus* (9) that is more similar to human, mouse, and rat PAR1 than to human PAR2, PAR3, or PAR4 (10). These findings indicate that a PAR1-like gene developed in a lower organism before the divergence of mammals and amphibians. The amino acid sequence of human PAR4 is only ~33% identical to that of human PAR1, PAR2, and PAR3. Nevertheless, the amino acid sequence identities of PAR1, PAR2, PAR3, and PAR4 are 78%, 83%, 71%, and 77%, respectively, when the relevant mouse PAR is compared to its human counterpart. The protease-activation site within the N terminus of each PAR also is similar in different species (Table 1). Because human PAR1 is substantially more similar to mouse PAR1 than to human PAR2 and because four PAR genes are present in mice and humans, all four PAR genes apparently evolved more than 100 million years ago before the divergence of the two mammals. It now appears that an ancestral PAR1-like gene duplicated and the resulting two genes translocated to different chromosomes. The new gene that segregated to the genomic fragment that eventually became human chromosome 19 and mouse chromosome 8 failed to duplicate and became PAR4 in both species. However, the ancestral PAR-like gene that segregated to the genomic fragment that eventually became human chromosome 5 and mouse chromosome 13 duplicated two additional times; the resulting three genes then underwent substantial amino acid divergence to create the final PAR1, PAR2, and PAR3 genes in both

Table 1 Activation Domains of Various Protease-Activated Receptors

Human PAR1	LDPR⇓SFLLRN
Baboon PAR1	LDPR⇓SFLLRN
Mouse PAR1	VNPR⇓SFFLRN
Rat PAR1	PNPR⇓SFFLRN
Xenopus PAR1[a]	MTIK⇓TFRIFD
Human PAR2	SKGR⇓SLIGKV
Mouse PAR2	SKGR⇓SLIGRL
Rat PAR2	SKGR⇓SLIGRL
Human PAR3	LPIK⇓TFRGAP
Mouse PAR3	LTIK⇓SFNGGP
Human PAR4	PAPR⇓GYPGQV
Mouse PAR4	PNPR⇓GYPGKF

⇓ = cleavage site.

[a] Although the protease activation site of the *Xenopus* PAR is more similar to that of human PAR3 than human PAR1, the overall amino acid sequence of the *Xenopus* PAR is more similar to that of human PAR1 than human PAR3 (10).

species. All four PAR genes were maintained during the evolution of mice and humans. The biological significance of these genetic events is that most PAR data obtained in rodents should be directly relevant to humans.

Targeted disruption of the mouse PAR1 gene results in significantly smaller litters (11). Although this finding indicated that PAR1 is important in fetal development, those few PAR1-null mice that were born eventually reached maturity and resembled wild-type mice in all examined parameters. Cathepsin G can activate platelets in a PAR1-independent manner (12). The additional finding that the thrombin responses of PAR1-null mice were indistinguishable from those of wild-type mice (11) indicated that platelets must contain additional thrombin-like receptors. Although platelets express more PAR1 than PAR3, the latter receptor also is thrombin-susceptible, and the thrombin-mediated responses of platelets are delayed and diminished in PAR3-null mice (13). When transiently expressed in COS cells, PAR4 can be activated by thrombin or trypsin. Human platelets express PAR4, and PAR4-specific antibodies inhibit thrombin-mediated platelet secretion and aggregation (14,15). In terms of platelet activation, it is now thought that thrombin acts predominantly via PAR1 even though this multifunctional serine protease can also activate platelets directly via PAR4. Cathepsin G acts predominantly via PAR4, and PAR3 functions as a cofactor for the protease-mediated activation of PAR4 and possibly PAR1 (15,16).

Although thrombin is unable to activate PAR2, this receptor is susceptible to pancreatic trypsin (4), extrapancreatic trypsin 2 (17), and membrane-type serine protease 1 (18). As noted below, human tryptase βII or some related MC granule protease can either activate or inactivate PAR2 depending on where the protease cleaves the receptor (19). As assessed immunohistochemically, PAR2 is abundantly expressed in the peripheral nerves of the day 12 mouse embryo (20). However, by day 17, immunoreactive PAR2 is present in most mouse tissues. Despite this strong correlation with embryonic development, PAR2-null mice produce normal sized litters and the resulting mice phenotypically resemble wild-type mice in most parameters (21). Although these data indicate that PAR2 is not essential for embryonic development in the mouse as is PAR1, the PAR1-mediated cardiovascular responses generated in PAR2-null mice are modestly enhanced relative to those of wild-type mice. This latter finding suggests substantial cross talk among the varied PARs that can either enhance or suppress certain biological responses. As noted below, this PAR1/PAR2 cross talk appears to be of critical importance in the lung because it can lead to either bronchoconstriction or bronchorelaxation.

B. Activation, Internalization, and Turnover of Protease-Activated Receptors

Each PAR is expressed on the plasma membrane as an inactive precursor, seven-transmembrane, G protein–coupled receptor. The amino terminus of the PAR resides on the external side of the membrane. When PAR1 is irreversibly cleaved by thrombin between Arg[41] and Ser[42], the newly formed tethered ligand Ser-Phe-Leu-Leu-Arg-Asn is unmasked, thereby allowing it to physically interact predominantly with the extracellular loop 2 of the receptor (9). After the protease-mediated conformational change occurs, the activated receptor binds to a G protein on the cytosolic side of the plasma membrane. Some of the pleiotropic actions of PAR-mediated signaling events are thought to result from the activated receptor binding to different G proteins inside the cell, which in turn results in the stimulation of varied signal transduction pathways. Synthetic peptides of five or more amino acids having an amino acid sequence identical to that of the newly generated amino terminus can activate most PARs that have not been proteolytically processed. Thus, PAR1-, PAR2-, and PAR4-specific agonist peptides and their synthetic variants have been invaluable reagents for helping investigators evaluate the PAR-mediated signaling events that occur in cells that express more than one receptor type. Peptide and nonpeptide PAR antagonists are just being developed by the pharmaceutical industry (22–25), and it is anticipated that these inhibitors, as well as antibodies to the varied PARs (26–28), will help investigators understand the complexities of PAR-mediated signal transduction pathways in the lung and its resident cells.

After the amino terminal exodomain is cleaved during a protease-mediated signaling event, the activated PAR is rapidly internalized via a β-arrestin-1/clathrin coated pit-dependent mechanism (29) into early endosomes (30). Endocytosis is dependent on the PAR's cytoplasmic C-terminal tail (31). Because the internalized receptor is then degraded in primary lysosomes (30), PARs differ from most other activating surface receptors in that they are used only once. PAR-expressing cells generally have large intracellular pools of these receptors in order to compensate for their irreversible loss from the plasma membrane and to control the magnitude of the overall signal transduction event elucidated by the activated receptor. Because these intracellular pools are not accessible to extracellular proteases, the PAR-expressing cell is able to quickly replenish any receptors it loses from its surface as long as the cell is not chronically exposed to an activating protease.

Human PAR1, PAR2, PAR3, and PAR4 are cleaved between Arg[41] and Ser[42], Arg[34] and Ser[35], Lys[38] and Thr[39], and Arg[47] and Gly[48], respectively (Table 1). Although three of the four human receptors are susceptible to thrombin, it is important to note that the P1 residue of each human, mouse, rat, and *Xenopus* PAR is either Lys or Arg. Thus, in a disease setting such as a bacterial or viral infection of the lung, all tryptic-like proteases should be considered as potential activators of a PAR-expressing cell. Virtually all published PAR studies have focused on mammalian proteases acting on mammalian PARs. Although the PAR-mediated regulation of airway smooth muscle tone is similar in noninfected and influenza A virus–infected mice (32), it is only a matter of time before a tryptic-like protease produced by an infectious organism is found to be a potent activator of a mammalian PAR in the lung. In this regard, gingipain-R (the major Arg-specific proteinase produced by *Porphyromonas gingivalis*) is able to activate neutrophils in vitro via PAR2 (33). Many allergens are serine proteases, and the mite allergens Der p3 and Der p9 are able to activate lung epithelial cells via PAR2 (33a).

C. Protease-Activated Receptors and Lung Function

Mouse lung fibroblasts express PAR1, and analysis of PAR1-null mice revealed that this receptor is necessary and sufficient for the thrombin-induced proliferation and MAP kinase–induced activation of cultured lung fibroblasts (34) as well as the thrombin-mediated production of interleukin-8 (IL-8) (35) and connective tissue growth factor (36). Thrombin also induces lung fibroblasts to modestly increase their biosynthesis of type I collagen via PAR1 (37).

Vascular endothelial cells contain substantial amounts of PAR1 and lesser amounts of PAR3 (2,38–40). Although these cells additionally express PAR2, the levels of this surface receptor are dramatically upregulated when endothelial cells are exposed to tumor necrosis factor–α (TNF-α), IL-1α, or bacterial lipopolysaccharide (41). Thrombin induces the proliferation of endothelial cells; increases their surface expression of E-selectin, P-selectin, ICAM-1, VCAM-1, and decay-accelerating factor; and increases their release of von Willebrand factor, endothelin-1, GRO-α, IL-8, basic fibroblast growth factor, and varied matrix metalloproteinases (42–52). Thrombin induces pulmonary microvascular permeability and vasoconstriction, and these effects are mediated predominantly by PAR1 (53,54). Thrombin-treated macrophages also increase their production of endothelin-1, IL-1β, and elastase/matrix metalloproteinase-12 (55,56).

Airway epithelial cells express PAR2, and in vitro activation of epithelial cells via this surface receptor results in increased production of matrix metalloproteinase 9 (57). Bronchial and alveolar epithelial cells express PAR1, PAR3, and PAR4, and thrombin activation of PAR1 on the surface of these cells results in increased production of platelet-derived growth factor (58). Peripheral blood neutrophils are regularly recruited into inflamed airways. Neutrophils express PAR2, and trypsin and PAR2-specific peptide agonists are able to activate these granulocytes (59). Neutrophil extravasation into the peritoneal cavity is not diminished in thioglycolate-treated PAR2-null mice (60). Nevertheless, neutrophil rolling along venules is modestly diminished in PAR2-null mice. The constituents of the neutrophil's granules contribute to airway hyperreactivity in various in vivo model systems of inflammation (61,62). The PAR2-mediated activation of these recruited neutrophils eventually will adversely affect airway function if the level of α1-antitrypsin and other protease inhibitors in the lung falls below the threshold needed to inactivate the increased amounts of neutrophil-derived elastase. Although wounded skin is healed in a normal fashion in PAR1-null mice (63), the above studies suggest that one or more PARs could be important in the connective tissue remodeling of the lung that occurs in patients with chronic asthma.

Chow et al. (53) noted that smooth muscle segments isolated from rat trachea and bronchi underwent contraction when exposed to a PAR1-specific peptide agonist. In contrast, PAR2- and PAR4-specific peptide agonists stimulated bronchial relaxation. In guinea pig airway models, thrombin and a PAR1-specific peptide agonist induced bronchoconstriction (64). Trypsin and PAR2-specific peptide agonists contracted intrapulmonary bronchi. However, these same agents relaxed the trachea and main bronchi (65). Moreover, a PAR2-specific peptide agonist was able to reduce histamine-mediated bronchial hyperresponsiveness (66). Activation of PAR2 resulted in bronchorelaxation in mouse, rat, guinea pig, and human airways in other studies, and this effect was mediated predominantly by the release of cyclooxygenase products (32,67). Whereas it is possible that the altered PAR2-mediated response in different regions of the lung is mediated by the coupling of the receptor to various intracellular G proteins, PAR1 and PAR2 are able to transactivate each other in cultured cells (40); PAR3 and PAR4 also interact in platelets (16). Thus, the nature of the other proteins on the plasma membrane of the PAR-expressing cell may be just as important as the intracellular signal transduction pathway to which the PAR is coupled.

The accumulated data now suggest that during acute inflammation, PAR1 activation of resident lung cells adversely affects lung function in many ways, including inducing bronchoconstriction. In contrast, the acute activation of resident cells in the lung via PAR2 (and probably PAR4) generally results in bronchorelaxation. A very different situation probably occurs during chronic states of inflammation. In those instances when large numbers of PAR2$^+$ neutrophils and other immune cells are recruited into the lung, it is likely that PAR2 activation dominantly affects lung function in an adverse manner. These studies highlight the complexity of evaluating PAR-mediated effects in the lung in normal and diseased states. The failure of thrombin and trypsin to induce a biological response in Chow et al.'s trachea and bronchi studies (53) also indicates that the level of endogenous protease inhibitors in the lung needs to be considered when evaluating the physiological or pathological response of a protease and its susceptible PAR.

D. Protease-Activated Receptor-Mediated Activation of Mast Cells

Mouse (68–72) and rat (73,74) peritoneal MCs store at least five distinct serine proteases in their granules. However, these cells do not express thrombin. Schick et al. (75–77) noted that a complex protease preparation derived from the secretory granules of rat peritoneal MCs was able to induce peritoneal MCs to quickly increase their cellular levels of cAMP and calcium in vitro. This rapid autoactivation event led to the release of substantial amounts of the arachidonic acid metabolite prostaglandin D_2 and the granule mediators histamine, serotonin, and β-hexosaminidase. Pretreatment of the granule preparation with lima bean trypsin inhibitor or diisopropyl fluorophosphate abolished its activity. Thus, the MC-degranulating factor in the tested preparation was one or more enzymatically active serine proteases.

Because trypsin pretreatment of the peritoneal MCs was able to counteract the protease-mediated generation of mediators but not the IgE/antigen-mediated generation of mediators, it became apparent that the unknown protease was not activating this MC population via the high affinity IgE receptor FcεRI. The fact that a brief trypsin pretreatment actually desensitized the peritoneal MC to the unknown protease also suggested that the relevant receptor was not PAR2. Subsequent studies revealed that rat peritoneal MCs become activated when exposed to thrombin or the thrombin receptor agonist peptide (TRAP) 6 (78). These data indicate that the primary protease-responsive protein that Schick and coworkers initially identified on the surface of rat peritoneal MCs was probably PAR1.

The granule serine protease that activates these cells has been assumed to be rat MC protease 1 (rMCP-1) because, on a weight basis, rRMCP-1 is the major serine protease produced by peritoneal MCs (73). Nevertheless, it is now known that rat peritoneal MCs store lesser amounts of many different types of serine proteases in their secretory granules (74). Thus, because recombinant rMCP-1 was not used in the earlier studies, the MC granular protease that is capable of autoactivating this immune cell remains to be identified. In support of the conclusion that in vivo differentiated MCs express one or more thrombin-responsive PARs, thrombin was able to induce edema in the rat hind paw in an MC-dependent manner (79,80). Moreover, both thrombin and TRAP-6 induced the MCs residing in subcutaneous fat to release their granule mediator β-hexosaminidase in an in vivo model of wound healing (78).

As expected on the basis of the above data, Nishikawa et al. (81) reported that rat peritoneal MCs contain PAR1 mRNA but not PAR2 mRNA. Surprisingly, these investigators (81) and others (82) were unable to induce purified rat peritoneal MCs to degranulate using either thrombin or PAR1-specific peptide agonists. The reason some investigators are unable to activate rat peritoneal MCs with thrombin remains to be determined. Although it is possible that the PAR1-mediated signaling pathway is defective in the MCs of certain rodent strains, a more likely explanation is that the manner by which MCs are purified prior to thrombin exposure is of critical importance. Rather harsh conditions are often used to liberate MCs from connective tissues (83). Even when exogenous proteases are not used as is routinely done to purify peritoneal MCs, some of the MC's own granule proteases are spontaneously released during the density gradient step used to purify these cells. Assuming that a substantial portion of surface-localized PARs are lost during the trauma that always occurs during the isolation of in vivo differentiated MCs, purified MCs should always be allowed to recover from the shock of the isolation procedure before a PAR susceptibility experiment is carried out.

Glycoprotein 49B1 and other inhibitory receptors have been identified on the surface of MCs that dominantly suppress FcεRI-mediated activation of these cells (84). Thus, it is also possible that engagement of one or more of these inhibitory receptors dominantly suppresses the thrombin/PAR-mediated activation response of MCs. The report by Strukova et al. (85) that rat peritoneal MCs release their histamine when exposed to α-thrombin but not γ-thrombin additionally highlights the importance of the particular protease used in the PAR susceptibility study. Finally, the amount of protease used in the PAR experiment and the duration of exposure of the PAR-expressing cell to the activating protease are of critical importance because proteases such as trypsin that possess broad substrate specificities can cleave PARs at secondary sites. If this occurs before the signal transduction pathway is activated, the receptor is desensitized rather than activated. In this regard, not only does cathepsin G fail to activate PAR1, this serine protease actually irreversibly inactivates the receptor by cleaving the N-terminal domain at three distinct sites (86). This desensitization event can occur even with more restricted serine proteases such as human MC tryptases.

As assessed immunohistochemically, D'Andrea et al. (87) noted that the MCs in a number of human tissues express both PAR1 and PAR2. The Golgi apparatus appears to be the primary storage site of PAR2 in epithelial cells (30). Although some PAR1 and PAR2 were found on the MC's plasma membrane as expected, surprisingly many of the intracellular receptors colocalized to the MC's tryptase$^+$ secretory granules. These granules contain tremendous amounts of enzymatically active neutral proteases. Moreover, they contain numerous acid hydrolases that are ubiquitously present in primary lysosomes (88). Because unwanted PARs are routinely degraded in lysosomes, the possibility has not been ruled out that the PAR1- and PAR2-antigenic epitopes detected in the granules of certain human MCs are residual degradation products formed during the normal turnover of these surface receptors. However, if the receptors are functional and if they reach the surface during an FcεRI-mediated activation event, PAR1 and/or PAR2 might be able to amplify the generation and release of mediator when MCs are exposed to suboptimal concentrations of IgE and/or antigen followed by the PAR-activating protease.

The inability to detect PAR2 mRNA in rat peritoneal MCs and the inability to induce degranulation in this MC population with trypsin initially suggested that human MCs differ from rodent MCs in terms of their PAR2 expression. Nevertheless, Kawabata et al. (89) noted that a PAR2-specific peptide agonist enhanced vascular permeability and caused edema in the rat hind paw in an MC-dependent manner. It is now known that mouse (68–72,90–96), rat (73,74,97,98), and human (99–101) MCs are quite heterogeneous in terms of what proteases they store in their secretory granules. Mast cells are also heterogeneous in terms of what arachidonic acid metabolites they express when immunologically activated (102–104). These data raise the possibility that no two MCs in the body might be identical in terms of what panel of receptors they express on their cell surfaces. No MC has been found in any species to date that expresses PAR3 or PAR4. Nevertheless, because peritoneal and cutaneous MCs differ in their PAR2 expression and in what mediators they produce and because MCs exhibit reversible plasticity in their development (105–110), the possibility has not been ruled out that certain human, rat, and/or mouse MCs express PAR3 and/or PAR4.

Mast cells developed by culturing mouse bone marrow progenitors for approximately 3 weeks in the presence of IL-3 (111–113) have been used by many investigators to understand at the molecular level the recruitment, proliferation, differentiation, maturation, senescence, and function of MCs. Razin and coworkers (82,114) were the first to note that this MC population derived in vitro is thrombin-responsive. GeneChip analysis revealed that IL-3-developed mouse bone marrow–derived MCs (mBMMCs) contain PAR1 mRNA (Yang and Stevens, unpublished observation). This finding was confirmed using an expressed sequence tag approach (Yang and Stevens, unpublished observation). Of the approximately 2000 arbitrarily sequenced clones from a BALB/c mBMMC cDNA library, forty-one, six, three, two, one, and one of the clones corresponded to carboxypeptidase A, the α chain of FcεRI, PAR1, CD97, CD34, and CD37, respectively. None of the sequenced clones corresponded to PAR2, PAR3, or PAR4. These findings indicate that IL-3-developed mBMMCs contain moderate levels of PAR1 mRNA. If this MC population expresses PAR2, PAR3, or PAR4, the levels of their transcripts are extremely low.

The Cl.MC/C57.1 MC line resembles mBMMCs (115). Cl.MC/C57.1 MCs and mouse peritoneal MCs dramatically increase their constitutive production of IL-6 but not TNF-α when exposed to thrombin or a PAR1-specific peptide agonist (116). Thrombin was also able to enhance the FcεRI-mediated generation of IL-6 when these MCs were exposed to suboptimal levels of allergen. Studies carried out using various metabolic inhibitors indicated that the thrombin-mediated response was dependent on the phosphatidylinositol triphosphate–and sphingosine kinase–signaling pathways. Activation of PAR1 in platelets results in phosphorylation of the Rac guanyl exchange factor Vav (117). Large amounts of IL-6 are produced in MCs that have been activated via FcεRI (118–120), and Vav is a key early-signal-transducing protein in many FcεRI-mediated responses including the generation of IL-6 (121,122). These data indicate that it is likely that the production of IL-6 in PAR1-activated MCs is mediated, in part, by Vav. Immunologically activated mouse MCs release various combinations of ~50 cytokines and chemokines. It is not known how adjacent cells in an organ such as the lung know how to respond when exposed to so many factors being released from a single activated MC. Probably the most significant finding of the Gordon et al. study is that thrombin can dramatically restrict the number and type of cytokines (and presumably chemokines) released from an MC that has been concomitantly activated by PAR1 and FcεRI.

III. Mast-Cell Tryptases

A. Identification and Cloning of Mouse and Human Tryptases

Mouse MCs store in their secretory granules large amounts of various combinations of at least 14 neutral proteases. Eight related proteases have been cloned from human MCs. Except for MC carboxypeptidase A (91,123), all of these granular constituents are serine proteases. Three of the mouse MC proteases are tryptases [designated mMCP-6, mMCP-7, and transmembrane tryptase (mTMT) (68,69,72,94)], whereas five of the human MC proteases are tryptases [designated tryptases α, βI, βII, βIII, and hTMT/tryptase γ (72,124–127)]. The mouse tryptase genes are clustered on chromosome 17 at the interface between bands 17A3.3 and 17B1 (72,128,129). Blot analysis suggested the presence of at least two additional tryptase genes in the mouse genome, and one of these additional tryptase genes was recently cloned by Wong et al. (130). Unlike the other members of its family, mouse tryptase 4 (mT4) is selectively expressed in eosinophils and in the developing testes and ovaries.

The corresponding human tryptase genes are clustered on the syntenic region of chromosome 16p13.3 (72,127,131). An additional mMCP-7-like human tryptase gene [now designated as tryptase δ1 or serine protease-like (SPL) 1] has been identified at this locus (131), but its transcript has not been found in any cell and its gene is predicted to encode a truncated protease that is not enzymatically active. A gene that encodes a human serine protease that is 68% identical to mT4 was initially identified by Ricke and coworkers when these investigators sequenced the 36 kb cosmid clone 352F10. This gene (now designated as the hEsp-1/testisin gene) was subsequently found to reside at the chromosome 16p13.3 tryptase complex (132–134) along with the marapsin gene.

Probing of GenBank's EST database with various human tryptase cDNAs recently resulted in the identification of human tryptase ε (134a). Analysis of the draft sequence of the human genome revealed that the human tryptase ε gene resides on a 2.5 Mb region of chromosome 16p13.3 that contains 14 serine protease–like genes. At least seven of the genes at this complex encode enzymatically active tryptases. Thus, more serine protease–like genes are present at chromosome 16p13.3 than at any other region of the human genome except the kallikrein locus at chromosome 19q13.4. The tryptase ε gene was initially missed by Ricke and coworkers and other Human Genome Project investigators because its first two exons do not resemble those of other serine protease genes. This resulted in a failure to identify the first 47 amino acids in the translated product. The inability of investigators to clone a full-length tryptase ε cDNA contributed to the incorrect conclusion that the tryptase ε gene is a nonfunctional "pseudogene." Tryptase ε is functional and is expressed in the trachea, esophagus, and lung. At the cellular level, tryptase ε is a major product of airway epithelial cells rather than airway MCs or eosinophils. Tryptase ε also differs from human tryptases α, βI, βII, βIII,

TMT, and hEsp-1 in that it is constitutively secreted from its expressing cell. More important, functional studies carried out with recombinant material revealed that the substrate specificity of tryptase ε is very different from that of human tryptase βI even though the amino acid sequences of these two family members are 40% identical. Comparative protein modeling studies revealed that the differential substrate preference is caused by variations in the amino acid sequences residing in four of the seven loops that form the substrate-binding cleft of each tryptase. It is now apparent that a primordial serine protease duplicated repeatedly during evolution to give rise to multiple tryptic-like serine proteases in humans with distinct tissue distributions and substrate specificities. A BLAST search of all serine proteases in GenBank revealed that the *Xenopus* serine proteases Xepsin and Xesp-1 are both more similar to human tryptase ε than the other members of the chromosome 16p13.3 family. Based on this finding, the tryptase ε gene was probably the first protease gene to evolve on human chromosome 16p13.3.

B. Biosynthesis and Structural Analysis of Tryptases

All mouse and human tryptases are initially translated as ''prepro'' zymogens. For example, mMCP-7 is initially translated as an inactive precursor monomer consisting of a signal peptide of 18 residues, a propeptide of 10 residues, and a mature domain of 245 residues (94). mTMT, hTMT, mT4, and hEsp-1/testisin are slightly larger than mMCP-7 because these tryptases have additional membrane-spanning segments located at their C termini. Trypsin and most other serine proteases do not need to form multimeric structures to cleave their susceptible substrates. Nevertheless, certain human (135) and mouse (136) MC tryptases are enzymatically active only when they exist as tetramers.

Using a protein modeling approach, Johnson and Barton (137) noted that most MC tryptases contain Trp-, Tyr-, and Pro-rich domains on their surfaces. Analysis of the crystallographic structure of human tryptase βII revealed that the Tyr- and Pro-rich domains are conserved because the Tyr-rich domain residing on the surface of one monomer physically interacts with the Pro-rich domain residing on the surface of the adjacent monomer (138). In vitro studies carried out with recombinant pro-mMCP-7 monomer revealed that this tryptase spontaneously forms the favored tetramer unit when its propeptide is proteolytically removed (136). Circular dichroism spectra and expression/site-directed mutagenesis data indicated that a dramatic conformational change occurs during the maturation process that is exquisitely dependent on the conserved Trp-rich domain. Using an antibody that recognizes properly folded tryptase but not denatured tryptase, Schwartz et al. (139) noted that human tryptase tetramers also undergo substantial structural changes when they spontaneously dissociate into inactive monomers. Subsequent circular dichroism data suggested that this inactivation process is also Trp-dependent (140,141). Many, if not all, tryptases exist as glycoproteins (130,142–144). Expression/site-directed mutagenesis of the two Asn-X-Ser/Thr sites within mMCP-7 revealed that N-linked glycans enhance the thermal stability of this protease (136). These data suggest that the post-translational modification of a human tryptase can also dramatically affect its half-life and/or enzymatic activity.

Human tryptase ε, hTMT, mTMT, hEsp-1, and mT4 contain the Trp-rich domain but not the Tyr- and Pro-rich domains present in mMCP-7 and human tryptase βII. The presence of the Trp-rich domain suggests that the foregoing five tryptase zymogens are proteolytically activated in a manner somewhat analogous to that of the mMCP-7 and human tryptase βII zymogens. Nevertheless, one area of difference is the fate of the propeptide. Unlike mature human tryptase βII, which is a single-chain protease in its monomer form, it now appears that the propeptides of the non-tetramer-forming tryptases remain covalently bound to their mature domains once each protease is activated. For example, mature human tryptase ε is a two-chain protease because Cys^{-9} in its propeptide forms a disulfide bond with Cys^{112} in its catalytic domain before the protease zymogen is activated. The functional significance of retention of the propeptide in human tryptase ε has not been ascertained, but a similar situation occurs when plasminogen is converted to plasmin (145). This latter finding is relevant because the propeptide of tryptase ε zymogen most closely resembles that in plasminogen.

The absence of the Tyr- and Pro-rich domains in human tryptase ε, hTMT, mTMT, hEsp-1, and mT4 imply that these tryptases are unable to form the tetramer unit. The crystallographic structure of tryptase βII revealed that the active site of each monomer resides in the tetramer's buried 50 × 30 Å central pore (138). This structural feature is predicted to physically restrict the substrate specificity of human tryptase βII. Recombinant mMCP-6 (146) and human tryptase βI (147) prefer to cleave peptides having a Pro at residues P2 to P5 and a Lys or Arg at residue P1. Because Pro residues enhance peptide rigidity, it is likely that the upstream Pro residue is needed to facilitate the insertion of the susceptible substrate into the central pore of the tetramer. Because of the unique structural features of the pore that forms in tryptase tetramers, larger dibasic inhibitors have been synthesized that are able to span the entire pore, thereby inactivating all four monomers in the tetramer at once (148,149). As noted above, mTMT, hTMT, and mT4 are all predicted to exist as monomers rather than as tetramers. Thus, it is important to note that the second generation of tryptase inhibitors have not been designed to inactivate these membrane-associated proteases. Nothing is known about how the enzymatic activities of these tryptases are regulated in vivo.

C. Interaction of Mast Cell Tryptases with Serglycin Proteoglycans

All MCs express serglycin proteoglycans (150). However, the nature of the glycosaminoglycan chain attached to serglycin varies considerably depending on the combination of factors the MC encounters in its tissue microenvironment (105,151–154). mMCP-7 and all other MC proteases that are exocytosed from the cell's secretory granules contain at least one positively charged domain on their surface that forms only when the protease is properly folded (95,137,138,155–157). Expression/site-directed mutagenesis studies of recombinant mMCP-7 revealed that this domain is needed for the tryptase to ionically interact with serglycin proteoglycan. Thus, the positively charged domain appears to be used as a fail safe system to ensure that denatured proteases are not targeted and/or retained in the MC's secretory granules via the serglycin proteoglycan-dependent pathway. Most granule proteases fail to dissociate from serglycin proteoglycans when the protease/proteoglycan macromolecular complexes are exocytosed from activated MCs. The fact that the proteoglycan-binding domains of these proteases are Lys/Arg-rich appears to be the primary reason for the continued tight association of proteases and proteoglycans outside of the MC (155,157). Thus, one of the major functions of serglycin proteoglycans is to minimize the diffusion of exocytosed neutral proteases in connective tissues. mMCP-7 is an exception. When exocytosed, most of this tryptase rapidly dissociates from its proteoglycan and moves toward the endothelium of capillaries and veins (157). In the case of the V3 mastocytosis mouse undergoing systemic anaphylaxis, substantial amounts of exocytosed mMCP-7 tetramers are able to get into the circulation.

The proteoglycan-binding domain of mMCP-7 differs from that of the other mouse MC granule proteases in that it is His-rich (156). The pH of the MC's secretory granule is ~5.5 (158). Thus, mMCP-7 remains bound to serglycin proteoglycans inside the granules like the other neutral proteases. However, when exocytosed into an environment of pH > 6.5, the critical His residues lose their positive charge, thereby enabling the released mMCP-7 to dissociate from the proteoglycan (156,157). Analysis of tetramer formation in vitro using various molar ratios of recombinant mMCP-6 and mMCP-7 revealed that these two mouse tryptases prefer to exist as homotypic tetramers (136). Nevertheless, they can form heterotypic tetramers in vitro. The finding that a small amount of exocytosed mMCP-7 is retained in tissues for hours as do homotypic mMCP-6 tetramers (157) suggests that heterotypic mMCP-7/mMCP-6 tetramers are formed in vivo. Because recombinant mMCP-6 (146) and mMCP-7 (159) preferentially cleave very different peptide sequences, the ability to form tetramers containing different combinations of tryptase monomers might be a novel way the MC controls how extensively proteins are degraded in extracellular matrices. Human lung MCs express multiple tryptases that are all predicted to form tetramers. If heterotypic tryptase tetramers also occur in humans, it may not be possible to interpret any data generated from a functional study carried out with a complex tryptase preparation obtained from a tissue source.

Although heparin was initially reported to be essential for tryptases to form stable enzymatically active tetramers (160), Mirza et al. (161) were able to generate enzymatically active human tryptases α and βII in mammalian cells that do not express heparin. Pereira et al. (138) also were able to crystallize human tryptase βII in the absence of heparin. Moreover, mMCP-7 was found to circulate in the blood of the V3 mastocytoma mouse for >1 h as an enzymatically active, homotypic tetramer free of proteoglycan (157). More conclusive evidence that formation of the tryptase tetramer is not exclusively dependent on heparin was obtained with transgenic mice unable to express fully sulfated heparin due to targeted disruption of the *N*-deacetylase/*N*-sulfotransferase-2 (NDST-2) gene (162). mBMMCs developed from NDST-2-null mice contain normal levels of the transcripts that encode carboxypeptidase A, the chymase mMCP-5, and the two tryptases mMCP-6 and mMCP-7. Whereas the levels of carboxypeptidase A and mMCP-5 protein in the granules of NDST-2-null mBMMCs were below detection, these cells stored normal levels of enzymatically active tryptases in their granules. These and other data indicate that mouse MC tryptases can bind to proteoglycans containing either chondroitin sulfate E or heparin. Thus, disruption of heparin biosynthesis does not adversely affect tryptase expression and granule storage as long as the MC contains substantial amounts of chondroitin sulfate E proteoglycans to compensate for the loss of heparin proteoglycans. Although chondroitin sulfate E and heparin are the two most negatively charged molecules in the body, the structures of these glycosaminoglycans are very different. Virtually all functional studies have been carried out with protease–heparin macromolecular complexes. It has been shown that heparin dramatically restricts the substrate specificity of mMCP-6 (146) and rRMCP-1 (163). The tryptase$^+$ MCs in human lung express both heparin and chondroitin sulfate E (164,165). Because mBMMCs generated from NDST-2-null mice contain normal levels of mMCP-6 and mMCP-7 (162), the possible cofactor role of chondroitin sulfate E in tryptase function now needs to be evaluated.

D. Function of Human and Mouse Tryptases

Although mMCP-6 and mMCP-7 are 75% identical (68,69,94), in vivo studies carried out with recombinant mMCP-6 and mMCP-7 demonstrated that these homologous tryptases are functionally distinct (146,159). The overall amino acid sequences of human tryptases α and βII are 93% identical, and these two MC granule proteases differ in only 18 of their 245 residues (124–126). Interestingly, nine of the amino acid differences reside in their substrate-binding clefts. Moreover, many of the differences represent substantial changes. Thus, strong evolutionary pressure occurred during human development to increase the number of tryptase genes and then to selectively mutate their substrate-binding clefts. Structural modeling and amino acid alignment analysis revealed that Asp^{215} is present in loop 2 of the substrate-binding cleft of tryptase α, whereas the corresponding amino acid in all other human and mouse tryptases is Gly. By using an expression/site-directed mutagenesis approach, recombinant human tryptase α and βII were found to be functionally distinct in terms of their ability to cleave fibrinogen due to this single amino acid difference (166). Human tryptase α and βI also differ in their ability to induce neutrophil extravasation in the lung (147). Finally, human tryptase ε cleaves H-D-Leu-Thr-Arg-pNA much more effectively than tosyl-Gly-Pro-Arg-pNA, whereas recombinant human tryptase βI cleaves tosyl-Gly-Pro-Arg-pNA much more effectively than H-D-Leu-Thr-Arg-pNA (134a). Thus, like that in the mouse, it is now apparent that the varied human tryptases are functionally distinct.

Until recently, all studies designed to deduce the function of a human tryptase were carried out using protease preparations purified to varying degrees from tissues. MCs contain multiple proteases in their granules that are similar in terms of their biochemical properties. Moreover, it is now known that human eosinophils (132) and airway epithelial cells (134a) express distinct members of the chromosome 16p13.3 family of tryptases. Because of the nearly impossible task of purifying these neutral proteases to homogeneity, especially from a lung source containing large numbers of eosinophils, nearly all functional studies previously carried out with a human tryptase preparation contained multiple proteases. A recombinant tryptase expressed in an insect or COS cell could differ slightly from the native MC product due to an unusual MC-restricted post-translational modification event (e.g., phosphorylation, sulfation, or glycosylation). Nevertheless, the contamination problem encountered using tissue-derived tryptase preparations is so great that it is anticipated that all future functional studies will rely on recombinant tryptases.

Exocytosed mMCP-7 circulates in the blood of the V3 mastocytosis mouse for >1 h as an enzymatically active homotypic tetramer (157). This finding raised the possibility that one of the physiological substrates of mMCP-7 is a protein that normally resides in blood. SDS-PAGE analysis of the plasma of a V3 mastocytosis mouse undergoing systemic anaphylaxis revealed the preferential accumulation of fragments of the α chain of the fibrinogen (159). Trypsin, chymotrypsin, and many other serine proteases are able to degrade fibrinogen in vitro if the digestion reaction is carried out in the absence of serum. However, because >10% of the proteins in mouse blood consist of a diverse array of protease inhibitors, fibrinogen is rarely degraded by any of these proteases in vivo. Studies carried out in the V3 mastocytosis mouse indicated that native, MC-derived mMCP-7 is unusual in terms of its resistance to the spectrum of protease inhibitors present in mouse blood (157). This finding was subsequently confirmed with insect cell–derived mMCP-7 (159). Analysis of the substrate specificity of recombinant mMCP-7 with a phage-display peptide library revealed that mMCP-7 prefers an amino acid sequence that is nearly identical to that present in the C-terminal domain of the α chain of fibrinogen. mMCP-7 is therefore an immunoprivileged protease in terms of its ability to degrade fibrinogen in the presence of multiple protease inhibitors in the circulation. Fibrinogen is a major protein in blood, where its concentration approaches 3 mg/mL. Histamine-induced edema is considerable during an MC inflammatory response. Thus, it was unclear why large amounts of cross-linked fibrin are rarely deposited in tissues during an MC-mediated inflammatory response, especially when substantial amounts of fibrinogen and thrombin are also present. It now appears that the primary function of mMCP-7 is to help prevent clot formation in the mouse by rapidly inactivating fibrinogen before it can be converted into fibrin by thrombin at the blood/endothelium barrier. Recent studies revealed that mMCP-7 has a second function, namely the regulation of eosinophil extravasation into certain tissues (147). Although the mechanism by which mMCP-7 induces this immune response remains to be determined at the molecular level, a single injection of a small amount of recombinant mMCP-7 into the mouse's peritoneal cavity results in the preferential extravasation of eosinophils.

Recent in vivo and in vitro studies revealed that the primary function of mMCP-6 is to regulate neutrophil extravasation into tissues. When a small amount of insect cell–derived (146) or human embryonic kidney 293 cell–derived (167) recombinant mMCP-6 is injected once into the peritoneal cavities of various mouse strains, the number of neutrophils increases dramatically at the treated site. The mMCP-6-mediated peritonitis is highly unusual in terms of its duration and cell type specificity. When injected into the trachea, both mMCP-6 and human tryptase βI selectively induced neutrophil extravasation into the lungs (147). Recombinant mMCP-6 was unable to induce neutrophil chemotaxis in an in vitro assay (146), and very little mMCP-6 is able to make its way into the circulation during an MC-mediated anaphylaxis event to directly encounter a blood neutrophil (157). Thus, mMCP-6 must induce neutrophil extravasation in vivo in an indirect manner. Neutrophils express PAR2 (59). Because neutrophils do not increase their cellular motility when exposed to mMCP-6 in an in vitro chemotaxis assay (146) and because the preferred peptide sequences of mMCP-6 (146) are not present in the activation domains of either mouse or human PAR2 (4,5), it was concluded that mMCP-6 does not induce neutrophil extravasation directly by activating the neutrophil's PAR2. In support of this conclusion, recombinant mMCP-6 (when bound to heparin) was unable to activate $PAR1^+/PAR2^+/PAR3^+$ HEK-293T cells and $PAR1^+/PAR3^+/PAR4^+$ Dami cells in vitro (147).

In contrast to recombinant mMCP-7, recombinant mMCP-6 induces cultured human vascular endothelial cells to express large amounts of IL-8 (146). Although these data suggested that mMCP-6 induces neutrophil extravasation predominantly by inducing bystander cells to express large amounts of IL-8-like chemokines, both mMCP-6 and human tryptase βI were able to induce large numbers of neutrophils to extravasate into the lungs of transgenic mice that lack IL-8 receptors (147). The IL-8 family of cytokines could still be important in many tryptase-mediated responses in humans. However, the unexpected data obtained with IL-8 receptor–null transgenic mice indicate that the mMCP-6- and human tryptase βI–mediated influx of neutrophils into lungs and the peritoneal cavity is more complicated than previously appreciated. Although the mechanism by which mMCP-6 and human tryptase βI regulate neutrophil extravasation also remains to be determined at the molecular level, the functional relevance of the mMCP-6/tryptase βI–mediated immune response has been deduced. The primary function of neutrophils is to kill bacteria. Wershil et al. (168) noted that large numbers of neutrophils were selectively recruited into mouse skin during an IgE-dependent late-phase reaction. Using anti-TNF-α antibodies and MC-deficient *W/W*^{v} mice, these investigators concluded that ~50% of this MC-mediated immune response was dependent on TNF-α. The remaining activity was derived from an unknown factor presumably produced by the cutaneous MCs. MC-deficient *W/W*^{v} mice are unable to combat massive bacterial infections of their peritoneal cavities and lungs (169,170). Although TNF-α was initially reported to be the primary MC-derived factor in this innate immune response, a factor that is more restricted to the MCs in the peritoneal cavity, skin, and lung had to be involved to account for the exquisite MC dependence. The MCs in the mouse peritoneal cavity (68,69), skin (71,157), and lung (Friend and Stevens, unpublished observation) express substantial amounts of the MC-restricted tryptase mMCP-6. Injection of a small amount of either recombinant mMCP-6 or human tryptase βI into the lungs of *W/W*^{v} mice 24 h prior to inducing a pulmonary infection with *Klebsiella pneumoniae* rescued the animal's diminished inability to combat this bacterial strain (147). Probably the most significant aspect of this study was the discovery that mMCP-6 and human tryptase βI were both able to recruit bacteria-killing neutrophils into the lungs in a manner that did not adversely alter airway reactivity. These studies highlight a potential dangerous side effect when generic tryptase inhibitors are administered to humans. *Klebsiella pneumoniae* infection is a major health problem. If the primary function of human tryptase βI in the lung is to regulate neutrophil extravasation during acute bacterial infections, then the long-term administration of a relatively nonspecific tryptase inhibitor such as compound APC-366 to an asthma patient could lead to repetitive upper respiratory infections. Fortunately, the growing appreciation of the complexities of tryptase expression in humans has led to the development of the second and third generation of tryptase inhibitors that reportedly are more specific than APC-366 (171–174).

E. Tryptase Activation of Protease-Activated Receptor 2

Numerous in vitro studies have been carried out during the last decade to evaluate whether or not dog, mouse, and/or human MC tryptases can activate any cell type in the lung via one of the four known PARs (19,175–181). Depending on the study and the in vitro system examined, MC tryptases have been reported to either to have no effect on any PAR, to activate PAR2, or to inactivate PAR2. The central problem with most previously published studies is that it was not appreciated until recently that MCs express functionally distinct tryptases. Because of the failure to comprehend the complexities of protease expression in MCs, eosinophils, and the other types of cells residing in the lung, too many studies were carried out using tryptase preparations of questionable purity. Complicating this deficiency was the discovery that the first generation of tryptase inhibitors produced by the pharmaceutical industry turned out to be rather nonspecific. For example, the most studied low molecular weight tryptase inhibitor, APC-366, actually inhibits pancreatic trypsin better than a human lung MC tryptase (182). Schechter et al. (177) were able to activate PAR2$^+$ cells in vitro following exposure to a tryptase preparation purified from human skin in the absence of heparin. However, the magnitude of the cellular response was substantially less than that of the response obtained with comparable amounts of trypsin. This diminished response was reported to be due, in part, to the presence of an additional tryptase-susceptible domain in PAR2 that can quickly inactivate the receptor if high levels of tryptase are used (19).

Screening of a phage-display peptide library revealed that when bound to heparin, recombinant human tryptase βI has a favored Lys/Arg-Pro-X-Lys/Arg sequence (where X can be 0 to 3 noncharged amino acids) (147). In support of these peptide library data with recombinant material, Stack and Johnson (183) found that an enriched human MC tryptase preparation preferentially cleaved the Lys^{158}-Ile^{159} bond in the Arg-Pro-Arg-Phe-Lys-Ile sequence in pro-urokinase. The fact that no Pro amino acid is present in the activation domain of mouse and human PAR2 (4,5) (Table 1) coupled with the fact that the recombinant human tryptase βI was unable to activate PAR1$^+$/PAR2$^+$/PAR3$^+$ HEK-293T cells (147) now suggests that tryptase βI probably does not induce neutrophil extravasation into the lung via a PAR2-dependent mechanism as was first thought. In support of this conclusion, Vliagoftis et al. (57) noted that tryptase treatment of PAR2$^+$ airway epithelial cells did not result in increased expression of matrix metalloproteinase 9 as occurred when these same cells were exposed to trypsin or a PAR2-specific peptide agonist.

Mast cell activation enhances airway responsiveness to methacholine in the mouse (184). Low-molecular-weight inhibitors of tryptic-like enzymes block antigen-induced airway constriction and tissue inflammatory responses in sheep (182) and guinea pigs (185). In early clinical trials, repeated administration of APC-366 to 16 mild atopic asthma patients over a 4-day period did not alter bronchial hyperresponsiveness. However, the tryptase inhibitor modestly reduced the magnitude of an antigen-induced late asthmatic response (186). Secretory leukocyte protease inhibitor is expressed in the lung. This protease inhibitor inactivates certain MC tryptases, chymases, and other hematopoietic proteases, and it reduces early- and late-phase bronchoconstriction in animal models (185,187–190). A dog tryptase also enhances the histamine-mediated contractile response of smooth muscle in vitro (191). From these and other data, it was concluded that an undefined MC tryptase promotes bronchoconstriction. If the relevant tryptase is acting predominantly via PAR2 as many have concluded, these in vivo findings contradict the findings of others (53,66,67) who reported that PAR2 activation in the lung results in bronchorelaxation rather than bronchoconstriction. The most likely explanation for the conflicting data is that the individual human tryptases and/or their splice variants are functionally distinct in terms of their ability to activate the varied PARs. Alternatively, whether the tryptase is bound to heparin, chondroitin sulfate E, or some other cofactor is of critical importance in dictating whether or not the exocytosed tryptase can activate a PAR.

The airways are innervated by sensory and autonomic nerves (192). Although not the focus of this review, neurons express PAR1 and PAR2 and thrombin induces neurons to undergo apoptosis via a PAR1-dependent pathway (193–195). The interactions of MCs and nerves are well documented by Bienenstock et al. (196–198) and others. Because there is greater prevalence of apoptotic neurons and Schwann cells in the optic nerves of NDST-2-null mice (Li and Stevens, unpublished finding), one of the MC's tryptases or other granule proteases that fails to package in the secretory granules of these transgenic mice (162) could affect lung function by damaging the sensory nerves in this organ via a PAR-mediated pathway.

IV. Gene Linkage Studies Evaluating the Possible Relationship of Protease-Activated Receptors, Tryptases, and Bronchial Hyperresponsiveness

Various gene linkage studies have revealed that asthma is a polygenetic disorder. One gene linkage study mapped a bronchial hyperresponsiveness candidate gene to mouse chromosome 13. Although the mouse PAR1, PAR2, and PAR3 genes reside on this chromosome, it remains to be determined whether or not one of these receptors is the putative asthma susceptibility gene. Allelic variants of the varied PARs are just beginning to be identified in humans and mice. In the Korean population, six polymorphisms have been identified in the 5′ untranslated region of the PAR1 gene (199). Whether a specific polymorphism is associated with a pulmonary abnormality has not been evaluated. However, no PAR1 polymorphism has been found in patients with coronary artery disease. Although no evidence has been obtained for a genetic abnormality in the coding domain of the PAR1 gene, a genetic polymorphism of the human PAR2 gene has been identified that results in an altered extracellular loop 2 (200). Transfection experiments revealed that this Phe^{240}/Ser^{240} mutation in PAR2 results in an approximately fourfold reduction in the signaling capacity of the trypsin-activated receptor. Thus, genetic defects in PAR2 may influence protease-mediated changes in airway reactivity.

The C57BL/6 mouse is regularly used in various inflammatory models because immune responses obtained in this strain are often quite different from those obtained with other mouse strains. Gene linkage studies revealed a locus on mouse chromosome 17 where the tryptase genes reside (72,128–130) that influences airway reactivity in backcrosses of A/J and C57BL/6 mice (201). Although the relevant gene has not yet been identified conclusively, it probably encodes TMT because the injection of this recombinant protease into the trachea of a BALB/c mouse results in airway hyperresponsiveness (134a). TMT induces its pulmonary effects by activating an IL-3/IL-4 receptor α/STAT6-dependent pathway. Mouse strains can differ greatly in terms of what tryptases their MCs express. Although the MCs in the lungs of all mouse strains that have been examined to date express mMCP-6, the MCs in the C57BL/6 mouse cannot express mMCP-7 because of a point mutation at the exon 2/intron 2 splice site (202).

Another tryptase that is expressed in a strain-dependent manner in the mouse is mTMT. For example, the mTMT gene is abundantly expressed in the MCs of the C57BL/6 mouse but not the MCs of the BALB/c mouse (72). In terms of human tryptase expression, a putative allelic variant of hTMT (designated tryptase γII) has been identified that contains a Ser at residue 123 (127) rather than the Trp that is found in the TMT that is expressed in most mouse strains and in humans (72). Because this amino acid resides in the Trp-rich domain (137,138) that is required for the activation of other MC tryptase zymogens (136), the enzymatic activity of the Ser^{123} variant may be reduced relative to that of the Trp^{123} variant. Splice variants of different human tryptase transcripts have been identified that are predicted to encode proteases with altered substrate-binding clefts (203). Splice variant abnormalities are not normally identified in gene linkage studies. Nevertheless, this new finding raises the possibility that differential splicing events may result in the expression of functionally distinct tryptases even if there is no alteration in the tryptase's gene. Finally, it is needs to be emphasized that mouse strains also differ considerably in their expression of various serpins. For example, the C57BL/6 mouse strain expresses the α_1-protease inhibitor family member DOM5 but not the related member DOM6 (204). In contrast, the DBA mouse strain expresses DOM5 but not DOM3. The reactive centers of these two serpins are very different. Thus, genetic differences in protease inhibitor expression may affect in vivo studies carried out to evaluate the function of a serine protease or PAR in the lung.

V. Future Therapeutic Approaches

It remains to be determined whether or not the development of low molecular weight inhibitors that inactivate a specific PAR or MC granule protease ultimately will be beneficial in the long-term treatment of patients with asthma. Although mouse studies indicate that PAR1 is important in embryonic development, the general consensus is that the PAR1-mediated activation of the various cell types in the adult human lung adversely affects this organ. So many different cell types express PAR1 that it is currently not possible to predict what would happen if a PAR1-mediated signaling pathway in the human lung were to be pharmacologically inhibited in a long-term manner. Nevertheless, of the four PARs, the next generation of pharmaceutical agents that inhibit PAR1 expression and/or function may be the most beneficial in the treatment of various lung disorders.

Tryptase βI and its related family members are highly restricted to MCs. Even though these serine proteases are more attractive candidates for pharmacological intervention owing to their restricted cellular expression, recent studies carried out in the mouse revealed that some of these proteases actually are beneficial in innate and acquired immune responses. Thus, even if a human MC tryptase promotes bronchoconstriction as many believe, a potential deleterious side effect of inhibiting human tryptase βI might result in an increase in upper respiratory infections. Because a number of the cloned human tryptases are 93–98% identical, it is not widely appreciated that some of these homologous MC proteases are functionally distinct. Thus, more attention to the functional consequences of tryptase heterogeneity is required before the next level of MC protease-specific inhibitors are developed and used in humans.

Mast cell proteases are exocytosed bound to serglycin proteoglycans that contain structurally different glycosaminoglycans. Because heparin restricts the substrate specificity of at least one tryptase and at least one chymase, it is imperative that we understand the cofactor roles of serglycin proteoglycans in protease-mediated responses in the lung. Finally, very little attention has been placed on understanding the mechanisms the lung uses to inactivate the various neutral proteases that are exocytosed from activated MCs. A synthetic low molecular weight inhibitor that inactivates an MC tryptase in vitro could have toxic side effects in vivo, especially if the inhibitor diffuses to the liver and is metabolized into a toxin. Thus, a more attractive approach is to identify an endogenous inhibitor (e.g., secretory leukocyte protease inhibitor or inter-α trypsin inhibitor) in human lung that inactivates the tryptase of interest. Using biotechnological approaches, large amounts of the native protease inhibitor or a bioengineered derivative could be generated in vitro and then administered to humans to dampen the protease-mediated response in a more physiological manner.

References

1. Davey MG, Luscher EF. Biochemical aspects of platelet function and hemostasis. Semin Hematol 1968; 5:5–17.
2. Vu TK, Hung DT, Wheaton VI, Coughlin SR. Molecular cloning of a functional

thrombin receptor reveals a novel proteolytic mechanism of receptor activation. Cell 1991; 64:1057–1068.

3. Nystedt S, Emilsson K, Wahlestedt C, Sundelin J. Molecular cloning of a potential proteinase activated receptor. Proc Natl Acad Sci USA 1994; 91:9208–9212.
4. Nystedt S, Larsson AK, Aberg H, Sundelin J. The mouse proteinase-activated receptor-2 cDNA and gene: Molecular cloning and functional expression. J Biol Chem 1995; 270:5950–5955.
5. Nystedt S, Emilsson K, Larsson AK, Strombeck B, Sundelin J. Molecular cloning and functional expression of the gene encoding the human proteinase-activated receptor-2. Eur J Biochem 1995; 232:84–89.
6. Kahn M, Ishii K, Kuo WL, Piper M, Connolly A, Shi YP, Wu R, Lin CC, Coughlin SR. Conserved structure and adjacent location of the thrombin receptor and protease-activated receptor-2 genes define a protease-activated receptor gene cluster. Mol Med 1996; 2:349–357.
7. Xu WF, Andersen H, Whitmore TE, Presnell SR, Yee DP, Ching A, Gilbert T, Davie EW, Foster DC. Cloning and characterization of human protease-activated receptor-4. Proc Natl Acad Sci USA 1998; 95:6642–6646.
8. Kahn ML, Hammes SR, Botka C, Coughlin SR. Gene and locus structure and chromosomal localization of the protease-activated receptor gene family. J Biol Chem 1998; 273:23290–23296.
9. Gerszten RE, Chen J, Ishii M, Ishii K, Wang L, Nanevicz T, Turck CW, Vu TK, Coughlin SR. Specificity of the thrombin receptor for agonist peptide is defined by its extracellular surface. Nature 1994; 368:648–651.
10. Coughlin SR. How the protease thrombin talks to cells. Proc Natl Acad Sci USA 1999; 96:11023–11027.
11. Darrow AL, Fung-Leung WP, Ye RD, Santulli RJ, Cheung WM, Derian CK, Burns CL, Damiano BP, Zhou L, Keenan CM, Peterson PA, Andrade-Gordon P. Biological consequences of thrombin receptor deficiency in mice. Thromb Haemost 1996; 76:860–866.
12. Selak MA. Cathepsin G and thrombin: Evidence for two different platelet receptors. Biochem J 1994; 297(pt 2):269–275.
13. Kahn ML, Zheng YW, Huang W, Bigornia V, Zeng D, Moff S, Farese RV, Tam C, Coughlin SR. A dual thrombin receptor system for platelet activation. Nature 1998; 394:690–694.
14. Kahn ML, Nakanishi-Matsui M, Shapiro MJ, Ishihara H, Coughlin SR. Protease-activated receptors-1 and -4 mediate activation of human platelets by thrombin. J Clin Invest 1999; 103:879–887.
15. Sambrano GR, Huang W, Faruqi T, Mahrus S, Craik C, Coughlin SR. Cathepsin G activates protease-activated receptor-4 in human platelets. J Biol Chem 2000; 275:6819–6823.
16. Nakanishi-Matsui M, Zheng YW, Sulciner DJ, Weiss EJ, Ludeman MJ, Coughlin SR. PAR3 is a cofactor for PAR4 activation by thrombin. Nature 2000; 404:609–613.
17. Alm AK, Gagnemo-Persson R, Sorsa T, Sundelin J. Extrapancreatic trypsin-2 cleaves proteinase-activated receptor-2. Biochem Biophys Res Commun 2000; 275:77–83.

18. Takeuchi T, Harris JL, Huang W, Yan KW, Coughlin SR, Craik CS. Cellular localization of membrane-type serine protease 1 and identification of protease-activated receptor-2 and single-chain urokinase-type plasminogen activator as substrates. J Biol Chem 2000; 275:26333–26342.
19. Molino M, Barnathan ES, Numerof R, Clark J, Dreyer M, Cumashi A, Hoxie JA, Schechter N, Woolkalis M, Brass LF. Interactions of mast cell tryptase with thrombin receptors and PAR-2. J Biol Chem 1997; 272:4043–4049.
20. Jenkins AL, Chinni C, de Niese MR, Blackhart B, Mackie EJ. Expression of protease-activated receptor-2 during embryonic development. Dev Dyn 2000; 218:465–471.
21. Damiano BP, Cheung WM, Santulli RJ, Fung-Leung WP, Ngo K, Ye RD, Darrow AL, Derian CK, de Garavilla L, Andrade-Gordon P. Cardiovascular responses mediated by protease-activated receptor-2 (PAR-2) and thrombin receptor (PAR-1) are distinguished in mice deficient in PAR-2 or PAR-1. J Pharmacol Exp Ther 1999; 288:671–678.
22. Bernatowicz MS, Klimas CE, Hartl KS, Peluso M, Allegretto NJ, Seiler SM. Development of potent thrombin receptor antagonist peptides. J Med Chem 1996; 39: 4879–4887.
23. Kato Y, Kita Y, Nishio M, Hirasawa Y, Ito K, Yamanaka T, Motoyama Y, Seki J. In vitro antiplatelet profile of FR171113, a novel non-peptide thrombin receptor antagonist. Eur J Pharmacol 1999; 384:197–202.
24. Ahn HS, Arik L, Boykow G, Burnett DA, Caplen MA, Czarniecki M, Domalski MS, Foster C, Manna M, Stamford AW, Wu Y. Structure-activity relationships of pyrroloquinazolines as thrombin receptor antagonists. Bioorg Med Chem Lett 1999; 9:2073–2078.
25. Ahn HS, Foster C, Boykow G, Stamford A, Manna M, Graziano M. Inhibition of cellular action of thrombin by N3-cyclopropyl-7-[[4-(1-methylethyl)phenyl]-methyl]-7H-pyrrolo[3, 2-f]quinazoline-1,3-diamine (SCH 79797), a nonpeptide thrombin receptor antagonist. Biochem Pharmacol 2000; 60:1425–1434.
26. Hoxie JA, Ahuja M, Belmonte E, Pizarro S, Parton R, Brass LF. Internalization and recycling of activated thrombin receptors. J Biol Chem 1993; 268:13756–13763.
27. Brass LF, Pizarro S, Ahuja M, Belmonte E, Blanchard N, Stadel JM, Hoxie JA. Changes in the structure and function of the human thrombin receptor during receptor activation, internalization, and recycling. J Biol Chem 1994; 269:2943–2952.
28. Ishihara H, Zeng D, Connolly AJ, Tam C, Coughlin SR. Antibodies to protease-activated receptor 3 inhibit activation of mouse platelets by thrombin. Blood 1998; 91:4152–4157.
29. Dery O, Thoma MS, Wong H, Grady EF, Bunnett NW. Trafficking of proteinase-activated receptor-2 and β-arrestin-1 tagged with green fluorescent protein: β-Arrestin-dependent endocytosis of a proteinase receptor. J Biol Chem 1999; 274: 18524–18535.
30. Bohm SK, Khitin LM, Grady EF, Aponte G, Payan DG, Bunnett NW. Mechanisms of desensitization and resensitization of proteinase-activated receptor-2. J Biol Chem 1996; 271:22003–22016.
31. Shapiro MJ, Coughlin SR. Separate signals for agonist-independent and agonist-

triggered trafficking of protease-activated receptor-1. J Biol Chem 1998; 273: 29009–29014.

32. Lan RS, Stewart GA, Henry PJ. Modulation of airway smooth muscle tone by protease activated receptor-1, -2, -3, and -4 in trachea isolated from influenza A virus-infected mice. Br J Pharmacol 2000; 129:63–70.
33. Lourbakos A, Chinni C, Thompson P, Potempa J, Travis J, Mackie EJ, Pike RN. Cleavage and activation of proteinase-activated receptor-2 on human neutrophils by gingipain-R from Porphyromonas gingivalis. FEBS Lett 1998; 435:45–48.

33a. Sun G, Stacey MA, Schmidt M, Mori L, Mattoli S. Interaction of mite allergens Der p3 and Der p9 with protease-activated receptor-2 expressed by lung epithelial cells. J Immunol 2001; 167:1014–1021.

34. Trejo J, Connolly AJ, Coughlin SR. The cloned thrombin receptor is necessary and sufficient for activation of mitogen-activated protein kinase and mitogenesis in mouse lung fibroblasts: Loss of responses in fibroblasts from receptor knockout mice. J Biol Chem 1996; 271:21536–21541.
35. Ludwicka-Bradley A, Tourkina E, Suzuki S, Tyson E, Bonner M, Fenton JW, Hoffman S, Silver RM. Thrombin upregulates interleukin-8 in lung fibroblasts via cleavage of proteolytically activated receptor-1 and protein kinase C-γ activation. Am J Respir Cell Mol Biol 2000; 22:235–243.
36. Chambers RC, Leoni P, Blanc-Brude OP, Wembridge DE, Laurent GJ. Thrombin is a potent inducer of connective tissue growth factor production via proteolytic activation of protease-activated receptor-1. J Biol Chem 2000; 275:35584–35591.
37. Chambers RC, Dabbagh K, McAnulty RJ, Gray AJ, Blanc-Brude OP, Laurent GJ. Thrombin stimulates fibroblast procollagen production via proteolytic activation of protease-activated receptor-1. Biochem J 1998; 333:121–127.
38. Mirza H, Yatsula V, Bahou WF. The proteinase activated receptor-2 mediates mitogenic responses in human vascular endothelial cells. J Clin Invest 1996; 97:1705–1714.
39. Schmidt VA, Nierman WC, Maglott DR, Cupit LD, Moskowitz KA, Wainer JA, Bahou WF. The human proteinase-activated receptor-3 (PAR-3) gene: Identification within a PAR gene cluster and characterization in vascular endothelial cells and platelets. J Biol Chem 1998; 273:15061–15068.
40. O'Brien PJ, Prevost N, Molino M, Hollinger MK, Woolkalis MJ, Woulfe DS, Brass LF. Thrombin responses in human endothelial cells: Contributions from receptors other than PAR1 include the transactivation of PAR2 by thrombin-cleaved PAR1. J Biol Chem 2000; 275:13502–13509.
41. Nystedt S, Ramakrishnan V, Sundelin J. The proteinase-activated receptor-2 is induced by inflammatory mediators in human endothelial cells: Comparison with the thrombin receptor. J Biol Chem 1996; 271:14910–14915.
42. Schini VB, Hendrickson H, Heublein DM, Burnett JC, Vanhoutte PM. Thrombin enhances the release of endothelin from cultured porcine aortic endothelial cells. Eur J Pharmacol 1989; 165:333–334.
43. Weiss RH, Maduri M. The mitogenic effect of thrombin in vascular smooth muscle cells is largely due to basic fibroblast growth factor. J Biol Chem 1993; 268:5724–5727.
44. Herbert JM, Dupuy E, Laplace MC, Zini JM, Bar SR, Tobelem G. Thrombin in-

duces endothelial cell growth via both a proteolytic and a non-proteolytic pathway. Biochem J 1994; 303:227–231.

45. Sugama Y, Malik AB. Thrombin receptor 14-amino acid peptide mediates endothelial hyperadhesivity and neutrophil adhesion by P-selectin-dependent mechanism. Circ Res 1992; 71:1015–1019.
46. Murakami K, Ueno A, Yamanouchi K, Kondo T. Thrombin induces GROα/MGSA production in human umbilical vein endothelial cells. Thromb Res 1995; 79:387–394.
47. Storck J, Kusters B, Vahland M, Morys-Wortmann C, Zimmermann ER. Trypsin induced von Willebrand factor release from human endothelial cells is mediated by PAR-2 activation. Thromb Res 1996; 84:463–473.
48. Ueno A, Murakami K, Yamanouchi K, Watanabe M, Kondo T. Thrombin stimulates production of interleukin-8 in human umbilical vein endothelial cells. Immunology 1996; 88:76–81.
49. Kaplanski G, Fabrigoule M, Boulay V, Dinarello CA, Bongrand P, Kaplanski S, Farnarier C. Thrombin induces endothelial type II activation in vitro: IL-1 and TNF-α-independent IL-8 secretion and E-selectin expression. J Immunol 1997; 158:5435–5441.
50. Duhamel-Clerin E, Orvain C, Lanza F, Cazenave JP, Klein-Soyer C. Thrombin receptor-mediated increase of two matrix metalloproteinases, MMP-1 and MMP-3, in human endothelial cells. Arterioscler Thromb Vasc Biol 1997; 17:1931–1938.
51. Kaplanski G, Marin V, Fabrigoule M, Boulay V, Benoliel AM, Bongrand P, Kaplanski S, Farnarier C. Thrombin-activated human endothelial cells support monocyte adhesion in vitro following expression of intercellular adhesion molecule-1 (ICAM-1; CD54) and vascular cell adhesion molecule-1 (VCAM-1; CD106). Blood 1998; 92:1259–1267.
52. Lidington EA, Haskard DO, Mason JC. Induction of decay-accelerating factor by thrombin through a protease-activated receptor-1 and protein kinase C-dependent pathway protects vascular endothelial cells from complement-mediated injury. Blood 2000; 96:2784–2792.
53. Chow JM, Moffatt JD, Cocks TM. Effect of protease-activated receptor (PAR)-1, -2 and -4-activating peptides, thrombin and trypsin in rat isolated airways. Br J Pharmacol 2000; 131:1584–1591.
54. Vogel SM, Gao X, Mehta D, Ye RD, John TA, Andrade-Gordon P, Tiruppathi C, Malik AB. Abrogation of thrombin-induced increase in pulmonary microvascular permeability in PAR-1 knockout mice. Physiol Genomics 2000; 4:137–145.
55. Kobayashi Y, Sakamoto Y, Shibasaki M, Kimura I, Matsuo H. Human alveolar macrophages synthesize endothelins by thrombin. J Immunol 1997; 158:5442–5447.
56. Raza SL, Nehring LC, Shapiro SD, Cornelius LA. Proteinase-activated receptor-1 regulation of macrophage elastase (MMP-12) secretion by serine proteinases. J Biol Chem 2000; 275:41243–41250.
57. Vliagoftis H, Schwingshackl A, Milne CD, Duszyk M, Hollenberg MD, Wallace JL, Befus AD, Moqbel R. Proteinase-activated receptor-2-mediated matrix metalloproteinase-9 release from airway epithelial cells. J Allergy Clin Immunol 2000; 106:537–545.

58. Shimizu S, Gabazza EC, Hayashi T, Ido M, Adachi Y, Suzuki K. Thrombin stimulates the expression of PDGF in lung epithelial cells. Am J Physiol Lung Cell Mol Physiol 2000; 279:L503–L510.
59. Howells GL, Macey MG, Chinni C, Hou, L, Fox MT, Harriott P, Stone SR. Proteinase-activated receptor-2: Expression by human neutrophils. J Cell Sci 1997; 110: 881–887.
60. Lindner JR, Kahn ML, Coughlin SR, Sambrano GR, Schauble E, Bernstein D, Foy D, Hafezi-Moghadam A, Ley K. Delayed onset of inflammation in protease-activated receptor-2-deficient mice. J Immunol 2000; 165:6504–6510.
61. Nagai H, Tsuji F, Shimazawa T, Goto S, Yoshitake K, Koda A. Participation of collagenase and elastase in LPS-induced airway hyperresponsiveness in guinea pigs. Inflammation 1991; 15:317–330.
62. Lukacs NW, Lamm WJ, Strieter RM, Albert RK. Airway hyperreactivity is associated with specific leukocyte subset infiltration in a mouse model of allergic airway inflammation. Pathobiology 1996; 64:308–313.
63. Connolly AJ, Suh DY, Hunt TK, Coughlin SR. Mice lacking the thrombin receptor, PAR1, have normal skin wound healing. Am J Pathol 1997; 151:1199–1204.
64. Cicala C, Bucci M, De Dominicis G, Harriott P, Sorrentino L, Cirino G. Bronchoconstrictor effect of thrombin and thrombin receptor activating peptide in guinea pigs in vivo. Br J Pharmacol 1999; 126:478–484.
65. Ricciardolo FL, Steinhoff M, Amadesi S, Guerrini R, Tognetto M, Trevisani M, Creminon C, Bertrand C, Bunnett NW, Fabbri LM, Salvadori S, Geppetti P. Presence and bronchomotor activity of protease-activated receptor-2 in guinea pig airways. Am J Respir Crit Care Med 2000; 161:1672–1680.
66. Cicala C, Spina D, Keir SD, Severino B, Meli R, Page CP, Cirino G. Protective effect of a PAR2-activating peptide on histamine-induced bronchoconstriction in guinea pig. Br J Pharmacol 2001; 132:1229–1234.
67. Cocks TM, Fong B, Chow JM, Anderson GP, Frauman AG, Goldie RG, Henry PJ, Carr MJ, Hamilton JR, Moffatt JD. A protective role for protease-activated receptors in the airways. Nature 1999; 398:156–160.
68. Reynolds DS, Stevens RL, Lane WS, Carr MH, Austen KF, Serafin WE. Different mouse mast cell populations express various combinations of at least six distinct mast cell serine proteases. Proc Natl Acad Sci USA 1990; 87:3230–3234.
69. Reynolds DS, Gurley DS, Austen KF, Serafin WE. Cloning of the cDNA and gene of mouse mast cell protease 6: Transcription by progenitor mast cells and mast cells of the connective tissue subclass. J Biol Chem 1991; 266:3847–3853.
70. Serafin WE, Sullivan TP, Conder GA, Ebrahimi A, Marcham P, Johnson SS, Austen KF, Reynolds DS. Cloning of the cDNA and gene for mouse mast cell protease 4: Demonstration of its late transcription in mast cell subclasses and analysis of its homology to subclass-specific neutral proteases of the mouse and rat. J Biol Chem 1991; 266:1934–1941.
71. Stevens RL, Friend DS, McNeil HP, Schiller V, Ghildyal N, Austen KF. Strain-specific and tissue-specific expression of mouse mast cell secretory granule proteases. Proc Natl Acad Sci USA 1994; 91:128–132.
72. Wong GW, Tang Y, Feyfant E, Šali A, Li L, Li Y, Huang C, Friend DS, Krilis SA, Stevens RL. Identification of a new member of the tryptase family of mouse

and human mast cell proteases that possesses a novel COOH-terminal hydrophobic extension. J Biol Chem 1999; 274:30784–30793.

73. Le Trong H, Parmelee DC, Walsh KA, Neurath H, Woodbury RG. Amino acid sequence of rat mast cell protease I (chymase). Biochemistry 1987; 26:6988–6994.
74. Lützelschwab C, Pejler G, Aveskogh M, Hellman L. Secretory granule proteases in rat mast cells: Cloning of 10 different serine proteases and a carboxypeptidase A from various rat mast cell populations. J Exp Med 1997; 185:13–29.
75. Schick B, Austen KF, Schwartz LB. Activation of rat serosal mast cells by chymase, an endogenous secretory granule protease. J Immunol 1984; 132:2571–2577.
76. Schick B, Austen KF. Rat serosal mast cell degranulation mediated by chymase, an endogenous secretory granule protease: Active site-dependent initiation at 1°C. J Immunol 1986; 136:3812–3818.
77. Schick B, Austen KF. Modulation of chymase-mediated rat serosal mast cell degranulation by trypsin or diisopropyl fluorophosphate. Immunology 1989; 66:434–438.
78. Umarova BA, Dugina TN, Shestakova EV, Gluza E, Strukova SM. Activation of rat mast cells upon stimulation of protease-activated receptor-1. Bull Exp Biol Med 2000; 129:370–373.
79. Cirino G, Cicala C, Bucci MR, Sorrentino L, Maraganore JM, Stone SR. Thrombin functions as an inflammatory mediator through activation of its receptor. J Exp Med 1996; 183:821–827.
80. Vergnolle N, Hollenberg MD, Wallace JL. Pro- and anti-inflammatory actions of thrombin: A distinct role for proteinase-activated receptor-1. Br J Pharmacol 1999; 126:1262–1268.
81. Nishikawa H, Kawabata A, Kuroda R, Nishida M, Kawai K. Characterization of protease-activated receptors in rat peritoneal mast cells. Jpn J Pharmacol 2000; 82: 74–77.
82. Razin E, Baranes D, Marx G. Thrombin-mast cell interactions: Binding and cell activation. Exp Cell Res 1985; 160:380–386.
83. Paterson NAM, Wasserman SI, Said JW, Austen KF. Release of chemical mediators from partially purified human lung mast cells. J Immunol 1976; 117:1356–1362.
84. Katz HR, Vivier E, Castells MC, McCormick MJ, Chambers JM, Austen KF. Mouse mast cell gp49B1 contains two immunoreceptor tyrosine-based inhibition motifs and suppresses mast cell activation when coligated with the high-affinity Fc receptor for IgE. Proc Natl Acad Sci USA 1996; 93:10809–10814.
85. Strukova SM, Dugina TN, Khlgatian SV, Redkozubov AE, Redkozubova GP, Pinelis VG. Thrombin-mediated events implicated in mast cell activation. Semin Thromb Hemost 1996; 22:145–150.
86. Molino M, Blanchard N, Belmonte E, Tarver AP, Abrams C, Hoxie JA, Cerletti C, Brass LF. Proteolysis of the human platelet and endothelial cell thrombin receptor by neutrophil-derived cathepsin G. J Biol Chem 1995; 270:11168–11175.
87. D'Andrea MR, Rogahn CJ, Andrade-Gordon P. Localization of protease-activated receptors-1 and -2 in human mast cells: Indications for an amplified mast cell degranulation cascade. Biotech Histochem 2000; 75:85–90.

88. Schwartz LB, Austen KF. Acid hydrolases and other enzymes of rat and human mast cell secretory granules. Kroc Found Ser 1981; 14:103–121.
89. Kawabata A, Kuroda R, Minami T, Kataoka K, Taneda M. Increased vascular permeability by a specific agonist of protease-activated receptor-2 in rat hindpaw. Br J Pharmacol 1998; 125:419–422.
90. Le Trong H, Newlands GF, Miller HR, Charbonneau H, Neurath H, Woodbury RG. Amino acid sequence of a mouse mucosal mast cell protease. Biochemistry 1989; 28:391–395.
91. Reynolds DS, Stevens RL, Gurley DS, Lane WS, Austen KF, Serafin WE. Isolation and molecular cloning of mast cell carboxypeptidase A: A novel member of the carboxypeptidase gene family. J Biol Chem 1989; 264:20094–20099.
92. Serafin WE, Reynolds DS, Rogelj S, Lane WS, Conder GA, Johnson SS, Austen KF, Stevens RL. Identification and molecular cloning of a novel mouse mucosal mast cell serine protease. J Biol Chem 1990; 265:423–429.
93. McNeil HP, Austen KF, Somerville LL, Gurish MF, Stevens RL. Molecular cloning of the mouse mast cell protease-5 gene: A novel secretory granule protease expressed early in the differentiation of serosal mast cells. J Biol Chem 1991; 266: 20316–20322.
94. McNeil HP, Reynolds DS, Schiller V, Ghildyal N, Gurley DS, Austen KF, Stevens RL. Isolation, characterization, and transcription of the gene encoding mouse mast cell protease 7. Proc Natl Acad Sci USA 1992; 89:11174–11178.
95. Hunt JE, Friend DS, Gurish MF, Feyfant E, Šali A, Huang C, Ghildyal N, Stechschulte S, Austen KF, Stevens RL. Mouse mast cell protease 9, a novel member of the chromosome 14 family of serine proteases that is selectively expressed in uterine mast cells. J Biol Chem 1997; 272:29158–29166.
96. Lützelschwab C, Huang MR, Kullberg MC, Aveskogh M, Hellman L. Characterization of mouse mast cell protease-8, the first member of a novel subfamily of mouse mast cell serine proteases, distinct from both the classical chymases and tryptases. Eur J Immunol 1998; 28:1022–1033.
97. Woodbury RG, Katunuma N, Kobayashi K, Titani K, Neurath H, Anderson WF, Matthews BW. Covalent structure of a group-specific protease from rat small intestine. Biochemistry 1978; 17:811–819.
98. Cole KR, Kumar S, Trong HL, Woodbury RG, Walsh KA, Neurath H. Rat mast cell carboxypeptidase: Amino acid sequence and evidence of enzyme activity within mast cell granules. Biochemistry 1991; 30:648–655.
99. Irani AA, Schechter NM, Craig SS, DeBlois G, Schwartz LB. Two types of human mast cells that have distinct neutral protease compositions. Proc Natl Acad Sci USA 1986; 83:4464–4468.
100. Irani AM, Goldstein SM, Wintroub BU, Bradford T, Schwartz LB. Human mast cell carboxypeptidase: Selective localization to MC_{TC} cells. J Immunol 1991; 147: 247–253.
101. Weidner N, Austen KF. Heterogeneity of mast cells at multiple body sites: Fluorescent determination of avidin binding and immunofluorescent determination of chymase, tryptase, and carboxypeptidase content. Pathol Res Pract 1993; 189:156–162.
102. Lewis RA, Soter NA, Diamond PT, Austen KF, Oates JA, Roberts LJ. Prostaglan-

din D_2 generation after activation of rat and human mast cells with anti-IgE. J Immunol 1982; 129:1627–1631.
103. Razin E, Mencia-Huerta JM, Lewis RA, Corey EJ, Austen KF. Generation of leukotriene C_4 from a subclass of mast cells differentiated in vitro from mouse bone marrow. Proc Natl Acad Sci USA 1982; 79:4665–4667.
104. Heavey DJ, Ernst PB, Stevens RL, Befus AD, Bienenstock J, Austen KF. Generation of leukotriene C_4, leukotriene B_4, and prostaglandin D_2 by immunologically activated rat intestinal mucosa mast cells. J Immunol 1988; 140:1953–1957.
105. Levi-Schaffer F, Austen KF, Gravallese PM, Stevens RL. Coculture of interleukin 3-dependent mouse mast cells with fibroblasts results in a phenotypic change of the mast cells. Proc Natl Acad Sci USA 1986; 83:6485–6488.
106. Ghildyal N, Friend DS, Nicodemus CF, Austen KF, Stevens RL. Reversible expression of mouse mast cell protease 2 mRNA and protein in cultured mast cells exposed to IL-10. J Immunol 1993; 151:3206–3214.
107. Gurish MF, Pear WS, Stevens RL, Scott ML, Sokol K, Ghildyal N, Webster MJ, Hu X, Austen KF, Baltimore D. Tissue-regulated differentiation and maturation of a v-abl-immortalized mast cell-committed progenitor. Immunity 1995; 3:175–186.
108. Longley BJ, Tyrrell L, Lu S, Ma Y, Klump V, Murphy GF. Chronically c-kit-stimulated clonally-derived human mast cells show heterogeneity in different tissue microenvironments. J Invest Dermatol 1997; 108:792–796.
109. Friend DS, Ghildyal N, Gurish MF, Hunt J, Hu X, Austen KF, Stevens RL. Reversible expression of tryptases and chymases in the jejunal mast cells of mice infected with Trichinella spiralis. J Immunol 1998; 160:5537–5545.
110. Lee YM, Jippo T, Kim DK, Katsu Y, Tsujino K, Morii E, Kim HM, Adachi S, Nawa Y, Kitamura Y. Alteration of protease expression phenotype of mouse peritoneal mast cells by changing the microenvironment as demonstrated by in situ hybridization histochemistry. Am J Pathol 1998; 153:931–936.
111. Razin E, Cordon-Cardo C, Good RA. Growth of a pure population of mouse mast cells in vitro with conditioned medium derived from concanavalin A-stimulated splenocytes. Proc Natl Acad Sci USA 1981; 78:2559–2561.
112. Schrader JW, Lewis SJ, Clark-Lewis I, Culvenor JG. The persisting (P) cell: Histamine content, regulation by a T cell-derived factor, origin from a bone marrow precursor, and relationship to mast cells. Proc Natl Acad Sci USA 1981; 78:323–327.
113. Razin E, Ihle JN, Seldin D, Mencia-Huerta JM, Katz HR, LeBlanc PA, Hein A, Caulfield JP, Austen KF, Stevens RL. Interleukin 3: A differentiation and growth factor for the mouse mast cell that contains chondroitin sulfate E proteoglycan. J Immunol 1984; 132:1479–1486.
114. Razin E, Marx G. Thrombin-induced degranulation of cultured bone marrow-derived mast cells. J Immunol 1984; 133:3282–3285.
115. Gordon JR, Galli SJ. Release of both preformed and newly synthesized tumor necrosis factor α (TNF-α)/cachectin by mouse mast cells stimulated via FcεRI: A mechanism for the sustained action of mast cell-derived TNF-α during IgE-dependent biological responses. J Exp Med 1991; 174:103–107.
116. Gordon JR, Zhang X, Stevenson K, Cosford K. Thrombin induces IL-6 but not

TNF-α secretion by mouse mast cells: Threshold-level thrombin receptor and very low level FcεRI signaling synergistically enhance IL-6 secretion. Cell Immunol 2000; 205:128–135.

117. Cichowski K, Brugge JS, Brass LF. Thrombin receptor activation and integrin engagement stimulate tyrosine phosphorylation of the proto-oncogene product, p95 Vav, in platelets. J Biol Chem 1996; 271:7544–7550.
118. Burd PR, Rogers HW, Gordon JR, Martin CA, Jayaraman S, Wilson SD, Dvorak AM, Galli SJ, Dorf ME. Interleukin 3-dependent and -independent mast cells stimulated with IgE and antigen express multiple cytokines. J Exp Med 1989; 170: 245–257.
119. Plaut M, Pierce JH, Watson CJ, Hanley-Hyde J, Nordan RP, Paul WE. Mast cell lines produce lymphokines in response to cross-linkage of FcεRI or to calcium ionophores. Nature 1989; 339:64–67.
120. Gurish MF, Ghildyal N, Arm J, Austen KF, Avraham S, Reynolds D, Stevens RL. Cytokine mRNAs are preferentially increased relative to secretory granule protein mRNAs in mouse bone marrow-derived mast cells that have undergone IgE-mediated activation and degranulation. J Immunol 1991; 146:1527–1533.
121. Song JS, Gomez J, Stancato LF, Rivera J. Association of a p95 Vav-containing signaling complex with the FcεRI γ chain in the RBL-2H3 mast cell line: Evidence for a constitutive in vivo association of Vav with Grb2, Raf-1, and ERK2 in an active complex. J Biol Chem 1996; 271:26962–26970.
122. Song JS, Haleem-Smith H, Arudchandran R, Gomez J, Scott PM, Mill JF, Tan TH, Rivera J. Tyrosine phosphorylation of Vav stimulates IL-6 production in mast cells by a Rac/c-Jun N-terminal kinase-dependent pathway. J Immunol 1999; 163: 802–810.
123. Reynolds DS, Gurley DS, Stevens RL, Sugarbaker DJ, Austen KF, Serafin WE. Cloning of cDNAs that encode human mast cell carboxypeptidase A, and comparison of the protein with mouse mast cell carboxypeptidase A and rat pancreatic carboxypeptidases. Proc Natl Acad Sci USA 1989; 86:9480–9484.
124. Miller JS, Westin EH, Schwartz LB. Cloning and characterization of complementary DNA for human tryptase. J Clin Invest 1989; 84:1188–1195.
125. Miller JS, Moxley G, Schwartz LB. Cloning and characterization of a second complementary DNA for human tryptase. J Clin Invest 1990; 86:864–870.
126. Vanderslice P, Ballinger SM, Tam EK, Goldstein SM, Craik CS, Caughey GH. Human mast cell tryptase: Multiple cDNAs and genes reveal a multi-gene serine protease family. Proc Natl Acad Sci USA 1990; 87:3811–3815.
127. Caughey GH, Raymond WW, Blount JL, Hau LW, Pallaoro M, Wolters PJ, Verghese GM. Characterization of human γ-tryptases, novel members of the chromosome 16p mast cell tryptase and prostasin gene families. J Immunol 2000; 164: 6566–6575.
128. Gurish MF, Nadeau JH, Johnson KR, McNeil HP, Grattan KM, Austen KF, Stevens RL. A closely linked complex of mouse mast cell-specific chymase genes on chromosome 14. J Biol Chem 1993; 268:11372–11379.
129. Gurish MF, Johnson KR, Webster MJ, Stevens RL, Nadeau JH. Location of the mouse mast cell protease 7 gene (Mcpt7) to chromosome 17. Mamm Genome 1994; 5:656–657.

130. Wong GW, Li L, Madhusudhan MS, Krilis SA, Gurish MF, Rothenberg ME, Šali A, Stevens RL. Tryptase 4, a new member of the chromosome 17 family of mouse serine proteases. J Biol Chem 2001; 276:20648–20658.
131. Pallaoro M, Fejzo MS, Shayesteh L, Blount JL, Caughey GH. Characterization of genes encoding known and novel human mast cell tryptases on chromosome 16p13.3. J Biol Chem 1999; 274:3355–3362.
132. Inoue M, Kanbe N, Kurosawa M, Kido H. Cloning and tissue distribution of a novel serine protease Esp-1 from human eosinophils. Biochem Biophys Res Commun 1998; 252:307–312.
133. Inoue M, Isobe M, Itoyama T, Kido H. Structural analysis of Esp-1 gene. Biochem Biophys Res Commun 1999; 266:564–568.
134. Hooper JD, Nicol DL, Dickinson JL, Eyre HJ, Scarman AL, Normyle JF, Stuttgen MA, Douglas ML, Loveland KA, Sutherland GR, Antalis TM. Testisin, a new human serine proteinase expressed by premeiotic testicular germ cells and lost in testicular germ cell tumors. Cancer Res 1999; 59:3199–3205.
134a. Wong GW, Yasuda S, Madhusudhan MS, Li L, Yang Y, Krilis SA, Šali A, Stevens RL. Human tryptase epsilon (PRSS22): a new member of the chromosome 16p13.3 family of human serine proteases expressed in airway epithelial cells. J Biol Chem 2001; 276:49169–49182.
135. Schwartz LB, Lewis RA, Austen KF. Tryptase from human pulmonary mast cells: Purification and characterization. J Biol Chem 1981; 256:11939–11943.
136. Huang C, Morales G, Vagi A, Chanasyk K, Ferrazzi M, Burklow C, Qiu WT, Feyfant E, Šali A, Stevens RL. Formation of enzymatically active, homotypic, and heterotypic tetramers of mouse mast cell tryptases: Dependence on a conserved Trp-rich domain on the surface. J Biol Chem 2000; 275:351–358.
137. Johnson DA, Barton GJ. Mast cell tryptases: Examination of unusual characteristics by multiple sequence alignment and molecular modeling. Protein Sci 1992; 1:370–377.
138. Pereira PJ, Bergner A, Macedo-Ribeiro S, Huber R, Matschiner G, Fritz H, Sommerhoff CP, Bode W. Human β-tryptase is a ring-like tetramer with active sites facing a central pore. Nature 1998; 392:306–311.
139. Schwartz LB, Bradford TR, Lee DC, Chlebowski JF. Immunologic and physicochemical evidence for conformational changes occurring on conversion of human mast cell tryptase from active tetramer to inactive monomer: Production of monoclonal antibodies recognizing active tryptase. J Immunol 1990; 144:2304–2311.
140. Schechter NM, Eng GY, Selwood T, McCaslin DR. Structural changes associated with the spontaneous inactivation of the serine proteinase human tryptase. Biochemistry 1995; 34:10628–10638.
141. Erba F, Fiorucci L, Coletta M, Ascoli F. Bovine mast cell tryptase inactivation: Effect of temperature. Peptides 1998; 19:437–443.
142. Cromlish JA, Seidah NG, Marcinkiewicz M, Hamelin J, Johnson DA, Chretien M. Human pituitary tryptase: Molecular forms, NH_2-terminal sequence, immunocytochemical localization, and specificity with prohormone and fluorogenic substrates. J Biol Chem 1987; 262:1363–1373.
143. Benyon RC, Enciso JA, Befus AD. Analysis of human skin mast cell proteins

by two-dimensional gel electrophoresis: Identification of tryptase as a sialylated glycoprotein. J Immunol 1993; 151:2699–2706.
144. Ghildyal N, Friend DS, Freelund R, Austen KF, McNeil HP, Schiller V, Stevens RL. Lack of expression of the tryptase mouse mast cell protease 7 in mast cells of the C57BL/6J mouse. J Immunol 1994; 153:2624–2630.
145. Peisach E, Wang J, de los Santos T, Reich E, Ringe D. Crystal structure of the proenzyme domain of plasminogen. Biochemistry 1999; 38:11180–11188.
146. Huang C, Friend DS, Qiu WT, Wong GW, Morales G, Hunt J, Stevens RL. Induction of a selective and persistent extravasation of neutrophils into the peritoneal cavity by tryptase mouse mast cell protease 6. J Immunol 1998; 160:1910–1919.
147. Huang C, De Sanctis GT, O'Brien PJ, Mizgerd JP, Friend DS, Drazen JM, Brass LF, Stevens RL. Evaluation of the substrate specificity of human mast cell tryptase βI and demonstration of its importance in bacterial infections of the lung. J Biol Chem 2001; 276:26276–26284.
148. Rice KD, Gangloff AR, Kuo EY, Dener JM, Wang VR, Lum R, Newcomb WS, Havel C, Putnam D, Cregar L, Wong M, Warne RL. Dibasic inhibitors of human mast cell tryptase: Synthesis and optimization of a novel class of inhibitors. Bioorg Med Chem Lett 2000; 10:2357–2360.
149. Rice KD, Wang VR, Gangloff AR, Kuo EY, Dener JM, Newcomb WS, Young WB, Putnam D, Cregar L, Wong M, Simpson PJ. Dibasic inhibitors of human mast cell tryptase: Structure-activity relationships and requirements for potent activity. Bioorg Med Chem Lett 2000; 10:2361–2366.
150. Tantravahi RV, Stevens RL, Austen KF, Weis JH. A single gene in mast cells encodes the core peptides of heparin and chondroitin sulfate proteoglycans. Proc Natl Acad Sci USA 1986; 83:9207–9210.
151. Yurt RW, Leid RW Jr, Austen KF. Native heparin from rat peritoneal mast cells. J Biol Chem 1977; 252:518–521.
152. Razin E, Stevens RL, Akiyama F, Schmid K, Austen KF. Culture from mouse bone marrow of a subclass of mast cells possessing a distinct chondroitin sulfate proteoglycan with glycosaminoglycans rich in N-acetylgalactosamine-4,6-disulfate. J Biol Chem 1982; 257:7229–7236.
153. Seldin DC, Austen KF, Stevens RL. Purification and characterization of protease-resistant secretory granule proteoglycans containing chondroitin sulfate di-B and heparin-like glycosaminoglycans from rat basophilic leukemia cells. J Biol Chem 1985; 260:11131–11139.
154. Gurish MF, Ghildyal N, McNeil HP, Austen KF, Gillis S, Stevens RL. Differential expression of secretory granule proteases in mouse mast cells exposed to interleukin 3 and c-kit ligand. J Exp Med 1992; 175:1003–1012.
155. Šali A, Matsumoto R, McNeil HP, Karplus M, Stevens RL. Three-dimensional models of four mouse mast cell chymases: Identification of proteoglycan binding regions and protease-specific antigenic epitopes. J Biol Chem 1993; 268:9023–9034.
156. Matsumoto R, Šali A, Ghildyal N, Karplus M, Stevens RL. Packaging of proteases and proteoglycans in the granules of mast cells and other hematopoietic cells: A cluster of histidines on mouse mast cell protease 7 regulates its binding to heparin serglycin proteoglycans. J Biol Chem 1995; 270:19524–19531.

157. Ghildyal N, Friend DS, Stevens RL, Austen KF, Huang C, Penrose JF, Šali A, Gurish MF. Fate of two mast cell tryptases in V3 mastocytosis and normal BALB/c mice undergoing passive systemic anaphylaxis: Prolonged retention of exocytosed mMCP-6 in connective tissues, and rapid accumulation of enzymatically active mMCP-7 in the blood. J Exp Med 1996; 184:1061–1073.
158. De Young MB, Nemeth EF, Scarpa A. Measurement of the internal pH of mast cell granules using microvolumetric fluorescence and isotopic techniques. Arch Biochem Biophys 1987; 254:222–233.
159. Huang C, Wong GW, Ghildyal N, Gurish MF, Šali A, Matsumoto R, Qiu WT, Stevens RL. The tryptase, mouse mast cell protease 7, exhibits anticoagulant activity in vivo and in vitro due to its ability to degrade fibrinogen in the presence of the diverse array of protease inhibitors in plasma. J Biol Chem 1997; 272:31885–31893.
160. Schwartz LB, Bradford TR. Regulation of tryptase from human lung mast cells by heparin: Stabilization of the active tetramer. J Biol Chem 1986; 261:7372–7379.
161. Mirza H, Schmidt VA, Derian CK, Jesty J, Bahou WF. Mitogenic responses mediated through the proteinase-activated receptor-2 are induced by expressed forms of mast cell α or β tryptases. Blood 1997; 90:3914–3922.
162. Humphries DE, Wong GW, Friend DS, Gurish MF, Qiu WT, Huang C, Sharpe AH, Stevens RL. Heparin is essential for the storage of specific granule proteases in mast cells. Nature 1999; 400:769–772.
163. Le Trong H, Neurath H, Woodbury RG. Substrate specificity of the chymotrypsin-like protease in secretory granules isolated from rat mast cells. Proc Natl Acad Sci USA 1987; 84:364–367.
164. Stevens RL, Fox CC, Lichtenstein LM, Austen KF. Identification of chondroitin sulfate E proteoglycans and heparin proteoglycans in the secretory granules of human lung mast cells. Proc Natl Acad Sci USA 1988; 85:2284–2287.
165. Thompson HL, Schulman ES, Metcalfe DD. Identification of chondroitin sulfate E in human lung mast cells. J Immunol 1988; 140:2708–2713.
166. Huang C, Li L, Krilis SA, Chanasyk K, Tang Y, Li Z, Hunt JE, Stevens RL. Human tryptases α and βII are functionally distinct due, in part, to a single amino acid difference in one of the surface loops that forms the substrate-binding cleft. J Biol Chem 1999; 274:19670–19676.
167. Hallgren J, Karlson U, Poorafshar M, Hellman L, Pejler G. Mechanism for activation of mouse mast cell tryptase: Dependence on heparin and acidic pH for formation of active tetramers of mouse mast cell protease 6. Biochemistry 2000; 39: 13068–13077.
168. Wershil BK, Wang ZS, Gordon JR, Galli SJ. Recruitment of neutrophils during IgE-dependent cutaneous late phase reactions in the mouse is mast cell-dependent: Partial inhibition of the reaction with antiserum against tumor necrosis factor-α. J Clin Invest 1991; 87:446–453.
169. Echtenacher B, Männel DN, Hültner L. Critical protective role of mast cells in a model of acute septic peritonitis. Nature 1996; 381:75–77.
170. Malaviya R, Ikeda T, Ross E, Abraham SN. Mast cell modulation of neutrophil influx and bacterial clearance at sites of infection through TNF-α. Nature 1996; 381:77–80.

171. Katz BA, Clark JM, Finer-Moore JS, Jenkins TE, Johnson CR, Ross MJ, Luong C, Moore WR, Stroud RM. Design of potent selective zinc-mediated serine protease inhibitors. Nature 1998; 391:608–612.
172. Combrink KD, Gulgeze HB, Meanwell NA, Pearce BC, Zulan P, Bisacchi GS, Roberts DG, Stanley P, Seiler SM. 1,2-Benzisothiazol-3-one 1,1-dioxide inhibitors of human mast cell tryptase. J Med Chem 1998; 41:4854–4860.
173. Burgess LE, Newhouse BJ, Ibrahim P, Rizzi J, Kashem MA, Hartman A, Brandhuber BJ, Wright CD, Thomson DS, Vigers GP, Koch K. Potent selective nonpeptidic inhibitors of human lung tryptase. Proc Natl Acad Sci USA 1999; 96:8348–8352.
174. Wright CD, Havill AM, Middleton SC, Kashem MA, Dripps DJ, Abraham WM, Thomson DS, Burgess LE. Inhibition of allergen-induced pulmonary responses by the selective tryptase inhibitor 1,5-bis-[4-[(3-carbamimidoyl-benzenesulfonylamino)-methyl]-phenoxy]-pentane (AMG-126737). Biochem Pharmacol 1999; 58:1989–1996.
175. Hartmann T, Ruoss SJ, Raymond WW, Seuwen K, Caughey GH. Human tryptase as a potent, cell-specific mitogen: Role of signaling pathways in synergistic responses. Am J Physiol 1992; 262:L528–L534.
176. Corvera CU, Dery O, McConalogue K, Bohm SK, Khitin LM, Caughey GH, Payan DG, Bunnett NW. Mast cell tryptase regulates rat colonic myocytes through proteinase-activated receptor-2. J Clin Invest 1997; 100:1383–1393.
177. Schechter NM, Brass LF, Lavker RM, Jensen PJ. Reaction of mast cell proteases tryptase and chymase with protease activated receptors on keratinocytes and fibroblasts. J Cell Physiol 1998; 176:365–373.
178. Steinhoff M, Corvera CU, Thoma MS, Kong W, McAlpine BE, Caughey GH, Ansel JC, Bunnett NW. Proteinase-activated receptor-2 in human skin: Tissue distribution and activation of keratinocytes by mast cell tryptase. Exp Dermatol 1999; 8:282–294.
179. Corvera CU, Dery O, McConalogue K, Gamp P, Thoma M, Al Ani B, Caughey GH, Hollenberg MD, Bunnett NW. Thrombin and mast cell tryptase regulate guinea-pig myenteric neurons through proteinase-activated receptors-1 and -2. J Physiol 1999; 517:741–756.
180. Steinhoff M, Vergnolle N, Young SH, Tognetto M, Amadesi S, Ennes HS, Trevisani M, Hollenberg MD, Wallace JL, Caughey GH, Mitchell SE, Williams LM, Geppetti P, Mayer EA, Bunnett NW. Agonists of proteinase-activated receptor-2 induce inflammation by a neurogenic mechanism. Nat Med 2000; 6:151–158.
181. Akers IA, Parsons M, Hill MR, Hollenberg MD, Sanjar S, Laurent GJ, McAnulty RJ. Mast cell tryptase stimulates human lung fibroblast proliferation via protease-activated receptor-2. Am J Physiol Lung Cell Mol Physiol 2000; 278:L193–L201.
182. Clark JM, Abraham WM, Fishman CE, Forteza R, Ahmed A, Cortes A, Warne RL, Moore WR, Tanaka RD. Tryptase inhibitors block allergen-induced airway and inflammatory responses in allergic sheep. Am J Respir Crit Care Med 1995; 152:2076–2083.
183. Stack MS, Johnson DA. Human mast cell tryptase activates single-chain urinary-type plasminogen activator (pro-urokinase). J Biol Chem 1994; 269:9416–9419.

184. Martin TR, Takeishi T, Katz HR, Austen KF, Drazen JM, Galli SJ. Mast cell activation enhances airway responsiveness to methacholine in the mouse. J Clin Invest 1993; 91:1176–1182.
185. Barrios VE, Middleton SC, Kashem MA, Havill AM, Toombs CF, Wright CD. Tryptase mediates hyperresponsiveness in isolated guinea pig bronchi. Life Sci 1998; 63:2295–2303.
186. Krishna MT, Chauhan A, Little L, Sampson K, Hawksworth R, Mant T, Djukanovic R, Lee T, Holgate S. Inhibition of mast cell tryptase by inhaled APC 366 attenuates allergen-induced late-phase airway obstruction in asthma. J Allergy Clin Immunol 2001; 107:1039–1045.
187. Pemberton AD, Huntley JF, Miller HR. Differential inhibition of mast cell chymases by secretory leukocyte protease inhibitor. Biochim Biophys Acta 1998; 1379:29–34.
188. Fath MA, Wu X, Hileman RE, Linhardt RJ, Kashem MA, Nelson RM, Wright CD, Abraham WM. Interaction of secretory leukocyte protease inhibitor with heparin inhibits proteases involved in asthma. J Biol Chem 1998; 273:13563–13569.
189. Wright CD, Havill AM, Middleton SC, Kashem MA, Lee PA, Dripps DJ, O'Riordan TG, Bevilacqua MP, Abraham WM. Secretory leukocyte protease inhibitor prevents allergen-induced pulmonary responses in animal models of asthma. J Pharmacol Exp Ther 1999; 289:1007–1014.
190. Forteza RM, Ahmed A, Lee T, Abraham WM. Secretory leukocyte protease inhibitor, but not α1 protease inhibitor, blocks tryptase-induced bronchoconstriction. Pulm Pharmacol Ther 2001; 14:107–110.
191. Sekizawa K, Caughey GH, Lazarus SC, Gold WM, Nadel JA. Mast cell tryptase causes airway smooth muscle hyperresponsiveness in dogs. J Clin Invest 1989; 83: 175–179.
192. Undem BJ, McAlexander M, Hunter DD. Neurobiology of the upper and lower airways. Allergy 1999; 54(suppl 57):81–93.
193. Smirnova IV, Zhang SX, Citron BA, Arnold PM, Festoff BW. Thrombin is an extracellular signal that activates intracellular death protease pathways inducing apoptosis in model motor neurons. J Neurobiol 1998; 36:64–80.
194. Smirnova IV, Vamos S, Wiegmann T, Citron BA, Arnold PM, Festoff BW. Calcium mobilization and protease-activated receptor cleavage after thrombin stimulation in motor neurons. J Mol Neurosci 1998; 10:31–44.
195. Turgeon VL, Lloyd ED, Wang S, Festoff BW, Houenou LJ. Thrombin perturbs neurite outgrowth and induces apoptotic cell death in enriched chick spinal motoneuron cultures through caspase activation. J Neurosci 1998; 18:6882–6891.
196. Bienenstock J, Befus D, Denburg J, Goto T, Lee T, Otsuka H, Shanahan F. Comparative aspects of mast cell heterogeneity in different species and sites. Int Arch Allergy Appl Immunol 1985; 77:126–129.
197. Bienenstock J, Perdue M, Blennerhassett M, Stead R, Kakuta N, Sestini P, Vancheri C, Marshall J. Inflammatory cells and the epithelium: Mast cell/nerve interactions in the lung in vitro and in vivo. Am Rev Respir Dis 1988; 138:S31–S34.
198. Bienenstock J, MacQueen G, Sestini P, Marshall JS, Stead RH, Perdue MH. Mast cell/nerve interactions in vitro and in vivo. Am Rev Respir Dis 1991; 143:S55–S58.

199. Park HY, Nabika T, Jang Y, Kim D, Kim HS, Masuda J. Identification of new single-nucleotide polymorphisms in the thrombin receptor gene and their effects on coronary artery diseases in Koreans. Clin Exp Pharmacol Physiol 2000; 27: 690–693.
200. Compton SJ, Cairns JA, Palmer KJ, Al Ani B, Hollenberg MD, Walls AF. A polymorphic protease-activated receptor-2 displaying reduced sensitivity to trypsin and differential responses to PAR agonists. J Biol Chem 2000; 275:39207–39212.
201. De Sanctis GT, Merchant M, Beier DR, Dredge RD, Grobholz JK, Martin TR, Lander ES, Drazen JM. Quantitative locus analysis of airway hyperresponsiveness in A/J and C57BL/6J mice. Nat Genet 1995; 11:150–154.
202. Hunt JE, Stevens RL, Austen KF, Zhang J, Xia Z, Ghildyal N. Natural disruption of the mouse mast cell protease 7 gene in the C57BL/6 mouse. J Biol Chem 1996; 271:2851–2855.
203. Wang HW, McNeil HP, Thomas PS, Murphy B, Webster MJ, Hettiaratchi A, King G, Heywood G, Huang C, Hunt JE. Molecular cloning and characterization of novel human tryptase cDNAs and splice variants. FASEB J 2000; 14:A1239–A1239.
204. Goodwin RL, Barbour KW, Berger FG. Expression of the α1-proteinase inhibitor gene family during evolution of the genus Mus. Mol Biol Evol 1997; 14:420–427.

6

Interleukin-4 Inhibition for the Treatment of Asthma

LARRY BORISH and JOHN W. STEINKE

University of Virginia Health System
Charlottesville, Virginia

BRUCE DAVIDSON

Bayer Pharmaceutical Corporation
West Haven, Connecticut

RICHARD S. SHAMES

Protein Design Labs, Inc.
Fremont, California

JAN M. AGOSTI

Immunex Corporation
Seattle, Washington

I. Introduction

Interleukin-4 (IL-4) mediates important proinflammatory functions in asthma including Th2 lymphocyte differentiation, induction of IgE production, upregulation of IgE receptors, expression of VCAM-1, promotion of eosinophil transmigration into the lungs, inhibition of T-lymphocyte apoptosis, and mucus secretion. The role of IL-4 in the pathogenesis of asthma is further supported by identification of polymorphisms linked to asthma in the IL-4 gene promoter and proteins involved in IL-4 signaling.

Several approaches to IL-4 antagonism are in clinical development, including soluble recombinant human IL-4 receptor, IL-4 mutein, humanized anti-interleukin-4 monoclonal antibody, and human anti-interleukin-4 receptor monoclonal antibody. Soluble recombinant human IL-4 receptor (sIL-4R) lacks the transmembrane and cytoplasmic activating domains of the cell-surface receptor and can therefore sequester IL-4 without mediating cellular activation. Early-phase clinical trials have demonstrated the safety and clinical efficacy of this IL-4 antagonist as a therapeutic agent in asthma. BAY 16-9996, a double mutein with both IL-4 and IL-13 antagonist activity, has shown efficacy in a cynomolgus monkey model of asthma.

Phase 1 studies showed safety and tolerance of multiple doses in humans. The humanized anti-IL-4 monoclonal antibody binds with high affinity to human IL-4, thus preventing interaction of IL-4 with its receptor. A phase 1 clinical study in asthma patients demonstrated that the antibody was well tolerated, was not immunogenic, and had a long half-life.

Human anti-interleukin-4 receptor monoclonal antibody is a cloned human antibody that blocks the IL-4α subunit. This subunit is contained in both the IL-4 and IL-13 receptors and acts as a dual inhibitor of IL-4 and IL-13 signaling.

II. Role of IL-4 in the Pathogenesis of Asthma

Interleukin-4 (IL-4) is a critical cytokine in the development of allergic inflammation. It plays a key central role in the initial differentiation of naive Th0 lymphocytes into the Th2 lymphocytes that drive the allergic phenotype (Fig. 1) (1,2). IL-4 acts via the IL-4 receptor on the surface of T lymphocytes and upregulates the expression of the IL-4 receptor in a positive autocrine loop (3). IL-13, which shares many biological activities with IL-4, is not able to promote Th2 differentiation, because IL-13 receptors are not expressed on T lymphocytes (4). Incubation of human T cells with IL-4 generates Th2-type lymphocyte clones and can be inhibited by anti-IL-4. These Th2-type cells secrete additional IL-4 as well as other Th2 cytokines, including IL-5, IL-9, and IL-13, and lose the ability to produce the Th1 cytokine interferon-γ (5).

Other important activities of IL-4 are induction of the IgE isotype switch, mitogenic stimulation of B-cell growth, and upregulation of class II MHC on B cells (6,7). The IgE-mediated immune responses are further enhanced by IL-4 through its ability to upregulate IgE receptors on the cell surface—both the low affinity IgE receptor (FcεRII; CD23) on B lymphocytes and mononuclear phagocytic cells and the high affinity IgE receptor (FcεRI) on mast cells and basophils (7). IgE-dependent mast cell activation induced by IL-4 plays a pivotal role in the development of immediate allergic reactions. Leukotriene mediators and their receptors are also increased by IL-4 exposure (8–10).

Interleukin-4 further promotes cellular inflammation in the asthmatic lung by the induction of vascular cell adhesion molecule (VCAM-1) on vascular endothelium (11). Through the interaction with VCAM-1, IL-4 directs the migration of T lymphocytes, monocytes, basophils, and eosinophils to inflammatory loci. In addition, IL-4 promotes eosinophilic inflammation by inducing eosinophil chemotaxis and activation and by inhibiting eosinophil apoptosis through increased expression of eotaxin (12).

In addition to driving the initial differentiation of Th0 lymphocytes toward a Th2 phenotype, IL-4 is important in maintaining allergic immune responses by preventing apoptosis of T lymphocytes. Activation of these cells results in rapid

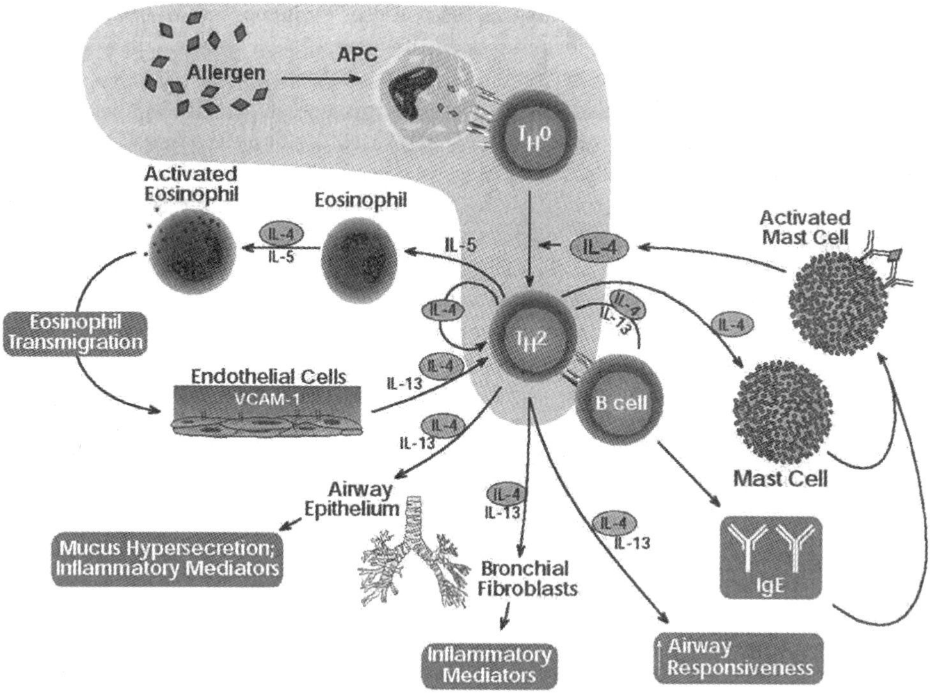

Figure 1 IL-4 plays a key central role in the pathogenesis of asthma. It is the only cytokine that causes the differentiation of naive Th0 cells into Th2 cells, which then leads to the release of IL-4 and other Th2 cytokines such as IL-5, IL-9, and IL-13. It also results in the isotype switch to IgE production, upregulation of IgE receptor, VCAM-1 expression leading to eosinophil transmigration into the lungs, inhibition of T-lymphocyte apoptosis, and mucus production.

proliferation and secretion of cytokines. In the absence of an appropriate signal, activated T-helper lymphocytes rapidly become apoptotic and are eliminated. Several cytokines, including IL-2, IL-4, IL-7, and IL-15, are effective in preventing the death of activated T cells. Of these, IL-4 and IL-15 are the most effective (13). Inhibition of apoptosis by IL-4 may be partially mediated by the ability of this cytokine to maintain levels of the survival-promoting, anti-apoptotic protein Bcl-2 in T cells (13). Apoptosis of T lymphocytes can be induced through signals mediated by FasL through the Fas (CD95) receptor expressed on these cells. T cells from asthmatic lungs show defective expression of Fas, which may give them increased resistance to apoptotic cell death. Coculture of T cells with IL-4 downregulates cell-surface Fas expression. The IL-4 in the asthmatic lung and secondary lack of Fas expression may explain a persistence of inflammatory cellular infiltrates in allergic asthma due to inhibition of apoptosis. Apoptosis of Th2 lymphocytes (and possibly eosinophils) could represent a pathway whereby IL-4 blockade will produce rapid clinical benefits in asthma.

Corticosteroids normally cause apoptosis of mature T-helper cell lines. Induction of cell death is prevented by IL-2 in Th1 cells and by IL-4 in Th2 cells (14). IL-2 and IL-4 synergize to render lymphocytes refractory to the anti-inflammatory influences of corticosteroids. This is a result of alternate splicing of glucocorticoid receptor (GCR) mRNA transcripts in the presence of IL-2 and IL-4, thereby generating GCR-β. GCR-β is unable to bind glucocorticoids but can bind to and antagonize the transactivation induced by GCR-α in the setting of glucocorticoid therapy. Through these mechanisms, the autocrine production of IL-4 by Th2 cells in the asthmatic lung may render these cells refractory to the anti-inflammatory influences of corticosteroids (15). Synergistic benefits of IL-4 inhibitory therapy and inhaled corticosteroids may be expected in patients with asthma. Furthermore, it has been demonstrated that glucocorticoid therapy induces a Th2 phenotype in patients (16). This provides an additional mechanism by which IL-4 inhibition may synergize with inhaled corticosteroids in the treatment of asthma.

Another mechanism by which IL-4 contributes to airway obstruction in asthma is through induction of mucin gene expression and mucus hypersecretion (17). IL-4-stimulated bronchial epithelial cell explants from asthmatic subjects but not normal controls release significantly increased transforming growth factor α, a growth factor that stimulates epithelial and fibroblast proliferation as well as mucus production (18). IL-4 increases the fibroblast expression of eotaxin, other inflammatory cytokines, and type I procollagen, which might contribute to inflammation and lung remodeling in chronic asthma (19,20).

III. Interleukin-4 Signaling

Optimal signaling by IL-4 (21–23) involves its interaction with a receptor complex that consists of a heterodimer of the high affinity IL-4Rα protein and either the common γ chain, shared with IL-2, IL-7, IL-9, and IL-15, or the IL-13Rα1 chain (Fig. 2). IL-4Rα chains are ubiquitously expressed. IL-13 mediates its biological activities through a heterodimer consisting of the IL-4Rα and IL-13Rα1 proteins. IL-13Rα1 expression is limited to hematopoietic cells, including B cells, mononuclear phagocytes, basophils, mast cells (but not T cells), and endothelial cells. This more limited distribution of IL-13Rα1 expression explains the pattern of shared biological activities of IL-4 and IL-13 but the unique ability of IL-4 to induce Th2 lymphocyte differentiation. The two IL-13Rα chains that have been described include the active form of the receptor IL-13Rα1 and a putative

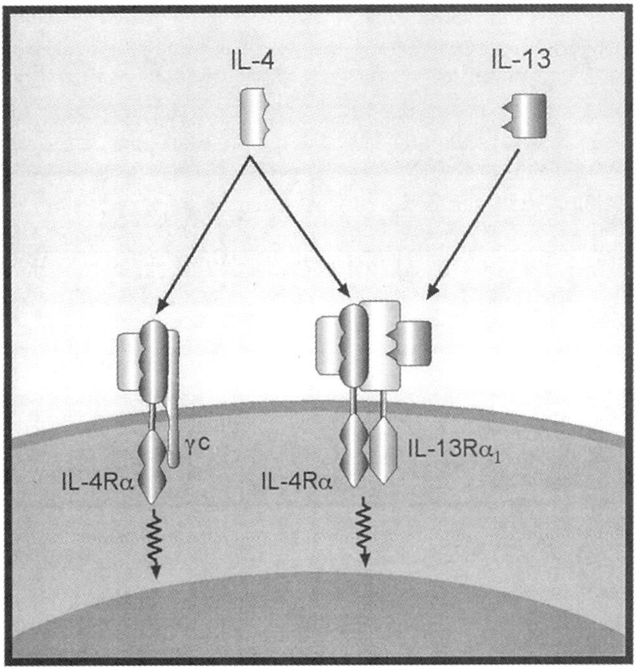

Figure 2 IL-4 signals via a heterodimeric receptor composed of high affinity IL-4Rα protein and the common γ chain (T cells) or the IL-13Rα1 chain (endothelial cells). IL-13 signals through the heterodimeric receptor consisting of IL-4α and IL-13α1. A putative inhibitory receptor for IL-13 has been described that consists of IL-4Rα and IL-13α2.

inhibitory receptor, IL-13α2, which lacks the motif required for the binding of Janus kinases (24).

Two tyrosine kinases, Jak1 and Jak3, constitutively associate with IL-4Rα and the γ chain, respectively. Engagement of the IL-4 receptor leads to the activation of Jak1 and phosphorylation of the IL-4 receptor cytoplasmic region, which in turn phosphorylates the signal transducer and activator of transcription 6 (Stat-6). After phosphorylation, Stat-6 molecules dimerize, then translocate to the nucleus, where they bind in the promoter region of responsive genes and activate gene transcription. Stat-6 is necessary for IL-4 dependent expression of IL-4Rα, ε heavy chain, MHC class II, CD23, and mucin (21,22). The phosphorylation of the IL-4Rα cytoplasmic region also provides a docking site for the insulin receptor substrate, IRS-1, and its homologe, IRS-2 (22,25). IRS-1 and IRS-2 regulate cellular proliferation and protect cells from apoptosis (21,22). Although the IRS-

1, 2 pathway is generally responsible for cell proliferation, and the Stat-6 pathway for regulation of gene expression, studies in Stat-6 knockout mice demonstrate that the altered expression of growth factors contributes to reduced proliferation of these cells in the presence of IL-4. IL-4 activates Stat-6, leading to the development of a Th2 response, whereas IL-12 activates Stat-4 and leads to a Th1 response (26). Inhibition of Stat-6 signaling offers a potential therapeutic opportunity; however, targeting an intracellular mediator is a challenge. There is an endogenous inhibitor of Stat-6 referred to as suppressor of cytokine signaling (SOCS-1) that inhibits IL-4 signaling (27). BCL-6 is a transcription factor that counteracts the stimulatory effects of Stat-6 by binding to Stat-6-responsive promoter elements, acting as a competitive inhibitor for Stat-6 binding, and suppressing gene transcription. BCL-6 suppresses Stat-6-dependent IL-4-induced IgE production (28). Inhibitors of intracellular signaling offer potential approaches to IL-4 inhibition.

Although the IL-13 receptor contains an IL-4Rα molecule, soluble IL-4R does not interrupt IL-13 signaling when tested in vitro (data on file, Immunex Corporation). Antibody directed against the IL-4Rα, however, blocks signaling of both IL-4 and IL-13. Similarly, the synthetic IL-4 mutein, by occupying the IL-4Rα molecule, will inhibit binding of both IL-4 and IL-13. Each of these approaches is being developed for therapy as a potential dual inhibitor of both IL-4 and IL-13.

IV. IL-4 Genetics and Asthma

Asthma is a complex genetic disorder (reviewed in Refs. 29 and 30). Abnormal production of IL-4 or hyperresponsiveness to this cytokine resulting from inherited defects may contribute to the pathophysiology of this disorder in a subset of asthmatic patients. In addition, individuals genetically programmed to be hyperresponsive to IL-4 may demonstrate enhanced treatment response to an IL-4 antagonist. Asthma has been associated with polymorphisms in the IL-4Rα, IL-13Rα1, Stat-6, and BCL-6 genes. The naturally occurring polymorphisms linked to atopy and asthma that may influence IL-4 production or IL-4 signaling are summarized in Table 1.

Genome searches and candidate gene approaches have each linked atopy and asthma to chromosome 5q31–33 (31–34), a locus for Th2 cytokines including IL-4 (31–34). We described a C/T exchange at −590 bp from the open reading frame of the IL-4 gene and correlated this with higher levels of total serum IgE and asthma (35–39). Other workers (39–42) subsequently confirmed this association in studies that included association of the 590T allele with asthma (37) and asthma severity (39). This variant is associated with enhanced IL-4 promoter strength and increased binding affinity by nuclear transcription factors

Table 1 Genes Associated with IL-4 and IL-4 Signaling Linked to Asthma and Allergies

Gene	Polymorphism	Location	Chromosome	Ref.
Interleukin-4 promoter	A-to-G	−81	5q31-33	43
	C-to-T	−285		43
	C-to-T	−590		35
Interleukin-4 receptor, α chain	Ile-to-Val	+50	16p12.1	51
	Ser-to-Pro	+503		59
	Gln-to-Arg	+576		49
Interleukin-13 receptor, α chain	A-to-G	+1398	Xq13	60
Stat-6	G-to-A	+2964 (3′ UTR)	12q13-14	62
BCL-6	HindIII	5′ UTR	3q27	91

to an NFAT site in the IL-4 promoter (38). Additional polymorphisms that may influence promoter activity have been reported within the IL-4 gene promoter (43). However, other investigators have been unable to confirm these latter polymorphisms in several populations, and their significance is unclear.

Candidate gene and genome-wide searches have also linked atopy to chromosome 16p12.1, which includes the IL-4Rα chain (44–47). Numerous polymorphisms have been identified in the IL-4R gene (48), and linkage to atopy and asthma are associated with three of them (Ile50Val, Gln576Arg, and Ser503Pro) (49,50). The isoleucine-to-valine mutation at amino acid 50 (Ile50Val) is associated with a higher prevalence of asthma (51). Ile50-bearing mononuclear cells demonstrate augmented IL-4-mediated CD23 expression, Stat-6 activation, T-cell proliferation, and transcriptional activity of the ε heavy chain promoter (51). The glutamine-to-arginine variant at amino acid 576 (Gln576Arg) lies in the cytoplasmic domain of IL-4Rα that is necessary for optimal activation of Stat-6 (49,52–54). Subjects with this mutation demonstrate enhanced phosphorylation of Stat-6 and CD23 induction in response to IL-4 (49). This mutation correlates with the presence of severe atopic eczema (49) and is a risk factor for decreased lung function in asthmatic subjects (55). However, these linkages have not been confirmed in other populations (51,56–58). It is possible that the reported associations of the Gln576Arg exchange represent linkage disequilibrium to the actual disease-causing mutation. Alternatively, these reported linkages might depend upon the presence of additional mutations in either IL-4Rα or one of its signaling molecules. The serine-to-proline polymorphism is present in the IRS-activating motif of the IL-4R (Ser503Pro) and associated with elevated total IgE levels (59).

The presence of this polymorphism—but only when there is also an additional Gln576Arg polymorphism—is associated with increased phosphorylation of IRS-1 and IRS-2. Increased phosphorylation of IRS-1 and IRS-2 could augment propagation signals mediated by IL-4, which would influence B-cell proliferation and IgE concentration.

In addition to the shared γ chain, IL-4Rα can form a functional receptor for IL-4 with IL-13Rα1 (21–23). A noncoding A/G exchange at +1398 of the IL-13Rα1 gene was associated with higher IgE levels (60). This association was not confirmed in a different cohort, and no association with asthma was detected in either population (60). The IL-13Rα gene is located on Xq13, which suggests X-linked inheritance of asthma and allergies and may explain some of the maternal influence in these conditions (61).

Aside from polymorphisms located in the IL-4 gene or its receptor, polymorphisms have been identified in the factors involved in signaling and transcription of genes activated in response to receptor engagement of IL-4. A G/A variant has been identified in the 3′ untranslated region of the Stat-6 gene, mapping to position +2964 from the transcription start site (62). There was a strong association of the alanine allele with mild atopic asthma in a Japanese cohort, but this association was not confirmed in a British population. The functional significance of this polymorphism in the 3′ untranslated region is unclear. It may influence mRNA stability, but if a true linkage is ultimately confirmed, the more likely explanation is that this polymorphism is in linkage disequilibrium with unidentified variants in either the regulatory or coding regions of the Stat-6 gene or other adjacent genes. Finally, a polymorphism described in a noncoding region of the BCL-6 gene has also been associated with the prevalence of allergy (63).

Many of these studies suffer from weak associations with allergy and asthma, lack of confirmation in unrelated populations, and the presence of polymorphisms in regions of the gene that would not be predicted to have a biological effect. Ultimately, many of these associations may be shown to be specious. However, it remains plausible that some polymorphisms are in linkage disequilibrium with either unidentified variants in important regulatory or coding regions or with variants in adjacent genes. An important weakness of these studies is that they examine single nucleotide polymorphisms (SNPs) in isolation. Genes typically have multiple polymorphisms, and it is the inheritance of a specific combination of these SNPs (the haplotype) that produces the genetic effect. Linkage studies based on examination of these haplotypes correct for errors mediated by linkage disequilibrium. More important, haplotype analysis takes into consideration the possible interaction of SNPs that may either have opposing influences on gene expression and function or need to interact to produce their biological effects. This approach has been applied to examine variations in the IL-4Rα gene (47). Eight SNPs were grouped into 17 haplotypes of which only eight were common to the three ethnic groups examined. Each cohort displayed evidence of an association with allergy or asthma; however, the haplotypes showing the strongest association differed between ethnic groups. These data confirm that the IL-4Rα gene is a susceptibility locus for allergy and asthma but also indicate that additional variation outside the coding region of the gene has important influences on susceptibility.

V. Animal Studies Demonstrating the Role of IL-4 Inhibition in Asthma Therapy

Neutralizing IL-4 with anti-IL-4 antibodies in mice inhibits development of allergen-specific IgE (64), reduces eosinophilic inflammation (64), and decreases airway reactivity (65). These results have been confirmed using mice deficient in IL-4 (IL-4 knockout mice). In addition to these effects, IL-4 knockout mice and mice that lack Stat-6 are characterized by marked attenuation of the production of Th2 lymphocytes (66,67). By inhibiting Th2-type lymphocyte differentiation and promoting the apoptosis of established Th2-type cells, IL-4 blockade will likely inhibit the biological activities of IL-4 and, equally important, reduce the production of Th2 cytokines such as IL-5. Nonetheless, IL-4 knockout mice maintain residual Th2 responses, which may explain the persistent low level expression of IL-5, eosinophilia, and airway hyperreactivity observed in some murine studies (4). Although there is a risk of overinterpreting data derived from animal models, these observations establish the role of IL-4 in asthma and allergic disorders.

VI. Clinical Observations of IL-4 in Allergic Disease

Interleukin-4 levels are increased in the serum and bronchoalveolar lavage (BAL) of allergic individuals (68,69), and BAL studies demonstrate increased numbers of T cells expressing mRNA for IL-4 (70). Peripheral blood mononuclear cells from atopic asthmatic subjects generate augmented IL-4 production in response to dust mite antigen (71,72). Nebulized administration of exogenous IL-4 to patients with mild asthma resulted in a significant increase in airway hyperresponsiveness that was associated with an influx of sputum eosinophils (73). A variety of findings suggest that atopic individuals have altered regulation of their IL-4 production. For example, $CD4^+$ T-cell clones from atopic individuals produce IL-4 and IL-5 in response to bacterial antigens, whereas $CD4^+$ T-cell clones from nonatopic individuals produce Th1 cytokines (74). Atopic subjects have a higher number of IL-4-producing T cells than normal subjects (75), and T-cell clones generated from cord blood lymphocytes of newborns with atopic parents produce higher IL-4 concentrations than neonatal lymphocytes of newborns with nonatopic parents (76).

VII. Therapeutic Approaches to Neutralizing IL-4 in Asthma

Several approaches are available to develop a biological therapy that interferes with the activity of IL-4 in asthma and other allergic diseases (Table 2). Soluble IL-4 receptor (Immunex Corporation), humanized anti-IL-4 antibody (Protein Design Labs, Inc., and GlaxoSmithKline), and mutated IL-4 (IL-4 mutein; Bayer Pharmaceutical Corporation) (77) are currently in human clinical trials and are discussed in detail below. Human anti-IL-4 receptor antibody (Immunex Corporation) is in preclinical studies. These agents have theoretical differences and advantages (Table 2). Soluble IL-4 receptor is a recombinant human protein, and because it has the same sequence as the human receptor it has a low likelihood of being immunogenic. This is in contrast to the humanized antibodies, which generally retain 3–5% murine amino acids, and the IL-4 double mutant, which has the potential to be immunogenic.

Another approach to producing therapeutic antibodies is to clone the human antibody in SCID mice that have been reconstituted with a human immune system. Human monoclonal antibodies, such as those against the IL-4α chain, no longer retain any murine sequences and are therefore predicted to be nonimmunogenic. Either human monoclonal antibody against the IL-4 receptor α chain (see later, Figs. 3 and 6) or the IL-4 mutein (see Fig. 5) has the advantage of being able to interfere with binding of IL-4 and IL-13 to their receptors. The active form of the IL-13 receptor consists of a heterodimer of IL-4Rα and IL-13Rα1, and engagement of the binding domain of these receptors by either the IL-4 mutein or an antibody directed against the IL-4Rα chain will block their activation by IL-13. Mutated ligands may act as mixed agonists/antagonists and inhibit only specific activities of the parent compound. Depending on the completeness of

Table 2 Pharmacological Agents with Potential Interleukin-4 Inhibitory Activity

	Soluble human IL-4 receptor	IL-4 double mutein (R121D, Y124D)	Humanized anti-IL-4 antibody	Human anti-IL-4 receptor antibody	IL-4 transcription inhibitors (RASONs, SOCS-1)
Inhibition of IL-4	Yes	Yes	Yes	Yes	Selective
Inhibition of IL-13	Unlikely	Yes	No	Yes	Possibly
Potential immunogenicity	Low	Low–moderate	Low	Low	Unknown
Half-life	5 days	4–6 h	18–21 days	—	—
Route of administration	Inhaled	Injection	Injection	—	—

the IL-4 inhibition mediated by the IL-4 mutein and the spectrum of activities inhibited, this could provide theoretical advantages or disadvantages. Another future theoretical approach to IL-4 blockade may be to inhibit IL-4 gene transcription with respirable antisense oligonucleotides (RASONs). Agents that interfere with IL-4 intracellular signaling, such as Stat-6 antagonists or IRS-1/IRS-2 antagonists, could also be developed and would block only selected biological activities of IL-4. Stat-6 is essential for IL-4- and IL-13-mediated induction of Th2 lymphocyte differentiation, IgE isotype switch, low-affinity IgE receptor (CD23) receptor expression, VCAM-1 induction, and mucin secretion. In contrast, antagonism of IRS-1 and -2 would modulate IL-4 influences on T- and B-cell proliferation and apoptosis. Members of a family of proteins termed the suppressors of cytokine signaling (SOCS) are naturally occurring inhibitors of Stat-6 (27). SOCS-1 can bind and inhibit the kinase activity of all four JAK family members. Overexpression of SOCS-1 inhibits IL-4 signaling, including the phosphorylation of JAK1 and Stat-6. Although these theoretical approaches offer the possibility of blockade of selective components of the biological activities of IL-4, the use of these signaling molecules tends to be degenerate, and their involvement in other pathways may limit their usefulness.

The route of administration is an additional difference among these various agents. Previously, large proteins could be administered only parenterally via injection. However, the technology now exists to deliver proteins via inhalation. It may also be plausible in the future to deliver smaller protein antagonists by mouth. Current trials of these agents vary in their routes of administration, including one inhaled preparation (soluble human IL-4 receptor) and several agents being developed in injectable formats (humanized anti-IL-4, IL-4 mutein, and human anti-IL-4 receptor). Depending on the degree of systemic absorption from the lung (or, alternatively, from the circulation to the airway), these delivery approaches may influence the biological effects of the agents. Thus, a topical agent may have more prominent influences on adhesion molecule expression, vascular permeability, apoptosis of airway epithelial cells, and other local inflammatory parameters, whereas a systemic agent could have broader influences on allergen-specific T-helper lymphocyte immune deviation. Inhaled and oral routes will have the advantage of increased patient acceptance and compliance compared to injected routes of administration.

A. Soluble Recombinant Human Interleukin-4 Receptor

The IL-4 receptor is a heterodimer consisting of a specific high affinity α chain that binds to IL-4 and a second chain that can either be the common gamma chain shared with multiple cytokine receptors or the IL-13 receptor α1 chain (Fig. 2) (22,25). Both chains mediate cellular activation, but only α-chain receptors are required for ligand interaction. Secreted forms of IL-4Rα occur naturally and are expressed in allergic inflammation (78). Soluble IL-4R is capable of interacting with IL-4 even though it lacks the transmembrane and cytoplasmic domains. Because soluble IL-4R does not induce cellular activation but instead binds and sequesters IL-4, it serves as an anti-inflammatory mechanism that can counter the effects of IL-4 and may represent an endogenous autoregulatory or homeostatic mechanism. Ability to act as a decoy to bind and neutralize circulating cytokine coupled with the high specificity and high affinity of binding for the cytokine makes the soluble receptor promising as a cytokine antagonist. Soluble recombinant human interleukin-4 receptor (IL-4R) (Fig. 3) (Immunex Corporation) is the extracellular portion of the alpha chain of the human receptor for IL-4 that has been cloned and produced in a mammalian expression system. Another soluble receptor, the soluble TNF receptor Enbrel (Immunex Corporation), has been dem-

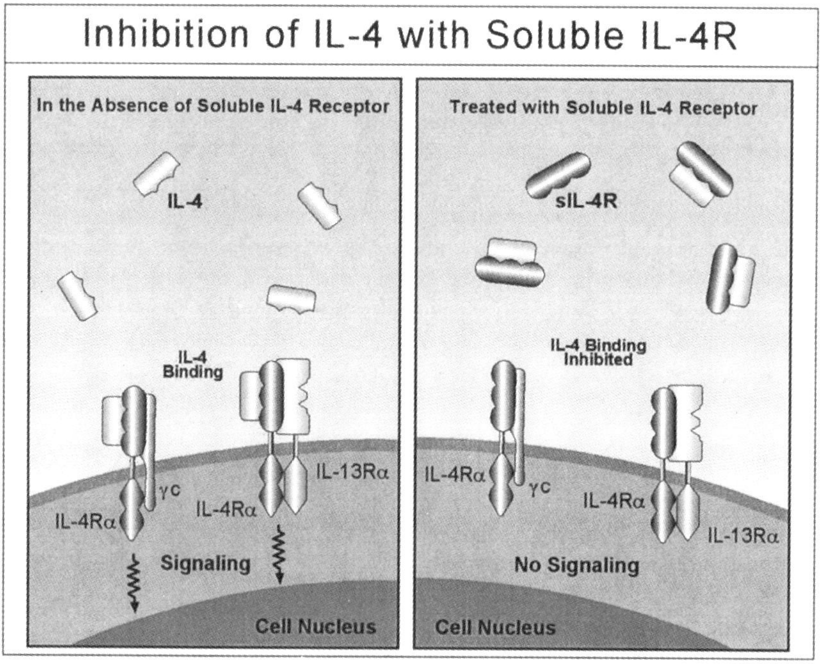

Figure 3 Soluble IL-4 receptor represents the extracellular region of the IL-4 receptor α chain. It retains the ability to bind IL-4 with high affinity and high specificity. Because it does not induce cellular activation but instead binds and sequesters IL-4, soluble IL-4R serves as an anti-inflammatory mechanism that may counter the effects of IL-4 in asthma.

onstrated to be safe and highly effective for long-term treatment of rheumatoid arthritis in adults and children.

Preclinical Studies

Recombinant murine soluble IL-4 receptor, which acts as a decoy for IL-4 binding and neutralizes IL-4 activity, has been shown in murine ovalbumin models to block total and allergen-specific IgE production, eosinophilia, and airway hyperreactivity (66) and to inhibit VCAM-1 expression, eosinophil influx, and excessive mucus production (67).

Clinical Studies with IL-4R

The promising data in preclinical studies led to preliminary investigations in which IL-4R proved safe and effective in the treatment of patients with asthma (79,80). In a phase 1 study, subjects with mild or moderate persistent asthma were withdrawn from inhaled corticosteroids and randomly assigned to receive placebo or IL-4R at 0.5 mg or 1.5 mg by nebulizer (79). There were no significant adverse events related to the study drug, and no patients developed antibodies to IL-4R. Pharmacokinetic analysis demonstrated systemic delivery and a serum half-life of approximately 5 days, making once weekly therapy feasible. Following sudden discontinuation of inhaled corticosteroids, no subject in the IL-4R 1.5 mg group withdrew for asthma exacerbations, compared with three of eight in the IL-4R 0.5 mg group and two of eight in the placebo group. Treatment with 1.5 mg IL-4R was associated with significantly better FEV_1 2 h after treatment and on days 2, 4, and 15 ($p < 0.05$). Statistically significant differences in asthma symptom score ($p < 0.05$) and β_2-agonist use ($p < 0.05$) were associated with IL-4R treatment. Scores on the third section of the AQLQ (patient's perception of general health and physical functioning) worsened in the placebo group and improved in the IL-4R 1.5 mg group ($p < 0.05$). Methacholine testing showed decreased sensitivity in six out of eight patients in the 1.5 mg group. Exhaled nitric oxide scores were significantly improved among patients receiving IL-4R ($p < 0.05$), consistent with an anti-inflammatory effect.

In the phase 1/2 double blind, placebo-controlled study of IL-4R, 62 patients with moderate persistent asthma were randomized to 12 weekly nebulizations of 0.75, 1.5, or 3.0 mg of IL-4R or placebo (80). Prestudy, patients documented dependence on inhaled corticosteroids by an exacerbation in asthma induced by stepwise 50% reductions in inhaled corticosteroid dose at 2-week intervals. After being restabilized on inhaled corticosteroids for 2 weeks, patients discontinued inhaled corticosteroids and began study medication. IL-4R was safe and well tolerated. Antibodies to IL-4R occurred in one patient, but they did not have neutralizing activity and produced no symptoms. In the absence of inhaled

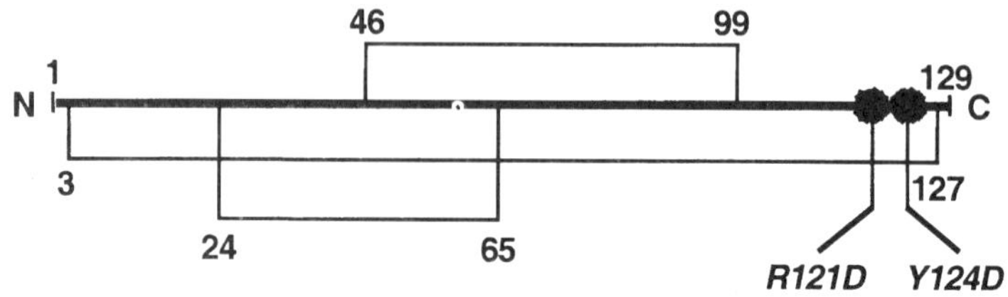

Figure 4 Primary structure of the IL-4 mutein IL4-R121D/Y124D, BAY 16-9996.

corticosteroids, patients receiving IL-4R had a stable FEV_1 (−0.09 L, −2% predicted) compared to the significant decline observed in the placebo group (−0.35 L, −13% predicted; $p = 0.05$ over the 3-month treatment period). Efficacy was demonstrated by a nearly stable daily morning FEV_1 measured at home by handheld device (−0.1 L, −4% predicted) compared to the significant decline in the placebo group (−0.5 L, −18% predicted; $p = 0.02$ over the 3-month treatment period). The evening FEV_1 also improved significantly at the highest dose and was 19% better than placebo. The efficacy of IL-4R was further confirmed by the absence of increase in asthma symptom score (Δ 0.1) in the 3.0 mg treatment group compared to the placebo group (Δ 1.4 over 1 month; $p = 0.075$).

More recently, two studies in asthma patients receiving only β-agonists evaluated soluble IL-4 receptor with weekly or daily doses by nebulizer and did not demonstrate clinical efficacy. In these two studies, the patient population or the drug regimen evaluated may not have been optimal to demonstrate the clinical effects of IL-4 inhibition. An ongoing phase 2 study is evaluating patients receiving inhaled corticosteroids for clinical efficacy of inhaled IL-4R.

B. Interleukin-4 Mutein

InterPenkin-4 (BAY 16-9996) is a competitive IL-4 and IL-13 receptor antagonist under development for the treatment of asthma (Bayer Pharmaceutical Corporation). It is expressed in *E. coli* K12, as a 15 kDa double mutant (mutein) in which arginine 121 and tyrosine 124 are both replaced by aspartic acid residues. The primary structure of BAY 16-9996 is presented in Figure 4 and the tertiary structure in Figure 5. The molecule retains high affinity binding to the IL-4Rα chain, which is a component of both the IL-4 and IL-13 receptors. However, BAY 16-9996 has no discernible agonist activity. The molecule is a full antagonist for all analyzed cellular responses, including IL-13-dependent B-cell responses (Refs. 81 and 82 and data on file, Bayer Pharmaceutical Corporation). Some of the

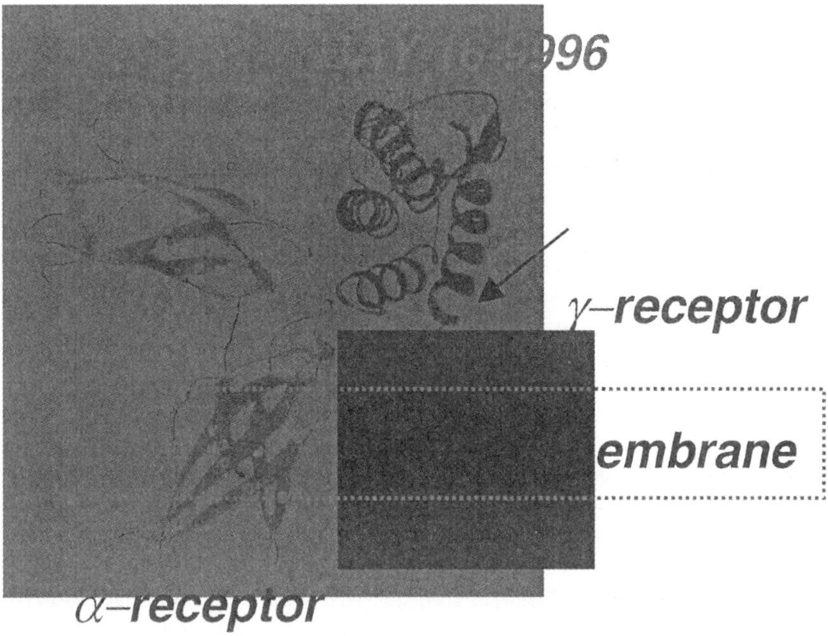

Figure 5 Tertiary structure of BAY 16-9996 and proposed holocomplex of BAY 16-9996 with the α and γ(c) chains of the IL-4 receptor. The secondary structure of BAY 16-9996 (red) is almost identical to that of IL-4. BAY 16-9996 is mostly α-helical (spirals) with very little β-folded structure (broad arrows). The black arrow indicates the position of the two amino acid replacements (R121D and Y124D) within the D helix of the C terminus of BAY 16-9996. These replacements lead to a surface charge mismatch that inhibits the receptor γc chain (blue) from binding to the BAY 16-9996/receptor α-chain complex. The structure of the receptor γc chain (blue) has not yet been fully elucidated.

biological activities of IL-4 are shared by IL-13, and both IL-4 and IL-13 antagonism may be required for optimal inhibition of the disease process in asthma.

Preclinical Studies

Repeated administration of BAY 16-9996 to cynomolgus monkeys prevented the induction of antigen-induced airway hyperresponsiveness and airway inflammation. Bay 16-9996 had an ED_{50} of approximately 0.1 mg/kg^{-1} day^{-1}. Repeated administration of BAY 16-9996 was subsequently shown to substantially reverse established antigen-induced airway hyperresponsiveness by 79% and decrease BAL eosinophil count (83). Administration of BAY 16-9996 prior to antigen challenge on days 3, 5, and 7 provided significant (97%) protection against antigen-induced airway hyperresponsiveness on day 10. This benefit was still evident on days 17 and 24 (59% and 62%, respectively; p = N.S.). Airway eosinophilia was also significantly reduced at day 10, but this effect was lost by day 17 (84,85). Long-term administration of BAY 16-9996 reduced cutaneous wheal-and-flare response and circulating levels of antigen-specific IgE. Loss of effect of BAY 16-9996 was temporally associated with the appearance of a blocking factor (possibly monkey anti-human antibody) in the plasma of treated animals (data on file, Bayer Pharmaceutical Corporation).

Clinical Experience with IL-4 Mutein

BAY 16-9996 phase 1 clinical trials are being completed. Two clinical studies enrolled a total of 116 adult patients with stable mild to moderate allergic asthma. Stable use of low-dose inhaled corticosteroids and monitored β agonist were permitted; other asthma therapies were excluded. An initial dose-ranging (0.07–20 mg) study investigated single subcutaneous injections of BAY 16-9996. A second study investigated multiple doses of BAY 16-9996 in patients over an extended period (20 mg SC every other day for three doses followed by weekly injections for 3 weeks). Initial data from the two studies indicate that BAY 16-9996 is safe and well tolerated at single and multiple doses. Based upon the safety and preclinical efficacy profile of BAY 16-9996, additional testing of this novel asthma therapy is in progress.

C. Humanized Antibodies (SB 240683 Anti-IL-4 Monoclonal Antibody)

SB 240683 is a humanized anti-IL-4 monoclonal (IgG_1) antibody that is being developed for the treatment of asthma (Protein Design Labs, Inc., GlaxoSmith Kline). SB 240683 targets human IL-4, thus blocking interaction of IL-4 with its receptor and inhibiting early-phase events of chronic asthma. As a humanized monoclonal antibody, SB 240683 is expected to have high binding affinity, low immunogenicity, and a long half-life; thus, dosing requirements may be infrequent.

SB 240683 was constructed using conventional molecular techniques to graft the complementarity-determining regions (CDRs) from the parent murine antibody, 3B9, into human heavy- and light-chain frameworks. SB 240683 and 3B9 are highly specific for a conformational epitope on human IL-4 and do not recognize bovine or murine IL-4. In pharmacological studies, SB 240683 has been shown to bind to human IL-4 with a high affinity (K_d = 45 pM at 25°C with an off rate of $2 \times 10^{-4} s^{-1}$).

Biological activity of the anti-IL-4 antibody has been demonstrated in laboratory studies. IL-5 synthesis by human peripheral blood mononuclear cells (PBMCs) stimulated with a recall antigen (tetanus toxoid) is significantly increased in the presence of exogenous recombinant human IL-4. In this model, antigen-driven, IL-4-dependent IL-5 synthesis is inhibited by mAb 3B9 (IC_{50} = 730 pM), providing evidence that antibody neutralization of IL-4 can downregulate Th2 cell cytokine production (GlaxoSmithKline, data on file).

Preclinical Studies

Inhibition of IgE production by the 3B9 mouse monoclonal antibody was examined in a SCID mouse model. Reconstitution of SCID mice with PMBCs from atopic donors, followed by daily injections of human IL-4, resulted in a significant increase in serum IgE levels. Treatment of mice with mAb 3B9 at the time of reconstitution inhibited IgE production in a dose-dependent manner without affecting serum IgG levels (GlaxoSmithKline; data on file).

Clinical Experience with SB 240683

A phase 1 randomized, double-blind, placebo-controlled dose-escalation study was conducted to determine the safety and pharmacokinetics of single-dose intravenous administration of SB 240683 in adult patients with asthma (86). Twenty-four asthmatic patients age 19–45 years (mean $\pm$ std dev, 30.3 $\pm$ 8.6 years) with mild to moderate asthma were administered a single intravenous dose of SB 240683 at one of four dose levels (0.5, 1.5, 4.5, or 10 mg/kg) or a single intravenous dose of placebo. In each dose cohort, five patients were randomized to active drug and one patient was randomized to placebo infusion. Patients were followed for 55 days after infusion. SB 240683 was safe and well tolerated with no dose-limiting adverse events. The elimination half-life ($T_{1/2}$) was 18–21 days. There were no neutralizing antibodies against SB 240683 up to day 55 in all dose cohorts and no evidence of antibodies in the high dose group after 5 months of infusion. Additional studies continue to evaluate safety and preliminary activity of the antibody.

D. Human Anti-IL-4 Receptor Alpha Monoclonal Antibody

Because both the IL-4 and IL-13 receptors contain an IL-4Rα subunit, monoclonal antibody directed against IL-4Rα will inhibit signaling of both IL-4 and IL-13 (Fig. 6) (Immunex Corporation). Studies in a murine asthma model have demonstrated inhibition of eosinophil influx, airway hyperreactivity, and Th2 cytokine production in treated mice (87). Additional preclinical studies are being conducted.

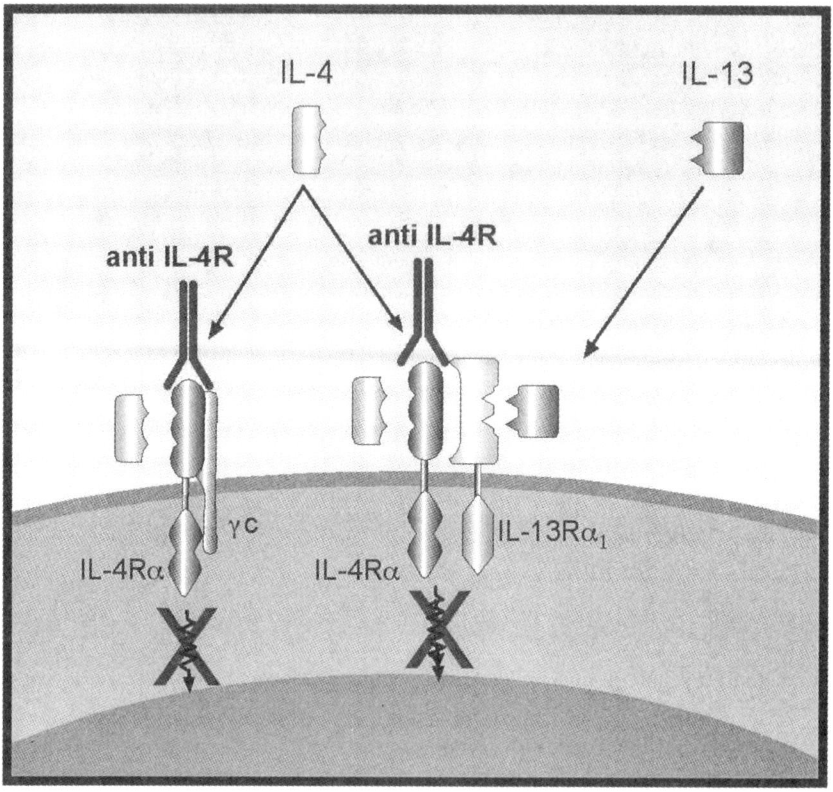

Figure 6 Antibody directed against the IL-4 receptor alpha chain will block signaling of both IL-4 and IL-13 through their receptors.

VIII. Theoretical Adverse Effects of IL-4 Inhibition

Inhibition of the biological activity of IL-4 offers obvious potential as a therapeutic approach to asthma and other allergic diseases. As a principle of immunomodulation, it is preferable to neutralize an existing biological mediator such as IL-4 rather than use a biological agent that may provide the desired immune deviation but may produce unacceptable side effects. Such active addition of a biological agent may directly mediate undesired activities or produce other unexpected downstream immune effects. For example, Th2 lymphocyte–derived IL-4 could in theory be reduced by agents designed to promote Th1-type lymphocyte differentiation, such as IFN-γ, IL-12, IL-18, or immunostimulatory DNA sequences (CpG vaccines). However, this approach ignores the established presence of Th1-type immune responses in asthma and the evidence that Th1-type lymphocytes also contribute to the presence and severity of asthma (88). Stimulation of a Th1 response does not necessarily block Th2 differentiation. Furthermore, anti-inflammatory cytokines such as IL-10 and TGF-β may be useful through their ability to inhibit Th2-type cells and IL-4 production; however, these cytokines have numerous untoward effects, including their activation of humoral immune responses, cytotoxic T cells, and fibrosis.

There remains a theoretical concern regarding the consequence to the immune system of inhibiting IL-4. IL-4 is thought to be important in the immune defense against parasitic diseases. However, IL-4-deficient mice do not demonstrate increased susceptibility to parasitic disease, possibly reflecting in part the IL-4-independent pathway for Th2 lymphocyte differentiation and non-Th2-dependent mechanisms for protection against parasites (89,90). Whether or not this will extend to humans is less important because asthma tends to be most prevalent in regions of the world where parasitic disease is not endemic. IL-4 is expressed in the placenta, where it is thought to contribute to maintaining the state of immune privilege. Normal reproduction in Stat-6-deficient mice suggests that this is not a significant issue. IL-4 knockout mice, IL-4R knockout mice, and transgenic IL-4R overexpressor mice had normal growth, lifespan, and reproduction without evidence of disease. IL-4 was originally cloned as a cofactor involved in B-cell proliferation and through its induction of Th2-type responses may be important in humoral immunity. IL-4-deficient mice do not demonstrate diminished humoral responses. In the clinical trials with soluble IL-4 receptor described previously, subjects immunized with tetanus booster during the study showed no inhibition of IgG response. Finally, there is a theoretical concern that IL-4 antagonism might promote an immune deviation from Th2-to Th1-type responses and that this could act to exacerbate autoimmune diseases such as rheumatoid arthritis, systemic lupus erythematosus, or multiple sclerosis (MS). In the murine model of MS, experimental allergic encephalitis, the use of an IL-4 antagonist did not augment the disease manifestations or worsen the outcome (data on file, Immunex Corporation).

IX. Conclusions

The understanding of the clinical value of IL-4 antagonism as a therapeutic modality in asthma has been enhanced through studies of new molecules. New approaches may provide potentially safe and effective treatments for asthma while minimizing the use of corticosteroids. Clinical trials will further clarify the target population of IL-4-based therapeutic agents for optimal inhibition of IL-4. The potential capacity for infrequent dosing of some IL-4 antagonists currently in development may improve patient compliance, which represents one of the greatest challenges to the effective treatment of asthma. By inhibiting inflammation at a key central regulatory point, IL-4 antagonism may impact long-term disease progression in asthma. These approaches should also be effective in patients with nonatopic forms of asthma. Although patients with nonatopic asthma do not demonstrate allergen-specific IgE, the presence of eosinophilic inflammation and elevated total IgE suggests the differentiation of Th2-type lymphocytes, which are responsible for the production of IL-5 and other cytokines that promote the development of eosinophilia. According to our current knowledge of the differentiation of IL-5-producing Th2-type lymphocytes, this process is IL-4-dependent and should be susceptible to suppression by IL-4-directed therapy. Other atopic disorders such as allergic rhinitis and atopic dermatitis are thought to be mediated by IL-4 also and represent areas for future investigation.

References

1. Hsieh CS, Heimberger AB, Gold JS, O'Garra A, Murphy KM. Differential regulation of T helper phenotype development by interleukins 4 and 10 in an alpha beta T-cell-receptor transgenic system. Proc Natl Acad Sci USA 1992; 89:6065–6069.
2. Seder RA, Paul WE, Davis MM, Fazekas de St. Groth B. The presence of interleukin 4 during in vitro priming determines the lymphokine-producing potential of CD4+ T cells from T cell receptor transgenic mice. J Exp Med 1992; 176:1091–1098.
3. Ohara J, Paul WE. Up-regulation of interleukin 4/B-cell stimulatory factor 1 receptor expression. Proc Natl Acad Sci USA 1988; 85:8221–8225.
4. Kopf M, Le Gros G, Bachmann M, Lamers MC, Bluethmann H, Kohler G. Disruption of the murine IL-4 gene blocks Th2 cytokine responses. Nature 1993; 362:245–248.
5. Jutel M, Pichler WJ, Skrbic D, Urwyler A, Dahinden C, Muller UR. Bee venom immunotherapy results in decrease of IL-4 and IL-5 and increase of IFN-gamma secretion in specific allergen-stimulated T cell cultures. J Immunol 1995; 154:4187–4194.
6. Coffman RL, Ohara J, Bond MW, Carty J, Zlotnik A, Paul WE. B cell stimulatory factor- 1 enhances the IgE response of lipopolysaccharide-activated B cells. J Immunol 1986; 136:4538–4541.
7. Pawankar R, Okuda M, Yssel H, Okumura K, Ra C. Nasal mast cells in perennial allergic rhinitis exhibit increased expression of the Fc epsilon RI, CD40L, IL-4, and IL-13, and can induce IgE synthesis in B cells. J Clin Invest 1997; 99:1492–1499.
8. Zaitsu M, Hamasaki Y, Matsuo M, Kukita A, Tsuji K, Miyazaki M, Hayasaki R, Muro E, Yamamoto S, Kobayashi I, Ichimaru T, Kohashi O, Miyazaki S. New induction of leukotriene A(4) hydrolase by interleukin-4 and interleukin- 13 in human polymorphonuclear leukocytes. Blood 2000; 96:601–609.
9. Hsieh FH, Lam BK, Penrose JF, Austen KF, Boyce JA. T helper cell type 2 cytokines coordinately regulate immunoglobulin E-dependent cysteinyl leukotriene production by human cord blood-derived mast cells: Profound induction of leukotriene C(4) synthase expression by interleukin 4. J Exp Med 2001; 193:123–133.

10. Rola-Pleszczynski M, Thivierge M, Stankova J. Upregulation of CysLT1 receptor expression by Th2 cytokine in human monocytes and macrophages. J Allergy Clin Immunol 2001; 107:S63.
11. Moser R, Fehr J, Bruijnzeel PL. IL-4 controls the selective endothelium-driven transmigration of eosinophils from allergic individuals. J Immunol 1992; 149:1432–1438.
12. Hoontrakoon R, Kailey J, Bratton D. IL-4 and TNF-alpha synergize to enhance eosinophil survival. J Allergy Clin Immunol 1999; 103:A239.
13. Vella A, Teague TK, Ihle J, Kappler J, Marrack P. Interleukin 4 (IL-4) or IL-7 prevents the death of resting T cells: Stat-6 is probably not required for the effect of IL-4. J Exp Med 1997; 186:325–330.
14. Xie H, Seward RJ, Huber BT. Cytokine rescue from glucocorticoid induced apoptosis in T cells is mediated through inhibition of IkappaBalpha. Mol Immunol 1997; 34:987–994.
15. Leung DYM, Hamid Q, Vottero A, Szefler SJ, Surs W, Minshall E, Chrousos GP, Klemm DJ. Association of glucocorticoid insensitivity with increased expression of glucocorticoid receptor beta. J Exp Med 1997; 186:1567–1574.
16. DeKruyff RH, Fang Y, Umetsu DT. Corticosteroids enhance the capacity of macrophages to induce Th2 cytokine synthesis in CD4+ lymphocytes by inhibiting IL-12 production. J Immunol 1998; 160:2231–2237.
17. Dabbagh K, Takeyama K, Lee HM, Ueki IF, Lausier JA, Nadel JA. IL-4 induces mucin gene expression and goblet cell metaplasia in vitro and in vivo. J Immunol 1999; 162:6233–6237.
18. Lordon J, Bucchieri F, Richter A, Holloway J, Beghe B, Konstantinidis A, Buchanan D, Wilson S, Djukanovic R, Holgate S, Davies D. The combined effects of Der p allergen and IL-4 or IL-13 on cytokine release by bronchial epithelial cell cultures of allergic asthmatics. J Allergy Clin Immunol 2001; 107:S63.
19. Doucet C, Brouty-Boye D, Pottin-Clemenceau C, Jasmin C, Canonica GW, Azzarone B. IL-4 and IL-13 specifically increase adhesion molecule and inflammatory cytokine expression in human lung fibroblasts. Int Immunol 1998; 10:1421–1433.
20. Chakir J, Page N, Barbeau B, Bergeron C. Interleukin-4, a Th2 cytokine, stimulates collagen 1 promoter activity in asthmatic bronchial fibroblasts. J Allergy Clin Immunol 2001; 107:S37.
21. Izuhara K, Shirakawa T. Signal transduction via the interleukin-4 receptor and its correlation with atopy. Int J Mol Med 1999; 3:3–10.
22. Jiang H, Harris MB, Rothman P. IL-4/IL-13 signaling beyond JAK/STAT. J Allergy Clin Immunol 2000; 105:1063–1070.
23. Leonard WJ, Lin JX. Cytokine receptor signaling pathways. J Allergy Clin Immunol 2000; 105:877–888.
24. Donaldson DD, Whitters MJ, Fitz LJ, Neben TY, Finnerty H, Henderson SL, O'Hara RM, Beier DR, Turner KJ, Wood CR, Collins M. The murine IL-13 receptor alpha 2: Molecular cloning, characterization, and comparison with murine IL-13 receptor alpha 1. J Immunol 1998; 161:2317–2324.
25. Nelms K, Keegan AD, Zamorano J, Ryan JJ, Paul WE. The IL-4 receptor: Signaling mechanisms and biologic functions. Annu Rev Immunol 1999; 17:701–738.
26. Jacobson NG, Szabo SJ, Weber-Nordt RM, Zhong Z, Schreiber RD, Darnell JE Jr,

Murphy KM. Interleukin 12 signaling in T helper type 1 (Th1) cells involves tyrosine phosphorylation of signal transducer and activator of transcription (Stat)3 and Stat4. J Exp Med 1995; 181:1755–1762.

27. Losman JA, Chen XP, Hilton D, Rothman P. Cutting edge: SOCS-1 is a potent inhibitor of IL-4 signal transduction. J Immunol 1999; 162:3770–3774.
28. Harris MB, Chang CC, Berton MT, Danial NN, Zhang J, Kuehner D, Ye BH, Kvatyuk M, Pandolfi PP, Cattoretti G, Dalla-Favera R, Rothman PB. Transcriptional repression of Stat6-dependent interleukin-4-induced genes by BCL-6: Specific regulation of iepsilon transcription and immunoglobulin E switching. Mol Cell Biol 1999; 19:7264–7275.
29. Borish L. Genetics of allergy and asthma. Ann Allergy Asthma Immunol 1999; 82: 413–424, 424–426.
30. Gao P-S, Mao X-Q, Hopkin JM, Adra CN, Yang X, Shirakawa T. Functional significance of polymorphisms of the interleukin-4 and interleukin-13 receptors in allergic disease. Clin Exp Allergy 2000; 30:1672–1675.
31. Marsh DG, Neely JD, Breazeale DR, Ghosh B, Freidhoff LR, Ehrlich-Kautzky E, Schou C, Krishnaswamy G, Beaty TH. Linkage analysis of IL4 and other chromosome 5q31.1 markers and total serum immunoglobulin E concentrations. Science 1994; 264:1152–1156.
32. Meyers DA, Postma DS, Panhuysen CI, Xu J, Amelung PJ, Levitt RC, Bleecker ER. Evidence for a locus regulating total serum IgE levels mapping to chromosome 5. Genomics 1994; 23:464–470.
33. Postma DS, Bleecker ER, Amelung PJ, Holroyd KJ, Xu J, Panhuysen CI, Meyers DA, Levitt RC. Genetic susceptibility to asthma: Bronchial hyperresponsiveness coinherited with a major gene for atopy. N Engl J Med 1995; 333:894–900.
34. Noguchi E, Shibasaki M, Arinami T, Takeda K, Maki T, Miyamoto T, Kawashima T, Kobayashi K, Hamaguchi H. Evidence for linkage between asthma/atopy in childhood and chromosome 5q31–q33 in a Japanese population. Am J Respir Crit Care Med 1997; 156:1390–1393.
35. Borish L, Mascali JJ, Klinnert M, Leppert M, Rosenwasser LJ. SSC polymorphisms in interleukin genes. Hum Mol Gen 1994; 3:1710.
36. Rosenwasser LJ, Klemm DJ, Dresback JK, Inamura H, Mascali JJ, Klinnert M, Borish L. Promoter polymorphisms in the chromosome 5 gene cluster in asthma and atopy. Clin Exp Allergy 1995; 25:74–78; discussion 95–96.
37. Walley AJ, Cookson WO. Investigation of an interleukin-4 promoter polymorphism for associations with asthma and atopy. J Med Genet 1996; 33:689–692.
38. Rosenwasser LJ, Borish L. Genetics of atopy and asthma: The rationale behind promoter-based candidate gene studies (IL-4 and IL-10). Am J Respir Crit Care Med 1997; 156:S152–S155.
39. Burchard EG, Silverman EK, Rosenwasser LJ, Borish L, Yandava C, Pillari A, Weiss ST, Hasday J, Lilly CM, Ford JG, Drazen JM. Association between a sequence variant in the IL-4 gene promoter and FEV_1 in asthma. Am J Respir Crit Care Med 1999; 160:919–922.
40. Boyer S, Pereira E, Plamer L, Rye J, Goldblatt J, Sanderson C, Le Souef PL. Confirmation of the presence of a polymorphism in the interleukin 4 promoter in an asthmatic cohort. Am J Respir Crit Care Med 1995; 151:A470.

41. Noguchi E, Shibasaki M, Arinami T, Takeda K, Yokouchi Y, Kawashima T, Yanagi H, Matsui A, Hamaguchi H. Association of asthma and the interleukin-4 promoter gene in Japanese. Clin Exp Allergy 1998; 28:449–453.
42. Dizier MH, Sandford A, Walley A, Philippi A, Cookson W, Demenais F. Indication of linkage of serum IgE levels to the interleukin-4 gene and exclusion of the contribution of the (−590 C to T) interleukin-4 promoter polymorphism to IgE variation. Genet Epidemiol 1999; 16:84–94.
43. Song Z, Casolaro V, Chen R, Georas SN, Monos D, Ono SJ. Polymorphic nucleotides within the human IL-4 promoter that mediate overexpression of the gene. J Immunol 1996; 156:424–429.
44. Daniels SE, Bhattacharrya S, James A, Leaves NI, Young A, Hill MR, Faux JA, Ryan GF, le Souef PN, Lathrop GM, Musk AW, Cookson WO. A genome-wide search for quantitative trait loci underlying asthma. Nature 1996; 383:247–250.
45. Deichmann KA, Heinzmann A, Forster J, Dischinger S, Mehl C, Brueggenolte E, Hildebrandt F, Moseler M, Kuehr J. Linkage and allelic association of atopy and markers flanking the IL4-receptor gene. Clin Exp Allergy 1998; 28:151–155.
46. Ober C, Cox NJ, Abney M, Di Rienzo A, Lander ES, Changyaleket B, Gidley H, Kurtz B, Lee J, Nance M, Pettersson A, Prescott J, Richardson A, Schlenker E, Summerhill E, Willadsen S, Parry R. Genome-wide search for asthma susceptibility loci in a founder population. The Collaborative Study on the Genetics of Asthma. Hum Mol Gen 1998; 7:1393–1398.
47. Ober C, Leavitt SA, Tsalenko A, Howard TD, Hoki DM, Daniel R, Newman DL, Wu X, Parry R, Lester LA, Solway J, Blumenthal M, King RA, Xu J, Meyers DA, Bleecker ER, Cox NJ. Variation in the interleukin 4-receptor alpha gene confers susceptibility to asthma and atopy in ethnically diverse populations. Am J Hum Genet 2000; 66:517–526.
48. Deichmann K, Bardutzky J, Forster J, Heinzmann A, Kuehr J. Common polymorphisms in the coding part of the IL4-receptor gene. Biochem Biophys Res Commun 1997; 231:696–697.
49. Hershey GKK, Friedrich MF, Esswein LA, Thomas ML, Chatila TA. The association of atopy with a gain-of-function mutation in the alpha subunit of the interleukin-4 receptor. N Engl J Med 1997; 337:1720–1725.
50. Mitsuyasu H, Izuhara K, Mao XQ, Gao PS, Arinobu Y, Enomoto T, Kawai M, Sasaki S, Dake Y, Hamasaki N, Shirakawa T, Hopkin JM. Ile50Val variant of IL4R alpha upregulates IgE synthesis and associates with atopic asthma [letter]. Nat Genet 1998; 19:119–120.
51. Mitsuyasu H, Yanagihara Y, Mao XQ, Gao PS, Arinobu Y, Ihara K, Takabayashi A, Hara T, Enomoto T, Sasaki S, Kawai M, Hamasaki N, Shirakawa T, Hopkin JM, Izuhara K. Cutting edge: Dominant effect of Ile50Val variant of the human IL-4 receptor alpha-chain in IgE synthesis. J Immunol 1999; 162:1227–1231.
52. Ryan JJ, McReynolds LJ, Keegan A, Wang LH, Garfein E, Rothman P, Nelms K, Paul WE. Growth and gene expression are predominantly controlled by distinct regions of the human IL-4 receptor. Immunity 1996; 4:123–132.
53. Wang HY, Paul WE, Keegan AD. IL-4 function can be transferred to the IL-2 receptor by tyrosine containing sequences found in the IL-4 receptor alpha chain. Immunity 1996; 4:113–121.

54. Ryan JJ, McReynolds LJ, Huang H, Nelms K, Paul WE. Characterization of a mobile Stat6 activation motif in the human IL-4 receptor. J Immunol 1998; 161:1811–1821.
55. Sandford AJ, Chagani T, Zhu S, Weir TD, Bai TR, Spinelli JJ, Fitzgerald JM, Behbehani NA, Tan WC, Pare PD. Polymorphisms in the IL4, IL4RA, and FCERIB genes and asthma severity. J Allergy Clin Immunol 2000; 106:135–140.
56. Noguchi E, Shibasaki M, Arinami T, Takeda K, Yokouchi Y, Kobayashi K, Imoto N, Nakahara S, Matsui A, Hamaguchi H. Lack of association of atopy/asthma and the interleukin-4 receptor alpha gene in Japanese. Clin Exp Allergy 1999; 29:228–233.
57. Wang HY, Shelburne CP, Zamorano J, Kelly AE, Ryan JJ, Keegan AD. Cutting edge: Effects of an allergy-associated mutation in the human IL-4R alpha (Q576R) on human IL-4-induced signal transduction. J Immunol 1999; 162:4385–4389.
58. Patuzzo C, Trabetti E, Malerba G, Martinati LC, Boner AL, Pescollderungg L, Zanoni G, Pignatti PF. No linkage or association of the IL-4R alpha gene Q576R mutation with atopic asthma in Italian families [letter]. J Med Genet 2000; 37:382–384.
59. Kruse S, Japha T, Tedner M, Sparholt SH, Forster J, Kuehr J, Deichmann KA. The polymorphisms S503P and Q576R in the interleukin-4 receptor alpha gene are associated with atopy and influence the signal transduction. Immunology 1999; 96:365–371.
60. Heinzmann A, Mao XQ, Akaiwa M, Kreomer RT, Gao PS, Ohshima K, Umeshita R, Abe Y, Braun S, Yamashita T, Roberts MH, Sugimoto R, Arima K, Arinobu Y, Yu B, Kruse S, Enomoto T, Dake Y, Kawai M, Shimazu S, Sasaki S, Adra CN, Kitaichi M, Inoue H, Yamauchi K, Tomichi N, Kurimoto F, Hamasaki N, Hopkin JM, Izuhara K, Shirakawa T, Deichmann KA. Genetic variants of IL-13 signalling and human asthma and atopy. Hum Mol Gen 2000; 9:549–559.
61. Shirakawa T, Li A, Dubowitz M, Dekker JW, Shaw AE, Faux JA, Ra C, Cookson WO, Hopkin JM. Association between atopy and variants of the beta subunit of the high-affinity immunoglobulin E receptor [see comments]. Nat Genet 1994; 7:125–129.
62. Gao PS, Mao XQ, Roberts MH, Arinobu Y, Akaiwa M, Enomoto T, Dake Y, Kawai M, Sasaki S, Hamasaki N, Izuhara K, Shirakawa T, Hopkin JM. Variants of STAT6 (signal transducer and activator of transcription 6) in atopic asthma [letter]. J Med Genet 2000; 37:380–382.
63. Adra CN, Gao PS, Mao XQ, Baron BW, Pauker S, Miki T, Shirakawa T, Hopkin JM. Variants of B cell lymphoma 6 (BCL6) and marked atopy [letter]. Clin Genet 1998; 54:362–364.
64. Coyle AJ, Le Gros G, Bertrand C, Tsuyuki S, Heusser CH, Kopf M, Anderson GP. Interleukin-4 is required for the induction of lung Th2 mucosal immunity. Am J Respir Cell Mol Biol 1995; 13:54–59.
65. Corry DB, Folkesson HG, Warnock ML, Erle DJ, Matthay MA, Wiener-Kronish JP, Locksley RM. Interleukin 4, but not interleukin 5 or eosinophils, is required in a murine model of acute airway hyperreactivity. J Exp Med 1996; 183:109–117.
66. Renz H, Bradley K, Enssle K, Loader JE, Larsen GL, Gelfand EW. Prevention of the development of immediate hypersensitivity and airway hyperresposiveness fol-

lowing in vivo treatment with soluble IL-4 receptor. Int Arch Allergy Immunol 1996; 109:167–176.
67. Henderson WR Jr, Chi EY, Maliszewski CR. Soluble IL-4 receptor inhibits airway inflammation following allergen challenge in a mouse model of asthma. J Immunol 2000; 164:1086–1095.
68. Walker C, Bauer W, Braun RK, Menz G, Braun P, Schwarz F, Hansel TT, Villiger B. Activated T cells and cytokines in bronchoalveolar lavages from patients with various lung diseases associated with eosinophilia. Am J Respir Crit Care Med 1994; 150:1038–1048.
69. Daher S, Santos LM, Sole D, De Lima MG, Naspitz CK, Musatti CC. Interleukin-4 and soluble CD23 serum levels in asthmatic atopic children. J Invest Allergol Clin Immunol 1995; 5:251–254.
70. Robinson DS, Hamid Q, Ying S, Tsicopoulos A, Barkans J, Bentley AM, Corrigan C, Durham SR, Kay AB. Predominant TH2-like bronchoalveolar T-lymphocyte population in atopic asthma. N Engl J Med 1992; 326:298–304.
71. Leonard C, Tormey V, Burke C, Poulter LW. Allergen-induced cytokine production in atopic disease and its relationship to disease severity. Am J Respir Crit Care Med 1997; 17:368–375.
72. Smart J, Horak E, Roberts M, Lanigan A, Kemp A. Melbourne study of childhood asthma: Allergen-specific cytokine responses according to clinical outcome at 42 years. J Allergy Clin Immunol 2001; 107:S64.
73. Shi HZ, Deng JM, Xu H, Nong ZX, Xiao CQ, Liu ZM, Qin SM, Jiang HX, Liu GN, Chen YQ. Effect of inhaled interleukin-4 on airway hyperreactivity in asthmatics. Am J Respir Crit Care Med 1998; 157:1818–1821.
74. Parronchi P, De Carli M, Manetti R, Simonelli C, Piccinni MP, Macchia D, Maggi E, Del Prete G, Ricci M, Romagnani S. Aberrant interleukin (IL)-4 and IL-5 production in vitro by CD4+ helper T cells from atopic subjects. Eur J Immunol 1992; 22:1615–1620.
75. Chan SC, Brown MA, Willcox TM, Li SH, Stevens SR, Tara D, Hanifin JM. Abnormal IL-4 gene expression by atopic dermatitis T lymphocytes is reflected in altered nuclear protein interactions with IL-4 transcriptional regulatory element. J Invest Dermatol 1996; 106:1131–1136.
76. Piccinni MP, Beloni L, Giannarini L, Livi C, Scarselli G, Romagnani S, Maggi E. Abnormal production of T helper 2 cytokines interleukin-4 and interleukin-5 by T cells from newborns with atopic parents. Eur J Immunol 1996; 26:2293–2298.
77. Grunewald SM, Werthmann A, Schnarr B, Klein CE, Brocker EB, Mohrs M, Brombacher F, Sebald W, Duschl A. An antagonistic IL-4 mutant prevents type I allergy in the mouse: Inhibition of the IL-4/IL-13 receptor system completely abrogates humoral immune response to allergen and development of allergic symptoms in vivo. J Immunol 1998; 160:4004–4009.
78. Benson M, Strannegard IL, Wennergren G, Strannegard O. Cytokines in nasal fluids from school children with seasonal allergic rhinitis. Pediatr Allergy Immunol 1997; 8:143–149.
79. Borish LC, Nelson HS, Lanz MJ, Claussen L, Whitmore JB, Agosti JM, Garrison L. Interleukin-4 receptor in moderate atopic asthma. A phase I/II randomized, placebo-controlled trial. Am J Respir Crit Care Med 1999; 160:1816–1823.

80. Borish L, Nelson H, Corren J, Bensch G, Busse W, Whitmore J, Agosti J. Efficacy of soluble interleukin-4 receptor for the treatment of adults with asthma. J Allergy Clin Immunol 2001; 107:963–970.
81. Snell N. Interleukin-4 as a therapeutic target in allergic disorders. Curr Opin Anti-Inflam Immunomod Invest Drug 2000; 2:99.
82. Shanafelt M, Harris P, Neyer L, Moy J, Barrientos J, Gundel R. Mechanism of action of an IL-4 receptor antagonist (BAY 16-9996) in the primate model of asthma. Am J Respir Crit Care Med 2000; 161:A201.
83. Harris P, Lindell D, Fitch N, Gundel R. The IL-4 receptor antagonist (BAY 16-9996) reverses airway hyperresponsiveness in a primate model of asthma. Am J Respir Crit Care Med 1999; 159:A230.
84. Fitch N, Harris P, Lindell D. Evaluation of a dual IL-4 and IL-13 receptor antagonist in a primate model of asthma. Submitted for publication.
85. Gundel R, Morton M, Bowden A, Fitch N, Shanafelt M, Shanafelt A, Wetzel G, Moy J, Gibbons J, Terrell T. Preclinical evaluation of BAY 16-9996 a dual IL-4/IL-13 receptor antagonist. Eur Respir J 2000; 16:564.
86. Shames R, Vexler V, Lane N, McClellan M, Shi J, Keller S, Young D, Nieman R, Hart T. The safety and pharmacokinetics of SSB240683 (anti-IL-4 humanized monoclonal antibody) in patients with mild to moderate asthma. J Allergy Clin Immunol 2001; 107:S317.
87. Tocker J, Raminfar L, Barone C. Effects of an antibody to IL-4R in a mouse asthma model. Am J Respir Crit Care Med 2001; 163:A523.
88. Hansen G, Berry G, DeKruyff RH, Umetsu DT. Allergen-specific Th1 cells fail to counterbalance Th2 cell-induced airway hyperreactivity but cause severe airway inflammation. J Clin Invest 1999; 103:175–183.
89. Finkelman FD, Shea-Donohue T, Goldhill J, Sullivan CA, Morris SC, Madden KB, Gause WC, Urban JF Jr. Cytokine regulation of host defense against parasitic gastrointestinal nematodes: Lessons from studies with rodent models. Annu Rev Immunol 1997; 15:505–533.
90. Urban JFJ, Noben-Trauth N, Donaldson D, Madden KB, Morris SC, Collins M, Finkelman FD. IL-13, IL-4R alpha and Stat6 are required for expulsion of the gastrointestinal nematode parasite Nippostrongylus brasiliensis. Immunity 1998; 8:255–264.
91. Baron BW, Billstrand C, Madronero L, McKeithan TW. HindIII polymorphism in the BCL6 gene. Hum Mol Gen 1993; 2:1513.

7

Immunobiology of Asthma

Biotherapeutic Management

FRANCIS M. CUSS

Schering-Plough Research Institute
Kenilworth, New Jersey

I. Introduction

Herbal remedies were the mainstays of asthma treatment before the beginning of the twentieth century, but with the birth of academic pharmacology and industrial chemistry, the active principles of many of these herbs were identified, characterized, and prescribed as medicines. Improvements in the potency, selectivity, pharmacokinetics, and delivery of medications such as beta-agonists, corticosteroids, and methyl xanthines during the twentieth century led to many of the asthma treatments widely used today. Over the last 25 years, there has been an enormous increase in our understanding of the pathological processes underlying asthma. Characterization of the interaction between host genetic factors and environmental stimuli and elucidation of subsequent events has led to identification of many novel drug targets and potential new therapies. The first class of drugs to come from these research efforts and reach the market are the leukotriene inhibitors. New theories of asthma pathogenesis, such as the concept that pulmonary inflammation underlies the signs and symptoms of asthma, have led to new treatment strategies (1).

One of the most influential hypotheses concerning the pathobiology of inflammation was proposed by Mosmann and Coffman, from the DNAX Research

Institute, in the mid-1980s (2). They hypothesized that $CD4^+$ T-helper cells differentiated into two distinct types, recognizable by their different patterns of lymphokine secretion and with distinct functional properties. They proposed that T-helper type 1 (Th1) cells produce predominantly interleukin-2 (IL-2) and interferon gamma (IFN-γ) and initiate mechanisms important in host defense to bacteria and viruses, whereas Th2 cells produce cytokines such as interleukins 4, 5, 9, 10, and 13 and are involved in allergic responses and parasitic infestation. Subsequent studies into the workings of the cytokine network have provided enormous opportunities for drug research in inflammation, and this chapter focuses on three Th2 cytokines, interleukins 5, 9, and 10, and how they may be involved in the asthmatic process.

II. Interleukin-5

A. Introduction

The association of worsening asthma, increased sputum cellularity, and eosin-staining material in sputum and lung tissues was noted in the late nineteenth century by von Leyden (3). He related his observations to Charcot's earlier description of long, thin crystalline rods in sputum, which subsequently became known as Charcot-Leyden crystals and later were recognized as products of activated eosinophils (4). Eosinophils, together with Charcot-Leyden crystals and other eosinophilic products (5), have long been recognized as prominent features of asthmatic sputum, becoming more numerous and degenerate as asthma worsens and improving with treatment. Studies in the late 1950s of tissue biopsies from patients who had died of asthma (6), and also those with chronic asthma (7), showed eosinophils and their products in the lung tissue. In the early 1980s, Gleich and colleagues at the Mayo Clinic rekindled interest in the eosinophil as an important effector cell in asthma by showing that eosinophil products, such as major basic protein (MBP), are cytotoxic in animals (8) and are closely associated with airway damage in biopsies from asthmatic patients (9). Concomitant with the resurgence of interest in the cytotoxic potential of eosinophils and their products in the pathogenesis of asthma, new insights developed into the immunoinflammatory mechanisms underlying asthma. The discovery that protein factors secreted by immune cells form a network controlling the growth, maturation, activation, and migration of inflammatory cells, including eosinophils, revolutionized our understanding of cellular inflammation in asthma.

Originally described as a T-cell replacement factor and as B-cell growth factor II (10), the cloned protein named interleukin-5 (IL-5) (11) was found to be identical to the protein factor that Warren and Sanderson (12) termed eosinophil differentiation factor. IL-5 is a cytokine comprehensively and selectively involved in eosinophilic development (12–16), and in humans, in comparison to mice, the B-cell effects of IL-5 are limited and eosinophil effects predominate (17). This makes IL-5 a potentially very attractive target for attenuating eosinophil inflammation in asthma. Although there are several different potential therapeutic approaches to the selective inhibition of IL-5, the most advanced and the one most likely to determine of the role of IL-5 and eosinophils in asthma is an anti-IL-5 monoclonal antibody (18–21).

B. Discovery and Characterization of IL-5

Murine IL-5 was cloned in 1986 and then used as a probe to isolate human IL-5 (hIL-5) from a human T-cell leukemic line (11,22). For IL-5, there is 77% homology between the mouse and human nucleotide sequences and 70% between the amino acid sequences. There is greater homology at the C terminal than at the N terminal, probably reflecting the presence of the active site in that region (23). IL-5 and other T-helper type 2 cytokines are clustered on chromosome 5q (24), suggesting a close evolutionary relationship. Positional cloning has shown this chromosomal region to have a significant linkage to asthmatic traits (25,26), and the cytokine IL-9 also has a significant linkage in this area (27). Although the IL-5 gene is not closely homologous to other cytokines, there are conserved sequences in its promoter region that are identical to sequences in the promoter region of the IL-3, IL-4, and GM-CSF genes (24,28), thereby implying coordinated control of the hematopoietic growth factors. IL-5 is a homodimer with variable reported molecular weights (45–60 kDa) that are a result of differential glycosylation (29), although glycosylation is not required for activity.

Three-dimensional modeling of IL-5 shows it to have a tertiary structure similar to that of GM-CSF, IL-3, and IL-4 (30). The IL-5 receptor, a type 1 cytokine family member (31), comprises two subunits (32). The α chain is unique to IL-5, whereas the β chain is shared with the GM-CSF and IL-3 receptors (32), again emphasizing the close evolutionary and functional relationship of these cytokines. IL-5 binds to the α chain with a K_D of about 1 nM (33) but signals only through the β subunit (32). The interaction of IL-5 and the high affinity receptor has a K_D of 250 nM (32), which marks the upper limit of the affinity for an effective neutralizing monoclonal antibody. The limited expression of the α chain of IL-5 restricts the functional effects of IL-5 to a small number of cell types (33). A soluble IL-5 receptor, without the transmembrane motif, has been shown to bind IL-5 and inhibit its function and may be part of a homeostatic control mechanism for eosinophil production (34).

Binding of IL-5 to the receptor complex leads to intracellular signaling through the JAK and STAT pathways (35,36). Binding of the beta chain activates JAK2, leading to tyrosine phosphorylation of STAT5, which translocates to the nucleus and binds to DNA, thereby modulating gene transcription (35,37). IL-5 is produced by several different cells including $CD4^+$ T cells (38), mast cells

(39), and eosinophils (40). IL-5 biosynthesis results from gene transcription (41) and can be blocked completely by corticosteroids (42) and partially by cyclosporin (43). In mice at least, it appears that T cells are the predominant source of IL-5 (44), because T-cell deletion results in reduced eosinophilia after challenge. In humans, $CD4^+$ cell lines raised from asthmatic BAL samples secrete more IL-5 than those derived from normal subjects (45).

In mice, IL-5 has prominent effects on B cells as well as eosinophils and basophils, whereas in humans the B-cell effects are absent (13,46,47). IL-5 has effects on eosinophil growth and maturation (14,15,47), migration (47–49), activation and degranulation (47,50,51), and survival (52). IL-3 and GM-CSF do not stimulate every stage of eosinophil development as IL-5 does and have growth effects on other hematopoietic cells such as neutrophils and mast cells (47). Corticosteroids antagonize IL-5-induced eosinophil survival and induce eosinophil apoptosis, and this may contribute to their antiasthmatic activity (53).

The cytotoxic effects of activated eosinophils are a result of the synthesis and release of mediators and preformed proteins such as peroxidases, proteinases, and cationic proteins unique to eosinophils (54–58). These low-molecular-weight cationic proteins include major basic protein (MBP), eosinophilic cationic protein (ECP), and eosinophilic derived neurotoxin (EDN) and are very cytotoxic (58). They are a good marker of eosinophilic inflammation and are seen in sputum (4,5) and associated with tissue damage (6–9) during asthma attacks and after death from asthma (6). Thus the comprehensive but selective effect of IL-5 on growth, maturation, and activation of eosinophils makes it an attractive drug target for the attenuation of eosinophilic inflammation.

C. Scientific Rationale for the Use of Inhibitors of IL-5 in Asthma

Administration of antigen to the lungs of sensitized animals or humans leads to airway inflammation and changes in airway caliber and responsiveness. It is a valuable means of confirming that drug effects observed in vitro are relevant in a more complex system in vivo and a useful model to analyze antigen-induced inflammation and its functional sequelae. Much of the scientific support for IL-5 as an important mediator of asthma comes from studies of pulmonary antigen challenge in animals with specific IL-5 inhibitors. However, because antigen challenge reflects only a subset of the features of human asthma, it may offer only limited predictive value in terms of drug efficacy in asthma.

There is considerable evidence of involvement of eosinophils and IL-5 in antigen-induced inflammation. Activated $CD4^+$ Th2 cells (59), eosinophils and their products, and VCAM (60), an integrin associated with eosinophil trafficking, are seen in the BAL after antigen challenge in humans (61–64), particularly in subjects exhibiting late antigen responses. Expression of IL-5 mRNA (65) and protein (66,67) are seen in the BAL, together with eosinophil products such as MBP (68), in patients with both early and late responses (60). Many of these features can be reproduced by direct administration of IL-5 into human airways. In atopic subjects, topical hIL-5 induces eosinophilia in bronchial biopsies and BAL samples (69), whereas in asthmatic subjects hIL-5 causes increases in airway responsiveness and sputum eosinophilia (70). In ''wild-type'' asthma, activated eosinophils and T-helper cells are seen in BAL and lung biopsies, and their numbers correlate with measures of airway responsiveness (71,72). Expression of IL-5 mRNA is increased in asthma compared to normal subjects (65,73), and its levels also correlate with the degree of symptomatic improvement and airway responsiveness (74). IL-5 protein measured in serum is higher in symptomatic patients than in asymptomatic patients (75) and when the asthma is severe (76). When an exacerbation improves, the concentration of IL-5 drops (76), and reduction in IL-5 is also associated with treatment with corticosteroids (77) and theophylline (78).

Antigen challenge in animals has been used extensively to explore the therapeutic effects of IL-5 inhibitors in allergic inflammation. In guinea pigs, antigen challenge induces eosinophilic infiltration and increases in airway responsiveness (79,80), which are blocked by an anti-IL-5 monoclonal antibody (80). Interestingly, the concentration of antibody needed to block airway responsiveness is considerably higher than that needed to block eosinophilia (80), suggesting a disassociation between inflammation and airway responsiveness in this animal model. It has been speculated that IL-5 may be modulating airway responsiveness in this system through a mechanism that is independent of eosinophils and their cytotoxic products (80,81). If sensitized airway smooth muscle from asthmatic subjects is treated with IL-5 in vitro, the contractile response to acetylcholine is significantly enhanced compared to untreated tissue (82). In this system, IL-5 administration leads to increased expression of IL-1β mRNA and protein, and the increased airway responsiveness can be inhibited by blocking the activity of IL-1. It is possible that following antigen challenge in guinea pigs, release of IL-5 leads to eosinophilic inflammation through chemotaxis of eosinophils but to airway responsiveness through direct effects on airway smooth muscle. When IL-5 is administered to the lungs of unsensitized guinea pigs, there is induction of an inflammatory response involving eosinophils and neutrophils but no increase in bronchial responsiveness (81). The differential effects of anti-IL-5 monoclonal antibodies in guinea pig studies may reflect differences in sensitivity of these mechanisms to IL-5 inhibition.

Mice are useful in characterizing cytokine biology, because their immune system is extremely well characterized, murine reagents are readily available, and breeding of genetically manipulated mice is relatively easy and fast. As with guinea pigs, antigen challenge in sensitized mice leads to eosinophilic inflammation in the lungs (83–85) and increase in airway responsiveness (84,85), and these are inhibited by pretreatment with IL-5 monoclonal antibodies (84–88) but not antibodies to IgE (88).

Expression of mRNA for IL-4 and IL-5 is increased in the lungs of these mice (89), and although T cells appear to be the dominant source of IL-5 following long-term antigen administration (90), mast cells appear to be an important source of IL-5 after a single challenge (91). Mice with overexpression of IL-5 in the lung show exuberant lung eosinophilia and increases in airway responsiveness even in the absence of antigen challenge (92). Mice in whom the IL-5 gene has been "knocked out" (IL-5$^{-/-}$ mice) have reduced circulating eosinophils, normal IgE (93), and normal B- and T-cell responses (94). Pulmonary antigen challenge in sensitized IL-5$^{-/-}$ mice has no effect compared to wild-type animals, which show the usual increases in eosinophilia and airway responsiveness (93). When IL-5 is reconstituted with delivery via an adenoviral vector to the lungs of IL-5$^{-/-}$ mice, antigen-induced pulmonary responses return (93). In some studies of IL-5 inhibitors in murine allergic inflammation, eosinophilic inflammation and airway responsiveness appear uncoupled from one another. For instance, despite blockade of antigen-induced eosinophilia by an anti-IL-5 monoclonal antibody, antigen-induced airway responsiveness is unchanged compared to vehicle-treated mice (95,96). It is not clear why these studies differ from studies where IL-5 monoclonal antibodies blocks both inflammation and airway responsiveness. It is possible that technical differences in the conduct of the study or in mouse strains may contribute to the different results or, as seen in a guinea pig study, increased concentrations of anti-IL-5 monoclonal antibody may be required (80). Hogan et al. (97), using combinations of different knockout mice and cytokine-neutralizing antibodies, suggest that airway inflammation and lung damage are linked to the expression of IL-5 and eosinophilic infiltration, and that airway responsiveness requires the presence of CD4^{+} T cells but not IL-5 and eosinophils. Tournoy et al. (98) also showed that increased airway responsiveness after antigen challenge does not require eosinophilic inflammation. Administration of anti-IL-5 monoclonal antibodies before antigen challenge prevents the release of eosinophils from the bone marrow and migration through the blood stream to the lungs (86). Because IL-5 enhances the survival of eosinophils in vitro (99), removal of IL-5 from the system could theoretically lead to necrosis of eosinophils in the lung and release of cytotoxic proteins. However, when an IL-5 monoclonal antibody is administered during an ongoing allergic response, there is no evidence of worsening inflammation (86).

Interleukin-5-deficient mice have also been used to study the host response to parasitic infestation. The worm burden is no different in *Mesocestoides corti* infection (94) or schistosomiasis (100,101), but the number and fertility of worms is increased in *Strongyloides ratti* infections (102). Interestingly, the lung damage and eosinophilic inflammation associated with *Toxocara canis* infection in wild-type mice is reduced in the IL-5$^{-/-}$ mice, suggesting that the toxocara-induced eosinophilic response is a detrimental host response. There does not appear to be any increased duration of infestation or reduction in response to a second infection in these IL-5-deficient mice compared to the wild-type animals. Even though infestation of mice with human helminthic parasites may not fully represent the natural history of human parasitosis, it is reassuring that the reduction in IL-5 production and tissue eosinophilia seen in IL-5$^{-/-}$ mice is not associated with dramatic deterioration of host defenses.

Sensitized monkeys respond to administration of antigen similarly to rodents and humans, with eosinophilic inflammation, early and late pulmonary responses, and increased airway hyperresponsiveness (103,104). Treatment with an anti-mIL-5 monoclonal antibody (TRFK5) blocks airway inflammation and increases in airway responsiveness (103), and this inhibition lasts for 3 months after a single dose (103). SCH 55700, a humanized anti-hIL-5 monoclonal antibody, blocks antigen-induced pulmonary eosinophilia in cynomolgus monkeys for up to 6 months, although airway responsiveness was not measured in this study (105). SB240563, another humanized anti-hIL-5 monoclonal antibody, has a half-life of 13 days in monkeys and shows an 81–96% reduction in baseline eosinophil count after subcutaneous dosing (106). Interestingly, the maximal effect observed on circulatory eosinophils is at 3 weeks, and the maximal concentration of monoclonal antibody is seen at about 2 days (106). Administration of multiple doses of rhIL-2 to cynomolgus monkeys causes a large increase in blood eosinophilia, mediated by IL-5, in control animals, whereas pretreatment with SB240563 causes a prolonged inhibition of eosinophilia (107).

There is strong circumstantial evidence that eosinophils cause significant damage in human asthma and that IL-5 is a key mediator in their control. Animal studies show that IL-5 inhibition prevents many of the asthma-like sequelae of antigen-induced pulmonary inflammation. Careful analysis of the numerous antigen challenge animal studies suggests that just blocking eosinophilic inflammation may be insufficient to prevent airway responsiveness in these acute models. Other evidence suggests that IL-5 may have direct effects on smooth muscle, thereby inducing airway responsiveness. The definitive proof of concept awaits the results of IL-5 inhibition in patients with wild-type asthma.

D. Effect of IL-5 Inhibitors in Clinical Studies

Two different anti-IL-5 monoclonal antibodies, SCH 55700 (reslizumab) (20) and SB240563 (mepolizumab) (21), are being studied in the clinic. Reslizumab is a humanized monoclonal antibody with an affinity of 81 pM, which is significantly higher than the affinity of IL-5 for its receptor (32), and with neutralizing activity against IL-5-induced cell proliferation. Reslizumab has prolonged anti-IL-5 activity in a number of species including mice, guinea pigs, and monkeys

(105). Even after prednisolone administration, reslizumab shows additive inhibition of antigenic responses in allergic mice (105). It shows a dose-related prolongation of inhibition of pulmonary eosinophilia up to 8 weeks in challenged mice (10 mg/kg) and 6 months in monkeys (0.3 mg/kg) (105). Mepolizumab is effective in a monkey model of eosinophilia (107) and induces a prolonged reduction in circulating eosinophils reflecting the 13 day half-life of the antibody (106,107).

The first study of SB240563 in humans was recently reported (21). The safety of a single dose (either 2.5 or 10 mg/kg) of SB240563 in eight patients per group with mild asthma was compared to a placebo injection over a 16-week period. Additionally, the effects of SB240563 on the sequelae of inhaled antigen challenge at 1 and 4 weeks were also characterized. A significant reduction in circulating eosinophils and sputum eosinophilia was recorded, but no changes in the early or late pulmonary responses or bronchial responsiveness were seen with SB240563. SB240563 was well tolerated. The first study of SCH 55700 was conducted in 32 patients with symptomatic, severe persistent asthma treated with high-dose inhaled or oral corticosteroids (20). A single dose of SCH 55700 or placebo was administered intravenously to asthmatic patients who were followed for 90 days. Circulating eosinophils were reduced by 80–90% within 24–48 h, and the duration of attenuation was dose-related and correlated with plasma concentrations. At the highest dose (1 mg/kg), the circulating eosinophil levels were still below baseline at the 90-day time point. FEV_1 was improved in all groups at 30 days, and there was a trend toward greater improvement in the two highest doses compared to placebo (0.3 and 1 mg/kg), although the differences in FEV_1 (4%, 11.2%, and 8.6% in the placebo, 0.3 mg/kg, and 1 mg/kg groups, respectively) between treatments did not reach statistical significance. SCH 55700 persisted for a prolonged period in the circulation and was well tolerated (20).

Despite different designs and patient populations, these studies show that single doses of anti-IL-5 monoclonal antibodies are well tolerated and have biological activity against IL-5. They significantly reduce, but do not abolish, circulating eosinophils for prolonged periods in a dose-dependent manner but do not show what would be considered clinically significant functional effects. This may be because IL-5 and eosinophils are actually not important in clinical asthma, or it may just reflect technological limitations in these small early-phase studies. Definitive proof of the activity of IL-5 inhibitors awaits larger scale studies.

E. Strategies for Inhibition of IL-5

The scientific rationale for the use of IL-5 inhibitors in asthma is strong, and the processes involved in the production, release, circulation, and action of IL-5 offer several potential targets for inhibition. Corticosteroids (42) and cyclosporin (41,43) are able to block IL-5 synthesis with a reasonable degree of selectivity, so it should be possible to identify potent, selective small-molecule biosynthesis inhibitors (108). When IL-5 is released into the circulation, it is possible to neutralize its effects with a monoclonal antibody (19) or a soluble alpha-chain receptor (109). Antagonizing the IL-5 receptor complex with small molecules has proven difficult, although peptide antagonists without homology to IL-5 have been identified (110). Blocking the synthesis of the IL-5R alpha chain should also reduce the effect of IL-5 on eosinophils, and this has been shown to work by the use of antisense oligonucleotides (111). The JAK-STAT pathway, which is activated by IL-5 binding to its receptor complex, is another potential site for IL-5 inhibitors. Because it has been possible to identify selective inhibitors of kinases involved in cell signaling in cancer cells, and they are presently undergoing clinical trials (112), this approach may also be possible in other cells such as eosinophils. Monoclonal antibodies are the first IL-5 inhibitors to enter clinical testing, and therefore the value of IL-5 inhibition in asthma and the practicality and safety of long-term administration of an anti-IL-5 monoclonal antibody in asthma will likely be determined in the near future.

III. Interleukin-9

A. Introduction

Interleukin-9 (IL-9) is one of several Th2 cytokines discovered in the last 15 years that may play a role in the pathogenesis of asthma. Suggestions that IL-9 might be a susceptibility gene in asthma generated considerable interest in its biology. IL-9 appears to be involved in mast cell and IgE biology and may be an attractive target in atopic asthma.

B. Discovery and Characterization of IL-9

Interleukin-9 was first identified as a factor derived from murine T-helper cells, with antigen-independent effects on $CD4^+$ T cells (113) by researchers from the Ludwig Institute. Subsequently shown to be identical to an antigen-dependent T cell (114) and a mast cell growth factor (115), the human cDNA was cloned by cross-hybridization with the mouse homolog (116). There is 69% homology between the mouse and human genes at the nucleotide level and 55% at the protein level (117). IL-9 maps to mouse chromosome 13 and human chromosome 5 (118). The IL-9 receptor is a member of the hematopoietin receptor superfamily, and there is 53% homology between the mouse and human receptors (119,120). A number of splice variants of the IL-9R have been identified from mRNAs that lack the membrane and intracellular portions of the molecule, but it is not clear if these represent circulating soluble receptors (119,121). IL-9 binds to the IL-2 receptor gamma chain, which is shared with several other cytokine receptors, and to its own IL-9 receptor chain (122). IL-9 shares several functions with these other cytokines but also has unique effects suggesting both redundant and highly controlled cellular signaling (123). JAK1 is associated with IL-9R and JAK2 with IL-2Rγ (122,124), thereby activating STAT1, STAT3, and STAT5 (125).

Interleukin-9 is a pleotrophic cytokine with a number of effects on different cell types (123), but reports of a significant genetic linkage between the cytokine cluster region on chromosome 5q, where the IL-9 gene resides, and airway responsiveness (25,26) focused interest on IL-9 as a potential target for the treatment of asthma. Studying IL-9 as a candidate asthma gene, Doull et al. (27) showed a significant association between the IL-9 locus and total IgE in a randomly acquired population. In a study in mice, linkage was also noted between the murine homolog of the human 5q region, containing the murine IL-9 gene, and airway responsiveness in different strains of mice (126), suggesting a causal role for IL-9 in the murine system.

Originally identified as a lymphokine produced by activated Th2 cells (113), both in vitro and in vivo, it is now clear that a significant amount of IL-9 is also produced by mast cells (127,128) and human eosinophils (129). IL-1 significantly enhances IL-9 production (128), particularly when IL-10 or kit ligand (127) are concomitantly present, suggesting an amplification mechanism during an inflammatory response that could be of importance during parasitic infections. Despite its early identification as a lymphokine, the role of IL-9 in T-cell responses is not as well defined as its effects on other types of cells such as mast cells (115,130), B cells (131), erythroid progenitors (132), and epithelial cells (133). IL-9 promotes the differentiation and proliferation of mast cells in vitro (130) and in transgenic mice (134,135). IL-9 enhances IL-4-induced immunoglobulin release from murine (136) and human (137) B lymphocytes but has no activity on its own. In an IL-9 transgenic mouse model (131), an expansion of the B1 cell population was noted. In vitro epithelial cell cultures treated with IL-9 express chemokines, and increased levels are also present in IL-9 overexpressing transgenic mice (133). Following direct installation of IL-9 into the airways of mice, eosinophil infiltration into the airways (138) and increased expression of the IL-5 receptor alpha chain are seen. Thus, it is probable that IL-9-induced eosinophilia is due to enhanced chemokine production and increased sensitivity of eosinophils to IL-5. Furthermore, these mechanisms may explain the enhanced eosinophil infiltration noted after lung antigen challenge (139) and intraperitoneal administration of thioglycolate (140) in IL-9 transgenic mice. IL-9 directly enhances mucin production in epithelial cells in vitro (141,142), and in vivo upregulation of mucin expression is seen in the airways of IL-9 overexpressing transgenic mice (142).

C. Scientific Rationale for Use of IL-9 Inhibitors in Asthma

The initial interest for targeting IL-9 in asthma arose from genetic studies in humans (25–27) and in mice (126). The human chromosonal region 5q31–q33, where the human IL-9 gene cluster resides, has been shown in several studies to be linked to asthma traits in humans (25,26), and the murine IL-9 gene on chromosome 13, to airway hyperresponsiveness (126). The human IL-9 receptor gene also shows significant linkage to asthma traits (143). Subsequently, several studies were performed to better characterize the association between IL-9 and asthma. IL-9 mRNA expression in mice strains with high airway responsiveness is higher (126), as is IL-9R as measured by Northern analysis, in the airways of patients with asthma (144). Immunohistochemical staining and in situ hybridization showed IL-9 mRNA to be significantly higher in asthmatic tissues than in normal controls and other chronic lung diseases, with IL-9 mRNA being predominantly seen in $CD3^+$ lymphocytes (68%) and MBP+ eosinophils (16%) (145). Mutations identified in the promoter region of IL-9 may explain the greater expression of IL-9 in asthma (146).

The hypothesis that the IL-9 system is associated with susceptibility for asthma has focused research on the elements of IL-9's biology that appear relevant to the pathogenesis of asthma. For instance, in vitro IL-9 increases IgE production from B cells (137), proliferation of mast cells (130), and mucin production (141), all of which may contribute to the asthma phenotype.

Several studies with transgenic mice have also shown asthma-like effects, although the relevance of these observations is difficult to determine because of the nonphysiological nature of constitutive cytokine expression, particularly when expression is generalized. Transgenic mice with generalized expression show baseline eosinophilia and increased expression of eotoxin and MCP-5 mRNA in cultured lung cells (133) and increased BAL eosinophilia, IgE concentration, and airway responsiveness after antigen challenge (139) compared to wild-type controls. There is a dramatic increase in mast cells in the gastrointestinal tract, kidneys, and lungs (134). Targeted and conditional overexpression models or "knockout" mice are generally more informative. In a mouse where the IL-9 gene was targeted to the lungs, with the Clara cell 10 promoter, there was an increase in mast cells in the lung epithelia and a large influx of eosinophils and lymphocytes (135), and although basal airway tone was normal, airway responsiveness was increased (135). In a granuloma model in the IL-$9^{-/-}$ mouse, goblet cell hyperplasia and increased mast cell numbers were seen, but eosinophilia and T-cell responses were unaffected (147). An anti-IL-9 monoclonal antibody has been tested in a murine model of antigen-induced lung inflammation by Kung et al. (148). Two therapeutic regimes were employed for administration of the antibody, either four times during the antigen sensitization period or as a single dose before antigen challenge. When administered during the sensitization period, the anti-IL-9 monoclonal antibody significantly reduced pulmonary eosinophilia, circulating IgE, goblet cell hyperplasia, airway damage, and measures of airway responsiveness compared to placebo-treated animals. The antibody did not affect the expression of IL-4, IL-5, or IL-13 mRNA in the lungs. In contrast, a single dose of anti-IL-9 just before challenge had no effect (148).

Thus, inhibition of IL-9 in asthma may prevent the activation and proliferation of mast cells, production of IgE, and mucin expression. It may have a profile similar to that of an inhibitor of IgE.

D. Strategies for Inhibition of IL-9

The targets for inhibition of IL-9's production, secretion, receptor binding, and signaling are similar to those described for IL-5 in the previous section. As for IL-5, the most expeditious route to test proof of concept of an IL-9 inhibitor in humans is probably through generation of a neutralizing monoclonal antibody or soluble receptor. To date there are no reports of clinical studies with an IL-9 inhibitor.

IV. Interleukin-10

A. Introduction

Interleukin-10 (IL-10) is a pleotrophic cytokine with effects on a number of lymphoid and myeloid cells, and like most cytokines its effects may be very dependent on the local cytokine milieu. It is a potent inhibitor of the effector function of macrophages, T cells, and NK cells and is considered to be an important regulator of inflammatory responses. There is some evidence to suggest that individuals with certain polymorphisms in the promoter region of the IL-10 gene may produce less IL-10 on stimulation, with the subsequent risk of inflammation becoming more severe or longer lasting. In contrast to IL-5 and IL-9, discussed in the preceding sections, IL-10 has the potential to be therapeutic in its own right.

B. Discovery and Biological Characterization of IL-10

As part of their hypothesis on functionally dichotomous Th cells, Mosmann and Coffman at DNAX (2) speculated that these cells were mutually regulating and that there should be a protein factor expressed by Th2 clones that inhibited Th1 clone activity. Using supernatants from murine Th2 cells, they identified an activity that inhibited IFN-γ production from mouse Th1 clones (149), subsequently cloning murine IL-10 in 1990. A year later, Mosmann and colleagues (150) cloned human IL-10, identifying it as a homodimer of approximately 18 kDa. Murine and human IL-10 genes are located on chromosomes 1 (151). Human IL-10 shows 81% homology at the nucleotide level and 73% at the protein level with mIL-10. Interestingly hIL-10 shows a strong homology to an open reading frame in the Epstein-Barr virus genome, the protein product of which is termed viral IL-10 (vIL-10) (150,152). Viral IL-10 has predominantly immunosuppressive effects, and its presence in the EB virus genome is probably an example of a virus hijacking a gene to evade host defenses. The IL-10 receptor is part of the interferon receptor family and was originally identified on murine and human cells by cross-linking studies (153). Subsequently, both chains of the human IL-10 receptor were cloned (154,155). vIL-10 associates with both murine and human receptors, whereas hIL-10 binds only to hIL-10. In a similar fashion to other cytokines, the intracellular signaling pathway for the IL-10 receptor involves the JAK–STAT transduction pathway. JAK1 and Tyk2, associated with IL-10R1 and IL-10R2, respectively, are phosphorylated when IL-10 binds the receptor, and then STAT1, STAT3, and in some cases STAT5 are activated (156). Differential IL-10 receptor expression is very important in determining the relative immunostimulatory and immunoinhibitory effects of IL-10 and vIL-10 on different tissues (157).

Interleukin-10 has been shown to be expressed by a large number of different immune cells, in addition to $CD4^+$. Th2 cells, including B cells (158), activated macrophages, monocytes (159), mast cells (160), and, interestingly, bronchial epithelium (161). In vitro IL-10 has various activities on different types of cells, but most prominently and probably the most therapeutically useful is its inhibition of cytokine release from monocytes (162). Administration of IL-10 prevents LPS-induced secretion of TNF, IL-1 and IL-6 in vitro and protects against LPS-induced lethality in vivo (163–165). Furthermore, IL-10 downregulates MHC class II expression on antigen-presenting cells, thereby reducing proliferation (166) and cytokine production by Th1 cells (167). Production of the chemokine IL-8 by activated neutrophils is blocked by IL-10 (168). Of particular relevance to the potential value of IL-10 in asthma is that it inhibits B7/CD28-dependent IL-5 production by human T cells (169) and LPS-induced cytokine production from and survival of human peripheral blood eosinophils in vitro (170). In addition to these anti-inflammatory and immunosuppressive effects, IL-10 also stimulates B cells, causing immunoglobulin production (171) and proliferation of pure CTLs (172), NK cells (173), and mast cells. IL-10's action on B cells could enhance IgE production, which may be detrimental in atopic asthma.

An indication of the possible therapeutic value of IL-10 emerged with the characterization of the phenotype of IL-10 knockout ($IL\text{-}10^{-/-}$) mice (174). Many $IL\text{-}10^{-/-}$ mice are runted and anemic, with indices of a blood loss pattern and rectal prolapse. Investigations of these animals determined that they have widespread inflammatory bowel disease with chronic blood loss. Starting in the cecum, the inflammation progresses to the transverse and ascending colon, and even the small intestine, if the animals survive into old age (175). Interestingly, animals raised in a pathogen-free environment do not get inflammatory changes in the gut, suggesting that the absence of IL-10 permits gut flora-induced inflammation in the gastrointestinal tract to become chronic. Administration of exogenous IL-10 to $IL\text{-}10^{-/-}$ mice early in life completely prevents these changes, and in older mice IL-10 administration acts therapeutically (176). In other immunological models of inflammatory bowel disease (IBD), IL-10 administration is also therapeutic. Adoptive transfer of lamina propria lymphocytes from IL-$10^{-/-}$ into Rag$2^{-/-}$ mice causes IBD (177), and treatment of IL-$10^{-/-}$ mice with anti-IFN-α monoclonal antibody reduces the inflammation, suggesting that T-helper type 1 lymphocytes are playing a pivotal role in these inflammatory responses. These studies strongly suggest that endogenous IL-10 is playing an immunomodulatory and anti-inflammatory role in response to noxious stimuli. It is tempting to speculate that impairment of the compensatory IL-10 production in predisposed individuals during a minor proinflammatory insult, as seen in the IL-$10^{-/-}$ mice, may lead to the chronic inflammation seen in asthma and that administration of exogenous hIL-10 might be therapeutic in these circumstances.

C. Scientific Rationale for Use of IL-10 in Asthma

The anti-inflammatory properties of IL-10 in vitro and the predisposition of IL-10 knockout mice to IBD stimulated interest in IL-10's effects on chronic inflammation in the lung. In 1995, Zuany-Amorim et al. (178) demonstrated that concurrent intranasal instillation of mIL-10 protein with administration of antigen inhibits infiltration of eosinophils and neutrophils and the secretion of TNF into the BAL of sensitized mice. Treatment with mIL-10 one or more hours after challenge had no effect (178). Systemic administration of mIL-10 at the same time as ragweed allergen challenge in sensitized mice produces significant reductions in BAL concentrations of IL-4, IL-5, and IFN-γ compared to control animals (179), but airway responsiveness to methacholine increases in the mIL-10-treated animals. Increases in airway responsiveness were not seen in sham-challenged naive or sensitized mice treated with IL-10. Administration of the IL-10 gene directly into the airways of sensitized and challenged mice attenuates both TNF, IL-4, and IL-5 in BAL and reduces airway responsiveness (180).

Three studies of allergic lung inflammation in IL-$10^{-/-}$ mice have been reported (181–183). IL-$10^{-/-}$ mice show an increase in pulmonary inflammation after antigen challenge compared to wild-type mice. IgE concentrations and IL-4 production are unaffected in the IL-$10^{-/-}$ animals, but IL-5 in the BAL is reduced compared to wild-type controls (181,182). Baseline airway responsiveness was increased in one study of IL-$10^{-/-}$ mice, but no differences in airway responsiveness were seen between IL-$10^{-/-}$ and wild-type mice after challenge (181). In another study Makela et al. (183) showed a loss of airway responsiveness in the IL-10-deficient mice that returned after reconstitution with IL-10 gene therapy. Production of Th1 cytokines, namely IL-12 and IFN-γ, was increased in the IL-$10^{-/-}$ mice (182). Taken as a whole, these data suggest that endogenously produced IL-10 may be important in modulation of allergic inflammation in the lung although its role in the generation of airway responsiveness remains unclear. One difference between these studies that may explain some of the apparently conflicting data is the method of administration, with topically administered IL-

10 appearing more effective than parenteral IL-10. Because, under normal conditions, cytokines function locally, this may have important therapeutic implications.

Because reduced or absent IL-10 is permissive of exaggerated allergic inflammation in animals, genetically determined reductions in IL-10 expression may predispose to asthma in humans. Comparison of the concentrations of IL-10 in BAL between asthmatic and normal subjects shows reduced IL-10 protein in the asthmatic group (184). Furthermore, constitutive and stimulated production of IL-10 from ex vivo monocytes in the asthmatic group is also reduced. A study of differentiation of monocytes in vitro shows that IL-10 is essential for generating a ''suppressive'' phenotype in macrophage and that this phenotype is reduced in asthmatic patients (185). John et al. (186) confirmed reduced IL-10 production from blood monocytes and alveolar macrophages in chronic asthma but much higher concentrations after 4 weeks of inhaled budesonide. In contrast, Zeibecoglou et al. (187) found an increase in IL-10 mRNA positive cells, 80% of which were macrophages, in atopic asthma compared to nonatopic asthma, and Colavita et al. (188) showed a prolonged increase in BAL IL-10 protein after antigen challenge in subjects with dual antigen responses compared to normals. Treatment of ex vivo BAL macrophages with dexamethasone had no effect on IL-10 production in this study (188). A number of polymorphisms are present in the IL-10 gene and its promoter, and there is a significant association of low IL-10 haplotypes with more severely asthmatic (189) patients in one study and with those with increased concentrations of IgE (190) in another. The authors speculate that local differences in IL-10 secretion may be influencing the asthma phenotype. IL-10 concentrations are also reduced in patients with chronic obstructive lung disease compared to controls (191) and in those patients who smoke compared to nonsmokers (191).

D. Effect of IL-10 in Human Studies

Administration of IL-10 intravenously to normal volunteers has a marked effect on white blood cell numbers. The intravenous half-life of IL-10 is 2 h (192), but IL-10-induced changes in white blood cells continue for 1–2 days (193). Neutrophil numbers increase, and both $CD4^+$ and $CD8^+$ lymphocytes are reduced (194). Lipopolysaccharide (LPS) induces cytokine production (TNF-α and IL-1β) from peripheral blood mononuclear cells sampled from normal subjects, but cytokine release is much reduced and IL-IRA is increased if the subjects are treated with IL-10 (192,193) before blood sampling. When LPS is injected directly into human volunteers, systemic proinflammatory cytokines increase and radiolabeled neutrophils are sequestered in the lungs, as measured by gamma camera scans (195). Pretreatment with systemic IL-10 attenuates cytokine release, neutrophil sequestration in the lung, and indirect measures of neutrophil degranulation (195).

Extrapolating from animal studies, IL-10 would also be expected to have an inhibitory effect on antigen-induced pulmonary responses in humans, and so the effect of pretreatment with systemic IL-10 in pulmonary antigen challenge in mild asthmatic subjects has been studied. A single parenteral dose of IL-10, sufficient to inhibit LPS responses (195), had no significant effect on early or late pulmonary responses or on bronchial responsiveness (S. Lim and P. J. Barnes, personal communication). There were small reductions in neutrophils and eosinophils measured in the bronchoalveolar lavage, but the changes did not reach statistical significance. It is possible that topical administration of IL-10 or larger and more frequent parenteral doses may show an effect, but it is also possible that IL-10 is ineffective in human antigen challenge. The results of a study of another potential antiasthmatic cytokine, IL-12 (196), was considered disappointing in this model and brings into question the predictive value of antigen challenge in animals for human studies.

E. Strategies for the Development of IL-10 in Asthma

The biology of IL-10 suggests that it could be an important endogenous modulator of inflammation and that reduction of its expression could exacerbate ongoing inflammation in a number of diseases including asthma. Even if asthma is not due to IL-10 deficiency, it is possible that administration of exogenous IL-10 may ameliorate the pulmonary inflammation seen in asthma. IL-10 is different from the cytokines discussed in the preceding sections because it is a pleotrophic cytokine with potential as a therapeutic modality in its own right. IL-10 is a potent cytokine with many inhibitory and stimulating effects in vitro and in vivo. These many potential activities make its characterization as a human therapeutic agent both extensive and challenging, with a development paradigm more similar to that of cytokines such as interferon than to those of specific growth factors such as erythropoietin. For instance, the biological profile of interferon promised several possible therapeutic opportunities in the treatment of infectious and malignant diseases, but it took many years to identify the diseases that were treatable with interferons and the most appropriate dosing regimens. In contrast, the biological effects of growth factors such as erythropoietin are specific, and the choice of therapeutic target is more limited, the major question being the clinical relevance of the increases in hematopoietic cells induced by the growth factor. The development program of the latter was significantly shorter. The challenge in the clinical development of pleotrophic cytokines such as IL-10 is the achievement of useful therapeutic effects at doses that do not induce unacceptable mechanism based side effects. In asthma this has been achieved for drugs with narrow therapeutic indices, such as corticosteroids, by their direct administration to the lungs by inhalation. Because in life cytokines are released locally to mediate local effects and there are suggestions in animals that IL-10 is more effective when delivered topically, inhaled delivery may be the preferred approach for IL-10 in asthma.

V. Development of Biological Therapeutic Agents

In this chapter there is considerable discussion concerning the scientific validation of individual cytokines as targets or therapeutic agents and the kind of evidence needed to move biotherapeutic agents into clinical testing. In the context of having a drug available for patients, the most important information is confirmation of the biotherapeutic agent as a medically and commercially viable product. Many different factors need to be considered to make a comprehensive assessment, and some of the development challenges posed by biotherapeutics are discussed in this section.

Interleukins-5, -9, and -10 represent different asthma targets and different approaches to the treatment of asthma. The major activity of IL-5 is related to eosinophils, their cytotoxicity for lung tissue, and their effects on the signs and symptoms of asthma and airway remodeling. IL-9's predominant activity appears to be on mast cells, IgE production, and mucin gene transcription, and IL-9 may therefore be more involved in the atopic aspects of asthma. Specific inhibition of these cytokines would be expected to have beneficial effects on these particular processes either alone or, more likely, in combination with other asthma medication. IL-10 may represent another therapeutic strategy where more widespread anti-inflammatory properties could provide better clinical efficacy and more general use.

The aim of drug discovery is to find a therapeutic agent that attenuates a pathological process and has minimal effects on healthy individuals. Ideally the targeted mechanism should be pivotal in the pathogenic process and only one element of a broader homeostatic mechanism in the normal individual. Thus an inhibitor should attenuate the pathology but leave normal function unimpaired. Sometimes, however, there is also considerable redundancy in the disease process itself and a very specific inhibitor has little if any clinical effect because many different inflammatory mechanisms are proceeding in parallel. Unfortunately, this lack of efficacy may become apparent only late in a program when the new therapeutic agent has been tested in large clinical studies. Some asthma experts favor new drugs with broad pharmacological profiles because such drugs would inhibit multiple inflammatory pathways and are more likely to be effective. These researchers support this view with the premise that corticosteroids, which have multiple anti-inflammatory mechanisms, are the most effective drug for the treatment of asthma. The potential downside of a broad pharmacological profile is demonstrated by the well-recognized side effects of long-term use of oral corticosteroids. Furthermore, with increasing doses of corticosteroids, their immunosuppressive effects become more evident. It is clear that broad and potent inhibition of many immune processes will eventually lead to significant impairment of host defenses. A degree of functional selectivity is achieved for corticosteroids by delivery by inhalation directly to the lungs, and this could be an attractive option for a pleotrophic cytokine like IL-10. The key success factor for a therapeutic cytokine with multiple actions will be its therapeutic index, but this may not become fully evident until late in the clinical testing.

A challenge in the development of new drugs for chronic diseases, and well illustrated in this chapter on biotherapeutics for asthma, is that there is neither a reliably predictive animal model nor a validated biomarker of clinical efficacy to aid the development process. This means that several years will pass between identification of the target, its validation in animal studies, and the final proof of concept in humans. Validation of the therapeutic target involves many elements that are discussed in the preceding sections. It is clear from the multitude of published animal studies that lung antigen challenge has become a popular model to define and analyze the effects of potential antiasthma medications. Asthma is nowadays defined as changes in airway caliber over time, increased bronchial responsiveness, and airway inflammation. Because antigen administration in sensitized animals leads to allergic inflammation, changes in airway caliber, and increased responsiveness, the attraction of antigen challenge as a surrogate for clinical asthma is obvious. The underlying hypothesis is that airway inflammation induced by antigen is directly responsible for the reduction in pulmonary function and increase in airway responsiveness. Therefore, it is proposed that if a potential anti-inflammatory therapeutic agent blocks the antigen-induced cellular inflammation and its sequelae it should also act on the cardinal features of asthma. However, as mechanism-based inhibitors have become more specific and scientists have carefully dissected the sequelae of antigen challenge, it has become clear that inhibition or induction of airway responsiveness may be independent of airway inflammation, at least in the context of an acute antigen challenge. If bronchial inflammation and airway responsiveness are induced by different processes in antigen-challenged animals, is this also the case in asthma, or can chronic asthmatic inflammation induce hyperresponsiveness in its own right? If so, could biotherapeutic agents that block inflammation in challenged animals but have no effect on airway responsiveness still have therapeutic value in humans because of long-term effects on inflammation? There is no answer to this question yet, but it is clear that a definitive proof of concept in asthma for a biotherapeutic agent can be definitively determined only in ''wild-type'' asthma. However, even this approach can lead to equivocal results because of differences in patient response, choice of endpoint, and duration of therapy. If the biotherapeutic agent has effects on lung function in a large proportion of the population, it is relatively easy to confirm efficacy. If, however, only a subgroup of asthmatic patients are likely to benefit and the effect is modest or takes months to be evident, a beneficial effect may be missed in small or short-term studies.

This chapter encompasses two distinct types of therapeutic proteins, namely monoclonal antibodies and cytokines. Monoclonal antibodies have the advantage of great selectivity for their protein targets and are relatively easy to generate with high affinity. On the other hand, they have high molecular weight, need to be given in large doses to neutralize their target, and have to be administered parenterally. Parenteral administration of any exogenous protein can induce antibody formation and an immune response to the protein. Humanized or fully human monoclonal antibodies infrequently elicit strong immune responses and have half-lives comparable to those of native immunoglobulins, giving them the advantage of prolonged duration in the systemic circulation (12). Conventional recombinant monoclonal antibodies are manufactured in human cells and have doses in the milligram range. In contrast, cytokines can be manufactured in bacteria and because of their lower molecular weight and potency require dosing only in microgram quantities. They too require dosing parenterally but because of their shorter half-lives, usually measured in hours, need to be dosed more frequently than monoclonal antibodies. An immune response can also occur with human cytokines, and if the host antibodies generated against the cytokine are neutralizing this can significantly reduce the therapeutic effect of the cytokine.

With better understanding of pathological processes and the advent of the genomics era, there has been a rapid expansion of potential drug targets in many diseases. Even with the dramatic improvements in small-molecule drug discovery, many of these targets are approachable only by protein therapeutic agents. Thus, it is likely that in the next few years one or more biotherapeutic agents will find a place in the management of asthma.

Acknowledgment

I thank Mrs. Carolyn Steinmeyer for preparing the manuscript and for bibliographic services.

References

1. Barnes PJ. A new approach to the treatment of asthma. N Engl J Med 1989; 321: 1517–1527.
2. Mosmann TR, Coffman RL. TH1 and TH2 cells: Different patterns of lymphokine secretion lead to different functional properties. Annu Rev Immunol 1989; 7:145–173.
3. von Leyden E. Üeber Bronchialasthma. Deut Militärärztl Z 1886; 15:515.
4. Sanerkin NG, Evans DMD. The sputum in bronchial asthma: Pathognomonic patterns. J Pathol Bacteriol 1965; 89:535–541.
5. Frigas E, Loegering DA, Solley GO, Farrow GM, Gleich GJ. Elevated levels of the eosinophil granule major basic protein in the sputum of patients with bronchial asthma. Mayo Clin Proc 1981; 56:345–353.

6. Dunnill MS. The pathology of asthma, with special reference to changes in the bronchial musosa. J Clin Pathol 1960; 13:27.
7. Glynn AA, Michaels L. Bronchial biopsy in chronic bronchitis and asthma. Thorax 1960; 15:142.
8. Frigas E, Loegering DA, Gleich GJ. Cytotoxic effects of guinea-pig eosinophil major basic protein on tracheal epithelium. Lab Invest 1980; 42:35–43.
9. Filley WV, Holley KE, Kephart GM, Gleich GJ. Identification by immunofluorescence of eosinophil granule major basic protein in lung tissues of patients with bronchial asthma. Lancet 1982; I:11–15.
10. Yokata T, Coffman RL, Hagiwara H, Rennick DM, Takebe Y, Yokata K, Gemmell L, Schrader B, Yang G, Meyerson P, Luh J, Hoy P, Pene J, Briere F, Spits H, Banchereau J, deVries J, Lee FP, Arai N, Arai K. Isolation and characterization of lymphokine cDNA clones encoding mouse and human IgA-enhancing factor and eosinophil colony-stimulating factor activities: Relationship to interleukin 5. Proc Natl Acad Sci USA 1987; 84:7388.
11. Kinashi T, Harada N, Severinson E, Tanabe T, Sideras P, Konishi M, Azuma C, Tominaga A, Bergstedt-Lindqvist S, Takahashi M. Cloning of complementary DNA encoding T-cell replacing factor and identity with B-cell growth factor II. Nature 1986; 324:70–73.
12. Warren DJ, Sanderson CJ. Production of a T-cell hybrid producing a lymphokine stimulating eosinophil differentiation. Immunology 1985; 54:615–623.
13. Clutterbuck E, Shields JG, Gorden J, Smith SH, Boyd A, Callard RE, Campbell HD, Young IG, Sandeson CJ. Recombinant human interleukin-5 is an eosinophil differentiation factor but has no activity in standard human B cell growth factor assays. Eur J Immunol 1987; 17:1743–1750.
14. Clutterbuck EK, Hirst EMA, Sanderson CJ. Human interleukin-5 (IL-5) regulates the production of eosinophils in human bone marrow cultures: Comparison and interaction with IL-1, IL-3, IL-6 and GM-CSF. Blood 1989; 73:1504–1512.
15. Clutterbuck EJ, Sanderson CJ. Regulation of human eosinophil precursor production by cytokines: A comparison of recombinant human interleukin-1 (rhIL-1), rhIL-3, rhIL-5, rhIL-6 and rh granulocyte-macrophage colony stimulating factor. Blood 1990; 75:1774–1779.
16. McKenzie ANJ, Ely B, Sanderson CJ. Mutated interleukin-5 monomers are biologically inactive. Mol Immunol 1991; 28:155–158.
17. Sanderson CJ, Campbell HD, Young IG. Molecular and cellular biology of eosinophil differentiation factor (interleukin-5) and its effects on human and mouse B cells. Immunol Rev 1988; 102:29–50.
18. Abrams JS, Roncarolo MG, Yssel H, Andersson U, Gleich GJ, Silver JE. Strategies of anti-cytokine monoclonal antibody development: Immunoassay of IL-10 and IL-5 in clinical samples. Immunol Rev 1992; 127:5–27.
19. Danzig M, Cuss F. Inhibition of interleukin-5 with a monoclonal antibody. Allergy 1997; 52:787–794.
20. Kips JC, O'Connor BJ, Langley SJ, Woodcock A, Kerstjens HAM, Postma DS, Danzig M, Cuss F, Pauwels RA. Results of a phase I trial with SCH55700, a humanized anti-IL-5 antibody, in severe persistent asthma. Am J Respir Crit Care Med 2000; 161:A505.

21. Leckie MJ, ten Brinke A, Khan J, Diamant Z, O'Connor BJ, Walls CM, Mathur AK, Cowley H, Chung KF, Djukanovic R, Hansel TT, Holgate ST, Sterk PJ, Barnes PJ. Effects of an interleukin-5 blocking monoclonal antibody on eosinophils, airway hyperresponsiveness, and the late asthmatic response. Lancet 2000; 356:2144–2148.
22. Azuma C, Tanabe T, Konishi M, Kinashi T, Noma T, Matsuda F, Yaoita Y, Takatsu K, Hammarstrom L, Edvard Smith Cl, Severinson E, Honio T. Cloning of CDNA for human T-cell replacing factor (interleukin-5) and comparison with the murine homologue. Nucl Acids Res 1986; 14:9149–9158.
23. Kodama S, Tsuruoka N, Tsujimoto M. Role of the C-terminus in the biological activity of human interleukin 5. Biochem Biophys Res Commun 1991; 178:514–519.
24. van Leeuwen BH, Martinson ME, Webb GC, Young IG. Molecular organization of the cytokine gene cluster, involving the human IL-3, IL-4, IL-5, and GM-CSF genes, on human chromosome 5. Blood 1989; 73:1142–1148.
25. Postma DS, Bleecker ER, Amelung PJ, Holroyd KJ, Xu J, Panhuysen CI, Meyers DA, Levitt RC. Genetic susceptibility to asthma: Bronchial hyperresponsiveness coinherited with a major gene for atopy. N Engl J Med 1995; 333:894–900.
26. Collaborative Study Group. A genome-wide search for asthma susceptibility loci in ethnically diverse populations. The Collaborative Study on the Genetics of Asthma (CSGA). Nat Genet 1997; 15:389–392.
27. Doull IJ, Lawrence S, Watson M, Begishvili T, Beasley RW, Lampe F, Holgate T, Morton NE. Allelic association of gene markers on chromosomes 5q and 11q with atopy and bronchial hyperresponsiveness. Am J Respir Crit Care Med 1996; 153:1280–1284.
28. Miyatake S, Shlomai J, Ken-Ichi A, Ari N. Characterization of the mouse granulocyte macrophage colony-stimulating factor (GM-CSF) gene promoter: Nuclear factors that interact with an element shared by three lymphokine genes—those for GM-CSF, interleukin-4 (IL-4) and IL-5. Mol Cell Biol 1991; 12:5894–5901.
29. Tominaga A, Takahashi T, Kikuchi Y, Mita S, Naomi S, Harada N, Yamaguchi N, Takatsu K. Role of carbohydrate moiety of IL-5. J Immunol 1990; 144:1345–1352.
30. Milburn MV, Hassell AM, Lambert MH, Jordan SR, Proudfoot AEI, Graber P, Wells TNC. A novel dimer configuration revealed by the crystal structure at 24A resolution of human interleukin-5. Nature 1993; 363:172–176.
31. Bazan JF. Structural design and molecular evaluation of a cytokine receptor superfamily. Proc Natl Acad Sci USA 1990; 87:6934–6938.
32. Tavernier J, Devos R, Cornelis S, Tuypens T, van der Heyden J, Fiers W, Plaetinck G. A human high affinity interleukin-5 receptor (IL5R) is composed of an IL5 specific α chain and a β chain shared with the receptor for GM-CSF. Cell 1991; 66:1175–1184.
33. Murata Y, Takaki S, Migita M, Kikuchi Y, Tominaga A, Takatsu K. Molecular cloning and expression of the human interleukin 5 receptor. J Exp Med 1992; 175: 341–351.
34. Travernier J, Tuypens T, Plaetinck G, Verhee A, Fiers W, Devos R. Molecular basis of the membrane-anchored and two soluble isoforms of the human interleukin-5 receptor α subunit. Proc Natl Acad Sci USA 1992; 89:7041–7045.

35. Ihle JN, Witthuhn BA, Quelle FW, Yamamoto K, Thierfelder WE, Kreider B. Silvennoinen O. Signaling by the cytokine receptor superfamily: JAKs and STATs. Trends Biochem Sci 1994; 19:222–227.
36. Darnell JE Jr, Kerr AM, Stark GR. Jak-STAT pathways and transcriptional activation in response to IFNs and other extracellular signaling proteins. Science 1994; 262:1415–1420.
37. Mul Al-F, Wakao H, O'Farrell A-M, Harada N, Miyajima A. Interleukin-3, granulocyte-macrophage colony stimulating factor and interleukin-5 transduce signals through two STAT5 homologues. EMBO J 1995; 14:1166–1175.
38. Altman A, Coggeshall KM, Mustelin T. Molecular events mediating T cell activation. Adv Immunol 1990; 48:227–360.
39. Bradding P, Roberts JA, Britten KM, Montefort S, Dujukanovic R, Mueller R, Heusser CH, Howarth PH, Holgate ST. Interleukin-4, -5, and -6 and tumor necrosis factor-α in normal and asthmatic airways: Evidence for the human mast cell as a source of these cytokines. Am J Respir Cell Mol Biol 1994; 10:471–478.
40. Dubucquoi S, Desreumaux P, Janin A, Klein O, Goldman M. Travernier J, Capron A, Capron M. Interleukin 5 synthesis by eosinophils: Association with granules and immunoglobulin-dependent secretion. J Exp Med 1994; 179:703–708.
41. van Straaten JFM, Dokter WHA, Stulp BK, Vellenga BK. The regulation of interleukin-5 and interleukin-3 gene expression in human T cells. Cytokine 1994; 6: 229–234.
42. Rolfe FG, Hughes JM, Armour CL, Sewell WA. Inhibition of interleukin-5 gene expression by dexamethasone. Immunology 1992; 77:494–499.
43. Umland SP, Shah H, Jakway JP, Shortall J, Razac S, Garlisi CF, Falcone A, Kung TT, Stelts D, Hegde V, Patel M, Billah MM, Egan RW. Effects of cyclosporin A and dinactin on T-cell proliferation, interleukin-5 production, and murine pulmonary inflammation. Am J Respir Cell Mol Biol 1999; 20:481–492.
44. Garlisi CG, Falcone A, Kung TT, Stelts D, Pennline KG, Beavis AJ, Smith SR, Egan RW, Umland SP. T cells are necessary for TH2 cytokine production and eosinophil accumulation in airways of antigen-challenged allergic mice. Clin Immunol Immunopathol 1995; 75:75–83.
45. Till S, Li B, Durham S, Humbert M, Assoufi B, Huston D, Dickason R, Jeannin P, Kay AB, Corrigan C. Secretion of the eosinophil-active cytokines interleukin-5, granulocyte/macrophage colony-stimulating factor and interleukin-3 by bronchoalveolar lavage CD4+ and CD8+ T cell lines in atopic asthmatics, and atopic and non-atopic controls. Eur J Immunol 1995; 25:2727–2731.
46. Hirai K, Yamaguchi M, Misaki Y, Takaishi T, Ohta K, Morita Y, Ito K, Miyamoto T. Enhancement of human basophil histamine release by interleukin 5. J Exp Med 1990; 172:1525–1528.
47. Lopez AF, Shannon MF, Chia MM, Park L, Vadas MA. Regulation of human eosinophil production and function by interleukin-5. Immunol Ser 1992; 57:549–571.
48. Resnick MB, Weller PF. Mechanisms of eosinophil recruitment. Am J Respir Cell Mol Biol 1993; 8:349–355.
49. Warringa RA, Schweizer RC, Maikoe T, Kuijper PH, Bruijnzeel PL, Koendermann L. Modulation of eosinophil chemotaxis by interleukin-5. Am J Respir Cell Mol Biol 1992; 7:631–636.

50. Carlson M, Peterson C, Venge P. The influence of IL-3, IL-5, and GM-CSF on normal human eosinophil and neutrophil C3b-induced degranulation. Allergy 1993; 48:437–442.
51. Kita H, Weiler DA, Abu-Ghazaleh R, Sanderson CJ, Gleich GJ. Release of granule proteins from eosinophils cultured with IL-5. J Immunol 1992; 149:629–635.
52. Yamaguchi Y, Suda T, Ohta S, Tominaga K, Miura Y, Kasahara T. Analysis of the survival of mature human eosinophils: Interleukin-5 prevents apoptosis in mature human eosinophils. Blood 1991; 78:2542–2547.
53. Wallen N, Kita H, Weiler D, Gleich GJ. Glucocorticoids inhibit cytokine-mediated eosinophil survival. J Immunol 1991; 147:3490–3495.
54. Abu-Ghazaleh RI, Fujisawa T, Mestecky J, Kyle RA, Gleich GJ. IgA-induced eosinophil degranulation. J Immunol 1989; 142:2393–2400.
55. Minnicozzi M, Anthes JC, Siegel MI, Billah MM, Egan RW. Activation of phospholipase D in normodense human eosinophils. Biochem Biophys Res Commun 1990; 170:540–547.
56. Petreccia DC, Nauseef WM, Clark RA. Respiratory burst of normal human eosinophils. J Leuk Biol 1987; 41:283–288.
57. Bruynzeel PLB, Kok PTM, Hamelink ML, Kijne AM, Verhagen J. Exclusive leukotrine C4 synthesis by purified human eosinophils induced by opsonized zymosan. FEBS Lett 1985; 189:350–354.
58. Gleich GJ, Adolphson CR. The eosinophilic leukocyte: Structure and function. Adv Immunol 1986; 39:177–253.
59. Robinson D, Hamid Q, Bentley A, Ying S, Kay AB, Durham SR. Activation of CD4+ T cells, increased TH2-type cytokine mRNA expression, and eosinophil recruitment in bronchoalveolar lavage after allergen inhalation challenge in patients with atopic asthma. J Allergy Clin Immunol 1993; 92:313–324.
60. Zangrilli JG, Shaver JR, Cirelli RA, Cho SK, Garlisi CG, Falcone A, Cuss FM, Fish JE, Peters SP. sVCAM-1 levels after segmental antigen challenge correlate with eosinophil influx, IL-4 and IL-5 production, and the late phase response. Am J Respir Crit Care Med 1995; 151:1346–1353.
61. Durham SR, Kay AB. Eosinophils, bronchial hyperreactivity and late phase asthmatic reactions. Clin Allergy 1985; 13:411–418.
62. Wardlaw AJ, Dunnett S, Gleich GJ, Collins JV, Kay AB. Eosinophils and mast cells in bronchoalveolar lavage in subjects with mild asthma: Relationship to bronchial hyperreactivity. Am Rev Respir Dis 1988; 137:62–69.
63. DeMonchy JG, Kauffman HF, Venge P, Koeter GH, Jansen HM, Sluiter HJ, De Vries K. Bronchoalveolar eosinophilia during allergen-induced late asthmatic reactions. Am Rev Respir Dis 1985; 131:373–376.
64. Bentley AM, Meng Q, Robinson DS, Hamid Q, Kasy AB, Durham SR. Increases in activated T lymphocytes, eosinophils, and cytokine mRNA expression for interleukin-5 and granulocyte/machrophage colony-stimulated factor in bronchial biopsies after allergen inhalation challenge in atopic asthmatics. Am J Respir Cell Mol Biol 1993; 8:35–42.
65. Marini M, Avoni E, Hollemborg J, Mattoli S. Cytokine mRNA profile and cell activation in bronchoalveolar lavage fluid from nonatopic patients with symptomatic asthma. Chest 1992; 102:661–669.

66. Sedgwick JB, Calhoun WC, Gleich GJ, Kita H, Abrams JS, Schwartz LB, Volovitz B, Ben-Yaakov M, Busse W. Immediate and late airway response of allergic rhinitis patients to segmental antigen challenge. Characterization of eosinophil and mast cell mediators. Am Rev Respir Dis 1991; 144:1274–1281.
67. Ohnishi T, Kita H, Weiler D, Sur S, Sedgwick JB, Calhoun WJ, Busse WW, Abrams JS, Gleich GJ. IL-5 is the predominant eosinophil-active cytokine in the antigen-induced pulmonary late-phase reaction. Am Rev Respir Dis 1993; 147: 901–907.
68. Diaz P, Gonzalez MC, Galleguillos FR, Ancic P, Cromwell O, Shepherd D, Durham SR, Gleich GJ, Kay AB. Leokocytes and mediators in bronchoalveolar lavage during allergen-induced late-phase asthmatic reactions. Am Rev Respir Dis 1989; 139: 1383–1389.
69. Shi H, Qin S, Huang G, Chen Y, Xiao C, Xu H, Liang G, Xie Z, Qin X, Wu J, Li G, Zhang C. Infiltration of eosinophils into the asthmatic airways caused by interleukin 5. Am J Respir Cell Mol Biol 1997; 16:220–224.
70. Shi HZ, Xiao CQ, Zhong D, Qin SM, Liu Y, Liang GR, Xu H, Chen YQ, Long XM, Xie ZF. Effect of inhaled interleukin-5 on airway hyperreactivity and eosinophilia in asthmatics. Am J Respir Crit Care 1998; 157:204–209.
71. Robinson DS, Hamid Q, Ying S, Tsicopoulos A, Barkans J, Bentley AM, Corrigan C, Durham SR, Kay AB. Predominant TH2-like bronchoalveolar T-lymphocyte population in atopic asthma. N Engl J Med 1992; 326:298–304.
72. Bentley AM, Menz G, Storz C, Robinson DS, Bradley B, Jeffery PK, Durham SR, Kay AB. Identification of T lympocytes, macrophages, and activated eosinophils in the bronchial mucosa in intrinsic asthma. Relationship to symptoms and bronchial responsiveness. Am Rev Respir Dis 1992; 146:500–506.
73. Hamid Q, Azzawi M, Ying S, Moqbel R, Wardlaw AJ, Corrigan CJ, Bradley B, Durham SR, Collins JV, Jeffery PK, Quint DJ, Kay AB. Expression of mRNA for interleukin-5 in mucosal bronchial biopsies from asthma. J Clin Invest 1991; 87: 1541–1546.
74. Robinson DS, Ying S, Bentley AM, Meng Q, North J, Durham SR, Kay AB, Hamid Q. Relationships among numbers of bronchoalveolar lavage cells expressing messenger ribonucleic acid for cytokines, asthma symptoms, and airway methacholine responsiveness in atopic asthma. J Allergy Clin Immunol 1993; 92:397–403.
75. Sur S, Gleich GJ, Swanson MC, Bartemes KR, Broide DH. Eosinophilic inflammation is associated with the elevation of interleukin-5 in the airways of patients with spontaneous symptomatic asthma. J Allergy Clin Immunol 1995; 96:661–668.
76. Motojima S, Akutsu I, Fukuda T, Makino S, Takatsu K. Clinical significance of measuring levels of sputum and serum ECP and serum IL-5 in bronchial asthma. Allergy 1993; 48:98–106.
77. Robinson D, Hamid Q, Ying S, Bentley A, Assoufi B, Durham S, Kay AB. Prednisolone treatment in asthma is associated with modulation of bronchoalveolar lavage cell interleukin-4, interleukin-5, and interferon-gamma cytokine gene expression. Am Rev Respir Dis 1993; 148:401–406.
78. Kosmas EN, Michaelides SA, Polychronaki A, Roussou T, Toukmatzi S, Polychronopoulos V, Baxevanis CN. Theophylline induces a reduction in circulating interleukin-4 and interleukin-5 in atopic asthmatics. Eur Respir J 1999; 13:53–58.

79. Gulbenkian AR, Egan RW, Fernandez X, Jones H, Kreutner W, Kung TT, Payvandi F, Sullivan L, Zurcher JA, Watnick AS. Interleukin-5 modulates eosinophil accumulation in allergic guinea pig lung. Am Rev Respir Dis 1992; 146:263–265.
80. Mauser PJ, Pitman A, Witt A, Fernandez X, Zurcher J, Kung T, Jones H, Watnick AS, Egan RW, Kreutner W, Adams GK III. Inhibitory effect of the TRFK-5 anti-IL-5 antibody in a guinea pig model of asthma. Am Rev Respir Dis 1993; 148: 1623–1627.
81. Lilly CM, Chapman RW, Sehring SJ, Mauser PJ, Showell HJ, Egan RW, Drazen JM. Effects of interleukin 5-induced pulmonary eosinophilia on airway reactivity in the guinea pig. Am J Physiol 1996; 270:L368–L375.
82. Hakonarson H, Maskeri N, Carter C, Chuang S, Grunstein MM. Autocrine interaction between IL-5 and IL-1β mediates altered responsiveness of atopic asthmatic sensitized airway smooth muscle. J Clin Invest 1999; 104:657–667.
83. Kung TT, Jones H, Adams GK III, Umland SP, Kreutner W, Egan RW, Chapman RW, Watnick AS. Characterization of a murine model of allergic pulmonary inflammation. Int Arch Allergy Immunol 1994; 105:83–90.
84. Hamelmann E, Oshiba A, Loader J, Larsen GL, Gleich G, Lee J, Gelfand EW. Antiinterleukin-5 antibody prevents airway hyperresponsiveness in a murine model of airway sensitization. Am J Respir Crit Care Med 1997; 155:819–825.
85. Hogan SP, Koshinen A, Foster PS. Interleukin-5 and eosinophils induce airway damage and bronchial hyperreactivity during allergic airway inflammation in BALB/c mice. Immunol Cell Biol 1997; 75:284–288.
86. Kung TT, Stelts DM, Zurcher JA, Adams GK III, Egan RW, Kreutner W, Watnick AS, Jones H, Chapman RW. Involvement of IL-5 in a murine model of allergic pulmonary inflammation: Prophylactic and therapeutic effect of an anti-IL-5 antibody. Am J Respir Cell Mol Biol 1995; 13:360–365.
87. Murali DS, Kumar A, Choi H, Bansal NK, Fink JN, Kurup VP. Aspergillus fumigatus antigen induced eosinophilia in mice is abrogated by anti-IL-5 antibody. J Leuk Biol 1993; 53:264–267.
88. Hamelmann E, Cieslewicz G, Schwarze J, Ishizuka T, Joetham A, Heusser C, Gelfand EW. Anti-interleukin 5 but not anti-IgE prevents airway inflammation and airway hyperresponsiveness. Am J Respir Crit Care Med 1999; 160:934–941.
89. Garlisi CG, Falcone A, Kung TT, Stelts D, Pennline KG, Beavis AJ, Smith SR, Egan RW, Umland SP. T cells are necessary for TH2 cytokine production and eosinophil accumulation in airways of antigen-challenged allergic mice. Clin Immunol Immunopathol 1995; 75:75–83.
90. Brusselle GG, Kips JC, Tavernier JH, van der Heyden JG, Cavelier CA, Pauwels RA, Bluethmann H. Attenuation of allergic airway inflammation in IL-4 deficient mice. Clin Exp Allergy 1994; 24:73–80.
91. Kung TT, Stelts D, Zurcher JA, Jones H, Umland SP, Kreutner W, Egan RW, Chapman RW. Mast cells modulate allergic pulmonary eosinophilia in mice. Am J Respir Cell Biol 1995; 12:404–409.
92. Lee JJ, McGarry MP, Farmer SC, Denzler KL, Larson KA, Carrigan PE, Brenneise IE, Horton MA, Haczku A, Gelfand EW, Leikauf GD, Lee NA. Interleukin-5 expression in the lung epithelium of transgenic mice leads to pulmonary changes pathognomonic of asthma. J Exp Med 1997; 185:2143–2156.

93. Foster PS, Hogan SP, Ramsay AJ, Matthaei KI, Young IG. Interleukin 5 deficiency abolishes eosinophilia, airways hyperreactivity, and lung damage in a mouse asthma model. J Exp Med 1996; 183:195–201.
94. Kopf M, Brombacher F, Hodgkin PD, Ramsay AJ, Milbourne EA, Dai WJ, Ovington KS, Behm CA, Kohler G, Young IG, Matthaei KI. IL-5-deficient mice have a developmental defect in CD5+ B-1 cells and lack eosinophilia but have normal antibody and cytotoxic T cell responses. Immunity 1996; 4:15–24.
95. Nagai H, Yamaguchi S, Inagaki N, Tsuruoka N, Hitoshi Y, Takatsu K. Effect of anti-IL-5 monoclonal antibody on allergic bronchial eosinophil and airway hyperresponsiveness in mice. Life Sci 1993; 53:243–247.
96. Corry DB, Folkesson HG, Warnock ML, Erle DJ, Matthay MA, Wierner-Kronish JP, Locksley RM. Interleukin 4, but not interleukin 5 or eosinophils, is required in a murine model of acute airway hyperreactivity. J Exp Med 1996; 183:109–117.
97. Hogan SP, Matthaei KI, Young JM, Koskinen A, Young IG, Foster PS. A novel T cell-regulated mechanism modulating allergen-induced airways hyperreactivity in BALB/c mice independently of IL-4 and IL-5. J Immunol 1998; 61:1501–1509.
98. Tournoy KG, Kips JC, Schou C, Pauwels RA. Airway eosinophilia is not a requirement for allergen-induced airway hyperresponsiveness. Clin Exp Allergy 2000; 30: 79–85.
99. Ohnishi T, Sur S, Collins DS, Fish JE, Gleich GJ, Peters SP. Eosinophil survival activity identified as interleukin-5 is associated with eosinophil recruitment and degranulation and lung injury twenty-four hours after segmental antigen lung challenge. J Allergy Clin Immunol 1993; 92:607–615.
100. Brunet LR, Sabin EA, Cheever AW, Kopf MA, Pearce EJ. Interleukin 5 (IL-5) is not required for expression of a Th2 response or host resistance mechanisms during murine Schistosomiasis mansoni but does play a role in development of IL-4-producing non-T, non-B cells. Infect Immun 1999; 67:3014–3018.
101. Takamoto M, Ovington KS, Behm CA, Sugane K, Young IG, Matthaei KI. Eosinophilia, parasite burden and lung damage in Toxocara canis infection in C57B1/6 mice genetically deficient in IL-5. Immunology 1997; 90:511–517.
102. Ovington KS, McKie K, Matthaei KI, Young IG, Behm CA. Regulation of primary Strongyloides ratti infections in mice: A role for interleukin-5. Immunology 1998; 95:488–493.
103. Mauser PJ, Pitman AM, Fernandez X, Foran SK, Adams GK III, Kreutner W, Egan RW, Chapman RW. Effects of an antibody to IL-5 in a monkey model of asthma. Am J Respir Crit Care Med 1995; 152:467–472.
104. Gundel RH, Wegner CD, Letts LG. Antigen-induced acute and late-phase responses in primates. Am Rev Respir Dis 1992; 146:369–373.
105. Egan RW, Athwal E, Bodmer MW, Carter JM, Chapman RW, Chou C-C, Cox MA, Emtage JS, Fernandez X, Genatt N, Indelicato SR, Jenh C-H, Kreutner W, Kung TT, Mauser PJ, Minnicozzi M, Murgolo NJ, Narula SK, Petro ME, Schilling A, Sehring S, Stelts D, Stephens S, Taremi SS, Weiner SH, Zavodny PJ, Zurcher J. Effect of SCH 55700, a humanized monoclonal antibody to human interleukin-5, on eosinophilic responses and bronchial hyperreactivity. Arzneimittel-Forschung 1999; 49:779–790.
106. Zia-Amirhosseini P, Minthorn E, Benincosa LJ, Hart TK, Hottenstein CS, Tobia

LAP, Davis CB. Pharmacokinetics and pharmacodynamics of SB-240563, a humanized monoclonal antibody directed to human interleukin-5, in monkeys. J Pharm Exp Ther 1999; 291:1060–1067.

107. Hart TK, Cook RM, Herzyk DJ, Zia-Amirhosseini P, Williams DM, Bugelski PJ. Inhibition of eosinophilia in monkeys with SB-240563, a humanized anti-human IL-5 monoclonal antibody. Am J Respir Crit Care Med 1998; 157:A744.
108. Van Wauwe J, Aerts F, Cools M, Deroose F, Freyne E, Goossens J, Hermans B, Lacrampe J, Van Genechten H, Van Gerven F, Van Nyen G. Identification of R146225 as a novel, orally active inhibitor of interleukin-5 biosynthesis. J Pharmacol Exp Ther 2000; 295:655–661.
109. Cameron L, Christodoulopoulos P, Lavigne F, Nakamura Y, Eidelman D, McEuen A, Walls A, Tavernier J, Minshall E, Moqbel R, Hamid Q. Evidence for local eosinophil differentiation within allergic nasal mucosa: Inhibition with soluble IL-5 receptor. J Immunol 2000; 164:1538–1545.
110. England BP, Balasubramanian P, Uings I, Bethell S, Chen MJ, Schatz PJ, Yin Q, Chen YF, Whitehorn EA, Tsavaler A, Martens CL, Barrett RW, McKinnon M. A potent dimeric peptide antagonist of interleukin-5 that binds two interleukin-5 receptor alpha chains. Proc Natl Acad Sci USA 2000; 97:6862–6867.
111. Lach-Trifilieff E, McKay RA, Monia BP, Karras JG, Walker C. In vitro and in vivo inhibition of interleukin (IL)-5-mediated eosinopoiesis by murine IL-5ralpha antisense oligonucleotide. Am J Respir Cell Mol Biol 2001; 24:116–122.
112. Al-Obeidi FA, Lam KS. Development of inhibitors for protein tyrosine kinases. Oncogene 2000; 19:5690–5701.
113. Van Snick J, Goethals A, Renauld JC, Van Roost E, Uyttenhove C, Rubira MR, Moritz RL, Simpson RJ. Cloning and characterization of a cDNA for a new mouse T cell growth factor (P40). J Exp Med 1989; 169:363–368.
114. Schmitt E, Van Brandwijk R, Van Snick J, Siebold B, Rude E. TCGF III/P40 is produced by naive murine CD4+ T cells but is not a general T cell growth factor. Eur J Immunol 1989; 19:2167–2170.
115. Hultner L, Druez C, Moeller J, Uyttenhove C, Schmitt E, Rude E, Dormer P, Van Snick J. Mast cell growth-enhancing activity (MEA) is structurally related and functionally identical to the novel mouse T cell growth factor P40/TCGFIII (interleukin 9). Eur J Immunol 1990; 20:1413–1416.
116. Renauld JC, Goethals A, Houssiau F, Van Roost E, Van Snick J. Cloning and expression of a cDNA for the human homolog of mouse T cell and mast cell growth factor P40. Cytokine 1990; 2:9–12.
117. Renauld JC, Goethals A, Houssiau F, Merz H, Van Roost E, Van Snick J. Human P40/IL-9. Expression in activated CD4+ T cells, genomic organization, and comparison with the mouse gene. J Immunol 1990; 144:4235–4241.
118. Mock BA, Krall M, Kozak CA, Nesbitt MN, McBride OW, Renauld JC, Van Snick J. IL9 maps to mouse chromosome 13 and human chromosome 5. Immunogenetics 1990; 31:265–270.
119. Renauld JC, Druez C, Kermouni A, Houssiau F, Uyttenhove C, Van Roost E, Van Snick J. Expression cloning of the murine and human interleukin 9 receptor cDNAs. Proc Natl Acad Sci USA 1992; 89:5690–5694.
120. Idzerda RL, March CJ, Mosley B, Lyman SD, Vanden Bos T, Gimpel SD, Din

WS, Grabstein KH, Widmer MB, Park LS, Cosman D, Beckmann MP. Human interleukin 4 receptor confers biological responsiveness and defines a novel receptor superfamily. J Exp Med 1990; 171:861–873.

121. Grasso L, Huang M, Sullivan CD, Messler CJ, Kiser MB, Dragwa CR, Holroyd KJ, Renauld JC, Levitt RC, Nicolaides NC. Molecular analysis of human interleukin-9 receptor transcripts in peripheral blood mononuclear cells. Identification of a splice variant encoding for a nonfunctional cell surface receptor. J Biol Chem 1998; 273: 24016–24024.

122. Russell SM, Johnston JA, Noguchi M, Kawamura M, Bacon CM, Friedmann M, Berg M, McVicar DW, Witthuhn BA, Silvennoinen O, Goldman AS, Schmalstieg FC, Ihle JN, O'Shea JJ, Leonard WJ. Interaction of IL-2R beta and gamma c chains with Jak1 and Jak3: Implications for XSCID and XCID. Science 1994; 266:1042–1045.

123. Demoulin JB, Renauld JC. Interleukin 9 and its receptor: An overview of structure and function. Int Rev Immunol 1998; 16:345–364.

124. Demoulin JB, Uyttenhove C, Van Roost E, DeLestre B, Donckers D, Van Snick J, Renauld JC. A single tyrosine of the interleukin-9 (IL-9) receptor is required for STAT activation, antiapoptotic activity, and growth regulation by IL-9. Mol Cell Biol 1996; 16:4710–4716.

125. Demoulin JB, Van Roost E, Stevens M, Groner B, Renauld JC. Distinct roles for STAT1, STAT3, and STAT5 in differentiation gene induction and apoptosis inhibition by interleukin-9. J Biol Chem 1999; 274:25855–25861.

126. Nicolaides NC, Holroyd KJ, Ewart SL, Eleff SM, Kiser MB, Dragwa CR, Sullivan CD, Grasso L, Zhang LY, Messler CJ, Zhou T, Kleeberger SR, Buetow KH, Levitt RC. Interleukin 9: A candidate gene for asthma. Proc Natl Acad Sci USA 1997; 94:13175–13180.

127. Stassen M, Arnold M, Hultner L, Muller C, Neudorfl C, Reineke T, Schmitt E. Murine bone marrow-derived mast cells as potent producers of IL-9: Costimulatory function of IL-10 and kit ligand in the presence of IL-1. J Immunol 2000; 164: 5549–5555.

128. Hultner L, Kolsch S, Stassen M, Kaspers U, Kremer JP, Mailhammer R, Moeller J, Broszeit H, Schmitt E. In activated mast cells, IL-1 up-regulates the production of several Th2-related cytokines including IL-9. J Immunol 2000; 164:5556–5563.

129. Gounni AS, Nutku E, Koussih L, Aris F, Louahed J, Levitt RC, Nicolaides NC, Hamid Q. IL-9 expression by human eosinophils: Regulation by IL-1beta and TNF-alpha. J Allergy Clin Immunol 2000; 106:460–466.

130. Renauld JC, Kermouni A, Vink A, Louahed J, Van Snick J. Interleukin-9 and its receptor: Involvement in mast cell differentiation and T cell oncogenesis. J Leukoc Biol 1995; 57:353–360.

131. Vink A, Warnier G, Brombacher F, Renauld JC. Interleukin 9-induced in vivo expansion of the B-1 lymphocyte population. J Exp Med 1999; 189:1413–1423.

132. Bourette RP, Royet J, Mouchiroud G, Schmitt E, Blanchet JP. Murine interleukin 9 stimulates the proliferation of mouse erythroid progenitor cells and favors the erythroid differentiation of multipotent FDCP-mix cells. Exp Hematol 1992; 20: 868–873.

133. Dong Q, Louahed J, Vink A, Sullivan CD, Messler CJ, Zhou Y, Haczku A, Huaux

F, Arras M, Holroyd KJ, Renauld JC, Levitt RC, Nicolaides NC. IL-9 induces chemokine expression in lung epithelial cells and baseline airway eosinophilia in transgenic mice. Eur J Immunol 1999; 29:2130–2139.
134. Godfraind C, Louahed J, Faulkner H, Vink A, Warnier G, Grencis R, Renauld JC. Intraepithelial infiltration by mast cells with both connective tissue-type and mucosal-type characteristics in gut, trachea, and kidneys of IL-9 transgenic mice. J Immunol 1998; 160:3989–3996.
135. Temann UA, Geba GP, Rankin JA, Flavell RA. Expression of interleukin 9 in the lungs of transgenic mice causes airway inflammation, mast cell hyperplasia, and bronchial hyperresponsiveness. J Exp Med 1998; 188:1307–1320.
136. Petit-Frere C, Dugas B, Braquet P, Mencia-Huerta JM. Interleukin-9 potentiates the interleukin-4-induced IgE and IgG1 release from murine B lymphocytes. Immunology 1993; 79:146–151.
137. Dugas B, Renauld JC, Pene J, Bonnefoy JY, Peti-Frere C, Braquet P, Bousquet J, Van Snick J, Mencia-Huerta JM. Interleukin-9 potentiates the interleukin-4-induced immunoglobulin (IgG, IgM and IgE) production by normal human B lymphocytes. Eur J Immunol 1993; 23:1687–1692.
138. Levitt RC, McLane MP, MacDonald D, Ferrante V, Weiss C, Zhou T, Holroyd KJ, Nicolaides NC. IL-9 pathway in asthma: New therapeutic targets for allergic inflammatory disorders. J Allergy Clin Immunol 1999; 103:S485–S491.
139. McLane MP, Haczku A, van de Rijn M, Weiss C, Ferrante V, MacDonald D, Renauld JC, Nicolaides NC, Holroyd KJ, Levitt RC. Interleukin-9 promotes allergen-induced eosinophilic inflammation and airway hyperresponsiveness in transgenic mice. Am J Respir Cell Mol Biol 1998; 19:713–720.
140. Louahed J, Zhou Y, Maloy WL, Rani PU, Weiss C, Tomer Y, Vink A, Renauld JC, Van Snick J, Nicolaides NC, Levitt RC, Haczku A. Interleukin 9 promotes influx and local maturation of eosinophils. Blood 2001; 97:1035–1042.
141. Longphre M, Li D, Gallup M, Drori E, Ordonez CL, Redman T, Wenzel S, Bice DE, Fahy JV, Basbaum C. Allergen-induced IL-9 directly stimulates mucin transcription in respiratory epithelial cells. J Clin Invest 1999; 104:1375–1382.
142. Louahed J, Toda M, Jen J, Hamid Q, Renauld JC, Levitt RC, Nicolaides NC. Interleukin-9 upregulates mucus expression in the airways. Am J Respir Cell Mol Biol 2000; 22:649–656.
143. Holroyd KJ, Martinati LC, Trabetti E, Scherpbier T, Eleff SM, Boner AL, Pignatti PF, Kiser MB, Dragwa CR, Hubbard F, Sullivan CD, Grasso L, Messler CJ, Huang M, Hu Y, Nicolaides NC, Buetow KH, Levitt RC. Asthma and bronchial hyperresponsiveness linked to the XY long arm pseudoautosomal region. Genomics 1998; 52:233–235.
144. Bhathena PR, Comhair SA, Holroyd KJ, Erzurum SC. Interleukin-9 receptor expression in asthmatic airways in vivo. Lung 2000; 178:149–160.
145. Shimbara A, Christodoulopoulos P, Soussi-Gounni A, Olivenstein R, Nakamura Y, Levitt RC, Nicolaides NC, Holroyd KJ, Tsicopoulos A, Lafitte JJ, Wallaert B, Hamid QA. IL-9 and its receptor in allergic and nonallergic lung disease: Increased expression in asthma. J Allergy Clin Immunol 2000; 1051:108–115.
146. Rosenwasser LJ. Promoter polymorphism in the candidate genes, IL-4, IL-9, TGF-beta1, for atopy and asthma. Int Arch Allergy Immunol 1999; 118:268–270.

147. Townsend JM, Fallon GP, Matthews JD, Smith P, Jolin EH, McKenzie NA. IL-9 deficient mice establish fundamental roles for IL-9 in pulmonary mastocytosis and goblet cell hyperplasia but not T cell development. Immunity 2000; 13:573–583.
148. Kung TT, Luo B, Crawley Y, Garlisi CG, Sheridon K, Minnicozzi M, Egan RW, Kreutner W, Chapman RW. Effect of anti-mIL-9 antibody on the development of pulmonary inflammation and airway hyperresponsiveness in allergic mice. Am J Respir Cell Mol Biol 2001; 25:600–605.
149. Fiorentino DF, Bond M, Mosmann TR. Two types of mouse helper T cell. IV. Th2 clones secrete a factor that inhibits cytokine production by Th1 clones. J Exp Med 1989; 170:2081–2095.
150. Vieira P, de Waal-Malefyt R, Dang MN, Johnson KE, Kastelein R, Fiorentino DF, de Vries JE, Roncarolo MG, Mosmann TR, Moore KW. Isolation and expression of human cytokine synthesis inhibitory factor cDNA clones: Homology to Epstein-Barr virus open reading frame BCRFI. Proc Natl Acad Sci USA 1990; 88:1172–1176.
151. Kim JM, Brannan CI, Copeland NG, Jenkins NA, Khan TA, Moore KW. Structure of the mouse IL-10 gene and chromosomal localization of the mouse and human genes. J Immunol 1992; 148:3618–3623.
152. Moore KV, Vieira P, Fiorentino DF, Trounstine ML, Khan TA, Mosmann TR. Homology of cytokine synthesis inhibitor factor (IL-10) to the Epstein-Barr virus gene BCRFI. Science 1990; 248:1230–1234.
153. Ho AS-Y, Liu Y, Khan TA, Hsu DH, Bazan JF, Moore KW. A receptor in interleukin-10 is related to interferon receptors. Proc Natl Acad Sci USA 1993; 90:11267–11271.
154. Liu Y, Wei SH-Y, Ho AS-Y, de Waal-Malefyt R, Moore KW. Expression cloning and characterization of a human interleukin-10 receptor. J Immunol 1994; 152: 1821–1829.
155. Kotenko S, Krause C, Izotova LS, Pollack BP, Wu W, Pestka S. Identification and function characterization of a second chain of the interleukin-10 receptor complex. EMBO J 1997; 16:5894–5903.
156. Riley JK, Takeda K, Akira S, Schreiber RD. Interleukin-10 receptor signaling through the JAK-STAT pathway. Requirement for two distinct receptor-derived signals for anti-inflammatory action. J Biol Chem 1999; 27:16513–16521.
157. Ding Y, Qin L, Tarcsafalvi A, Kotenko S, Pestka S, Moore K, Bromberg JS. Differential IL-10R1 expression plays a critical role in IL-10-mediated immune regulation. J Immunol 2001; 167:6884–6892.
158. O'Garra A, Stapleton G, Dhar V, Pearce M, Schumacher J, Rugo H, Barbis D, Stall A, Cupp J, Moore K. Production of cytokines by mouse B cells: B lymphomas and normal B cells produce interleukin-10. Int Immunol 1990; 2:821–832.
159. Enk AH, Katz SI. Identification and induction of keratinocyte-derived IL-10. J Immunol 1992; 149:92–95.
160. Fiorentino DF, Zlotnik A, Mosmann TR, Howard M, O'Garra A. IL-10 inhibits cytokine production by activated macrophages. J Immunol 1991; 147:3815–3822.
161. Bonfield TL, Konstan MW, Burfeind P, Panuska JR, Hilliard JB, Berger M. Normal bronchial epithelial cells constitutively produce the anti-inflammatory cytokine IL-10 which is down-regulated in cystic fibrosis. Am J Respir Cell Mol Biol 1995; 13:257–261.

162. de Waal-Malefyt R, Abrams J, Bennett B, Figdor CG, de Vries JE. IL-10 inhibits cytokine synthesis by human monocytes: An autoregulatory role of IL-10 produced by monocytes. J Exp Med 1991; 174:1209–1220.
163. Smith SR, Terminelli C, Kenworthy-Bott L, Calzetta A, Donkin J. The cooperative effects of TNF-alpha and IFN-gamma are determining factors in the ability of IL-10 to protect mice from lethal endotoxemia. J Leukoc Biol 1994; 55:711–718.
164. Howard M, Muchamuel T, Andrade S. Interleukin 10 protects mice from lethal endotoxemia. J Exp Med 1993; 177:1205–1208.
165. Gerard C, Bruyns C, Marchant A, Abramowicz D, Vandenabeele P, Delvaux A, Fiers W, Goldman M, Velu T. IL-10 reduces the release of tumor necrosis factor and prevents lethality in experimental endotoxemia. J Exp Med 1993; 177:547–550.
166. de Waal-Malefyt R, Haanen J, Spits H, Roncarolo MG, te Velde A, Figdor C, Johnson K, Kastelein R, Yssel H, de Vries JE. IL-10 and viral IL-10 strongly reduce antigen-specific human T cell proliferation by diminishing the antigen-pressenting capacity of monocytes via downregulation of class II MHC expression. J Exp Med 1991; 174:915–924.
167. Fiorentino DF, Zlotnik A, Vieira P, Mosmann TR, Howard M, Moore KW, O'Garra A. IL-10 acts on the antigen presenting cell to inhibit cytokine production by Th1 cells. J Immunol 1991; 146:3444–3451.
168. Bazzoni F, Cassatella MA, Rossi F, Ceska M, Dewald B, Baggiolini M. Phagocytosing neutrophils produce and release high amounts of the neutrophil activating peptide 1/interleukin 8. J Exp Med 1991; 173:771–774.
169. Schandene L, Alonso-Vega C, Willems F, Gerard C, Delvaux A, Velu T, Devos R, de Boer M, Goldman M. B7/CD28-dependent IL-5 production by human resting T cells is inhibited by IL-10. J Immunol 1994; 152:4368–4374.
170. Takanaski S, Nonaka R, Xing Z, O'Byrne P, Dolovich J, Jordana M. Interleukin 10 inhibits lipopolysaccharide-induced survival and cytokine production by human peripheral blood eosinophils. J Exp Med 1994; 179:711–715.
171. Rousset F, Garcia E, DeFrance T, Peronne C, Vezzio N, Hsu DH, Kastelein R, Moore KW, Banchereau J. Interleukin-10 is a potent growth and differentiation factor for activated human B cells. Proc Natl Acad Sci USA 1992; 89:1890–1893.
172. Chen W-F, Zlotnik A. IL-10: A novel cytotoxic T cell differentiation factor. J Immunol 1991; 47:528–534.
173. Schwarz M, Hamilton L, Tardelli L, Narula S, Sullivan L. Stimulation of cytolytic activity by interleukin-10. J Immunother 1994; 16:95–104.
174. Kuhn R, Lohler J, Rennick D, Rajewsky K, Muller W. Interleukin-10 deficient mice develop chronic enterocolitis. Cell 1993; 75:263–274.
175. Berg DJ, Davidson N, Kuhn R, Muller W, Menon S, Holland G, Thompson-Snipes L, Leach MW, Rennick D. Enterocolitis and colon cancer in interleukin-10-deficient mice are associated with aberrant cytokine production and CD4+ TH1-like responses. J Clin Invest 1996; 98:1010–1020.
176. Powrie F, Leach MW, Mauze S, Menon S, Caddle LB, Coffman RL. Inhibition of Th1 responses prevents inflammatory bowel disease in SCID mice reconstituted with CD45 RB high CD-4+ T cells. Immunity 1994; 1:553–562.
177. Davidson NJ, Leach MW, Fort MM, Thompson-Snipes L, Kuhn W, Berg DJ, Ren-

nick DM. T helper cell 1-type CD 4+ T cells, but not B cells, mediate colitis in interleukin 10-deficient mice. J Exp Med 1996; 184:241–251.

178. Zuany-Amorim C, Haile S, Leduc D, Dumarey C, Huerre M, Vargaftig BB, Pretolani M. Interleukin-10 inhibits antigen-induced cellular recruitment into the airways of sensitized mice. J Clin Invest 1995; 95:2644–2651.

179. van Scott MR, Justice JP, Bradfield JF, Enright E, Sigounas A, Sur S. IL-10 reduces TH2 cytokine production and eosinophilia but augments airway reactivity in allergic mice. Am J Physiol Lung Cell Mol Physiol 2000; 278:L667–L674.

180. Stampfli MR, Cwiartka M, Gajewska BU, Alvarez D, Ritz SA, Inman MD, Xing Z, Jordana M. Interleukin-10 gene transfer to the airway regulates allergic mucosal sensitization in mice. Am J Respir Cell Mol Biol 1999; 21:586–596.

181. Tournoy KG, Kips JC, Pauwels RA. Endogenous interleukin-10 suppresses allergen-induced airway inflammation and nonspecific airway responsiveness. Clin Exp Allergy 2000; 30:775–783.

182. Yang X, Wang S, Fan Y, Han X. IL-10 deficiency prevents IL-5 overproduction and eosinophilic inflammation in a murine model of asthma-like reaction. Eur J Immunol 2000; 30:382–391.

183. Makela MJ, Kanehiro A, Borish L, Dakhama A, Loader J, Joetham A, Xing Z, Jordana M, Larsen GL, Gelfand EW. IL-10 is necessary for the expression of airway hyperresponsiveness but not pulmonary inflammation after allergic sensitization. Proc Natl Acad Sci USA 2000; 23:97:6007–6012.

184. Borish L, Aarons A, Rumbyrt J, Cvietusa P, Negri J, Wenzel S. Interleukin-10 regulation in normal subjects and patients with asthma. J Allergy Clin Immunol 1996; 97:1288–1296.

185. Tormey VJ, Leonard C, Faul J, Bernard S, Burke CM, Poulter LW. Dysregulation of monocyte differentiation in asthmatic subjects is reversed by IL-10. Clin Exp Allergy 1998; 28:992–998.

186. John M, Lim S, Seybold J, Jose P, Robichaud A, O'Connor B, Barnes PJ, Chung KF. Inhaled corticosteroids increase interleukin-10 but reduce macrophage inflammatory protein-1 alpha, granulocyte-macrophage colony-stimulating factor, and interferon-gamma release from alveolar macrophages in asthma. Am J Respir Crit Care Med 1998; 157:256–262.

187. Zeibecoglou K, Ying S, Meng Q, Poulter LW, Robinson DS, Kay AB. Macrophage subpopulations and macrophage-derived cytokines in sputum of atopic and nonatopic asthmatic subjects and atopic and normal control subjects. J Allergy Clin Immunol 2000; 106:697–704.

188. Colavita AM, Hastie AT, Musani AI, Pascual RM, Reinach AJ, Lustine HT, Galati SA, Zangrilli JG, Fish JE, Peters SP. Kinetics of IL-10 production after segmental antigen challenge of atopic asthmatic subjects. J Allergy Clin Immunol 2000; 106:880–886.

189. Lim S, Crawley E, Woo P, Barnes PJ. Haplotype associated with low interleukin-10 production in patients with severe asthma. Lancet 1998; 352:113.

190. Hobbs K, Negri J, Klinnert M, Rosenwasser LJ, Borish L. Interleukin-10 and transforming growth factor-beta promoter polymorphisms in allergies and asthma. Am J Respir Crit Care Med 1998; 158:1958–1962.

191. Takanashi S, Hasegawa Y, Kanehira Y, Yamamoto K, Fujimoto K, Satoh K, Oka-

mura K. Interleukin-10 level in sputum is reduced in bronchial asthma, COPD and in smokers. Eur Respir J 1999; 14:309–314.

192. Radwanski E, Chakraborty A, Van Wart S, Huhn RD, Cutler DL, Affrime MB, Jusko WJ. Pharmacokinetics and leukocyte responses of recombinant human interleukin-10. Pharm Res 1998; 15:1895–1901.
193. Huhn RD, Radwanski E, Gallo J, Affrime MB, Sabo R, Gonyo G, Monge A, Cutler DL. Pharmacodynamics of subcutaneous recombinant human interleukin-10 in healthy volunteers. Clin Pharmacol Ther 1997; 62:171–180.
194. Huhn RD, Pennline K, Radwanski E, Clarke L, Sabo R, Cutler DL. Effects of single intravenous doses of recombinant human interleukin-10 on subsets of circulating leukocytes in humans. Immunopharmacology 1999; 41:109–117.
195. Pajkrt D, Camoglio L, Tiel-van Buul MC, de Bruin D, Cutler DL, Affrime MB, Rikken G, van der Poll T, ten Cate JW, van Deventer SJ. Attenuation of proinflammatory response by recombinant human IL-10 in human endotoxemia: Effect of timing of recombinant human IL-10 administration. J Immunol 1997; 158:3971–3977.
196. Bryan SA, O' Connor BJ, Matti S, Leckie MJ, Kanabar V, Khan J, Warrington SJ, Renzetti L, Rames A, Bock JA, Boyce MJ, Hansel TT, Holgate ST, Barnes PJ. Effects of recombinant human interleukin-12 on eosinophils, airway hyper-responsiveness, and the late asthmatic response. Lancet 2000; 356:2149–2153.

8

Therapeutic Targeting of Chemokines and Chemokine Receptors

NIVES ZIMMERMANN

Children's Hospital Medical Center
Cincinnati, Ohio

MARC E. ROTHENBERG

University of Cincinnati College of Medicine
and Children's Hospital Medical Center
Cincinnati, Ohio

I. Introduction

One of the hallmarks of asthma is the accumulation of an abnormally large number of leukocytes including eosinophils, neutrophils, lymphocytes, basophils, and macrophages in the lung (1). There is now substantial evidence that inflammatory cells are major effector cells in the pathogenesis of asthma. Therefore, understanding the mechanisms by which leukocytes accumulate is of fundamental relevance to allergic diseases. Another characteristic of allergic inflammation is the activation of leukocytes, resulting in the release of biologically active mediators such as histamine from mast cells and basophils. It is now apparent that chemokines are potent leukocyte chemoattractants, cellular activating factors, histamine-releasing factors, and regulators of homeostatic immunity, making them particularly important in the pathogenesis of airway inflammation in asthma (2). In this regard, chemokines are attractive new therapeutic targets for the treatment of allergic disease. This chapter focuses on recently emerging data on the importance of chemokines and their receptors in allergic airway inflammation as well as on the potential for pharmacologically targeting these pathways.

II. Chemokine Family

Chemokines are a large family of chemotactic cytokines that have been divided into four groups, designated CXC, CC, C, and CX3C, depending upon the spacing of conserved cysteines (where X is any amino acid) (Fig. 1). The CXC and CC groups, in contrast to the C and CX3C chemokines, contain many members and have been studied in greatest detail. The CXC chemokines mainly target neutrophils whereas the CC chemokines target a variety of cell types including macrophages, eosinophils, and basophils. Owing to the complexity of the system, a new nomenclature has recently been proposed (3). This nomenclature is based on the chemokine receptor nomenclature currently used, which uses CC, CXC, XC, or CX3C (to designate the chemokine group) followed by R (for receptor) and then a number. The new chemokine nomenclature substitutes the R with L (for ligand), and the number is derived from the one already assigned to the gene encoding the chemokine from the small secreted cytokine (SCY) nomenclature. Thus, a given gene has the same number as its protein ligand (for example, the gene encoding eotaxin-1 is SCYA11 and the chemokine is referred to as CCL11). Table 1 summarizes the chemokine family utilizing this nomenclature.

This review concentrates on CC chemokines because the members of this family primarily stimulate the movement of cells associated with allergic responses (including eosinophils, basophils, T cells, and monocytes). CC chemokines are divided into several structure subgroups including a group composed of the macrophage chemoattractant proteins (MCPs) and eotaxin (also known as eotaxin-1) (4) (Fig. 1). Members of the MCP and eotaxin subfamily of chemokines share structural and functional features and have been strongly implicated in asthma and other allergic diseases. The four human MCP proteins (MCP-1,

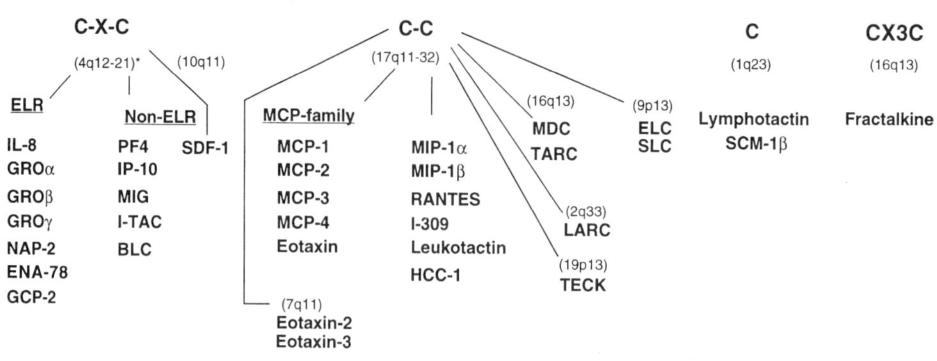

Figure 1 Human chemokine family. The chromosomal position in the human genome is indicated in parentheses.

Table 1 Chemokine Ligands[a]

Systematic name	Human ligand	Mouse ligand
CXC family		
CXCL1	GROα/MGSA-α	GRO/KC?*
CXCL2	GROβ/MGSA-β	GRO/KC?
CXCL3	GROγ/MGSA-γ	GRO/KC?
CXCL4	PF4	PF4
CXCL5	ENA-78	LIX?
CXCL6	GCP-2	Ckα-3
CXCL7	NAP-2	?
CXCL8	IL-8	?
CXCL9	Mig	Mig
CXCL10	IP-10	IP-10
CXCL11	I-TAC	?
CXCL12	SDF-1α/B	SDF-1
CXCL13	BLC/BCA-1	BLC/BCA-1
CXCL14	BRAK/bolekine	BRAK
CXCL15	?	Lungkine
CC family		
CCL1	I-309	TCA-3, P500
CCL2	MCP-1/MCAF	JE ?
CCL3	MIP-1α/LD78α	MIP-1α
CCL4	MIP-1β	MIP-1β
CCL5	RANTES	RANTES
CCL6	?	C10, MRP-1
CCL7	MCP-3	MARC?
CCL8	MCP-2	MCP-2?
CCL9/10	?	MRP-2, CCF18, MIP-1γ
CCL11	Eotaxin	Eotaxin
CCL12	?	MCP-5
CCL13	MCP-4	?
CCL14	HCC-1	?
CCL15	HCC-2/Lkn-1/MIP-1δ	?
CCL16	HCC-4/LEC	LCC-1
CCL17	TARC	TARC
CCL18	DC-CK1/PARC/AMAC-1	?
CCL19	MIP-3β/ELC/exodus-3	MIP-3β/ELC/exodus-3
CCL20	MIP-3α/LARC/exodus-1	MIP-3α/LARC/exodus-1
CCL21	6Ckine/SLC/exodus-2	6Ckine/SLC/exodus-2/TCA-4
CCL22	MDC/STCP-1	ABCD-1
CCL23	MPIF-1	?
CCL24	MPIF-2/Eotaxin-2	Eotaxin-2
CCL25	TECK	TECK
CCL26	Eotaxin-3	?
CCL27	CTACK/ILC	ALP/CTACK/ILC/ESkine
CCL28	MEC	MEC
C family		
XCL1	Lymphotactin/SCM-1α/ATAC	Lymphotactin
XCL2	SCM-1β	?
CX3C family		
CX3CL1	Fractalkine	Neurotactin

[a] A question mark indicates that the mouse and human homologs are ambiguous.

-2, -3, -4) share ~65% amino acid identity. In addition, eotaxin-1 also shares ~65% amino acid identity with the MCP proteins. Comparison of the amino acid sequences has revealed some striking similarities and differences in this family of chemokines. For example, all members of this family have a highly conserved 23-amino-acid leader sequence. In addition to the four conserved cysteines, several other residues are highly conserved between all members of the family, such as the serine-tyrosine residues between the second and third cysteines and the region around the fourth cysteine (4). In contrast to the majority of the MCPs, eotaxin-1 and murine MCP-3 contain one- to five-amino-acid gaps resulting in a shorter amino terminus preceding the first cysteine in the mature protein. Recently, human and murine eotaxin-2 and human eotaxin-3 have been cloned (5–9). Although eotaxin-2 and eotaxin-3 share only ~35% amino acid identity with eotaxin-1 and the MCP proteins, a phylogenetic tree analysis has placed them in the MCP branch of CC chemokines (8).

A. Three-Dimensional Structure

Although members of the different chemokine subfamilies have only weak homology and display nonoverlapping receptor binding, investigations solving the three-dimensional structure of chemokines have revealed that they share the same basic characteristics (10–14). A disordered amino terminus is linked to the rest of the molecule by the two amino-terminal cysteines. This is followed by an extended loop that leads into three antiparallel β-pleated sheets, which provides a flat base over which the carboxy-terminal α helix lies.

B. Genomic Organization

Chemokines have a conserved intron–exon structure generally organized into three exons and two introns (15–18). For example, in the MCP/eotaxin subfamily, the positions of the splice sites within the codons is conserved, suggesting that this subfamily arose from a common ancestral gene. In support of this concept, related chemokines are located in a similar chromosomal position (Fig. 1), suggesting that chemokine diversity may be the product of gene duplication. For example, most CXC chemokines are located on human chromosome 4q in two separate clusters: CXC chemokines that mainly act on neutrophils (through receptors CXCR1 and CXCR2) are clustered at 4q12–13, and those highly specific for T lymphocytes (ligands of CXCR3, such as monokine induced by interferon gamma (MIG), 10 kDa interferon-inducible protein (IP-10), and interferon-inducible T-cell alpha chemoattractant (I-TAC), are located in a separate minicluster at 4q21. Additionally, most CC chemokines are located on human chromosome 17q11–32. The MCPs and eotaxin were found to be contained on the same yeast artificial chromosome clone containing human chromosome 17q11 (19). According to the National Center for Biotechnology Information (NCBI;

www.ncbi.nlm.nih.gov), 11 of the CC chemokine genes are clustered within 2 Mbp on human chromosome 17q11. In distinction to other CC chemokines, eotaxin-2 and eotaxin-3 have been mapped to human 7q11.23 (8,20).

C. Regulation of Chemokine Production and Activity

The main stimuli for secretion of chemokines are the early proinflammatory cytokines, such as interleukin-1 (IL-1) and tumor necrosis factor alpha (TNF-α), bacterial products such as lipopolysaccharide (LPS), and viral infection (21–23). In addition, products of both Th1 and Th2 cells, interferon-gamma (IFN-γ) and IL-4, respectively, can also induce the production of chemokines independently and in synergy with IL-1 and TNF-α. Although there are many similarities in the regulation of chemokines, important differences that may have implications for asthma are beginning to be appreciated. For example, in the healthy lung, epithelial cells are the primary source of chemokines; however, in the inflamed lung infiltrating cells within the submucosa are a major cellular source of chemokines (24). Furthermore, the induced expression of eotaxin and MCP-4 by TNF-α or IL-1 treatment of epithelial cells is suppressed by the steroid dexamethasone (25). This may be relevant to the clinical effectiveness of inhaled glucocorticoids at decreasing the eosinophil-rich inflammatory exudate characteristically seen in the respiratory tract of individuals with asthma. Recent studies have shown that the selectivity and production of chemokines can be regulated by a concentration-dependent mechanism. For example, TNF-α is a potent inducer of a variety of chemokines including RANTES (regulated upon activation, normal T cell expressed and secreted), MCP-4, and eotaxin. However, the level of TNF-α required to activate RANTES production (>100 U/mL) is 100-fold higher than is required to activate MCP-4 and eotaxin production (23,25,26). Various proinflammatory mediators also possess the ability to regulate chemokine production by modulation in a cell-specific manner. For example, IL-3 activates eotaxin production in eosinophils (22), and IgE cross-linking activates mast cells to produce MCP-3 (27).

Chemokines also undergo substantial post-translational modification, which can influence their biological activity and function. For example, the CXC chemokines connective tissue-activating peptide (CTAP)-III, β-thromboglobulin, and neutrophil-activating protein-2 (NAP-2) arise from the amino-terminal processing of a common precursor platelet basic protein. Furthermore, mature chemokines may also undergo enzymatic modification, which results in the generation of chemokine derivatives with unique receptor usage and functional activity. For example, cleavage of the first two amino acids of RANTES by dipeptidyl peptidase IV (CD26) results in a truncated form of RANTES that loses its functional activity on CCR1 but retains it on CCR5 (28). Additionally, modification of eotaxin-1 by CD26 results in a truncated eotaxin-1 that is not capable of transmitting positive signals through CCR3 but can desensitize the receptor to subsequent signaling by intact eotaxin-1 (29). Interestingly, infectious organisms appear to have developed pathways to metabolize chemokines. For example, products of the parasite *Necator americanus* enzymatically inactivate eotaxin-1 (30). This process may be a mechanism to curtail antihelminth immunity (30).

D. Chemokine Promoter Analysis

Analysis of the 5′ flanking regions of most chemokines reveals several conserved regulatory elements that may explain the observed regulation of the chemokine genes by cytokines and glucocorticoids (17,31). Of note, nuclear factor (NF)-κB, glucocorticoid response element (GRE), gamma interferon response element (γIRE), Sp1, and E2A binding site motifs are well conserved in both human and mouse chemokine promoters. For example, the eotaxin promoter in mice and humans has NF-κB and signal transducer and activator of transcription (STAT)-6 sequences; mutation of the NF-κB and STAT-6 site impairs eotaxin promoter activity in response to TNF-α and IL-4, respectively (32). NF-κB is a nuclear factor that is activated following stimulation of cells with various immunological agents such as LPS, IL-1, and TNF-α. NF-κB has been shown to be important for the transcriptional activation of selected chemokines. For example, a single NF-κB binding site is essential for TNF-α- and IL-1-induced expression of the MCP-1 (33) and growth-regulated oncogene-α (GRO-α) (34) genes and LPS-induced expression of the macrophage inflammatory protein (MIP)-2 gene (35). GRE mediates glucocorticoid regulation of transcription (36). Interestingly, IL-5, an eosinophil-specific growth and differentiation factor, and the chemokine IL-8 also contain a GRE sequence in their promoters. Furthermore, deletion analysis of the GRE from the IL-8 promoter revealed that this element participated in dexamethasone suppression of IL-8 expression (37). In vitro, the glucocorticoid budesonide inhibits eotaxin promoter-driven reporter gene activity and accelerates the decay of eotaxin mRNA (38). These studies indicate that glucocorticoids inhibit chemokine expression through multiple mechanisms of action. Finally, Bcl-6 appears to be a repressor of the transcription of several chemokines in vitro, including MCP-1, MCP-3, and macrophage inflammatory protein-related protein-1 (MRP-1) (39). This correlates in vivo with the STAT-6-independent Th2-type inflammation found in Bcl-6-deficient mice, thus providing a potential novel mechanism for the regulation of Th2-type inflammation.

III. Chemokine Receptor Family

Chemokines induce leukocyte migration and activation by binding to specific G protein-coupled seven-transmembrane-spanning cell-surface receptors (GPCRs) (40). Although chemokine receptors are similar to many GPCRs, they have unique structural motifs such as the amino acid sequence DRYLAIV in the second intracellular domain (40,41). Five CXCR receptors have been identified, which are referred to as CXCR1–CXCR5 and 11 human CC chemokine receptor genes have been cloned, which are known as CCR1–CCR11. The chemokine and leukocyte selectivity of chemokine receptors overlap extensively; a given leukocyte often expresses multiple chemokine receptors, and more than one chemokine typically binds to the same receptor (Fig. 2). For example, monocytes express the CC chemokine receptors CCR1, CCR2, CCR4, and CCR5; eosinophils express CCR1 and CCR3; and basophils express CCR1, CCR2, and CCR3. All of the MCP proteins characterized to date are ligands for CCR2. In addition, MCP-2, -3, and -4 are also ligands for CCR3. In contrast, the eotaxin chemokines signal only through CCR3.

Further complexity is added in that chemokine receptors can be constitutively expressed on some cells, whereas they are inducible on others. For example, CCR1 and CCR2 are constitutively expressed on monocytes but are expressed on lymphocytes only following IL-2 stimulation (42,43). Activated lymphocytes are then responsive to multiple CC chemokines that use these receptors, including the MCPs. In addition, some constitutive receptors can be downmodulated by biological response modifiers. For example, IL-10 modifies the

CCR1	CCR2	CCR3	CCR4	CCR5	CCR6	CCR7	CCR8	CCR9	CCR10	CCR11
CCL3 CCL5 CCL7 CCL14 CCL15 CCL23	CCL2 CCL7 CCL8 CCL13	CCL5 CCL7 CCL8 CCL11 CCL13 CCL15 CCL24 CCL26 CCL28	CCL17 CCL22	CCL3 CCL4 CCL5	CCL20	CCL19 CCL21	CCL1	CCL25	CCL27 CCL28	CCL2 CCL7 CCL8 CCL13 CCL11

(a)

CXCR1	CXCR2	CXCR3	CXCR4	CXCR5
CXCL6 CXCL8	CXCL1 CXCL2 CXCL3 CXCL5 CXCL6 CXCL7 CXCL8	CXCL9 CXCL10 CXCL11	CXCL12	CXCL13

(b)

Figure 2 Ligands for (a) CC and (b) CXC receptor families.

activity of CCR1, CCR2, and CCR5 on dendritic cells and monocytes (44). Normally, dendritic cells mature in response to inflammatory stimuli and shift from expressing CCR1, CCR2, and CCR5 to expressing CCR7. However, IL-10 blocks the chemokine receptor switch. Notably, although CCR1, CCR2, and CCR5 remain detectable on the cell surface and bind appropriate ligands, they do not signal in calcium mobilization and chemotaxis assays. Thus, IL-10 converts chemokine receptors to functional decoy receptors, thereby serving a downregulatory function.

Chemokines have two main sites for interaction with their receptors: one in the amino-terminal region and the other in the exposed loop of the backbone between the second and third cysteine (45). Site-directed mutagenesis has indicated that the loop region is important for receptor binding and the amino terminus is important for receptor activation (46–48). Based on these observations, a "two-step" model has been proposed for chemokine receptor activation (47,49–51). In the first step, the loop region of the chemokine binds to the amino-terminal region of the receptor. In the second step, the amino terminus of the chemokine binds to a second site on the receptor, presumably located between or close to the transmembrane helices, inducing a conformational change of the receptor and consequent transmembrane signaling. In addition to mutagenesis studies, the first step of this model is supported by observations of direct interaction of the CXC chemokine IL-8, the CX3C chemokine fractalkine, and CC chemokines eotaxin-1 and eotaxin-2, with peptides corresponding to the N-terminal regions of their respective receptors (14,52–54).

A. Eosinophil Chemokine Receptors

Because eosinophilia is a hallmark feature of allergic inflammation, a large body of research has focused on the analysis of chemokine receptors and signaling pathways on eosinophils. Eosinophils from most healthy donors express CCR3 at the highest level (4,55,56) and have significantly lower levels of CCR1 (Fig. 3). Consistent with the expression of CCR1 and CCR3, eosinophils respond to MIP-1α, RANTES, MCP-2, MCP-3, MCP-4, eotaxin-1, eotaxin-2, and eotaxin-3. Leukotactin (HCC2) has been demonstrated to be a ligand for CCR1 and CCR3, but its activity on eosinophils has not yet been reported (57,58). CCR3 appears to function as the predominant eosinophil chemokine receptor because CCR3 ligands are generally more potent eosinophil chemoattractants. Furthermore, an inhibitory monoclonal antibody specific for CCR3 blocks the activity of RANTES, a chemokine that could signal through CCR1 or CCR3 in eosinophils (59). Additionally, cytokine-primed human eosinophils respond to IL-8 (60), and eosinophils have the capacity to express CXCR2, the low affinity IL-8 receptor, when they are cultured in IL-5 (59). IL-5 also primes eosinophils to respond to CCR3 ligands (61). The mechanism by which IL-5 primes the response of eosinophils to chemotactic signals remains to be elucidated, because

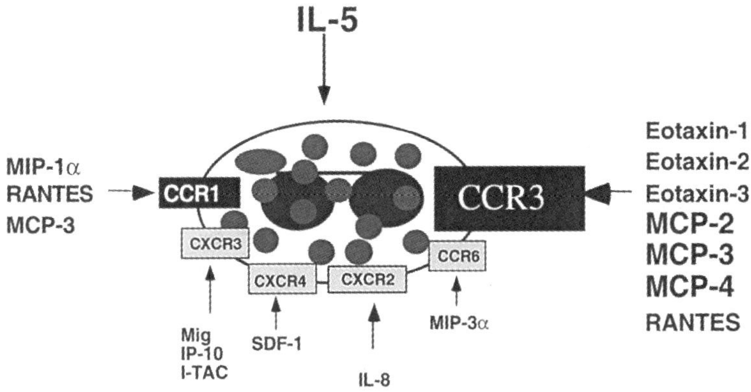

Figure 3 Eosinophil chemokine receptors and some of their ligands. The main chemokine receptors on eosinophils (CCR1 and CCR3) are depicted with black rectangles. Other chemokine receptors present on eosinophil subpopulations or under select conditions are shown in gray rectangles. Representative corresponding ligands are shown. IL-5 is also indicated because this chemokine primes eosinophils to respond to chemokines.

IL-5 does not merely increase the expression of CCR3 on mature eosinophils. Finally, eosinophils have recently been shown to express or respond to ligands of CCR6, CXCR3, and CXCR4 (62–64). For instance, eosinophils isolated from allergic donors responded to MIP-3α in chemotaxis and calcium mobilization assays; FACS analysis reveals that ~20% of eosinophils express low levels of CCR6. Notably, eosinophils isolated from nonallergic donors fail to respond to MIP-3α (62). In contrast, 50% of eosinophils from nonallergic donors express CXCR3 by FACS analysis, and these cells respond in functional assays. Interestingly, IL-2 is capable of upregulating CXCR3 on the nonexpressing eosinophils, and IL-10 completely downregulates the receptor on cells already expressing CXCR3 (64). Additionally, eosinophils isolated from nonallergic donors express CXCR4 on their surface following incubation in vitro for 24 h at 37°C. Notably, incubation of eosinophils in the presence of IL-4 or IL-5 inhibits the increase in CXCR4 expression (63). Additionally, dexamethasone specifically upregulates the expression of CXCR4 on eosinophils (65), and cells expressing CXCR4 respond in functional assays to stromal cell derived factor-1 alpha (SDF-1α), the ligand for CXCR4. The significance of these chemokine receptors in eosinophil accumulation in health and disease remains to be elucidated.

B. Signal Transduction

Chemokine receptor signal transduction mechanisms have not been extensively examined, and most studies have been conducted in nonhematopoietic cells transfected with chemokine receptors (40). Chemokine receptors are, for the most part, inhibited by pertussis toxin, indicating that they are primarily coupled to Gi proteins (40). However, in freshly isolated cells such as neutrophils and eosinophils and in an eosinophilic cell line, direct inhibition of adenylate cyclase activity has not been routinely observed (66,67). Receptor activation leads to a cascade of intracellular signaling events leading to activation of phosphatidylinositol-specific phospholipase C, protein kinase C, small GTPases, Src-related tyrosine kinases, phosphatidylinositol-3-OH kinases, and protein kinase B. Phospholipase C delivers two secondary messengers, inositol-1,4,5-triphosphate, which releases intracellular calcium, and diacylglycerol, which activates protein kinase C. Multiple phosphorylation events are triggered by chemokines. Phosphatidylinositol-3-OH kinase can be activated by the Bγ subunit of G proteins, small GTPases, or Src-related tyrosine kinases. Phosphorylation of the tyrosine kinase RAFTK (related adhesion focal tyrosine kinase), a member of the focal adhesion kinase family, has been shown to be induced by signaling through CCR5 (68). Recently, mitogen-activated protein kinases have also been shown to be phosphorylated and activated within 1 min after exposure of eosinophils to CCR3 ligands (69,70). This activation was required for eotaxin-induced eosinophil chemotaxis, actin polymerization, and degranulation (69,70). Additionally, Src family kinases Hck and c-Fgr have been shown to associate with CCR3 following eotaxin stimulation (71). In addition to triggering intracellular events, engagement with ligand induces rapid chemokine receptor internalization. For example, in human eosinophils, following only 15 min of exposure to eotaxin or RANTES, CCR3 expression is reduced to only 20–40% of the original level. Internalized CCR3 enters an early endosome compartment shared with the transferrin receptor and is subsequently recycled or targeted to the lysozyme for protein degradation. Interestingly, long-term exposure to RANTES results in prolonged receptor internalization for at least 18 h (72). Ligand-induced internalization of most chemokine receptors occurs independently of calcium transients, G-protein coupling, and protein kinase C, indicating a different mechanism compared with induction of chemotaxis. Thus, chemokine receptor internalization may provide a mechanism for chemokines to also halt leukocyte trafficking in vivo.

C. Genetic Organization and Polymorphisms in Chemokine Receptors

The genes for CCR1–CCR5 are located on human chromosome 3p21–24. Specifically, CCR1, 2, 3 and 5 are clustered on 3p21 within about 300 kb (73). Similarly to other chemoattractant receptor genes, CCR genes are composed of a single coding exon, and the 5′ untranslated region is separated by at least one large intron (40). Several chemokine receptors, including CXCR2, CCR5, and CCR3, have a complex genomic organization with multiple 5′ untranslated exons differentially used by alternative splicing and/or the use of different promoters (74–76). For instance, the CCR3 gene consists of four exons that give rise to multiple mRNA species by alternative splicing (Fig. 4). Exon 1 is present in all transcripts, whereas exon 2 or 3 is present at low frequency (<10%). The function of the untranslated exons is related to transcription. For example, exon 1 of CCR3 acts as an enhancer for the endogenous promoter (76). The open reading frame of the human CCR3 gene (exon 4) is polymorphic and contains four nucleotide variants; two of these encode for an amino acid substitution. One variant (G824A, allele frequency = 0.01) encodes for a change of arginine to glutamine in position

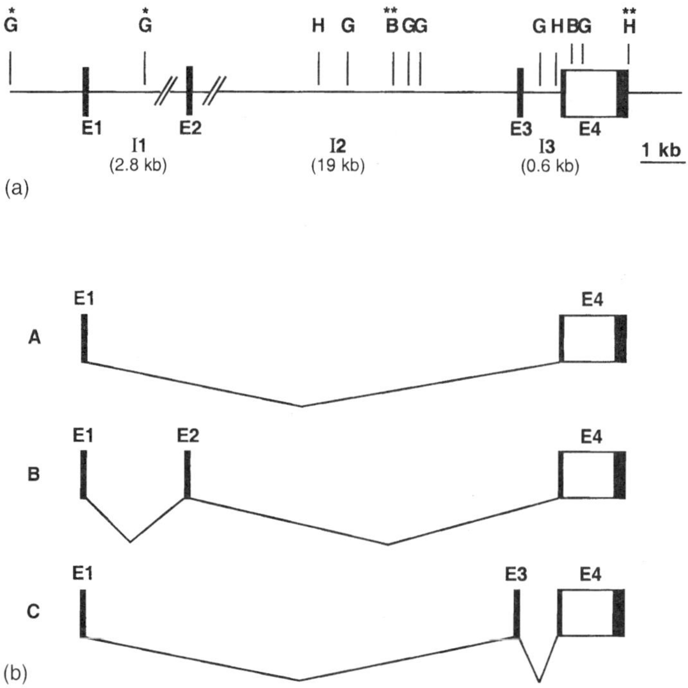

Figure 4 (a) Genomic organization and (b) mRNA processing of the CCR3 gene. (a) A schematic diagram of the organization of the CCR3 gene. The translated DNA area is depicted as an open rectangle, and untranslated DNA is shown as shaded rectangles. Restriction enzymes are labeled as follows: G = Bgl II; B = Bam HI, H = Hind III. Exons are labeled E1–E4; introns, I1–I3. DNA fragments flanked by a single asterisk (*) and double asterisk (**) were fully sequenced (Genbank accession numbers AF237380, U51241, and AF237381). (b) The corresponding mRNA species. A: The majority of mRNA species contain only exons 1 and 4; B and C show the use of exon 1 with exons 2 or 3, respectively. (Adapted from Ref. 76.)

275 of the protein; this is a nonconservative amino acid change in the third extracellular domain of the receptor, a region implicated in ligand binding to CCR3 (77). Stratification of DNA samples into a population with asthma suggested no change in this allele's frequency, but the frequency may change in other inflammatory conditions (78). Another polymorphism (T1052C, allele frequency = 0.005) encodes for a leucine-to-proline substitution at position 351 in the serine/threonine-rich cytoplasmic tail (78). This occurs in a putative G-protein-coupled receptor kinase (GRK)-2 phosphorylation site and therefore may have consequences for receptor signaling. A recent study reported an additional genetic polymorphism (C218S) found at low frequency (0.001) (79). The promoter region and exon 1 have also been screened for polymorphisms. Surprisingly, only one polymorphism was found in 19 tested individuals. This mutation, C-37T, disrupts a CREB (cAMP response element-binding protein) DNA-binding consensus sequence and may affect CCR3 transcription regulation (76). Genetic polymorphisms have been found in other chemokine receptors and appear to have an effect on human disease. For instance, chemokine receptors were identified as coreceptors for the entry of HIV-1 into cells (80). Whereas CXCR4 serves as a coreceptor for T-cell-trophic HIV strains, CCR5 can function as a coreceptor for macrophage (M)-trophic strains of the virus. CCR2b and CCR3 also serve as receptors for some M-trophic strains, and administration of a CCR3-specific ligand such as eotaxin blocks the entry of selected strains of HIV-1 into cells in vitro (81). Interestingly, genetic polymorphisms in the CCR2 and CCR5 gene confer protection from HIV infection (82–86). A small study has suggested that individuals carrying the CCR5Δ32 polymorphism may be protected from developing asthma (87). Thus, chemokine receptors contain several genetic variations that may have consequences in disease processes.

IV. Chemokine and Chemokine Receptor Gene–Deficient Mice

Research using chemokine and chemokine receptor gene disruptions have substantially contributed to the current understanding of the pleiotropic functions of these molecules. A summary of chemokine gene-targeted mice is presented in Table 2. The first chemokine gene deletion to be reported was the targeted disruption of the MIP-1α chemokine (88). Mice deficient in MIP-1α had a marked impairment in inflammatory responses following virus-induced myocarditis and pneumonitis. This demonstrates the essential role for MIP-1α in the development of antiviral immunity. The SDF-1 gene was the second chemokine to be gene-targeted in mice (89). This targeted disruption resulted in embryonic lethality owing to the surprising essential role of SDF-1 in cardiac development. Immunological analysis of embryonic blood also revealed defects in hematopoiesis in

Table 2 Phenotype of Chemokine Gene-Deleted Mice

Chemokine	Phenotype
MIP-1α	Impaired inflammatory responses to viral infections
SDF-1	Embryonic lethality due to impaired cardiac development and defects in hematopoiesis
Eotaxin	Impaired early recruitment of eosinophils to the lung following allergen challenge; reduced levels of eosinophils in tissues at baseline; protection from gastrointestinal allergy
MCP-1	Impaired macrophage recruitment; Th1/Th2 imbalance
Lungkine	Impaired neutrophil recruitment into the airspace and increased susceptibility to *Klebsiella pneumoniae infection*

these animals (89). Eotaxin was the third chemokine gene to be deleted from mice (90). As discussed below, eotaxin-deficient mice had an impairment in the early recruitment of eosinophils to the lung following allergen challenge. Additionally, they had a marked deficiency in the levels of tissue eosinophils, indicating the critical importance of eotaxin as a homeostatic chemokine that regulates eosinophil homing to nonhematopoietic tissues (91). MCP-1-deficient mice were developed and found to have a marked impairment in macrophage recruitment in response to peritoneal injection of thioglycolate (92). Additionally, they had an imbalance in Th1 versus Th2 cytokines. Recently, lungkine-deficient mice were developed and demonstrated increased susceptibility to *Klebsiella pneumoniae* infection, which correlated with reduced neutrophil recruitment into the airspace (93).

Several chemokine receptors have been genetically deleted (Table 3). The first chemokine receptor to be gene-deleted in mice was the low affinity receptor for IL-8 (CXCR2) (94). These mice had no overt abnormalities, but they had an impairment in neutrophil recruitment in response to thioglycolate. Additionally, they had a surprising increase in myelopoiesis and marked lymphadenopathy due to B-cell expansion when housed in conventional animal facilities. The second chemokine receptor to be gene-targeted was CXCR5 (95). These gene-deleted mice lacked inguinal lymph nodes and possessed markedly reduced and abnormal Peyer's patches. Furthermore, the migration of B lymphocytes into the spleen was abnormal, resulting in no functional germinal centers in these mice. These results indicated the critical role of CXCR5 in B-cell homing into lymphoid compartments. Next, CCR1- and CCR2-deficient mice were generated (96–98). CCR1-deficient mice have dysregulated trafficking of mature leukocytes into hematopoietic tissues during both steady states and inflammatory conditions. Additionally, mature neutrophils in these mice failed to respond to MIP-1α, indicating that the predominant receptor for MIP-1α in neutrophils was CCR1. CCR1-

Table 3 Chemokine Receptor Gene–Deleted Mice

Chemokine receptor	Phenotype
CXCR2	Splenomegaly, bone marrow myeloid hyperplasia, neutrophilia, and an increase in B cells (these abnormalities do not develop in germ-free facilities).
	Delayed wound healing.
	Impaired resistance to multiple microbial pathogens.
CXCR3	Delayed or absent allograft rejection.
CXCR4	Lethal phenotype with hematopoietic and cardiac defects.
CXCR5	Lack of inguinal lymph nodes and reduced or abnormal Peyer's patches.
	Lack of functional germinal centers.
CCR1	Impaired neutrophil-mediated host defense mechanisms.
	Dysregulation of Th1/Th2 balance.
	Reduced airway remodeling in asthma model.
CCR2	Failure to clear infection by *Listeria monocytogenes*.
	Failure to recruit macrophages into the peritoneum in response to thioglycolate.
	Variable effect in asthma model.
CCR4	Decreased mortality in LPS-induced endotoxic shock.
CCR5	Reduced clearance of *Listeria monocytogenes*.
	Enhanced delayed-type hypersensitivity (DTH) reaction and increased humoral responses.
CCR6	Absence of CD11c-positive dendritic cells in the subepithelial dome of the Peyer's patches.
	Impaired humoral responses.
	Increased T-cell populations within the intestinal mucosa.
CCR7	Reduced trafficking of T cells to lymph nodes.
CCR8	Impaired Th2 responses (reduced production of Th2 cytokines and diminished eosinophilia).
	No effect on Th1 immune responses.
DARC	Exaggerated response to endotoxin with significantly increased inflammatory infiltrates in lung and liver.

deficient mice have impaired clearance of *Aspergillus fumigatus* that appears to result from an imbalanced Th1 response compared to a Th2 response in wild-type mice. These data suggest that chemokines and their receptors have a role in inducing these types of immune responses (Th1 vs. Th2). CCR2-deficient mice develop normally and have no impairment in hematopoiesis. However, they failed to clear the intracellular pathogen *Listeria monocytogenes* and to recruit macrophages into the peritoneum in response to thioglycolate (97,98). Both CCR1- and

CCR2-deficient mice have been tested in allergic airway inflammation models. In a model of eosinophilic inflammation of the lungs in response to *Aspergillus fumigatus*, CCR1-deficient animals were found to have significantly fewer goblet cells and subepithelial fibrosis, implicating CCR1 in airway remodeling (99). In the same model, CCR2-deficient animals exhibited an increase of eosinophils and lymphocytes in the airways, serum IgE, Th2 cytokines, and Th2-induced chemokines, airway hyperresponsiveness, and fibrosis compared to wild-type mice (100). However, in an ovalbumin-induced model of allergic airway inflammation, CCR2-deficient mice displayed no difference in pulmonary eosinophilia, Th2 cytokine levels, or airway hyperresponsiveness compared to wild-type mice (101). CCR8-deficient mice have been developed and tested in models of Th2 immune responses, such as *Schistosoma mansoni* soluble egg antigen-induced granuloma formation as well as OVA and cockroach antigen-induced allergic airway inflammation. In these mice, Th2 immune responses were defective, with impaired Th2 cytokine production and reduced eosinophilia, whereas the Th1 response to *Mycobacterium bovis* purified protein derivative was unaffected (102). Additionally, gene targeting of CXCR4 resulted in a lethal phenotype with hematopoietic and cardiac defects reminiscent of those observed in SDF-1-targeted mice (103,104). Recently, mice deficient in CCR4, CCR5, CCR6, CCR7, CXCR3, and DARC (Duffy antigen/receptor for chemokines) were generated and displayed various immunological defects (Table 3) (105–110). For instance, the CCR4-deficient mice displayed decreased mortality in LPS-induced endotoxic shock. Whereas humans carrying the CCR5Δ32 polymorphism appear to be healthy despite their lack of CCR5 expression, mice deficient in CCR5 display reduced clearance of *Listeria monocytogenes*, enhanced delayed-type hypersensitivity (DTH) reactions, and increased humoral responses. CCR6- and CCR7-deficient mice display defects in T-cell and dendritic cell trafficking as discussed below. Finally, CXCR3-deficient animals present with delayed or absent allograft rejection. The role of these defects in allergic airway inflammation remains to be elucidated.

Taken together, these studies indicate that despite the large number of chemokines and their receptors, there is likely to be a nonredundant role for each individual molecule. Similar gene-targeting approaches will provide essential information regarding the complexity and importance of chemokines and their receptors in allergic and other inflammatory states.

V. Pleiotropic Functions of Chemokines in Allergic Responses

Chemokines have been implicated in diverse functions, and the significance of these results as related to allergy is reviewed in this section. (See Table 4.)

Table 4 Pleiotropic Effects of Chemokines in Allergic Diseases

Cellular activation
Chemoattraction
Airway hyperreactivity
Histamine release
Modulation of dendritic cell function
Modulation of lymphocyte function
Regulation of hematopoiesis
Regulation of homeostatic immunity

A. Chemoattraction

The interaction between leukocytes in the circulation and endothelial cells lining blood vessels is a complex network of signaling events regulating trafficking of particular leukocyte subsets (111). The interaction is mediated by a multistep process that involves (1) leukocyte rolling (mediated by endothelial selection and specific leukocyte ligands), (2) rapid activation of leukocyte integrins, (3) firm adhesion to endothelial ligands through activated integrins, and (4) transmigration of leukocytes through the endothelial layer. Chemokines have a central role in the modulation of this multistep process by (1) activating both the leukocyte and the endothelium and (2) increasing leukocyte integrin and adhesion molecule interaction affinity. The rapidity of the chemokine-mediated signaling events in this multistep process (seconds to minutes) is important for leukocytes that dynamically roll through venules. Thus, the multistep chemokine signaling cascade must occur rapidly to allow for the leukocyte to reduce rolling velocity, mediate adherence, and extravasate into tissues in response to a chemokine gradient. In addition to mediating leukocyte movement from the bloodstream into tissues, chemokines follow similar steps to mediate leukocyte-directed motion across other tissue barriers such as the respiratory epithelium.

CXC chemokines containing ELR (Glu-Leu-Arg) (e.g., IL-8) are mainly chemoattractive for neutrophils, whereas non-ELR CXC chemokines (e.g., IP-10) chemoattract selected populations of lymphocytes. CC chemokines are active on a variety of leukocytes including dendritic cells, monocytes, basophils, lymphocytes, and eosinophils. As their names imply, all MCPs have strong chemoattractive activity for monocytes. However, they display partially overlapping chemoattractant activity on basophils and eosinophils. For example, MCP-2, MCP-3, and MCP-4 have basophil and eosinophil chemoattractive activity, but MCP-1 is active only on basophils. In contrast to the MCPs, eotaxin has limited activity on macrophages whereas it is a potent eosinophil and basophil chemoattractant (4,112). Similarly, eotaxin-2 is inactive on macrophages but is a potent lymphocyte and eosinophil chemoattractant (5). The entire MCP/eotaxin family has variable lymphocyte chemoattractive activity. Administration of eotaxin intranasally or subcutaneously revealed that eotaxin induced a rapid selective tissue accumulation of eosinophils in murine lung or skin, respectively, in the presence of high levels of IL-5, an eosinophil growth and activating cytokine (using IL-5 transgenic mice) (113). Cooperativity between eotaxin and IL-5 in promoting tissue eosinophilia has been reported by several groups (114,115). IL-5 collaborates with eotaxin in promoting tissue eosinophilia by (1) increasing the pool of circulating eosinophils (by stimulating eosinophilopoiesis and bone marrow release) and (2) priming eosinophils to have enhanced responsiveness to eotaxin. Additionally, synergy between eotaxin and the lipid mediator 5-oxo-6,8,11,14-eicosatetraenoic acid in inducing eosinophil chemotaxis has been demonstrated (116). Although eotaxin has been demonstrated to have activity on basophils in vitro, all administration studies in vivo have shown a selective eosinophil accumulation in guinea pigs (117), mice (113), and monkeys (118). This indicates that eotaxin's predominant role in leukocyte recruitment in vivo is restricted to eosinophils. It remains possible that eotaxin may promote the cellular accumulation of noneosinophils in vivo if the appropriate second signal is present. For example, eotaxin may promote basophil accumulation if coadministered with IL-3. The ability of two cytokines (IL-5 and eotaxin) that are relatively eosinophil-selective to cooperate in promoting tissue eosinophilia offers a molecular explanation for the occurrence of selective tissue eosinophilia in human allergic diseases.

B. Cellular Activation

In addition to promoting leukocyte accumulation, chemokines are potent cell activators. After binding to the appropriate G-protein-linked seven-transmembrane-spanning receptor, chemokines elicit transient intracellular calcium flux, actin polymerization, oxidative burst with release of superoxide free radicals, the exocytosis of secondary granule constituents, and increased avidity of integrins for their adhesion molecules (119–121). For example, in basophils, chemokine-induced cellular activation results in degranulation with the release of histamine and the de novo generation of leukotriene C4 (22,122,123). Basophil activation by chemokines requires cellular priming with IL-3, IL-5, or granulocyte monocyte colony stimulating factor (GM-CSF) for the maximal effect of each chemokine. Although all MCPs can induce histamine release in cytokine-primed basophils, there is marked variability between individual basophil donors. MCP-1 appears to be the most potent secretagogue for basophils, whereas eotaxin is weak. In eosinophils, CCR3 ligands induce degranulation, and this effect is amplified when cells are primed with IL-5 (124–126).

C. Hematopoiesis

In addition to being involved in leukocyte accumulation during inflammatory reactions, chemokines also have a role in regulating baseline hematopoiesis. These functions include (1) chemotaxis of hematopoietic progenitor cells (HPCs), (2) suppression and enhancement activity on HPC proliferation and differentiation, and (3) mobilization of HPCs to the peripheral blood (reviewed in Ref. 127). For example, SDF-1, a CXC chemokine, is critical for B-cell lymphopoiesis and bone marrow myelopoiesis as demonstrated by gene targeting (89). Furthermore, eotaxin has been shown to directly stimulate the release of eosinophilic progenitor cells and mature eosinophils from the bone marrow (128). Eotaxin synergizes with stem cell factor in stimulating yolk sac development into mast cells in vitro (129) and has been shown to function as a granulocyte-macrophage colony-stimulating factor following allergic challenge in the lungs (130). In contrast, MIP-1α appears to be an inhibitor of hematopoiesis (131).

D. Homeostatic Role

Chemokines have an important role in baseline leukocyte trafficking during development, differentiation, and immune surveillance (132,133). For example, several chemokines including thymus-expressed chemokine (TECK), SDF-1, secondary lymphoid organ chemokine (SLC), liver and activation regulated chemokine (LARC), and dendritic cell-derived CC chemokine (DC-CK-1) and eotaxin have been shown to be constitutively expressed at high levels in a broad range of tissues, including the thymus, lymph nodes, and gastrointestinal tract (134,135). Individual chemokines may also have multifunctional roles, modulating both cellular trafficking and differentiation. For example, SDF-1 has been shown to regulate B-cell trafficking into lymphoid organs and to also be crucial for B-cell development and differentiation (89). Recent studies in CXCR5-deficient mice suggest that chemokines also have a role in lymph organ architecture and compartmentalization. As described above, CXCR5-deficient mice are characterized by defective formation of primary and secondary follicles and germinal centers in the spleen and other lymphoid follicles (95). T-cell trafficking into lymph nodes is also dependent on chemokines, specifically SLC and ELC (Epstein-Barr virus-induced molecule ligand chemokine) and their receptor CCR7. SLC is expressed by high endothelial venules (HEV), which are the site of T-lymphocyte entry into lymph nodes. Both SLC and ELC are expressed by stromal cells within T-cell areas of lymph nodes, spleen, and Peyer's patches.

The role for SLC and ELC in T-cell migration into lymph nodes was suggested by the observation that mice bearing a spontaneous mutation, *plt* (paucity of lymph node T cells), have markedly reduced or absent SLC and ELC expression and have defective T-cell trafficking into lymph nodes as well as severely disturbed organization of cells in the T-cell areas (136,137). This was further supported by the demonstration that lymph nodes in CCR7-deficient mice have significantly reduced numbers of T cells (109). Collectively, these studies suggest that chemokines have an important role in B- and T-cell trafficking into lymph nodes and the structural organization of lymphoid tissues.

The role of chemokines in homeostatic leukocyte trafficking has important implications in allergic states because the leukocytes involved in allergic responses (e.g., mast cells and eosinophils) primarily reside in tissue locations rather than hematopoietic organs. The eosinophil-selective chemokine eotaxin is constitutively expressed in a variety of tissues, especially mucosal tissues in which eosinophils normally reside (24,138). Furthermore, mice deficient in eotaxin have a selective and marked reduction of tissue eosinophils in the gastrointestinal tract and thymus (91,139). This underscores the critical role of chemokines in establishing the location of allergic inflammatory cells at baseline.

E. Role in Allergen Uptake, Processing, and Presentation by Dendritic Cells

A central goal in allergy research is to understand the mechanism for initial allergen recognition in mucosal surfaces. Tissue-resident dendritic cells are believed to have a fundamental role in this process because they are able to efficiently take up, process, and deliver antigens to lymphoid tissues. The migration pattern of dendritic cells is complex and is thought to involve a coordinated chemokine signaling network. Dendritic cell progenitors from the bone marrow migrate into nonlymphoid tissues, where they develop into immature dendritic cells that play an active role in antigen uptake and processing. Antigen stimulation and the production of inflammatory cytokines promote the differentiation of immature ''processing stage'' dendritic cells into mature presenting dendritic cells and mobilizes these cells. This promotes trafficking from the periphery to regional lymph nodes via afferent lymphatics. Upon reaching the lymph nodes, dendritic cells home to T-cell-rich regions where they present the processed antigen to naive T cells and generate an antigen-specific primary T-cell response. As part of the maturation program, immature dendritic cells upregulate the expression of CCR7 and become responsive to ELC and SLC, chemokines responsible for their trafficking to lymph nodes. At the same time, they decrease the expression of CCR1, CCR2, and CCR5—the receptors for inflammatory chemokines (140–142). However, it is becoming apparent that there may be differences between distinct subsets of dendritic cells. For instance, in mice lacking CCR6, myeloid-derived dendritic cells (expressing CD11b and CD11c) are absent from the subepithelial dome of Peyer's patches. Additionally, these mice have impaired humoral immune responses and increased T-cell populations within the intestinal mucosa (110). Although the role of dendritic cells and the chemokines that regulate their trafficking in allergic responses has not been extensively evaluated, these processes are likely to have fundamental implications in understanding allergic responses. Recent studies indicate that dendritic cells are required for the development of eosinophilic airway inflammation in response to inhaled antigen (143). Importantly, adoptive transfer of antigen-pulsed dendritic cells has been shown to be sufficient for the induction of Th2 responses and eosinophilic airway inflammation to inhaled antigen (144).

F. Effector Function in Elicitation of End-Organ Damage

Chronic allergic inflammation is associated with end-organ damage including tissue remodeling and airway hyperreactivity (145,146). Chemokines have been shown to participate, directly and indirectly, in the pathogenesis of tissue damage by multiple mechanisms. For example, direct administration of selected chemokines to pulmonary tissue (e.g., MCP-1) in vivo is sufficient for the induction of rapid airway hyperreactivity (145,146). This effect may be mediated by a combination of processes including activation of allergic inflammatory cells (e.g., basophils) and by direct effects on structural tissue cells. Chemokines have also been shown to participate in wound healing and tissue remodeling because they can have direct effects on angiogenesis (132).

G. Modulation of T-Cell Immune Responses

Recently there has been rapid progress in understanding the effects of chemokines on T-lymphocyte biology (133). T lymphocytes have been shown to express a majority of chemokine receptors, thus being potentially responsive to a large number of different chemokines. Characterization of chemokine receptor expression has shown that T lymphocytes display a dynamic expression pattern of chemokine receptors, and it is the differential expression of receptors during T-lymphocyte maturation and differentiation that is thought to allow for individual chemokine specific functionality on T lymphocytes (133). As mentioned previously, CCR7 plays an important role in trafficking of naive T cells into lymph nodes (147). Upon activation, T cells may express an array of chemokine receptors including CCR1, CCR2, CCR5, CXCR1, and CXCR4. They thus become sensitive to inflammatory chemokines including MIP-1α, MIP-1β, MCP-3, and RANTES, which are thought to mediate T-cell trafficking to sites of inflammation (148). Additionally, specific subsets of memory T cells can be distinguished on the basis of their expression of CCR7 and their propensity to migrate into lymph nodes (149). Chemokines have an important role in the induction of inflammatory responses and are also central in selecting the type of immune response (Th1 vs. Th2). During bacterial or viral infections, IP-10, MIG, IL-8, and I-TAC production correlates with the presence of CD4$^+$ Th1-type T cells. In contrast, during allergic inflammatory responses, eotaxin, RANTES, MCP-2, MCP-3, and MCP-4 are induced and the majority of the CD4$^+$ T lymphocytes are of the Th2-type phenotype. Characterization of chemokine receptor expression on T lymphocytes suggests that this may be explained by the expression of CXCR3 and CCR5 predominantly on Th1-type T cells, whereas CCR3, CCR4, and CCR8 have been associated with Th2-type T cells (Fig. 5). Additionally, Th1 and Th2 cells secrete distinct chemokines (Fig. 5) (150). In mice, Th1 cells preferentially secrete RANTES and lymphotactin, whereas Th2 cells secrete monocyte-derived chemokine (MDC) and thymus-derived chemotactic agent (TCA)-3. Interestingly, supernatants from Th2 cells preferentially attract Th2 cells. These data suggest that the presence of specific patterns of chemokine receptors on T-cell subsets predicts which subset will be preferentially accumulated at sites of inflammation. Alternatively, chemokines may directly influence the differentiation of naive T cells to the Th1 or Th2 phenotype. MIP-1α and MCP-1 have been described as capable of inducing the differentiation of Th1 and Th2 cells (151), and MCP-1-deficient mice have defective Th2 responses (152). Consistent with this, animals deficient in Bcl-6, a transcriptional repressor described above, express high levels of chemokines, including MCP-1, and suffer from systemic Th2-type inflammation (39).

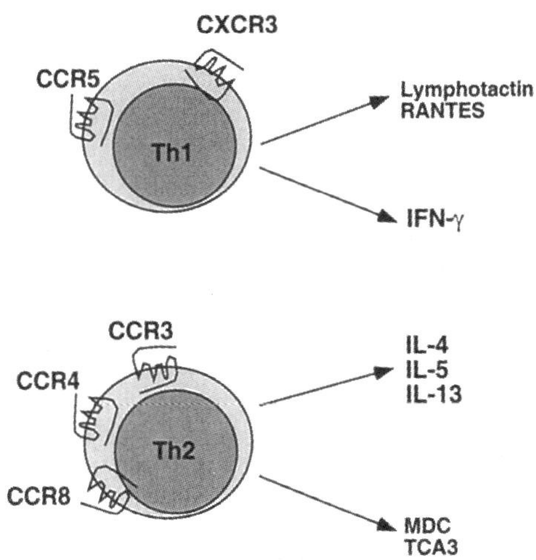

Figure 5 Chemokine and chemokine receptor expression by Th1 and Th2 cells. Th1 cells preferentially express CCR5 and CXCR3 whereas Th2 cells express CCR3, CCR4, and CCR8. In addition to expressing distinct cytokines (IL-4, IL-5, IL-13, and IFN-γ), murine T cells have recently been shown to express a unique panel of chemokines as indicated.

VI. Chemokines in Animal Models of Allergy

A. Animal Models

The importance of eosinophils in the pathogenesis of airway damage has been an active area of research in animals (153). Most studies use a model of eosinophilic pulmonary inflammation that is induced by challenging sensitized animals with antigen exposure in the lung. Although no one model mimics all the features of the human disease, they have been useful in dissecting the mechanisms required for the induction of allergic inflammation (154–156). These models involve sensitization of animals with systemic doses of antigen, typically ovalbumin (OVA), in the presence of an adjuvant such as alum. Although the use of an adjuvant is not necessary, it enhances the magnitude of the IgG1, IgE, and cellular responses. Following sensitization, the animals are mucosally exposed to antigen by direct intranasal application of antigen to anesthetized animals or by aerosolization of the antigen to conscious animals via a nebulizer. Alternatively, unsensitized animals are exposed to repeated doses of mucosal antigen, which induces sensitization and allergic inflammation. In each of these models, antigen challenge leads to a marked accumulation of inflammatory leukocytes in the lung primarily composed of eosinophils, lymphocytes, and, to a lesser extent, neutrophils. Most studies in guinea pigs and mice have shown that eosinophils and IL-5 are required for the induction of airway hyperresponsiveness; however, the mere presence of eosinophils in the airway does not always lead to hyperresponsiveness (157–160). This indicates that other signals in addition to those provided by IL-5, such as chemokines, are likely to be responsible for eosinophil-mediated tissue damage (161). A smaller set of experiments have clearly shown that pathways independent of eosinophils for the induction of allergic airway inflammation can also be operational (162,163). Recent studies have indicated that IL-13 is sufficient to induce many of the pathophysiological processes associated with asthma and, interestingly, that IL-13 is a potent activator of chemokine expression (164–167).

Models of allergic airway inflammation have proven useful for the study of chemokines. In fact, eotaxin was initially discovered as the chief chemoattractive activity released into the bronchoalveolar lavage fluid in a guinea pig model of allergic airway disease (117). These models have demonstrated rapid induction of chemokine mRNA expression following allergen challenge. For example, following OVA sensitization and challenge, eotaxin mRNA increased at 3 h in guinea pigs; in mice, eotaxin peaked at 3–6 h after OVA but remained elevated for at least 48 h (168). Additionally, the MCPs have been demonstrated to be induced by OVA and remain elevated for 3–48 h after antigen challenge (4). Likewise, repeated exposure of animals to intranasal *Aspergillus fumigatus* antigen resulted in ~60-fold increase in eotaxin lung mRNA at 18 h after the last antigen dose compared to saline-treated animals (4).

T lymphocytes have been demonstrated to be essential for the induction of eosinophilic allergic airway inflammation (153,169,170). Antigen-specific CD4$^+$ Th2 lymphocytes play a central role in eosinophil recruitment, because depletion of these cells (170,171) or their secreted products (IL-4 and IL-5) (158,169,172,173) significantly reduces pulmonary eosinophilia. The mechanism by which T cells assist in the recruitment of eosinophils to the lung in these models is not completely understood. As discussed earlier, T-cell products such as IL-5 cooperate with eotaxin in vivo. Treatment of allergen-challenged mice with a monoclonal antibody against CD3 inhibited the induction of eotaxin but not MIP-1α mRNA and significantly reduced eosinophil accumulation in the lung (168). In addition, antigen-specific antibody responses and mast cell degranulation following antigen challenge in sensitized mice were not affected by T-cell elimination (168). Thus, mast cell degranulation alone is not sufficient for the induction of eotaxin and pulmonary eosinophilia. These findings suggest that selective chemokines such as eotaxin may be molecular links between antigen-specific T-cell activation and the recruitment of eosinophils into the airways.

B. Role of Chemokines in Allergy Models

Multiple studies have demonstrated that a variety of chemokines are strongly induced in models of allergic inflammation and in human allergic disorders, but few studies have determined the relative importance of one chemokine over another in promoting the pathological events. Determining the significance of each chemokine has important implications for the design of therapeutic intervention aimed at blocking chemokine activity and suggests whether therapy should target individual chemokines or particular chemokine receptors. Because members of the chemokine family have apparent in vitro redundancy, it might be expected that no one chemokine would provide a critical signal for cell recruitment. However, a variety of approaches including antibody neutralization experiments and gene targeting have shown nonredundant specific roles for selected chemokines in allergic diseases. For example, eotaxin gene-deficient mice have been shown to have an impairment in the recruitment of eosinophils during the early part of the late-phase response in the lung and cornea in experimental models of asthma and keratitis (90). Additionally, employment of neutralizing antibodies against RANTES, MIP-1α, MCP-1, MCP-5, and eotaxin have indicated the individual importance of each of these chemokines in the development and regional localization of inflammatory cells during allergen-induced pulmonary inflammation and airway hyperreactivity (146). For instance, neutralization of eotaxin reduced eosinophil infiltration and airway hyperresponsiveness transiently after each allergen challenge, whereas neutralization of MCP-5 abolished airway hyperresponsiveness by altering the trafficking of eosinophils through the lung interstitium.

In contrast, neutralization of MCP-1 blocked the development of airway hyperresponsiveness even though eosinophil recruitment was unchanged in these mice (146). Taken together, these studies suggest that pharmacological therapy that targets chemokine and/or chemokine receptor pathways involved in allergic inflammation is a promising therapeutic strategy.

VII. Evidence for the Role of Chemokines in Patients with Asthma

Allergic diseases are thought to be polygenic diseases, with multiple genes contributing to the pathogenesis of the disease. In support of the complex polygenic nature of allergic diseases, genetic linkage analysis has identified multiple different candidate genes including the high-affinity IgE receptor, IL-4 receptor alpha chain, a locus that maps near the IL-4 and IL-5 cytokine gene cluster on chromosome 5q31–32, and, most relevant for this review, a locus that maps near the CC chemokine locus on chromosome 17q11.2 (174–181). Additionally, the occurrence of eosinophilia in atopic individuals has been genetically mapped to a locus near the class I genes of the major histocompatibility complex on chromosome 6. Finally, a familial form of the idiopathic hypereosinophilic syndrome with autosomal dominant inheritance has been genetically linked to the cytokine locus on chromosome 5q32 (182,183). Clinical and experimental investigations have shown that epithelial cells from bronchial biopsy specimens have an increased expression level of several chemokines, including eotaxin and MCPs (61,184). In support of these findings, the concentrations of MCP-1, MCP-4, MIP-1α, RANTES, IL-8, and eotaxin in the bronchoalveolar fluid are elevated in patients with mild asthma (185). Furthermore, an endobronchial challenge with allergen results in an increase in the level of chemokines in the bronchoalveolar lavage fluid. The chemoattractant activity of the lavage fluid from patients with asthma is partially inhibited by antibodies against RANTES, MCP-3, MCP-4, and eotaxin (61). For example, a combination of antibodies against eotaxin, MCP-4, and RANTES inhibits ~50% of the eosinophil chemotactic activity in the bronchoalveolar fluid (61). Recently, in a clinical study, an association between the plasma concentration of eotaxin and the incidence of asthma and reduced lung function was established (186). Experimental induction of cutaneous and pulmonary late-phase responses in humans has revealed that eotaxin is induced early (6 h) and correlates with early eosinophil recruitment; in contrast, eotaxin-2 and MCP-4 correlate with eosinophil accumulation at 24 h (187,188). Together, these studies indicate the importance of chemokines in the pathogenesis of airway inflammation in humans.

Polymorphisms in individual chemokines and chemokine receptor genes are likely to influence the course of asthma. As noted earlier, CCR5Δ32 appears to protect against asthma (87). Additionally, a polymorphism in the RANTES promoter (G → A at position −401) appears to have an effect on atopic dermatitis (189). The polymorphism confers higher transcriptional activity and a new GATA transcription binding site. Additionally, it is associated with increased susceptibility to atopic dermatitis, because the proportion of individuals carrying the mutant allele is higher in children with atopic dermatitis. Furthermore, the polymorphism has a higher frequency in individuals of African descent compared to Caucasian subjects and has recently been associated with increased susceptibility to both asthma and atopy, because the proportion of individuals carrying the mutant allele is higher in atopic and nonatopic asthma patients (190). Additionally, the polymorphism is associated with increased aeroallergen skin test positivity, and homozygosity is associated with increased risk of airway obstruction.

From a variety of clinical and experimental human studies the following generalizations can be made:

1. The mRNA and protein for selected chemokines (such as MCPs and eotaxin) are constitutively expressed in pulmonary tissue and primarily derived from epithelial cells.
2. Allergen challenge in atopic and nonatopic asthmatic patients promotes an increase in both protein and mRNA for selected chemokines (such as eotaxin and MCP-4) compared with saline challenge.
3. During pulmonary inflammation, macrophages and to a lesser extent eosinophils and lymphocytes localized to the subepithelial layer are significant sources of chemokines.
4. Allergen-induced chemokine expression during experimental late-phase responses reveals kinetic correlation between individual chemokines and infiltrating cell types.
5. Genetic polymorphisms in chemokines and their receptors are likely to influence disease risk and phenotype.

VIII. Therapeutic Approach to Interfering with Chemokines

One of the actions of glucocorticoids is to inhibit the transcription and/or stability of chemokine mRNA. However, the ideal pharmaceutical agent would interfere with the selective function of critical chemokines and/or their receptors in the pathophysiology of asthma but not in protective immune responses. CCR3 represents such a potential target, because preliminary studies indicate that it is likely to be critically involved in allergic inflammation and antagonizing CCR3 would selectively target eosinophils, basophils, and Th2 cells. Although the benefits of targeting eosinophils may be questioned with the results from preliminary clinical trials of antibody blockade of IL-5 in subjects with mild asthma (191), activity on Th2 cells may be important, because these cells contribute to airway hyperresponsiveness. Additionally, CCR4 and CCR8 may be potential targets, because both are reported to be Th2-specific and involved in recruitment of Th2 cells in allergic inflammation (102,192). CCR8 represents a potentially attractive target, because recent studies with CCR8-deficient mice have shown impaired antigen-driven Th2 responses and pulmonary eosinophilia (102). The impact of CCR3 targeting on physiological responses should also be considered. However, the cells that mainly express CCR3 (such as eosinophils and basophils) do not appear to have essential physiological roles, so targeting these cells would be unlikely to result in significant immunosuppression. The role of CCR3 on Th2 cells and other types of cells that may express this receptor is not fully understood. However, the impact of antagonists on physiological homeostasis will need to be evaluated.

Chemokine and/or chemokine receptor inhibition has thus been an active area of research. Studies have also been fueled by the finding that natural chemokine receptor mutations block the HIV coreceptor function of selected chemokine receptors (such as CCR2 and CCR5), suggesting that pharmaceutical targeting of chemokine receptors is a promising strategy for treatment of HIV infection (82,86). There are several potential approaches for blockade of chemokines and their receptors (Table 5). One approach is to develop humanized monoclonal antibodies against chemokines and/or their receptors, an approach already validated in animal models (193). Specifically, an antibody directed against CCR3

Table 5 Therapeutic Approaches to Inhibiting Chemokines and Their Receptors

Humanized monoclonal antibodies against chemokines and/or their receptors
Anti-CCR3
Induction of receptor desensitization and/or internalization
CCR3 receptor antagonists
Met-RANTES
AOP-RANTES
Met-Ckβ7
Small-molecule CCR3 inhibitors
UCB35625 (Banyu)
Hoffmann-La Roche compound
Merck compound
Signal transduction inhibitors
Transcriptional inhibitors
Antisense oligonucleotides
Transcription factor inhibitors

would offer an advantage over antibodies against chemokines, because actions of multiple chemokines through a single receptor would be affected. An antibody against human CCR3, designated 7B11, has been validated as a potent binding and functional antagonist in vitro (194). However, rodent-derived antibodies, such as 7B11, will have to be humanized before clinical trials are conducted. Another approach involves developing receptor antagonists based on chemokine protein modifications. One such agent has been derived by the addition of a single methionine to the amino terminus of RANTES (designated Met-RANTES; Serono) (195,196). This agent acts as a strong competitive inhibitor of CCR1, CCR3, and CCR5. In vivo studies have demonstrated significant reduction in eosinophil numbers following Met-RANTES administration in a murine model of allergic airway inflammation (197). The success of protein antagonists has already been recognized by viruses, some of which have developed their own chemokine antagonists. For example, the human herpes simplex virus-8 genome encodes for two chemokine-related proteins, and one of these, vMIP-II, is a potent broad-spectrum antagonist against both CXC and CC chemokine receptors (198,199). Another example is a potent CCR8 antagonist encoded by the poxvirus *Molluscum contagiosum*, termed MC148 (200). Additionally, small-molecule inhibitors of chemokine receptors have recently been described and display potent inhibition at nanomolar concentrations in vitro (201,202). Three companies (Banyu Pharmaceuticals, Hoffmann-La Roche, and Merck) have reported the development of small-molecule CCR3 antagonists (Fig. 6) (203,204). These compounds share the presence of a hydrophobic group some distance away from a basic nitrogen group. It has been postulated that the basic nitrogen group interacts with a key anionic residue in or near the seven-transmembrane region of the receptor, as found with antagonists of the monoamine receptors, which are seven-transmembrane-spanning receptors. However, no in vivo data are yet available.

An additional approach to inhibiting chemokines can be induction of prolonged desensitization to chemokine stimulation (205). It may be possible to induce cellular desensitization by promoting chemokine receptor internalization (72). Alternatively, the transcription or translation of specific chemokines or chemokine receptors could be blocked. For example, antisense oligonucleotides and transcription factor inhibitors specifically designed to interact with regulatory regions in the CCR3 gene (76) may have clinical utility. A more detailed understanding of the regulation of chemokine and chemokine receptor genes is necessary for the development of these approaches.

IX. Summary

Over the last decade, chemokines, in particular the MCP/eotaxin subfamily, have emerged as cytokines likely to be important in the regulation of allergic inflam-

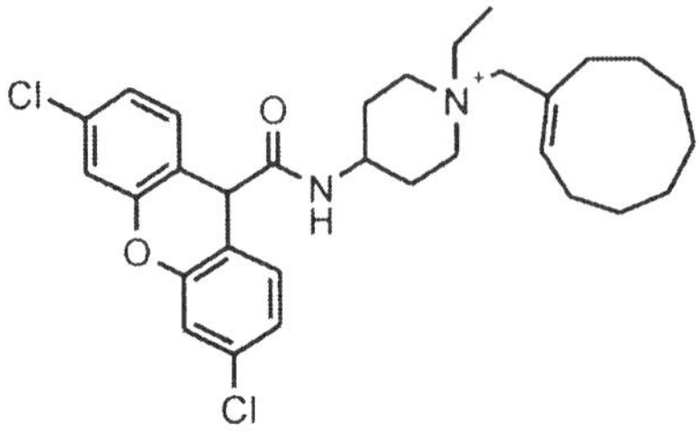

Formula I

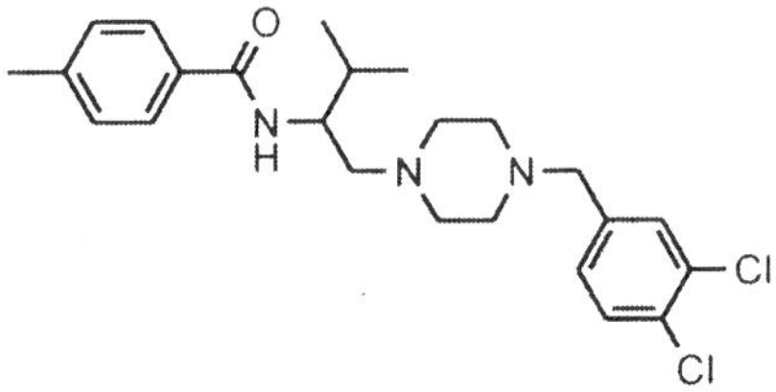

Formula II

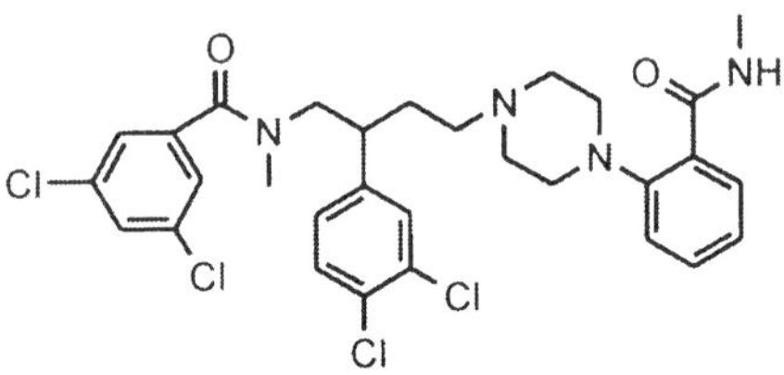

Formula III

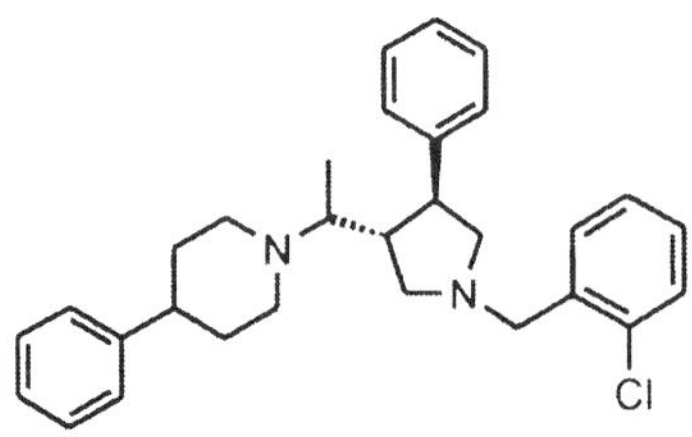

Formula IV

Figure 6 Chemical structure of CCR3 antagonists. Representative chemical structures of CCR3 antagonists from Banyu Pharmaceuticals (formula I), Hoffmann-La Roche (formula II), and Merck (formulas III and IV). (From Ref. 203.)

mation. A combination of mouse and human studies has been used to define the role of chemokines in allergic diseases and their potential as therapeutic targets. Through the use of targeted gene deletion and neutralizing antibodies, the role of individual chemokines in mouse models of inflammation has begun to be determined. Furthermore, murine studies have been used to understand the regulation of chemokine expression in vivo. These murine studies have been correlated with human studies aimed at determining which chemokines are relevant to distinct human disease processes such as asthma.

Although we are in the early phase of this type of analysis and there has been only partial identification of the molecules involved in allergic inflammation, some principles are emerging. First, chemokines collaborate with other cytokines in the generation of eosinophil-rich inflammatory exudates. This involves increasing the pool of circulating leukocytes, upregulating particular adhesion molecules, and increasing a leukocyte's responsiveness to chemokines. So while eotaxin may be induced in many situations where TNF-α and IL-1 are present, it is only in those situations where IL-5 is coproduced that significant pathological tissue eosinophilia occurs. Second, several chemokines appear to contribute to eosinophil recruitment in allergic inflammation in the lung. For example, the human genome contains three eosinophil-selective chemokines (eotaxin-1, eotaxin-2, and eotaxin-3), and gene-targeting eotaxin-1 has only a partial effect on allergen-induced lung inflammation. Likewise, in bronchoalveolar lavage fluid from patients with asthma, eotaxin and MCP-4 each contribute to the eosinophil chemotactic activity. Third, the partially overlapping activity of these chemokines in allergic inflammation is explained by the coexpression of multiple chemokines in allergic tissue and the fact that each recruited inflammatory cell expresses multiple promiscuous chemokine receptors. Fourth, we have seen that the role of chemokines varies in different tissues and during baseline or inflammatory states. So although eotaxin's role in the lung may be partially overlapping with other cytokines, in the gastrointestinal tract eotaxin has a more dominant role (91,139,206). This suggests that targeting allergic diseases of the lung may be best accomplished with more broad-spectrum agents (anti-CCR3 agents) whereas allergic diseases in the gastrointestinal tract may be amenable to anti-eotaxin therapeutics.

In conclusion, chemokines have now emerged as potentially critical cytokines involved in the pathogenesis of allergic airway inflammation. This has provided the rationale for increased scientific investigation in the field and for the development of antichemokine and anti-chemokine receptor therapeutics. The challenge for the future will be to understand the role of each chemokine and chemokine receptor and their polymorphic variants in the pathophysiology of allergic diseases. Once this is accomplished, neutralization of chemokine function is likely to have therapeutic value in the treatment of allergic diseases. However, the ultimate proof of these principles awaits the testing of these therapeutic agents in humans, which may not be too far in the future.

Acknowledgments

The editorial assistance of Andrea Lippelman is appreciated. This work was supported in part by NIH grant R01 AI42242 (to M.E.R.), a grant from the Human Frontier Science Program (to M.E.R.), and the American Heart Association Scientist Development Grant (to N.Z.). N.Z. is a Parker B. Francis fellow in pulmonary research. This manuscript was adapted and updated from our previous review (207).

References

1. Bousquet J, Chanez P, Lacoste JY, et al. Eosinophilic inflammation in asthma. N Engl J Med 1990; 323:1033–1039.

2. Baggiolini M, Dahinden CA. CC chemokines in allergic inflammation. Immunol Today 1994; 15:127–133.
3. Zlotnik A, Yoshie O. Chemokines: A new classification system and their role in immunity. Immunity 2000; 12:121–127.
4. Luster AD, Rothenberg ME. Role of monocyte chemoattractant protein and eotaxin subfamily of chemokines in allergic inflammation. J Leukoc Biol 1997; 62:620–633.
5. Patel VP, Kreider BL, Li Y, et al. Molecular and functional characterization of two novel human C-C chemokines as inhibitors of two distinct classes of myeloid progenitors. J Exp Med 1997; 185:1163–1172.
6. Forssmann U, Uguccioni M, Loetscher P, et al. Eotaxin-2, a novel CC chemokine that is selective for the chemokine receptor CCR3, and acts like eotaxin on human eosinophil and basophil leukocytes. J Exp Med 1997; 185:2171–2176.
7. Zimmermann N, Hogan SP, Mishra A, et al. Murine eotaxin-2: A constitutive eosinophil chemokine induced by allergen challenge and IL-4 overexpression. J Immunol 2000; 165:5839–5846.
8. Kitaura M, Suzuki N, Imai T, et al. Molecular cloning of a novel human CC chemokine (eotaxin-3) that is a functional ligand of CC chemokine receptor 3. J Biol Chem 1999; 274:27975–27980.
9. Shinkai A, Yoshisue H, Koike M, et al. A novel human CC chemokine, eotaxin-3, which is expressed in IL-4-stimulated vascular endothelial cells, exhibits potent activity toward eosinophils. J Immunol 1999; 163:1602–1610.
10. Clore GM, Gronenborn AM. Three-dimensional structures of alpha and beta chemokines. FASEB J 1995; 9:57–62.
11. Lodi PJ, Garrett DS, Kuszewski J, et al. High-resolution solution structure of the beta chemokine hMIP-1 beta by multidimensional NMR. Science 1994; 263:1762–1767.
12. Handel TM, Domaille PJ. Heteronuclear (^{1}H, ^{13}C, ^{15}N) NMR assignments and solution structure of the monocyte chemoattractant protein-1 (MCP-1) dimer. Biochemistry 1996; 35:6569–6584.
13. Stone MJ, Mayer KL. Three-dimensional structure of chemokines. In: Rothenberg ME, ed. Chemokines in Allergic Diseases. New York: Marcel Dekker, 1999:67–94.
14. Mayer KL, Stone MJ. NMR solution structure and receptor peptide binding of the CC chemokine eotaxin-2. Biochemistry 2000; 39:8382–8395.
15. Rothenberg ME, Luster AD, Leder P. Murine eotaxin: An eosinophil chemoattractant inducible in endothelial cells and in interleukin 4-induced tumor suppression. Proc Natl Acad Sci USA 1995; 92:8960–8964.
16. Garcia-Zepeda EA, Combadiere CC, Rothenberg ME, et al. Human monocyte chemoattractant protein (MCP)-4: A novel CC chemokine with activities on monocytes, eosinophils, and basophils induced in allergic and non-allergic inflammation that signals through the CC chemokine receptors CKR-2 and -3. J Immunol 1996; 157:5613–5626.
17. Garcia-Zepeda EA, Rothenberg ME, Weremowicz S, Sarafi MN, Morton CC, Luster AD. Genomic organization, complete sequence, and chromosomal location of

the gene for human eotaxin (SCYA11), an eosinophil-specific CC chemokine. Genomics 1997; 41:471–476.

18. Coillie EV, Fiten P, Nomiyama H, et al. The human MCP-2 Gene (Scya8): Cloning, sequence analysis, tissue expression, and assignment to the CC chemokine contig on chromosome 17q11.2. Genomics 1997; 40:323–331.
19. Naruse K, Ueno M, Satoh T, et al. A YAC contig of the human CC chemokine genes clustered on chromosome 17q11.2. Genomics 1996; 34:236–240.
20. Nomiyama H, Osborne LR, Imai T, et al. Assignment of the human CC chemokine MPIF-2/eotaxin-2 (SCYA24) to chromosome 7q11.23. Genomics 1998; 49:339–340.
21. Proost P, Wuyts A, Van Damme J. Human monocyte chemotactic proteins-2 and -3: Structural and functional comparison with MCP-1. J Leuk Biol 1996; 59:67–74.
22. Garcia-Zepeda EA, Rothenberg ME, Ownbey RT, Celestin J, Leder P, Luster AD. Human eotaxin is a specific chemoattractant for eosinophil cells and provides a new mechanism to explain tissue eosinophilia. Nat Med 1996; 2:449–456.
23. Stellato C, Collins P, Ponath PD, et al. Production of the novel C-C chemokine MCP-4 by airway cells and comparison of its biological activity to other C-C chemokines. J Clin Invest 1997; 99:926–936.
24. Minshall E, Cameron L, Levigne F, et al. Eotaxin mRNA expression in chronic sinusitis and allergen-induced nasal responses in seasonal allergic rhinitis. Am J Respir Cell Mol Biol 1997; 17:683–690.
25. Lilly CM, Nakamura H, Kesselman H, et al. Expression of eotaxin by human lung epithelial cells: Induction by cytokines and inhibition by glucocorticoids. J Clin Invest 1997; 99:1767–1773.
26. Kulmburg PA, Huber NE, Scheer BJ, Wrann M, Baumruker T. Immunoglobulin E plus antigen challenge induces a novel intercrine/chemokine in mouse mast cells. J Exp Med 1992; 176:1773–1778.
27. Burd PR, Rogers HW, Gordon JR, et al. Interleukin 3-dependent and -independent mast cells stimulated with IgE and antigen express multiple cytokines. J Exp Med 1989; 170:245–257.
28. Oravecz T, Pall M, Roderiquez G, et al. Regulation of the receptor specificity and function of the chemokine RANTES (regulated on activation, normal T cell expressed and secreted) by dipeptidyl peptidase IV (CD26)-mediated cleavage. J Exp Med 1997; 186:1865–1872.
29. Struyf S, Proost P, Schols D, et al. CD26/dipeptidyl-peptidase IV down-regulates the eosinophil chemotactic potency, but not the anti-HIV activity of human eotaxin by affecting its interaction with CC chemokine receptor 3. J Immunol 1999; 162: 4903–4909.
30. Culley FJ, Brown A, Conroy DM, Sabroe I, Pritchard DI, Williams TJ. Eotaxin is specifically cleaved by hookworm metalloproteases preventing its action in vitro and in vivo. J Immunol 2000; 165:6447–6453.
31. Nelson PJ, Kim HT, Manning WC, Goralski TJ, Krensky AM. Genomic organization and transcriptional regulation of the RANTES chemokine gene. J Immunol 1993; 151:2601–2612.

32. Matsukura S, Stellato C, Plitt JR, et al. Activation of eotaxin gene transcription by NF-kappa B and STAT6 in human airway epithelial cells. J Immunol 1999; 163: 6876–6883.
33. Ueda A, Okuda K, Ohno S, et al. NF-kappa B and Sp1 regulate transcription of the human monocyte chemoattractant protein-1 gene. J Immunol 1994; 153:2052–2063.
34. Anisowicz A, Messineo M, Lee SW, Sager R. An NF-kappa B-like transcription factor mediates IL-1/TNF-alpha induction of gro in human fibroblasts. J Immunol 1991; 147:520–527.
35. Widmer U, Manogue KR, Cerami A, Sherry B. Genomic cloning and promoter analysis of macrophage inflammatory protein (MIP)-2, MIP-1 alpha, and MIP-1 beta, members of the chemokine superfamily of proinflammatory cytokines. J Immunol 1993; 150:4996–5012.
36. Beato M. Gene regulation by steroid hormones. Cell 1989; 56:335–344.
37. Mukaida N, Gussella GL, Kasahara T, et al. Molecular analysis of the inhibition of interleukin-8 production by dexamethasone in a human fibrosarcoma cell line. Immunology 1992; 75:674–679.
38. Stellato C, Matsukura S, Fal A, et al. Differential regulation of epithelial-derived CC chemokine expression by IL-4 and the glucocorticoid budesonide. J Immunol 1999; 163:5624–5632.
39. Toney LM, Cattoretti G, Graf JA, et al. BCL-6 regulates chemokine gene transcription in macrophages. Nat Immunol 2000; 1:214–220.
40. Murphy PM. The molecular biology of leukoctye chemoattractant receptors. Annu Rev Immunol 1994; 12:593–633.
41. Gerard C, Gerard NP. The pro-inflammatory seven-transmembrane segment receptors of the leukocyte. Curr Opin Immunol 1994; 6:140–145.
42. Loetscher P, Seitz M, Baggiolini M, Moser B. Interleukin-2 regulates CC chemokine receptor expression and chemotactic responsiveness in T lymphocytes. J Exp Med 1996; 184:569–577.
43. Loetscher M, Gerber B, Loetscher P, et al. Chemokine receptor specific for IP10 and mig: Structure, function, and expression in activated T-lymphocytes. J Exp Med 1996; 184:963–969.
44. D'Amico G, Frascaroli G, Bianchi G, et al. Uncoupling of inflammatory chemokine receptors by IL-10: Generation of functional decoys. Nat Immunol 2000; 1:387–391.
45. Clark-Lewis I, Kim KS, Rajarathnam K, et al. Structure-activity relationships of chemokines. J Leukoc Biol 1995; 57:703–711.
46. Hebert CA, Vitangcol RV, Baker JB. Scanning mutagenesis of interleukin-8 identifies a cluster of residues required for receptor binding. J Biol Chem 1991; 266: 18989–18994.
47. Crump MP, Gong JH, Loetscher P, et al. Solution structure and basis for functional activity of stromal cell-derived factor-1; dissociation of CXCR4 activation from binding and inhibition of HIV-1. EMBO J 1997; 16:6996–7007.
48. Hemmerich S, Paavola C, Bloom A, et al. Identification of residues in the monocyte chemotactic protein-1 that contact the MCP-1 receptor, CCR2. Biochemistry 1999; 38:13013–13025.

49. Siciliano SJ, Rollins TE, DeMartino J, et al. Two-site binding of C5a by its receptor: An alternative binding paradigm for G protein-coupled receptors. Proc Natl Acad Sci USA 1994; 91:1214–1218.
50. Wells TNC, Guyecoulin F, Bacon KB. Peptides from the amino-terminus of RANTES cause chemotaxis of human T-lymphocytes. Biochem Biophys Res Commun 1995; 211:100–105.
51. Crump MP, Rajarathnam K, Kim KS, Clark-Lewis I, Sykes BD. Solution structure of eotaxin, a chemokine that selectively recruits eosinophils in allergic inflammation. J Biol Chem 1998; 273:22471–22479.
52. Clubb RT, Omichinski JG, Clore GM, Gronenborn AM. Mapping the binding surface of interleukin-8 complexes with an N-terminal fragment of the type 1 human interleukin-8 receptor. FEBS Lett 1994; 338:93–97.
53. Mizoue LS, Bazan JF, Johnson EC, Handel TM. Solution structure and dynamics of the CX3C chemokine domain of fractalkine and its interaction with an N-terminal fragment of CX3CR1. Biochemistry 1999; 38:1402–1414.
54. Ye J, Kohli LL, Stone MJ. Characterization of binding between the chemokine eotaxin and peptides derived from the chemokine receptor CCR3. J Biol Chem 2000.
55. Ponath PD, Qin S, Post TW, et al. Molecular cloning and characterization of a human eotaxin receptor expressed selectively on eosinophils. J Exp Med 1996; 183: 2437–2448.
56. Daugherty BL, Siciliano SJ, DeMartino JA, Malkowitz L, Sirotina A, Springer MS. Cloning, expression, and characterization of the human eosinophil eotaxin receptor. J Exp Med 1996; 183:2349–2354.
57. Youn BS, Zhang SM, Lee EK, et al. Molecular cloning of leukotactin-1: A novel human beta-chemokine, a chemoattractant for neutrophils, monocytes, and lymphocytes, and a potent agonist at CC chemokine receptors 1 and 3. J Immunol 1997; 159:5201–5205.
58. Zhang S, Youn BS, Gao JL, Murphy PM, Kwon BS. Differential effects of leukotactin-1 and macrophage inflammatory protein-1alpha on neutrophils mediated by CCR1. J Immunol 1999; 162:4938–4942.
59. Heath H, Qin SX, Rao P, et al. Chemokine receptor usage by human eosinophils: The importance of CCR3 demonstrated using an antagonistic monoclonal antibody. J Clin Invest 1997; 99:178–184.
60. Warringa RAJ, Koenderman L, Kok PTM, Kreukniet J, Bruijnzeel PLB. Modulation and induction of eosinophil chemotaxis by granulocyte-macrophage colony-stimulating factor and interleukin-3. Blood 1991; 77:2694–2700.
61. Lamkhioued B, Renzi PM, Abi-Younes S, et al. Increased expression of eotaxin in bronchoalveolar lavage and airways of asthmatics contributes to the chemotaxis of eosinophils to the site of inflammation. J Immunol 1997; 159:4593–4601.
62. Sullivan SK, McGrath DA, Liao F, Boehme SA, Farber JM, Bacon KB. MIP-3alpha induces human eosinophil migration and activation of the mitogen-activated protein kinases (p42/p44 MAPK). J Leukoc Biol 1999; 66:674–682.
63. Nagasė H, Miyamasu M, Yamaguchi M, et al. Expression of CXCR4 in eosinophils: Functional analyses and cytokine-mediated regulation. J Immunol 2000; 164:5935–5943.

64. Jinquan T, Jing C, Jacobi HH, et al. CXCR3 expression and activation of eosinophils: Role of IFN-gamma-inducible protein-10 and monokine induced by IFN-gamma. J Immunol 2000; 165:1548–1556.
65. Nagase H, Miyamasu M, Yamaguchi M, et al. Glucocorticoids preferentially upregulate functional CXCR4 expression in eosinophils. J Allergy Clin Immunol 2000; 106:1132–1139.
66. Uhing RJ, Gettys TW, Tomhave E, Synderman R, Didsbury JR. Differential regulation of cAMP by endogenous versus transfected formylpeptide chemoattractant receptors: Implications for Gi-coupled receptor signalling. Biochem Biophys Res Commun 1992; 183:1033–1039.
67. Zimmermann N, Daugherty BL, Stark JM, Rothenberg ME. Molecular analysis of CCR-3 events in eosinophilic cells. J Immunol 2000; 164:1055–1064.
68. Ganju RK, Dutt P, Wu L, et al. Beta-chemokine receptor CCR5 signals via the novel tyrosine kinase RAFTK. Blood 1998; 91:791–797.
69. Boehme SA, Sullivan SK, Crowe PD, et al. Activation of mitogen-activated protein kinase regulates eotaxin-induced eosinophil migration. J Immunol 1999; 163: 1611–1618.
70. Kampen GT, Stafford S, Adachi T, et al. Eotaxin induces degranulation and chemotaxis of eosinophils through the activation of ERK2 and p38 mitogen-activated protein kinases. Blood 2000; 95:1911–1917.
71. El-Shazly A, Yamaguchi N, Masuyama K, Suda T, Ishikawa T. Novel association of the src family kinases, hck and c-fgr, with CCR3 receptor stimulation: A possible mechanism for eotaxin-induced human eosinophil chemotaxis. Biochem Biophys Res Commun 1999; 264:163–170.
72. Zimmermann N, Conkright JJ, Rothenberg ME. CC chemokine receptor-3 undergoes prolonged ligand-induced internalization. J Biol Chem 1999; 274:12611–12618.
73. Daugherty BL, Springer MS. The beta-chemokine receptor genes CCR1 (CMKBR1), CCR2 (CMKBR2), and CCR3 (CMKBR3) cluster within 285 kb on human chromosome 3p21. Genomics 1997; 41:294–295.
74. Ahuja SK, Shetty A, Tiffany HL, Murphy PM. Comparison of the genomic organization and promoter function for human interleukin-8 receptors A and B. J Biol Chem 1994; 269:26381–26389.
75. Mummidi S, Ahuja SS, McDaniel BL, Ahuja SK. The human CC chemokine receptor 5 (CCR5) gene. Multiple transcripts with 5′-end heterogeneity, dual promoter usage, and evidence for polymorphisms within the regulatory regions and noncoding exons. J Biol Chem 1997; 272:30662–30671.
76. Zimmermann N, Daugherty BL, Kavanaugh JL, El-Awar FY, Moulton EA, Rothenberg ME. Analysis of the CC chemokine receptor 3 gene reveals a complex 5′ exon organization, a functional role for untranslated exon 1, and a broadly active promoter with eosinophil-selective elements. Blood 2000; 96:2346–2354.
77. Pease JE, Wang J, Ponath PD, Murphy PM. The N-terminal extracellular segments of the chemokine receptors CCR1 and CCR3 are determinants for MIP-1alpha and eotaxin binding, respectively, but a second domain is essential for efficient receptor activation. J Biol Chem 1998; 273:19972–19976.

78. Zimmermann N, Bernstein JA, Rothenberg ME. Polymorphisms in the human CC chemokine receptor-3 gene. Biochim Biophys Acta 1998; 1442:170–176.
79. Kato H, Tsuchiya N, Izumi S, et al. New variations of human CC-chemokine receptors CCR3 and CCR4. Genes Immun 1999; 1:97–104.
80. Bates P. Chemokine receptors and HIV-1: An attractive pair? Cell 1996; 86:1–3.
81. Choe H, Farzan M, Sun Y, et al. The beta-chemokine receptors CCR3 and CCR5 facilitate infection by primary HIV-1 isolates. Cell 1996; 85:1135–1148.
82. Dean M, Carrington M, Winkler C, et al. Genetic restriction of HIV-1 infection and progression to AIDS by a deletion allele of the CKR5 structural gene. Hemophilia Growth and Development Study, Multicenter AIDS Cohort Study, Multicenter Hemophilia Cohort Study, San Francisco City Cohort, ALIVE Study. Science 1996; 273:1856–1862.
83. Liu R, Paxton WA, Choe S, et al. Homozygous defect in HIV-1 coreceptor accounts for resistance of some multiply-exposed individuals to HIV-1 infection. Cell 1996; 86:367–377.
84. Samson M, Soularue P, Vassart G, Parmentier M. The genes encoding the human CC-chemokine receptors CC-CKR1 to CC-CKR5 (CMKBR1-CMKBR5) are clustered in the p21.3–p24 region of chromosome 3. Genomics 1996; 36:522–526.
85. Quillent C, Oberlin E, Braun J, et al. HIV-1-resistance phenotype conferred by combination of two separate inherited mutations of CCR-5 gene. Lancet 1998; 351: 14–18.
86. Smith MW, Dean M, Carrington M, et al. Contrasting genetic influence of CCR2 and CCR5 variants on HIV-1 infection and disease progression. Hemophilia Growth and Development Study (HGDS), Multicenter AIDS Cohort Study (MACS), Multicenter Hemophilia Cohort Study (MHCS), San Francisco City Cohort (SFCC), ALIVE Study. Science 1997; 277:959–965.
87. Gerard C, Rollins BJ. Chemokines and disease. Nat Immunol 2001; 2:108–115.
88. Cook DN, Beck MA, Coffman TM, et al. Requirement of MIP-1 alpha for an inflammatory response to viral infection. Science 1995; 269:1583–1585.
89. Nagasawa T, Hirota S, Tachibana K, et al. Defects of B-cell lymphopoiesis and bone-marrow myelopoiesis in mice lacking the CXC chemokine PBSF/SDF-1. Nature 1996; 382:635–638.
90. Rothenberg ME, MacLean JA, Pearlman E, Luster AD, Leder P. Targeted disruption of the chemokine eotaxin partially reduces antigen-induced tissue eosinophilia. J Exp Med 1997; 185:785–790.
91. Matthews AN, Friend DS, Zimmermann N, et al. Eotaxin is required for the baseline level of tissue eosinophils. Proc Natl Acad Sci USA 1998; 95:6273–6278.
92. Lu B, Rutledge BJ, Gu L, et al. Abnormalities in monocyte recruitment and cytokine expression in monocyte chemoattractant protein 1-deficient mice. J Exp Med 1998; 187:601–608.
93. Chen SC, Mehrad B, Deng JC, et al. Impaired pulmonary host defense in mice lacking expression of the CXC chemokine lungkine. J Immunol 2001; 166:3362–3368.
94. Cacalano G, Lee J, Kikly K, et al. Neutrophil and B cell expansion in mice that lack the murine IL-8 receptor homolog. Science 1994; 265:682–684.

95. Forster R, Mattis AE, Kremmer E, Wolf E, Brem G, Lipp M. A putative chemokine receptor, BLR1, directs B cell migration to defined lymphoid organs and specific anatomic compartments of the spleen. Cell 1996; 87:1037–1047.
96. Gao JL, Wynn TA, Chang Y, et al. Impaired host defense, hematopoiesis, granulomatous inflammation and type 1-type 2 cytokine balance in mice lacking CC chemokine receptor 1. J Exp Med 1997; 185:1959–1968.
97. Boring L, Gosling J, Chensue SW, et al. Impaired monocyte migration and reduced type 1 (Th1) cytokine responses in C-C chemokine receptor 2 knockout mice. J Clin Invest 1997; 100:2552–2261.
98. Kurihara T, Warr G, Loy J, Bravo R. Defects in macrophage recruitment and host defense in mice lacking the CCR2 chemokine receptor. J Exp Med 1997; 186: 1757–1762.
99. Blease K, Mehrad B, Standiford TJ, et al. Airway remodeling is absent in CCR1 −/− mice during chronic fungal allergic airway disease. J Immunol 2000; 165: 1564–1572.
100. Blease K, Mehrad B, Standiford TJ, et al. Enhanced pulmonary allergic responses to Aspergillus in CCR2 −/− mice. J Immunol 2000; 165:2603–2611.
101. MacLean JA, De Sanctis GT, Ackerman KG et al. CC chemokine receptor-2 is not essential for the development of antigen-induced pulmonary eosinophilia and airway hyperresponsiveness. J Immunol 2000; 165:6568–6575.
102. Chensue SW, Lukacs NW, Yang TY, et al. Aberrant in vivo T helper type 2 cell response and impaired eosinophil recruitment in CC chemokine receptor 8 knockout mice. J Exp Med 2001; 193:573–584.
103. Zou YR, Kottmann AH, Kuroda M, Taniuchi I, Littman DR. Function of the chemokine receptor CXCR4 in haematopoiesis and in cerebellar development. Nature 1998; 393:595–599.
104. Tachibana K, Hirota S, Iizasa H, et al. The chemokine receptor CXCR4 is essential for vascularization of the gastrointestinal tract. Nature 1998; 393:591–594.
105. Zhou Y, Kurihara T, Ryseck RP, et al. Impaired macrophage function and enhanced T cell-dependent immune response in mice lacking CCR5, the mouse homologue of the major HIV-1 coreceptor. J Immunol 1998; 160:4018–4025.
106. Chvatchko Y, Hoogewerf AJ, Meyer A, et al. A key role for CC chemokine receptor 4 in lipopolysaccharide-induced endotoxic shock. J Exp Med 2000; 191:1755–1764.
107. Dawson TC, Lentsch AB, Wang Z, et al. Exaggerated response to endotoxin in mice lacking the Duffy antigen/receptor for chemokines (DARC). Blood 2000; 96: 1681–1684.
108. Hancock WW, Lu B, Gao W, et al. Requirement of the chemokine receptor CXCR3 for acute allograft rejection. J Exp Med 2000; 192:1515–1520.
109. Forster R, Schubel A, Breitfeld D, et al. CCR7 coordinates the primary immune response by establishing functional microenvironments in secondary lymphoid organs. Cell 1999; 99:23–33.
110. Cook DN, Prosser DM, Forster R, et al. CCR6 mediates dendritic cell localization, lymphocyte homeostasis, and immune responses in mucosal tissue. Immunity 2000; 12:495–503.

111. Butcher EC. Leukocyte-endothelial cell recognition: Three (or more) steps to specificity and diversity. Cell 1991; 67:1033–1036.
112. Yamada H, Hirai K, Miyamasu M, et al. Eotaxin is a potent chemotaxin for human basophils. Biochem Biophys Res Commun 1997; 231:365–368.
113. Rothenberg ME, Ownbey R, Mehlhop PD, et al. Eotaxin triggers eosinophil-selective chemotaxis and calcium flux via a distinct receptor and induces pulmonary eosinophilia in the presence of interleukin 5 in mice. Mol Med 1996; 2:334–348.
114. Collins PD, Marleau S, Griffiths-Johnson DA, Jose PJ, Williams TJ. Cooperation between interleukin-5 and the chemokine eotaxin to induce eosinophil accumulation in vivo. J Exp Med 1995; 182:1169–1174.
115. Mould AW, Matthaei KI, Young IG, Foster PS. Relationship between interleukin-5 and eotaxin in regulating blood and tissue eosinophilia in mice. J Clin Invest 1997; 99:1064–1071.
116. Powell WS, Ahmed S, Gravel S, Rokach J. Eotaxin and RANTES enhance 5-oxo-6,8,11,14-eicosatetraenoic acid-induced eosinophil chemotaxis. J Allergy Clin Immunol 2001; 107:272–278.
117. Jose PJ, Griffiths-Johnson DA, Collins PD, et al. Eotaxin: A potent eosinophil chemoattractant cytokine detected in a guinea pig model of allergic airways inflammation. J Exp Med 1994; 179:881–887.
118. Ponath PD, Qin SX, Ringler DJ, et al. Cloning of the human eosinophil chemoattractant, eotaxin: Expression, receptor binding, and functional properties suggest a mechanism for the selective recruitment of eosinophils. J Clin Invest 1996; 97: 604–612.
119. Bischoff SC, Krieger M, Brunner T, Dahinden CA. Monocyte chemotactic protein 1 is a potent activator of human basophils. J Exp Med 1992; 175:1271–1275.
120. Dahinden CA, Geiser T, Brunner T, et al. Monocyte chemotactic protein 3 is a most effective basophil- and eosinophil-activating chemokine. J Exp Med 1994; 179:751–756.
121. Elsner J, Hochstetter R, Kimming D, Kapp A. Human eotaxin represents a potent activator of the respiratory burst of human eosinophils. Eur J Immunol 1996; 26: 1919–1925.
122. Alam R, Lett-Brown MA, Forsythe PA, et al. Monocyte chemotactic and activating factor is a potent histamine-releasing factor for basophils. J Clin Invest 1992; 89: 723–728.
123. Alam R, Forsythe P, Stafford S, et al. Monocyte chemotactic protein-2, monocyte chemotactic protein-3, and fibroblast-induced cytokine. Three new chemokines induce chemotaxis and activation of basophils. J Immunol 1994; 153:3155–3159.
124. Alam R, Stafford S, Forsythe P, et al. RANTES is a chemotactic and activating factor for human eosinophils. J Immunol 1993; 150:3442–3448.
125. El-Shazly A, Masuyama K, Nakano K, Eura M, Samejima Y, Ishikawa T. Human eotaxin induces eosinophil-derived neurotoxin release from normal human eosinophils. Int Arch Allergy Immunol 1998; 117(suppl 1):55–58.
126. Fujisawa T, Kato Y, Nagase H, et al. Chemokines induce eosinophil degranulation through CCR-3. J Allergy Clin Immunol 2000; 106:507–513.
127. Kim CH, Broxmeyer HE. Chemokines for immature blood cells: Effects on migra-

tion, proliferation, and differentiation. In: Rothenberg ME, ed. Chemokines in Allergic Diseases. New York: Marcel Dekker, 1999:227–262.
128. Palframan RT, Collins PD, Williams TJ, Rankin SM. Eotaxin induces a rapid release of eosinophils and their progenitors from the bone marrow. Blood 1998; 91: 2240–2248.
129. Quackenbush EJ, Aguirre V, Wershil BK, Gutierrez-Ramos JC. Eotaxin influences the development of embryonic hematopoietic progenitors in the mouse. J Leukoc Biol 1997; 62:661–666.
130. Peled A, Gonzalo JA, Lloyd C, Gutierrez-Ramos JC. The chemotactic cytokine eotaxin acts as a granulocyte-macrophage colony-stimulating factor during lung inflammation. Blood 1998; 91:1909–1916.
131. Graham GJ, Wright EG, Hewick R, et al. Identification and characterization of an inhibitor of haemopoietic stem cell proliferation. Nature 1990; 344:442–444.
132. Luster AD. Chemokines: Chemotactic cytokines that mediate inflammation. N Engl J Med 1998; 338:436–445.
133. Rollins BJ. Chemokines. Blood 1997; 90:909–928.
134. Hromas R, Kim CH, Klemsz M, et al. Isolation and characterization of Exodus-2, a novel C-C chemokine with a unique 37-amino acid carboxyl-terminal extension. J Immunol 1997; 159:2554–2558.
135. Imai T, Baba M, Nishimura M, Kakizaki M, Takagi S, Yoshie O. The T cell-directed CC chemokine TARC is a highly specific biological ligand for CC chemokine receptor 4. J Biol Chem 1997; 272:15036–15042.
136. Gunn MD, Kyuwa S, Tam C, et al. Mice lacking expression of secondary lymphoid organ chemokine have defects in lymphocyte homing and dendritic cell localization. J Exp Med 1999; 189:451–460.
137. Luther SA, Tang HL, Hyman PL, Farr AG, Cyster JG. Coexpression of the chemokines ELC and SLC by T zone stromal cells and deletion of the ELC gene in the plt/plt mouse. Proc Natl Acad Sci USA 2000; 97:12694–12699.
138. Stahl J, Cook E, Rothenberg ME, Graziano FM. Epithelial cells are a major cellular source of eotaxin mRNA in the guinea pig lung. J Allergy Clin Immunol 1997; 97:403a.
139. Mishra A, Hogan SP, Lee JJ, Foster PS, Rothenberg ME. Fundamental signals that regulate eosinophil homing to the gastrointestinal tract. J Clin Invest 1999; 103: 1719–1727.
140. Sallusto F, Schaerli P, Loetscher P, et al. Rapid and coordinated switch in chemokine receptor expression during dendritic cell maturation. Eur J Immunol 1998; 28: 2760–2769.
141. Sozzani S, Luini W, Borsatti A, et al. Receptor expression and responsiveness of human dendritic cells to a defined set of CC and CXC chemokines. J Immunol 1997; 159:1993–2000.
142. Dieu-Nosjean MC, Vicari A, Lebecque S, Caux C. Regulation of dendritic cell trafficking: A process that involves the participation of selective chemokines. J Leukoc Biol 1999; 66:252–262.
143. Lambrecht BN, Salomon B, Klatzmann D, Pauwels RA. Dendritic cells are required for the development of chronic eosinophilic airway inflammation in response to inhaled antigen in sensitized mice. J Immunol 1998; 160:4090–4097.

144. Lambrecht BN, De Veerman M, Coyle AJ, Gutierrez-Ramos JC, Thielemans K, Pauwels RA. Myeloid dendritic cells induce Th2 responses to inhaled antigen, leading to eosinophilic airway inflammation. J Clin Invest 2000; 106:551–559.
145. Lukacs NW, Strieter RM, Warmington K, Lincoln P, Chensue SW, Kunkel SL. Differential recruitment of leukocyte populations and alteration of airway hyperreactivity by C-C family chemokines in allergic airway inflammation. J Immunol 1997; 158:4398–4404.
146. Gonzalo JA, Lloyd CM, Wen D, et al. The coordinated action of CC chemokines in the lung orchestrates allergic inflammation and airway hyperresponsiveness. J Exp Med 1998; 188:157–167.
147. Gunn MD, Tangemann K, Tam C, Cyster JG, Rosen SD, Williams LT. A chemokine expressed in lymphoid high endothelial venules promotes the adhesion and chemotaxis of naive T lymphocytes. Proc Natl Acad Sci USA 1998; 95:258–263.
148. Ward SG, Bacon K, Westwick J. Chemokines and T lymphocytes: More than an attraction. Immunity 1998; 9:1–11.
149. Sallusto F, Lenig D, Forster R, Lipp M, Lanzavecchia A. Two subsets of memory T lymphocytes with distinct homing potentials and effector functions. Nature 1999; 401:708–712.
150. Zhang S, Lukacs NW, Lawless VA, Kunkel SL, Kaplan MH. Cutting edge: Differential expression of chemokines in Th1 and Th2 cells is dependent on Stat6 but not Stat4. J Immunol 2000; 165:10–14.
151. Karpus WJ, Kennedy KJ. MIP-1alpha and MCP-1 differentially regulate acute and relapsing autoimmune encephalomyelitis as well as Th1/Th2 lymphocyte differentiation. J Leukoc Biol 1997; 62:681–687.
152. Gu L, Tseng S, Horner RM, Tam C, Loda M, Rollins BJ. Control of TH2 polarization by the chemokine monocyte chemoattractant protein-1. Nature 2000; 404:407–411.
153. Hogan SP, Mould AW, Young JM, et al. Cellular and molecular regulation of eosinophil trafficking to the lung. Immunol Cell Biol 1998; 76:454–460.
154. Dunn CJ, Elliott GA, Oostveen JA, Richards IM. Development of a prolonged eosinophil-rich inflammatory leukocyte infiltration in the guinea-pig asthmatic response to ovalbumin inhalation. Am Rev Respir Dis 1988; 137:541–547.
155. Wegner CD, Gundel RH, Reilly P, Haynes N, Letts LG, Rothlein R. Intercellular adhesion molecule-1 (ICAM-1) in the pathogenesis of asthma. Science 1990; 247: 456–459.
156. Renz H, Smith HR, Henson JE, Ray BS, Irvin CG, Gelfand EW. Aerosolized antigen exposure without adjuvant causes increased IgE production and increased airway responsiveness in the mouse. J Allergy Clin Immunol 1992; 89:1127–1138.
157. Chand N, Harrison JE, Rooney S, et al. Anti-IL-5 monoclonal antibody inhibits allergic late phase bronchial eosinophilia in guinea pigs: A therapeutic approach. Eur J Pharmacol 1992; 211:121–123.
158. Foster PS, Hogan SP, Ramsay AJ, Matthaei KI, Young IG. Interleukin 5 deficiency abolishes eosinophilia, airways hyperreactivity, and lung damage in a mouse asthma model. J Exp Med 1996; 183:195–201.
159. Lefort J, Bachelet CM, Leduc D, Vargaftig BB. Effect of antigen provocation of

IL-5 transgenic mice on eosinophil mobilization and bronchial hyperresponsiveness. J Allergy Clin Immunol 1996; 97:788–799.
160. Lilly CM, Chapman RW, Sehring SJ, Mauser PJ, Egan RW, Drazen JM. Effects of interleukin 5-induced pulmonary eosinophilia on airway reactivity in the guinea pig. Am J Physiol 1996; 270:L368–L375.
161. Drazen JM, Arm JP, Austen KF. Sorting out the cytokines of asthma. J Exp Med 1996; 183:1–5.
162. Corry DB, Folkesson ML, Warnock DJ, et al. Interleukin 4, but not interleukin 5 or eosinophils, is required in a murine model of acute airway hyperreactivity. J Exp Med 1996; 183:109–117.
163. Hogan SP, Matthaei KI, Young JM, Koskinen A, Young IG, Foster PS. A novel T cell-regulated mechanism modulating allergen-induced airways hyperreactivity in BALB/c mice independently of IL-4 and IL-5. J Immunol 1998; 161:1501–1509.
164. Wills-Karp M, Luyimbazi J, Xu X et al. Interleukin-13: Central mediator of allergic asthma. Science 1998; 282:2258–2261.
165. Chiaramonte MG, Schopf LR, Neben TY, Cheever AW, Donaldson DD, Wynn TA. IL-13 is a key regulatory cytokine for Th2 cell-mediated pulmonary granuloma formation and IgE responses induced by Schistosoma mansoni eggs. J Immunol 1999; 162:920–930.
166. Grunig G, Warnock M, Wakil AE et al. Requirement for IL-13 independently of IL-4 in experimental asthma. Science 1998; 282:2261–2263.
167. Li L, Xia Y, Nguyen A, et al. Effects of Th2 cytokines on chemokine expression in the lung: IL-13 potently induces eotaxin expression by airway epithelial cells. J Immunol 1999; 162:2477–2487.
168. MacLean JA, Ownbey R, Luster AD. T cell-dependent regulation of eotaxin in antigen-induced pulmonary eosinophila. J Exp Med 1996; 184:1461–1469.
169. Nakajima H, Iwamoto I, Tomoe S, et al. CD4+ T-lymphocytes and interleukin-5 mediate antigen-induced eosinophil infiltration into the mouse trachea. Am Rev Respir Dis 1992; 146:374–377.
170. Gavett SH, Chen X, Finkelman F, Wills-Karp M. Depletion of murine CD4+ T lymphocytes prevents antigen-induced airway hyperreactivity and pulmonary eosinophilia. Am J Respir Cell Mol Biol 1994; 10:587–593.
171. Garlisi CG, Falcone A, Kung TT et al. T cells are necessary for Th2 cytokine production and eosinophil accumulation in airways of antigen-challenged allergic mice. Clin Immunol Immunopathol 1995; 75:75–83.
172. Iwamoto I, Tomoe S, Tomioka H, Takatsu K, Yoshida S. Role of CD4+ T lymphocytes and interleukin-5 in antigen-induced eosinophil recruitment into the site of cutaneous late-phase reaction in mice. J Leukoc Biol 1992; 52:572–578.
173. Lukacs NW, Strieter RM, Chensue SW, Kunkel SL. Interleukin-4-dependent pulmonary eosinophil infiltration in a murine model of asthma. Am J Respir Cell Mol Biol 1994; 10:526–532.
174. Marsh DG, Hsu SH, Roebber M. HLA-Dw2: A genetic marker for human immune response to short pollen allergen Ra5. I. Response resulting primarily from antigenic exposure. J Exp Med 1982; 155:1439–1451.
175. Reishaus E, Innis M, MacIntyre N, Liggett SB. Mutations in the gene encoding

for the β2-adrenergic receptor in normal and asthmatic subjects. Am J Respir Cell Mol Biol 1993; 8:334–339.
176. Young RP, Dekker JW, Wordsworth BP. HLA-DR and HLA-DP genotypes and immunoglobulin E responses to common major allergens. Clin Exp Allergy 1994; 24:431–439.
177. Shirakawa T, Li A, Dubowitz M, et al. Association between atopy and variants of the β subunit of the high-affinity IgE receptor. Nat Genet 1994; 7:125–129.
178. Meyers DA, Postma DS, Panhuysen CI, et al. Evidence for a locus regulating total serum IgE levels mapping to chromosome 5. Genomics 1994; 23:464–470.
179. Postma DS, Bleecker ER, Amelung PJ, et al. Genetic susceptibility to asthma: Bronchial hyperresponsiveness coinherited with a major gene for atopy. N Engl J Med 1995; 333:894–900.
180. Khurana Hershey GK, Friedrich MF, Esswein LA, Thomas ML, Chatila TA. Association of atopy with gain-of-function mutation in the interleukin-4 receptor alpha chain. N Engl J Med 1997; 337:1720.
181. Nickel R, Barnes KC, Sengler CA, et al. Evidence for linkage of chemokine polymorphisms to asthma in populations of African descent. J Allergy Clin Immunol 1999; 103:S174.
182. Lin AY, Nutman TB, Kaslow D, et al. Familial eosinophilia: Clinical and laboratory results on a U.S. kindred. Am J Med Genet 1998; 76:229–237.
183. Rioux JD, Stone VA, Daly MJ, et al. Familial eosinophilia maps to the cytokine gene cluster on human chromosomal region 5q31–q33. Am J Hum Genet 1998; 63:1086–1094.
184. Ying S, Robinson DS, Meng Q, et al. Enhanced expression of eotaxin and CCR3 mRNA and protein in atopic asthma. Association with airway hyperresponsiveness and predominant co-localization of mRNA to bronchial epithelial and endothelial cells. Eur J Immunol 1997; 27:3507–3516.
185. Alam R, York J, Boyars M, et al. Increased MCP-1, RANTES, and MIP-1alpha in bronchoalveolar lavage fluid of allergic asthmatic patients. Am J Respir Crit Care Med 1996; 153:1398–1404.
186. Lilly CM, Woodruff PG, Camargo CA Jr, et al. Elevated plasma eotaxin levels in patients with acute asthma. J Allergy Clin Immunol 1999; 104:786–790.
187. Ying S, Meng Q, Zeibecoglou K, et al. Eosinophil chemotactic chemokines (eotaxin, eotaxin-2, RANTES, monocyte chemoattractant protein-3 (MCP-3), and MCP-4), and C-C chemokine receptor 3 expression in bronchial biopsies from atopic and nonatopic (intrinsic) asthmatics. J Immunol 1999; 163:6321–6329.
188. Ying S, Robinson DS, Meng Q, et al. C-C chemokines in allergen-induced late-phase cutaneous responses in atopic subjects: Association of eotaxin with early 6-hour eosinophils, and of eotaxin-2 and monocyte chemoattractant protein-4 with the later 24-hour tissue eosinophilia, and relationship to basophils and other C-C chemokines (monocyte chemoattractant protein-3 and RANTES). J Immunol 1999; 163:3976–3984.
189. Nickel RG, Casolaro V, Wahn U, et al. Atopic dermatitis is associated with a functional mutation in the promoter of the C-C chemokine RANTES. J Immunol 2000; 164:1612–1616.
190. Fryer AA, Spiteri MA, Bianco A, et al. The −403 G → A promoter polymorphism

in the RANTES gene is associated with atopy and asthma. Genes Immun 2000; 1: 509–514.
191. Leckie MJ, ten Brinke A, Khan J, et al. Effects of an interleukin-5 blocking monoclonal antibody on eosinophils, airway hyper-responsiveness, and the late asthmatic response. Lancet 2000; 356:2144–2148.
192. Lloyd CM, Delaney T, Nguyen T, et al. CC chemokine receptor (CCR)3/eotaxin is followed by CCR4/monocyte-derived chemokine in mediating pulmonary T helper lymphocyte type 2 recruitment after serial antigen challenge in vivo. J Exp Med 2000; 191:265–274.
193. Sabroe I, Conroy DM, Gerard NP, et al. Cloning and characterization of the guinea pig eosinophil eotaxin receptor, C-C chemokine receptor-3: Blockade using a monoclonal antibody in vivo. J Immunol 1998; 161:6139–6147.
194. Heath H, Qin S, Rao P, et al. Chemokine receptor usage by human eosinophils. The importance of CCR3 demonstrated using an antagonistic monoclonal antibody. J Clin Invest 1997; 99:178–184.
195. Proudfoot AE, Power CA, Hoogewerf AJ, et al. Extension of recombinant human RANTES by the retention of the initiating methionine produces a potent antagonist. J Biol Chem 1996; 271:2599–2603.
196. Elsner J, Petering H, Hochstetter R, et al. The CC chemokine antagonist Met-RANTES inhibits eosinophil effector functions through the chemokine receptors CCR1 and CCR3. Eur J Immunol 1997; 27:2892–2898.
197. Kips J, Palmans E, Proudfoot A, et al. The effect of Met-RANTES on the allergen-induced airway eosinophilia in an in vivo mouse model. Am J Respir Crit Care Med 1997; 155:A733.
198. Moore PS, Boshoff C, Weiss RA, Chang Y. Molecular mimicry of human cytokine and cytokine response pathway genes by KSHV. Science 1996; 274:1739–1744.
199. Kledal TN, Rosenkilde MM, Coulin F, et al. A broad-spectrum chemokine antagonist encoded by Kaposi's sarcoma-associated herpesvirus. Science 1997; 277: 1656–1659.
200. Luttichau HR, Stine J, Boesen TP, et al. A highly selective CC chemokine receptor (CCR)8 antagonist encoded by the poxvirus Molluscum contagiosum. J Exp Med 2000; 191:171–180.
201. White JR, Lee JM, Young PR, et al. Identification of a potent, selective non-peptide CXCR2 antagonist that inhibits interleukin-8-induced neutrophil migration. J Biol Chem 1998; 273:10095–10098.
202. Hesselgesser J, Ng HP, Liang M, et al. Identification and characterization of small molecule functional antagonists of the CCR1 chemokine receptor. J Biol Chem 1998; 273:15687–15692.
203. Bertrand CP, Ponath PD. CCR3 blockade as a new therapy for asthma. Expert Opin Invest Drugs 2000; 9:43–52.
204. Sabroe I, Peck MJ, Van Keulen BJ, et al. A small molecule antagonist of chemokine receptors CCR1 and CCR3. Potent inhibition of eosinophil function and CCR3-mediated HIV-1 entry. J Biol Chem 2000; 275:25985–25992.
205. Rutledge BJ, Rayburn H, Rosenberg R, et al. High level monocyte chemoattractant protein-1 expression in transgenic mice increases their susceptibility to intracellular pathogens. J Immunol 1995; 155:4838–4843.

206. Hogan SP, Mishra A, Brandt EB, Foster PS, Rothenberg ME. A critical role for eotaxin in experimental oral antigen-induced eosinophilic gastrointestinal allergy. Proc Natl Acad Sci USA 2000; 97:6681–6686.
207. Rothenberg ME, Zimmermann N, Mishra A, et al. Chemokines and chemokine receptors: Their role in allergic airway disease. J Clin Immunol 1999; 19:250–265.

9

IL-13 Antagonism as a Therapeutic Strategy for the Treatment of Asthma

MARSHA WILLS-KARP

Children's Hospital Medical Center
Cincinnati, Ohio

I. Introduction

The prevalence, morbidity, and mortality of asthma have increased dramatically over the last few decades despite increased use of currently available therapies. These findings underscore the need for the development of novel therapies. Asthma is a complex inflammatory disease of the lung characterized by variable airflow obstruction, airway hyperresponsiveness, and airway inflammation. Although asthma is multifactorial in origin, the inflammatory process is believed to be a result of inappropriate immune responses to common aeroallergens in genetically susceptible individuals. As such it has been hypothesized that $CD4^+$ T cells that produce a Th2 pattern of cytokines (IL-4, IL-5, IL-13) play a pivotal role in the pathogenesis of disease. Activation of these cells results in the release of a plethora of inflammatory mediators that individually or in concert induce changes in airway wall geometry and produce the symptoms of the disease. Based on the importance of these lymphocytes, it has recently been postulated that inhibition of the development of the Th2 response or the actions of these cytokines may provide therapeutic benefit.

Attempts at identifying the mechanisms by which Th2 cytokines mediate allergic responses were initially focused on the paradigmatic Th2 cytokines IL-

4 and IL-5. However, recent studies suggest that these two cytokines are not obligatory for these processes. On the basis of similarities in structure and the sharing of receptor components with IL-4, it was hypothesized that interleukin-13 may play a pivotal role in the development of allergic responses. This assumption was confirmed in animal models of allergic disease. Furthermore, recent studies suggest that IL-13 is consistently overexpressed in the lungs of asthmatic humans and that indeed genetic polymorphisms in the IL-13 gene may contribute to susceptibility to asthma and related traits. Based on these observations, it has been postulated that blockade of IL-13 may provide a good target for therapeutic drug development. This chapter discusses our current understanding of the role of IL-13 in the pathogenesis of allergic asthma and potential approaches to the blockade of IL-13's actions in vivo.

II. Interleukin-13 and Its Receptors

Human IL-13 is a 17 kDa glycoprotein cloned from activated T cells (1). The human IL-13 gene is located on human chromosome 5q31 or mouse chromosome 11 in the cluster of genes encoding IL-4, IL-3, IL-5, IL-9, and GM-CSF. The gene encoding IL-13 is only 25 kilobases (kb) upstream of the IL-4 gene and in the same orientation, leading to speculation that these genes arose as a duplication event during evolution. Although the IL-13 protein has only approximately 25% homology with IL-4, it shares many structural characteristics with IL-4. Furthermore, it shares many but not all functional properties with IL-4. The similarities in the functional properties of IL-4 and IL-13 are due to the sharing of a receptor chain in their individual heterodimeric receptor complexes (2).

Two distinct IL-13 receptor chains have been cloned, and they are designated as IL-13Rα1 and IL-13RAα2 (3–5). The genes encoding both receptor chains are mapped to the X chromosome. IL-13Rα1 is a 68–70 kDa protein that binds IL-13 with low affinity (2–10 nM). The extracellular portion of IL-13Rα1 possesses the WSXWS motif, which is characteristic of the type 1 cytokine receptor superfamily. This receptor chain has an intracytoplasmic domain in which box 1 and box 3 motifs can be identified, suggesting that it may contribute to signaling. Several lines of evidence suggest that the functional IL-13 receptor is a heterodimeric complex composed of the IL-4Rα chain and the IL-13Rα1 chain, including the fact that cells do not respond to IL-13 unless both receptor chains are present (6). Moreover, disruption of IL-4Rα has been shown to impair IL-13-induced immune responses (7). Although the unique IL-4 receptor is composed of the IL-4Rα chain and the γc chain, IL-4 can also bind to the receptor complex formed by IL-4Rα and IL-13Rα1 in cells lacking the γc chain. The ability of both cytokines to bind this complex explains the redundancies in function observed between IL-4 and IL-13.

On the other hand, IL-13Rα2 binds IL-13, but not IL-4, with high affinity (0.5–1.2 nM). In contrast to IL-13Rα1, the short cytoplasmic domain of the IL-13Rα2 is devoid of box 1 and box 2 signaling motifs, suggesting that it does not have direct signaling capabilities. The exact function of the IL-13Rα2 chain is currently unknown; however, it does not appear to contribute to signaling, because transfection of cells with this subunit either alone or in combination with the IL-4Rα chain does not reconstitute IL-13 responsiveness of cells (8). Current speculation is that it either acts as a decoy receptor, possibly regulating IL-13 binding, or may combine with IL-13Rα1 to facilitate the formation of a high affinity signaling complex. In support of the decoy receptor theory, this receptor chain has been found in soluble form in murine serum and urine (9). The fact that the IL-13Rα2 chain binds IL-13, not IL-4, with high affinity has recently been exploited to probe the in vivo actions of IL-13 and to distinguish IL-13-mediated processes from those of IL-4. Donaldson and colleagues have generated a soluble form of the murine and human IL-13Rα2 receptor, sIL-13Rα2, by fusing the extracellular domain of the receptor to the Fc portion of human IgG1 (10). This molecule is a specific inhibitor of IL-13 in vitro and can inhibit the action of IL-13 in murine models of Th2-mediated immune responses in vivo (discussed below).

The IL-13R (IL-4Rα/IL-13Rα1) is expressed on both hematopoietic and nonhematopoietic cells such as B cells, monocyte/macrophages, dendritic cells, eosinophils, basophils, fibroblasts, and endothelial cells. IL-13Rα1 has also been shown in hair follicles, sweat glands, intestinal smooth muscle, cardiac myocytes, and hepatocytes. Of particular relevance to allergy and asthma, recent studies demonstrated the existence of the IL-13Rα1 on airway epithelial cells and airway smooth muscle cells (11,12). Interestingly, although the message for the IL-13Rα1 chain is present in T cells, there appears to be no surface expression of this chain on human or mouse T cells (13). Consequently, IL-13 is not thought to exert any control over T-cell function. Furthermore, whereas human B cells express the IL-13 receptor it has not been detected on mouse B cells. Although the expression of the IL-13Rα2 chain is less well characterized, it has been shown to be present in high quantities in testis, fibroblast, and airway smooth muscle cells.

Ligation of the IL-13/IL-4 receptor complex results in activation of a variety of signal transduction pathways (Fig. 1). Upon IL-13Rα1 dimerization with IL-4Rα, Janus-tyrosine kinases (JAK-1) and Tyk-2 kinases, which are consititutively associated with the receptors, become phosphorylated and activated, and subsequently phosphorylate tyrosine residues on the IL-4Rα and IL-13Rα1 chains. A number of signaling pathways are then activated. For example, monomers of STAT6 bind through their SH2 domains to phosphorylated tyrosine residues of IL-4Rα. Once bound, STAT6 is phosphorylated by JAK kinases (JAK1), whereupon it is released from the receptor. It then dimerizes with other phosphor-

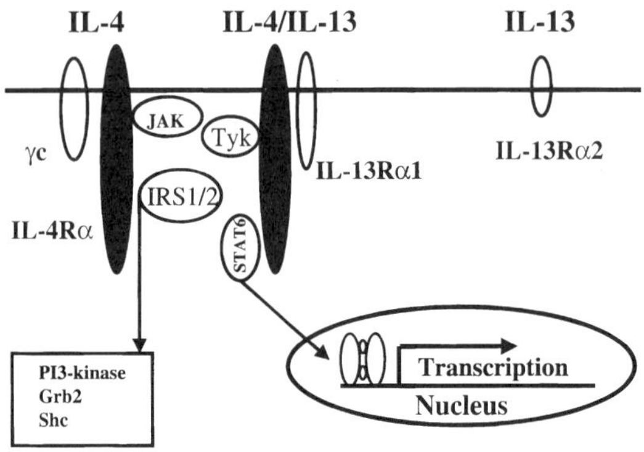

Figure 1 IL-13/IL-4 signal transduction pathways. The functional IL-13 receptor consists of a heterodimeric complex composed of the IL-4Rα and IL-13Rα1 chains. On the other hand, IL-4 can signal through a receptor complex composed of either IL-4Rα and γc or IL-4Rα and IL-13Rα1. Both cytokines (IL-13, IL-4) can induce heterodimerization of the IL-4Rα and IL-13RAα1 chains, and dimerization of both chains induces phosphorylation and activation of JAK kinases. Activated JAK kinases thus phosphorylate tyrosine residues of the IL-4Rα chain. IRS and STAT6 are attached with phosphorylated tyrosine via SH domains and phosphorylated by JAK kinases. Phosphorylated IRS1/2 is associated with several signal molecules such as P13-kinase, Grb2, and Shc that mediate downstream signals for growth and cell proliferation. Phosphorylated STAT6 proteins dimerize and translocate to the nucleus, where they bind to specific DNA sequences. The IL-13Rα2 chain binds only IL-13, not IL-4, with high affinity. Because it has a short cytoplasmic domain devoid of signaling motifs it is not thought to have direct signaling capabilities. The exact function of the IL-13Rα2 chain is currently unknown; however, current speculation is that either it acts as a decoy receptor possibly regulating IL-13 binding or it may combine with IL-13Rα1 to facilitate the formation of a high affinity signaling complex.

ylated STAT6 molecules and translocates to the nucleus, where it binds to specific consensus sequences found within the promoter regions of genes regulated by IL-13 and IL-4. Analyses of STAT6 KO mice have verified the necessity of STAT6 for several IL-4- and IL-13-mediated processes such as class switching of B cells (14). Furthermore, the development of the allergic phenotype in mouse models has been shown to be dependent on the STAT6 signaling pathway (15). Ligation of the IL-13/IL-4 receptor complex also results in tyrosine phosphorylation of the insulin receptor substrate (IRS) followed by activation of a number of signaling molecules including PI-3 kinase, Grb2, and Shc. Stimulation of these pathways is thought to be important in cell proliferation and cell growth. Recent studies also suggest that IL-13 activates STAT3 as well, although the exact consequences of this are currently unknown (16). Activation of these multiple signaling pathways may explain the plethora of actions mediated via IL-13 and IL-4.

III. Biological Actions of IL-13 Relevant to the Allergic Phenotype

Many types of inflammatory cells associated with the asthmatic phenotype, including Th2 cells, synthesize and secrete IL-13. It is produced at relatively high levels by both Th1 and Th2 $CD4^+$ T cells after activation. In addition, Th0 and $CD8^+$ T cells produce considerable quantities of IL-13. IL-13, unlike IL-4, is also produced by naive $CD45RA^+$ T cells. Thus, IL-13 does not behave as a classical Th2 cytokine. It is also produced by a number of non-T-cell populations such as keratinocytes and mast cells and in large quantities by basophils.

IL-13 is known to perform a number of actions relevant to the asthmatic diathesis such as regulation of isotype class switching in B cells to IgE synthesis, induction of MHC II and CD23 expression, induction of adhesion molecule expression on endothelial cells (VCAM-1), induction (eotaxin) or downregulation (MIP-1, MIP-B, and MCP-3) of chemokine production, activation of mast cells and eosinophils, and inhibition of proinflammatory gene expression (IL-1, TNF, and IL6) (see review, Ref. 17). Many of these functions are overlapping with those of IL-4 due to the sharing of the receptor chain in their individual heterodimeric complexes as discussed above (2). However, there are clear differences in their functions, such as the fact that in contrast to IL-4, IL-13 does not support proliferation of activated human and mouse T cells. More important, IL-13 is unable to directly drive differentiation of naive $CD4^+$ T cells toward a Th2 phenotype. This is likely because of the fact that functional IL-13 receptors have not been shown on T cells, although the message for the receptor has been detected in activated T cells. Even though IL-13 does not have direct effects on T cells, it may influence T-cell differentiation indirectly via downregulatory effects on production of proinflammatory cytokines, particularly on monocyte production of IL-12.

In addition to the effects on hematopoietic and immune cells described above, IL-13 has been shown to regulate enzymes of the arachidonic acid pathway, nitric oxide production, VCAM expression, chemokine secretion, and collagen production (17,18). These activities likely play a role in the ability of IL-13 to mediate the asthmatic phenotype.

IV. Role of IL-13 in Experimental Murine Models of Allergic Disease and Efficacy of sIL-13Rα2-Ig

Several recent studies suggest that IL-13 plays a pivotal role in the effector phase of the allergic response. Specifically, blockade of endogenous levels of IL-13 in antigen-sensitized mice by administration of a soluble form of the IL-13Rα2 chain, which binds only IL-13, completely reverses AHR and pulmonary mucus cell hyperplasia (19,20). Similarly, anti-IL-13 antibody treatment of mice after sensitization inhibited *A. fumigatus*-induced AHR, collagen deposition, and goblet cell hyperplasia (21). Interestingly, despite the similarities in function between IL-13 and IL-4, IL-4 blockade at the time of antigen challenge does not ablate airway hyperresponsiveness (22). This was further supported by the finding that transfer of Th2 cells derived from IL-4-deficient mice was still able to confer airway hyperresponsiveness (23).

Further evidence of its importance as an effector molecule in asthma is provided by the fact that short-term administration of IL-13 itself was sufficient to recreate many features of the allergic phenotype such as AHR, eosinophilic inflammation, and mucus cell hyperplasia in nonimmunized mice or RAG-deficient mice (19,20). Moreover, chronic expression of IL-13 in the murine lung results in development of these features as well as subepithelial fibrosis and the formation of Charcot-Leyden crystals (24). In contrast, overexpression of the IL-4 gene in the murine lung does not result in AHR or subepithelial fibrosis (25). From the above observations, it can be concluded that disruption of IL-13 production or signaling alone may have significant therapeutic potential in asthma and other allergic diseases.

V. Potential Mechanisms of IL-13-Induced Allergic Responses

Although the exact mechanisms by which IL-13 mediates allergic symptoms are currently not well understood, several hypotheses have been put forth. IL-13 may mediate its effects directly or via indirect effects on resident airway cells or infiltrating inflammatory cells (Fig. 2).

Although $CD4^+$ T cells are clearly required to initiate allergic responses, it appears that once IL-13 is produced by T cells, those cells are no longer required for development of the allergic phenotype. Evidence for this is presented in RAG −/− mice, which are deficient in functional T cells (20). In these mice IL-13 induces hyperreactivity similar to that observed in wild-type controls. This is not surprising given the lack of IL-13 receptors on T cells.

Interleukin-13 has been shown to regulate human B-cell function and IgE synthesis in vitro (17). Although IL-13 clearly regulates IgE synthesis in human B cells, the effect of IL-13 on mouse B cells is more complex. In vitro studies have failed to show induction of IgE production by mouse B cells exposed to IL-13 (1). However, IL-13 transgenic mice have elevated serum levels of IgE with normal levels of IgG isotypes (26). Furthermore, IL-4-deficient mice overexpressing IL-13 still have elevations in IgE, suggesting that indeed IL-13 is able to induce IgE class switching independently from IL-4. A role for IL-13 in IgE

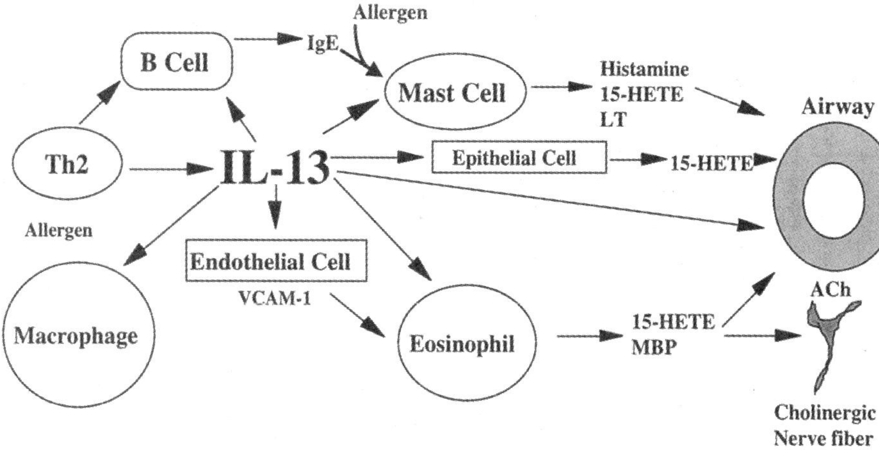

Figure 2 Potential mechanisms of IL-13's role in the effector phase of the allergic response. Interleukin 13 receptors are found on a number of cells relevant to the allergic airway response, including B cells, mast cells, eosinophils, epithelial cells, and airway smooth muscle cells. Binding of its receptor on these cells individually or in concert may induce the symptoms of asthma.

production has also been shown in IL-13-deficient mice (27). Whether the effects of IL-13 are direct or are due to modulation of other types of cells that influence IgE regulation is not clear at the present time. Nonetheless, regulation of IgE synthesis by IL-13 is likely to be important, because IgE-mediated processes play a pivotal role in human disease. In this regard, McKenzie and colleagues (28) recently demonstrated the importance of IL-13 in anaphylaxis in mice, which is presumably mediated via IgE.

IL-13 also plays a major role in allergic inflammation through regulation of recruitment, homing, and activation of inflammatory cells. It has been shown to have several actions relevant to the recruitment of T cells and eosinophils into the lung. Among these actions are its role in upregulation of vascular cell adhesion molecule-1 (VCAM-1) expression, its ability to prolong eosinophil survival, and its activity as an eosinophil activation and chemotactic agent. IL-13 has been shown to induce the expression of VCAM-1, resulting in preferential extrasavation of eosinophils into the airway spaces. In addition, IL-13 has been shown to induce eotaxin production in airway epithelial cells in vitro (29). In vivo confirmation of this finding has been provided in IL-13 transgenic mice (24). Despite the importance of IL-13 in eosinophil recruitment, preliminary reports suggest that eosinophil infiltration does not appear to be required for IL-13-induced AHR (Wills-Karp, unpublished data).

Another feature of the asthmatic airway that is thought to be mediated via IL-13 is subepithelial fibrosis. Overexpression of IL-13 in the murine lung induces a dramatic fibrotic response in the airway wall (24). Furthermore, IL-13 transgenic mice express matrix proteases such as MMP and cathepsins, which are thought to be important in the fibrotic response (30). A clear demarcation of function for IL-4 and IL-13 in fibrosis has been demonstrated in Th2-mediated pathology of *Schistosoma mansoni* infection in mice. Schistosome-induced collagen deposition is reduced in the lungs of STAT6-deficient animals but not in IL-4-deficient mice (18). Furthermore, sIL-13Rα2-Ig delivery completely prevented the fibrotic response in parasite-infected mice. Thus in several models of Th2-mediated fibrosis, blockade of IL-13 selectively inhibited fibrotic remodeling processes in the lung, suggesting that blockade of this cytokine may be beneficial in limiting the fibrotic response observed in the asthmatic lung.

Mucus hypersecretion is a consistent feature of the allergic phenotype. In fact, extensive plugging of the airway lumen has been associated with fatal episodes of asthma. Allergen challenge in murine models results in extensive mucus cell metaplasia. This response is a Th2 cell–dependent process because adoptive transfer of Th2 cells into the murine lung reconstitutes the effect of antigen challenge (23). Several lines of evidence suggest that mucus cell metaplasia is an IL-13-, not IL-4-, dependent process. For example, transfer of Th2 cells devoid of the IL-4 or IL-5 genes still induces extensive goblet cell metaplasia in the murine lung (23). However, blockade of the IL-4Rα chain or deficiency in STAT6 prevents the development of mucus cell metaplasia following allergen challenge, suggesting that IL-13 may be the ligand for the IL-4/STAT6 pathway in mucus cell changes (15,31). Indeed, administration of soluble IL-13Rα2 reversed the metaplastic response of goblet cells induced by allergen sensitization and challenge (19,20). Administration of rIL-13 in vivo or overexpression of the IL-13 gene recapitulates antigen effects on mucus production. Conversely, allergen-induced goblet cell metaplasia is significantly reduced in IL-13-deficient mice (32). This was not further reduced when IL-4 was blocked with neutralizing antibodies, suggesting that indeed IL-13 is the primary regulator in vivo of mucus cell hyperplasia.

Recent reports suggest that IL-13 may induce airway hyperresponsiveness by means of its direct effects on airway smooth muscle. In this regard, Laporte et al. (12) report that human airway smooth muscle cells express IL-4Rα, IL-13Rα1, and IL-13Rα2 chains. Moreover, they demonstrate that IL-13, but not IL-4, significantly reduces β-adrenoceptor-induced reduction in human airway smooth muscle cell stiffness through an MAP kinase–dependent pathway. These results suggest that IL-13 may have direct effects on airway smooth muscle that contribute at least in part to the airway narrowing observed in asthmatic individuals.

VI. IL-13 and Human Asthma

The importance of IL-13 in allergic disorders in humans is supported by numerous reports of exaggerated IL-13 production in asthma, atopic rhinitis, allergic dermatitis, and chronic sinusitis. In asthma in particular, both message and protein levels of IL-13 are elevated in bronchial biopsy specimens and BAL cells from allergic individuals compared with those of control subjects (33–35). Interestingly, elevations in IL-13 mRNA and protein levels appear to be more associated with asthma than with atopy because levels were increased in the lungs of atopic and nonatopic asthmatic patients but not in those of atopic nonasthmatic patients compared with normal subjects (34). IL-13 levels are strongly correlated with BAL eosinophils in allergic asthmatic subjects after local allergen challenge, whereas IL-4 levels are not (35). Conversely, IL-13 levels are reduced in patients undergoing allergen desensitization treatment regimes or steroid treatment (33).

In support of the notion that IL-13 is a central mediator of asthma, several groups recently reported associations of polymorphisms in the IL-13 gene with various features of the asthmatic phenotype (11,36,37). Of particular interest is the Arg130Gln substitution in the coding region of IL-13 noted by two groups and detected across multiple ethnic groups. Molecular modeling suggests potential biological impacts of this change including enhanced receptor binding and activation. Mutations in the putative promoter region could also explain elevations in tissue and serum IL-13 levels (36). Taken together with the accumulating biological evidence of the importance of IL-13 in the pathogenesis of asthma, these results support the contention that IL-13 is a major locus for atopy/asthma on chromosome 5q. Identification of variants of IL-13 signaling in the development of atopy/asthma in humans provides a focus for the development of novel diagnostic and therapeutic strategies for asthma.

VII. Advantages of IL-13 Antagonism in Treatment of Asthma

Because asthma is likely a disease of imbalance of the Th2–Th1 axis, the ideal therapeutic agent would restore this balance without further enhancing the Th1 response or impairing the beneficial actions of Th2 cytokines. Th2 cytokines serve as important brakes on Th1 cell–mediated immune responses, and without this brake tissue damage ensues, as is seen in diseases such as arthritis and diabetes. IL-4 and IL-13 are both potent inhibitors of the production of Th1-mediated inflammatory mediators such as nitric oxide, IL-1, TNF, and IL-6. The redundancy of IL-4 and IL-13 in this instance may be beneficial in that blockade of one of these cytokines would not completely impair their combined anti-inflammatory actions. However, it is likely that blockade of IL-4 will result in impairment of IL-13 production as well. The beneficial effect of blockade of the IL-4/IL-13 pathway in human disease has been demonstrated in clinical studies with the soluble IL-4 receptor (38). However, the long-term effects of IL-4 blockade have not been assessed. The primary advantage of IL-13 over IL-4 blockade is the lack of effect of IL-13 on T-cell differentiation and Th2 cell growth. IL-13 blockade will provide inhibition of the effector phase of the allergic response while leaving the ability to generate Th2 cells intact. Furthermore, studies in a chronic model of fungal asthma suggest that IL-13 neutralization is effective when initiated long after the induction of chronic asthma (21). More important, the therapeutic effects persisted even following cessation of IL-13 neutralization.

VIII. Therapeutic Approaches to IL-13 Blockade

Several approaches can be employed to antagonize IL-13 signaling including administration of soluble receptors (IL-13Rα2-Ig), anti-IL-13 monoclonal antibodies, antagonistic mutant proteins (39), and antireceptor antibodies. Suitable targets for small molecule antagonists of IL-13 include the IL-13 signaling receptor complex and signaling molecules such as STAT6. Identification of additional genes regulated by IL-13 and validation of their participation in individual aspects of asthma pathogenesis may provide further therapeutic opportunities for development of small molecules.

Potential advantages of the sIL-13Rα2Fc-Ig over other approaches include extended half-life in vivo and high-affinity binding to IL-13. Because the sIL-13Rα2 is a fully human peptide sequence and is found naturally in tissues, it should reduce the possibility of development of host antibodies against this molecule.

IX. Conclusion

Studies in human asthma and in animal models of disease have highlighted the role of IL-13 as a major mediator of the pathophysiology of asthma. The ability of IL-13 administration or overexpression to recapitulate all aspects of the asthmatic diathesis (i.e., airway hyperresponsiveness, mucus production, and remodeling) coupled with the compelling efficacy of IL-13 antagonism in animal models supports IL-13 antagonism as a viable therapeutic option for the treatment of asthma. Validation of the efficacy and safety of IL-13 antagonism in asthma awaits clinical trials in asthmatic patients.

References

1. Zurawski G, deVries J. Interleukin-13, an interleukin-4 like cytokine that acts on monocytes and B cells but not on T-cells. Immunol Today 1994; 15:19–26.
2. Zurawski SM, Vega F, Huyghe B, Zurawski G. Receptors for interleukin-13 and interleukin-4 are complex and share a novel component that functions in signal transduction. EMBO J 1993; 12:2663–2670.
3. Hilton DJ, Zhang J-G, Metcalf D, Alexander WS, Nicols NA, Wilson TA. Cloning and characterization of a binding subunit of the interleukin 13 receptor that is also a component of interleukin 4 receptor. Proc Natl Acad Sci USA 1996; 93:497–501.
4. Aman MJ, Tayebi N, Obii NI, Puri RK, Modi WS, Leonard WJ. CDNA cloning and characterization of the human interleukin-13 receptor alpha chain. J Biol Chem 1996; 271:29265–29270.
5. Caput D, Laurent P, Kaghad M, Lelias JM, Lefort S, Vita N, Ferrara P. Cloning and characterization of specific interleukin (IL)-13 binding protein and structurally related to the IL-5 receptor a chain. J Biol Chem 1996; 271:16921–16926.
6. Zurawski S, Chomarat P, Djossou O, Bidaudi C, McKenzie ANJ, Miossec P, Banchereau J, Zuawski G. The primary binding subunit of the human interleukin-4 receptor is also a component of the interleukin-13 receptor. J Biol Chem 1995; 270:13869–13878.
7. Urban, JF Jr, Noben-Trauth N, Donaldson DD, Madden KB, Morris SC, Collins M, Finkelman FD. IL-13, IL-4Ralpha and Stat6 are required for the expulsion of the gastrointestinal nematode parasite Nippostrongylus brasiliensis. Immunity 1998; 8: 255–264.
8. Murata T, Obiri NI, Puri K. Structure of and signal transduction through interleukin-4 and interleukin-13 receptors. Int J Mol Med 1998; 1:551–557.
9. Zhang, JG, Hilton DJ, Wilson TA, McFarane C, Roberts BA, Moritz RL, Simpson RJ, Alexander WS, Metcalf D, Nicola NA. Identification, purification, and characterization of a soluble interleukin (IL)-13-binding protein: Evidence that it is distinct from the cloned IL-13 receptor and IL-4 receptor a-chains. J Biol Chem 1997; 272: 9474–9480.
10. Donaldson DD, Whitters MJ, Fitz LJ, Neben TY, Finnerty H, Henderson SL, O'Hara RMJ, Beier DR, Turner KJ, Wood CR, Collins M. The murine IL-13 receptor alpha 2: Molecular cloning, characterization, and comparison with murine IL-13 receptor alpha 1. J Immunol 1998; 161:2317–2324.
11. Heinzmann A, Mao X-Q, Akaiwa M, et al. Genetic variants of IL-13 signalling and human asthma and atopy. Hum Mol Gen 2000; 9:549–559.
12. Laporte JC, Moore PE, Baraldo S, Jouvin M-H, Church TL, Schwartzman IN, Panettieri RA, Kinet J-P, Shore SA. Direct effects of interleukin-13 on signaling pathways for physiological responses in cultured human airway smooth muscle cells. Am J Respir Crit Care Med 2001; 164:141–148.
13. Graber P, Gretener D, Herren S, Aubry JP, Elson G, Poudrier J. The distribution of IL-13 receptor alpha 1 expression on B cells, T cells, and monocytes and its regulation by IL-13 and IL-4. Eur J Immunol 1998; 28:4286–4298.
14. Kaplan M, Schindler U, Smiley S, Grusby M. STAT6 is required for mediating

responses to IL-4 and for the development of Th2 cells. Immunity 1996; 4:313–319.

15. Kuperman D, Schofield B, Wills-Karp M, Grusby MJ. Signal transducer and activator of transcription factor 6 (Stat6)-deficient mice are protected from antigen-induced airway hyperresponsiveness and mucus production. J Exp Med 1998; 187:939–948.
16. Wery-Zennao S, Letourneur, David M, Bertoglio J, Piere J. Binding of IL-4 to the IL-13Ralpha(1)/IL-4Ralpha receptor complex leads to STAT3 phosphorylation but not to its nuclear translocation. FEBS Lett 1999; 464:91–96.
17. De Vries JE. The role of IL-13 and its receptor in allergy and inflammatory responses. J Allergy Clin Immunol 1998; 102:165–169.
18. Chiaramonte, MG, Donaldson DD, Cheever AW, Wynn TA. An IL-13 inhibitor blocks the development of hepatic fibrosis during a T-helper type 2-dominated inflammatory response. J Clin Invest 1999; 104:777–785.
19. Wills-Karp M, Luyimbazi J, Xu X, et al. Interleukin-13: Central mediator of allergic asthma. Science 1998; 282:2258–2261.
20. Grunig G, Warnock M, Wakil AE, Schofield B, Neben TY, Karp CL, Donaldson DD. Requirement for IL-13 independently of IL-4 in experimental asthma. Science 1998; 282:2261–2262.
21. Blease K, Jakubzic C, Westwick J, Lukacs N, Kunkel SL, Hogaboam CM. Therapeutic effect of IL-13 immunoneutralization during chronic experimental fungal asthma. J Immunol 2001; 166:5219–5224.
22. Coyle AJ, Le Gros G, Bertrand C, Tsuyuki S, Heusser CH, Kopf M, Anderson GP. Interleukin-4 is required for the induction of lung Th2 mucosal immunity. Am J Respir Cell Mol Biol 1995; 13:54–59.
23. Cohn L, Tepper JS, Bottomly K. Cutting edge: IL-4-independent induction of airway hyperresponsiveness by Th2, but not Th1, cells. J Immunol 1998; 161:3813–3816.
24. Zhu Z, Homer RJ, Wang Z, Chen Q, Geba GP, Want J, Zhang Y, Elias JA. Pulmonary expression of interleukin-13 causes inflammation, mucus hypersecretion, subepithelial fibrosis, physiologic abnormalities, and eotaxin production. J Clin Invest 1999; 102:779–788.
25. Rankin JA, Picarella DE, Geba GP, et al. Phenotypic and physiologic characterization of transgenic mice expressing interleukin 4 in the lung: Lymphocytic and eosinophilic inflammation without airway hyperreactivity. Proc Natl Acad Sci USA 1996; 93:7821–7825.
26. Emson CL, Bell SE, Jones A, Wisden W, McKenzie ANJ. Interleukin (IL)-4-independent induction of immunoglobulin (Ig)E, and perturbation of T cell development in transgenic mice expressing IL-13. J Exp Med 1998; 188:399–404.
27. McKenzie GJ, Emson CL, Bell SE, Anderson S, Fallon P, Zurawski G, Murray R, McKenzie ANJ. Impaired development of Th2 cells in IL-13 deficient mice. Immunity 1998; 9:423–432.
28. Fallon PG, Emson CL, Smith P, McKenzie ANJ. IL-13 overexpression predisposes to anaphylaxis following antigen sensitization. J Immunol 2001; 166:2712–2717.
29. Li L, Xia Y, Nguyen A, Lai YH, Feng L, Mosmann TR, Lo D. Effects of Th2 cytokines on chemokine expression in the lung: IL-13 potently induces eotaxin expression by airway epithelial cells. J Immunol 1999; 162:2477–2487.

30. Zheng T, Zhu Z, Want Z, Homer RJ, Ma B, Riese RJ, Chapman HA, Shapiro SD, Elias JA. Inducible targeting of IL-13 to the adult lung causes matrix metalloproteinase- and cathepsin-dependent emphysema. J Clin Invest 2000; 106:1081–1093.
31. Gavett SH, O'Hearn DJ, Karp CL, Patel EA, Schofield BH, Finkelman FD, Wills-Karp M. Interleukin-4 receptor blockade prevents airway responses induced by antigen challenge in mice. Am J Physiol Lung Cell Mol Physiol 1997; 272:L253–L261.
32. Webb DC, McKenzie ANJ, Koshinen AML, Yang M, Mattes J, Foster PS. Integrated signals between IL-13, IL-4, and IL-5 regulate airways hyperactivity. J Immunol 2000; 165:108–113.
33. Naseer T, Minshall EM, Leung DYM, Laberge S, Ernst P, Martin RJ, Hamid Q. Expression of IL-12 and IL-13 mRNA in asthma and their modulation in response to steroid therapy. Am J Respir Crit Care Med 1997; 155:845–851.
34. Humbert M, Durham SR, Kimmitt P, et al. Elevated expression of messenger ribonucleic acid encoding IL-13 in the bronchial mucosa of atopic and nonatopic subjects with asthma. J Allergy Clin Immunol 1997; 99:657–665.
35. Kroegel C, Julius P, Matthys H, Virchow JC Jr, Luttman W. Endobronchial secretion of interleukin-13 following local allergen challenge in atopic asthma: Relationship to interleukin-4 and eosinophil counts. Eur Respir J 1996; 9:899–904.
36. van der Pouw Kraan TCTM, van Veen A, Boeije LCM. An IL-13 promoter polymorphism associated with increased risk of allergic asthma. Genes Immunity 1999; 1: 61–65.
37. Graves PE, Kabesch M, Halonen M, et al. A cluster of seven tightly linked polymorphisms in the IL-13 gene is associated with total serum IgE levels in three populations of white children. J Allergy Clin Immunol 2000; 105:506–513.
38. Borish LC, Nelson HS, Corren J, Bensch G, Busse WW, Whitmore JB, Agosti JM; IL-4R Asthma Study Group. Efficacy of soluble IL-4 receptor for the treatment of adults with asthma. J Allergy Clin Immunol 2001; 107(6):963–970.
39. Grunewald SM, Werthmann A, Schnarr B, Klein CE, Brocker EB, Mohrs M, Brombacher F, Sebald W, Duschl A. An antagonistic IL-4 mutant prevents type I allergy in the mouse: Inhibition of the IL-4/IL-13 receptor system completely abrogates humoral immune response to allergen and development of allergic symptoms in vivo. J Immunol 1998; 160:4004–4009.

10

Tumor Necrosis Factor α and Interleukin-1β Inhibitory Therapies

JOHAN C. KIPS and ROMAIN A. PAUWELS

Ghent University Hospital
Ghent, Belgium

I. Introduction

The presence of a Th2-driven chronic inflammation of the lower airway mucosa is currently considered to be the central feature in the pathogenesis of asthma. This inflammatory process shows not only features characteristic of an acute inflammatory response such as vasodilatation, plasma exudation, or the presence of activated inflammatory cells but also characteristics of a more chronic phase of an inflammatory reaction that results in tissue remodeling (1). This inflammatory process is orchestrated and regulated by a complex network of mutually interacting cytokines and growth factors released not only from Th2 cells but from a wide range of inflammatory cells as well as structural tissue components. Tumor necrosis factor α (TNFα) and interleukin-1β (IL-1β) are among the cytokines that could play an important role within this network. Several studies have demonstrated increased amounts of TNFα and IL-1β at either the mRNA or protein level in sputum (2,3), BAL (4–6), or biopsies from asthmatic patients (7–10). Hence the interest in inhibitors of the these cytokines as a potential novel form of asthma treatment.

II. Tumor Necrosis Factor α

Tumor necrosis factor α (TNFα) is a homotrimer consisting of three 17 kDa 157-amino-acid polypeptides (11,12). Soluble TNF is obtained by proteolytic cleavage from its membrane-bound precursor (13) through the activity of the TNFα-converting enzyme (TACE) (14,15). TNFα can be produced in response to a range of stimuli by a variety of cells, including lymphocytes, mast cells, eosinophils, epithelial cells, fibroblasts, and airway smooth muscle cells (Fig. 1). The major source is the alveolar macrophage (16). The structurally and biologically related TNFβ or lymphotoxin α (LTα) is produced exclusively by lymphocytes and natural killer cells. The genes coding for TNFα and LTα are located on human chromosome 6 (17). Both TNFα and LTα exert their biological effects through binding with one of two surface receptors that belong to the TNF receptor gene family, TNFR-I (CD120a, 55 kDa) and TNFR-II (CD120b, 75 kDa) (18,19). Both receptors are ubiquitously expressed (20). Signals are induced by ligand-mediated clustering of monomeric TNFR (21). Both receptors are also released by proteolysis as soluble mediators capable of binding TNF.

To what extent TNFR-I and TNFR-II mediate distinct cellular responses remains somewhat unclear. It has been reported that the TNFR-I propagates both TNFα and LTα-induced effects, whereas the TNFR-II only mediates TNFα-induced activity and acts as a decoy receptor for LTα (22). In addition, it has been claimed that stimulation of the TNFR-I induces cytotoxic effects, whereas

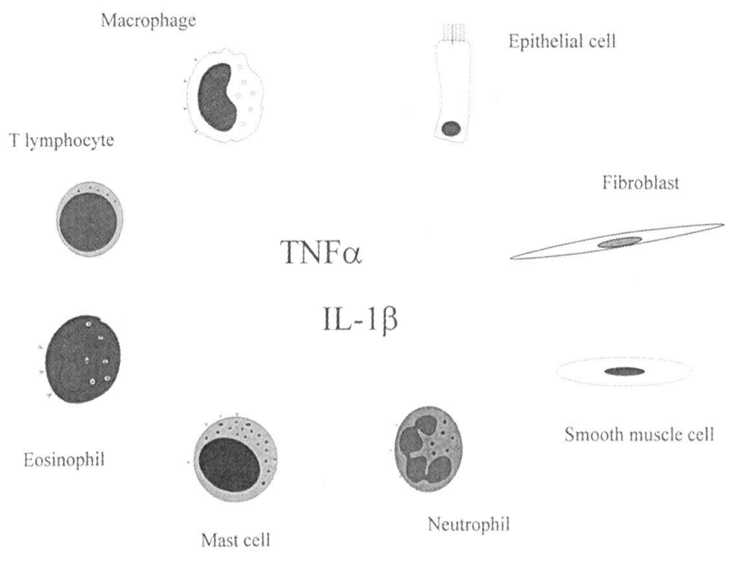

Figure 1 Cellular sources of TNFα and IL-1β.

TNFR-II activation results in cell proliferation (23). However, these findings have not been invariably confirmed. Others have shown that both receptors are important in mediating TNFα-induced effects (24). The concept has been proposed that TNFR-II passes on TNFα to the TNFR-I, which acts as the main signal transducer (25). A more recent alternative hypothesis is that enhancement of TNFR-I-dependent responses by TNFR-II, rather than involving ligand passing, is due to overlapping intracellular signaling (26,27). In vivo animal models using TNFR-I- and/or TNFR-II-deficient mice further illustrate the complexity of TNF signaling. TNFR-I$^{-/-}$ but not TNFR-II$^{-/-}$ mice are highly susceptible to infection by *Listeria monocytogenes* (28–30). Similar results were observed when mice were treated with specific antibodies against TNFR-I or TNFR-II (31). In mice, early resistance to this intracellular pathogen is critically dependent upon TNFα and IFNγ (32). This adds to the observation that TNFR-I$^{-/-}$ but not TNFR-II$^{-/-}$ mice are moderately resistant to the lethal effect of LPS whereas TNFR-II$^{-/-}$ mice are moderately resistant to the lethal effect of TNFα itself (28,29,33,34). These findings further confirm the importance of TNFR-I as the main signal transducer. In some models, however, TNFR-II, instead of enhancing TNFR-I signaling antagonized it. *M. faeni*-induced neutrophil recruitment in the lung is decreased in TNFR-I$^{-/-}$ but enhanced in TNFR-II$^{-/-}$ mice, illustrating that under certain experimental conditions TNFR-II signaling downregulates TNFR-I-mediated effects (28). A possible explanation for these findings is that endogenous production of soluble TNFR-II, which has been shown to exceed the production of soluble TNFR-I, prevents TNFα interaction with membrane-bound TNFR-I by binding free TNFα(35).

These animal models also illustrate that despite the redundancy between TNFα and LTα in in vitro systems, their in vivo effect can be different. In contrast to TNF$^{-/-}$ mice, LTα$^{-/-}$ mice lack lymph nodes (36). LTα forms not only a homotrimer but also a heteromer with lymphotoxin-β (37) that interacts with the LTβR (38). It would therefore seem that activation of LTβR is essential for normal lymph node development.

Another interesting observation emerging from these models is that although LPS-induced lethality is reduced in TNFR-I$^{-/-}$ and TNFR-II$^{-/-}$ mice, mortality to high doses of LPS and other LPS-induced effects, including PMN recruitment into the lungs, are not (28,39,40). This indicates the presence of TNFα-independent pathways, possibly involving chemokines such as MIP1α, that need to be taken into account when postulating as to the therapeutic role of TNFα antagonists in diseases associated with pulmonary inflammation.

A. TNFα in Asthma

The interaction between TNFα and TNFR activates two main signaling pathways (41,42). The first pathway leads to cell death and is mainly transduced though TNFR-I activation. It has been proposed that cells become sensitive to TNFα-

Table 1 Effects of TNFα and IL-1β Relevant to Asthma

Antigen presentation
Maturation and migration of dendritic cells
Development of airway inflammation
Upregulation of endothelial adhesion molecules
Increased production of cytokines (e.g., GM-CSF) and chemokines (CC, CXC)
Activation of inflammatory cells and release of inflammatory mediators
Increased expression of inducible NO synthase
Increase in bronchial responsiveness
Development of airway remodeling
Increased growth factor synthesis (e.g., PDGF, HB-EGF)
Upregulation of EGF receptor
Stimulation of fibroblast proliferation
Increased production of extracellular matrix proteins and matrix metalloproteinases
Stimulation of smooth muscle proliferation
Enhanced expression of adhesion molecules on smooth muscle cells

induced death only when new protein synthesis is inhibited, possibly through caspase activation (43). At present, the physiological role of TNFα-induced cell death remains to a large extent unknown. The second pathway leads to activation of gene transcription. Through a series of steps including TNF receptor–associated death domain protein (TRADD) and receptor-interacting protein (RIP), TNFα activates the transcription factors nuclear factor κb (NFκB) and activating protein-1 (AP-1). This induces important antiapoptotic and proinflammatory signals. As a result, at the cellular level, TNFα exerts a wide range of pleiotropic activities that could have an important impact at various stages in the pathogenesis of asthma (Table 1).

Antigen Presentation

The major antigen-presenting cell (APC) involved in the process of sensitization to aeroallergens is the dendritic cell (DC) present in the airway epithelium. Mucosal DCs have a high antigen-uptake capacity but low antigen-presenting capacity (44). During migration from the airway mucosa to the local lymph nodes, antigen-laden DCs mature, acquiring their full immunostimulatory phenotype. TNFα has been shown to promote migration and induce maturation of DC (45–47). It is thought that the effect of TNFα on the migration of DCs involves a time-ordered production of inflammatory and constitutive chemokines by DCs (48). In the lymph nodes naive T cells are then stimulated and differentiate toward a Th1 or Th2 phenotype. One of the main factors influencing the T-cell differentiation is the cytokine composition of the microenvironment, IL-12 having been identified as the necessary cofactor for Th1 cell development (49). In some experimental systems, TNFα has been shown to enhance the IL-12 production by APCs and thus to contribute to a preferential Th1 cell development (50,51). In other models, however, TNFα has similar effects on Th1 and Th2 cells (52). Of note is the observation that prolonged exposure to TNFα can reduce T-cell responses by interfering with signal transduction mechanisms (53).

Development of Airway Inflammation

An important feature of TNFα is its potential to induce an influx of inflammatory cells into the airway mucosa. TNFα is very effective at upregulating adhesion molecules such as VCAM-1 and ICAM-1 on vascular endothelium (54–56). This latter phenomenon is enhanced in the presence of IL-4 (57). At the same time, TNFα, in addition to having some chemotactic activity toward granulocytes, is a very potent inducer of CXC and CC chemokines (58–65). Through the combination of these effects, endogenous release of TNFα may substantially contribute to the recruitment of inflammatory cells into the airway mucosa. TNFα also has the potential to activate inflammatory cells and cause the release of a range of mediators, including platelet-activating factor (PAF), prostaglandins (PGs), and leukotrienes (LTs). As a result of these and other features, such as induction of NO synthase, TNFα could substantially contribute to the perpetuation of the antigen-induced inflammatory response (66) (Fig. 2).

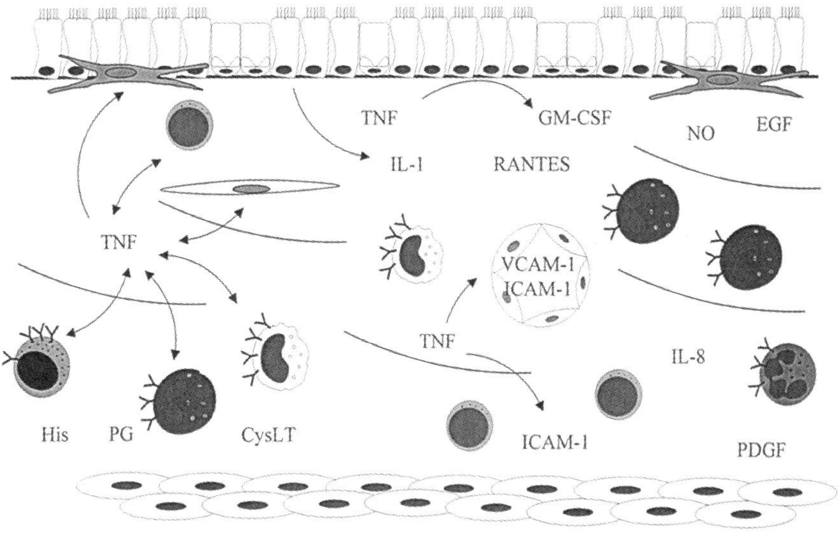

Figure 2 Schematic representation of TNFα- and IL-1β-mediated effects in asthma.

Airway Remodeling

The presence of structural airway changes or airway remodeling in asthmatic airways is increasingly recognized (67). TNFα and IL-1β might again be key elements in the induction of this process. TNFα is known to increase the transcription of genes encoding for growth factors such as platelet-derived growth factor (PDGF) or heparin-binding epithelial growth factor (HB-EGF) (68,69) and to upregulate expression of epithelial growth factor receptor (EGF-R)(70). The importance of the EGF system in the pathogenesis of remodeling has been highlighted (71). For example, among other effects, activation of EGFR by IL-13 causes goblet cell hyperplasia and mucus hypersecretion (72). TNFα also has the potential to stimulate proliferation of fibroblasts and to increase the production of extracellular matrix proteins including collagen and tenascin as well as matrix metalloproteinases (73–75). Experimental animal models of pulmonary fibrosis further illustrate the role of TNF in this process. Lung-specific expression of TNFα under the control of human surfactant protein SP-C in transgenic mice causes fibrosing alveolitis, whereas neutralization of TNFα largely reduces the fibrotic response to bleomycin or silica in murine lungs (76–79). Finally, TNFα also exerts various effects on airway smooth muscle cells, including stimulation of their proliferation or increased expression of adhesion molecules, which enhances interaction with inflammatory cells (80–84). In addition, by augmenting Gα protein expression TNFα has been shown to increase smooth muscle tone and to enhance the carbachol-induced inhibition of adenyl cyclase activity (85).

In view of this wide range of effects on inflammatory as well as structural tissue components, it is not surprising that TNFα can cause bronchial hyperresponsiveness, as has been demonstrated both in animals and in humans (86–88).

B. TNF as a Determinant of the Severity of Asthma

Circumstantial evidence illustrates the crucial role of Th2 cells in the induction of allergic airway inflammation (89). Concordant with these observations, sensitization and repeated allergen exposure are not abrogated in $TNF\alpha^{-/-}$ mice (90,91). However, once wild-type animals are sensitized, pretreatment with TNF antagonists attenuates the pulmonary response to further allergen challenge (92–94). This illustrates that although TNFα might not be essential for the development of allergic inflammation in the lower airways, through its pleiotropic effect on inflammatory cells and structural tissue components it could further enhance the airway response in established asthma to environmental stimuli, thus contributing to the severity of the disease. Several reports have highlighted the presence of increased numbers of neutrophils in the airways of patients with severe persistent asthma (95–97). Inhaled TNFα has been shown to increase sputum neutrophil counts in healthy volunteers, and TNFα levels in BAL are higher in symptomatic than in asymptomatic asthma (4,88). One of the most important stimuli of endogenous TNFα release is endotoxin. House dust contains measurable amounts of endotoxin (98). Moreover, it has been reported that in asthmatic subjects allergic to house dust mites, the severity of asthma is related to the concentration of endotoxin but not Der p1 in the home environment (99). Inhalation of LPS has been shown to augment airway responsiveness in asthmatic subjects and to increase neutrophil numbers in sputum and BAL fluid (100–102). In vivo animal models illustrate the TNFα dependency of airway neutrophilia and hyperresponsiveness induced by exposure to aerosolized or intranasally administered LPS (86,103). In addition, exposure to low levels of LPS enhances allergen-induced eosinophilic airway inflammation (104,105), possibly through a TNFα-mediated priming of eosinophil chemotaxis (106). Conversely, asthmatic subjects are more sensitive than normal volunteers to the bronchoconstrictor effect of endotoxin (100), and prior allergen challenge has been shown to augment the inflammatory response to inhaled endotoxin (107). LPS exerts its biological activity through binding with LPS-binding protein (LBP). The LPS–LBP complex then interacts with the cell-surface receptor CD14. Allergen inhalation has been shown to increase LBP level in BAL fluid of asthmatic individuals (108). Of note is the interindividual variability in the airway responsiveness to inhaled LPS (109). This suggests that genetically determined differences in the LPS–LBP–CD14–TNFα axis might be one of the features that contributes to asthma severity (110). One of the polymorphisms identified to date relates to position −308 in the promotor region of the TNFα gene. Allele 2 of the −308 TNFα promoter polymorphism consists of a substitution of guanine by adenosine and is characterized by increased releasability of TNFα in response to various stimuli (111). Albeit not consistently confirmed, it has been claimed that this −308TNFα promotor polymorphism is a risk factor for asthma and is even associated with the degree of bronchial hyperresponsiveness (112–115).

TNFα might not be only a determinant of severe persistent asthma, it could also be involved in the pathogenesis of exacerbations. Increased neutrophil numbers have been reported in sputum samples collected during acute exacerbations in an emergency department (116). Similarly, BAL fluid from patients requiring mechanical ventilation for a status asthmaticus were shown to contain increased numbers of neutrophils as well as increased IL-1β and TNFα bioactivity (117,118).

III. Interleukin-1β

Interleukin-1β (IL-1β) is another proinflammatory cytokine (119). Together with IL-1α and IL-1 receptor antagonist (IL-1ra), IL-1β belongs to the IL-1 family. In its mature form, IL-1β is a 17 kDa protein cleaved from a less active precursor by an intracellular protease, IL-1β-converting enzyme (ICE). Like TNFα, IL-1β is produced by a wide variety of cells in response to a range of stimuli, including endotoxin, other cytokines (TNF in particular), or antigens. IL-1β can bind with equal affinity to two IL-1 receptors, both of which have membrane-bound and soluble forms. Activation of the universally expressed membrane type I receptor (mIL-1RI) transduces the biological effects of IL-1β. In contrast, the type II receptor (mIL-1RII), which has been identified on B cells, neutrophils, monocytes, and bone marrow cells, acts as a decoy receptor, because binding with IL-1β does not transduce intracellular signals (120,121).

Asthmatic airways contain increased levels of IL-1β (10). IL-1β has been recognized as an important cofactor in the interaction between antigen-presenting cells and T-helper cells. Optimal T-cell activation and proliferation require the presence of IL-1. To what extent IL-1 influences the development of Th1 versus Th2 responses is debated (122). The main role of IL-1 in the pathogenesis of established asthma, however, is thought to relate to its proinflammatory effects, which are largely redundant with TNFα. Synergism between the two cytokines has even been observed, which might at least in part be explained by the ability of TNFα to induce IL-1β production and vice versa (123,124).

The biological activity of IL-1β is tightly regulated by naturally occurring antagonists. Both IL-1RI and IL-1RII have been found in soluble form in circulation. They bind IL-1β with equal affinity to mIL-1RI/II, neutralizing free circulating IL-1β. Another naturally occurring antagonist is IL-1ra, released together with IL-1α and IL-1β. IL-1ra binds to mIL-1RI without inducing biological activities, thus inhibiting IL-1β-mediated effects. Th2 cytokines have been reported to upregulate the synthesis of IL-1ra relative to IL-1β (125).

Of note is that activation of small numbers of mIL-1RI is sufficient to trigger an inflammatory response. As a result, IL-1ra will inhibit IL-1β-mediated effects only if it occupies nearly all mIL-1RI. This requires 100-fold to 10,000-fold molar excess of IL-1ra relative to IL-1β. This does not apply to soluble IL-1R type I and type II, which effectively neutralize IL-1β before it can bind to the surface receptor. Importantly, IL-1ra also binds to sIL-1RI but not to sIL-RII, implying that the inhibitory activity of IL-1ra is hindered in the presence of sIL-1RI but not sIL-1RII (126,127).

IV. TNF and IL-1β as Targets for Treatment in Asthma

From the various data discussed so far it would seem that inhibiting the effect of TNFα and/or IL-1β could prove beneficial in asthma. Various approaches can be considered in this respect (Table 2).

To date, two main strategies have been used to regulate TNF activity in humans: the use of either soluble TNFR or monoclonal antibodies against TNFα. As described above, naturally occurring soluble TNFR is a physiological regula-

Table 2 Approaches to Reduction in TNFα or IL-1β Activity

TNFα
Soluble TNF receptor (dimeric sTNFRII:FcIgG_1; etanercept)
PEGylated sTNFRI
Chimeric murine/human anti-TNF monoclonal antibody (infliximab)
Humanized anti-TNF monoclonal antibody (D2E7)
IL-1β
IL-1 receptor antagonist (IL-1ra)
Soluble IL-1 receptor type II (sIL-1RII)

tor of TNFα activity. It binds soluble and membrane-bound TNFα and LTα, thus inhibiting interaction with both membrane-bound TNFRs (128–130). Monomeric sTNFR has a short half-life and low affinity in vivo, precluding its therapeutic use. This problem has been circumvented by assembling a dimeric fusion protein composed of two soluble TNFR-II moieties, bound to the Fc portion of human IgG_1 (etanercept) (131). This has substantially improved the binding affinity and TNF-neutralizing capacity compared to monomeric sTNFR-II and has prolonged the pharmacokinetic half-life (to 4.8 days). There was theoretical concern that by stabilizing the trimeric structure of TNF the molecule might prolong TNF bioactivity and that it might fix complement because the IgG_1 Fc region contains the complement-binding domain (132). These concerns abated as data demonstrated that this did not occur. Another approach to stabilizing sTNFR has been to fuse monomeric TNFR-I to polyethylene glycol (PEG) (133). In comparison to monoclonal antibodies against TNF such as infliximab, which is 75% human and 25% murine, these sTNFR fusion proteins have the advantage of being fully human and thus relatively nonimmunogenic.

Etanercept has not been effective in the treatment of septic shock. It can be postulated that this disease entity is due to such an overwhelming cascade of events that a selective blockade of a single pathway is insufficient to halt the response (134). At present, the therapeutic potential of TNF monoclonal antibodies and sTNFR has been documented mainly in diseases that are thought to be largely Th1-driven, such as Crohn's disease (135,136), psoriatic arthropathy (137), and, especially, rheumatoid arthritis (RA). Initial 3–6-month studies showed the clinical benefit of repeated administration of infliximab or etanercept in patients with refractory rheumatoid arthritis (138–141). More recent studies illustrate the additional benefit of adding etanercept to methotrexate in severe RA (142). Finally, in patients with early rheumatoid arthritis, etanercept in monotherapy offered a more rapid improvement of symptoms than methotrexate. Of particular interest is that in this study etanercept also slowed joint damage. The compounds were well tolerated. The most frequently reported side effects were injection site reactions. Current safety recommendations are that patients with active infection should not be started on either compound and that in those who develop an infection, treatment should be discontinued. Before starting treatment, patients should in particular be evaluated for active and inactive tuberculosis. To date, serious infectious complications have been rarely reported (143). Because repeated administration of infliximab induced the formation of antiglobulin antibodies in 50% of patients, it has been recommended that this compound should be combined with methotrexate to decrease the formation of neutralizing antibodies (144).

To date, the clinical development of IL-1 antagonists has been very much in parallel to that of TNF antagonists. As for inhibition for TNFα, IL-1ra has no proven effects in the treatment of patients with the sepsis syndrome (145,146). In RA, however, repeated administration of IL-1ra is well tolerated, reduces symptoms, and inhibits radiographic progression of the disease (147–149). In view of the synergistic effect of the two cytokines, it can even be anticipated that the combination of an anti-TNF and anti-IL-1 approach might achieve additional benefit. This has been confirmed in an animal model of RA (150).

The therapeutic potential of IL-1 antagonists in allergic disorders has been illustrated by in vivo animal models (151,152). Of note also is an early study showing that the subcutaneous administration of soluble IL-1R type I inhibits the clinical manifestation of the cutaneous allergic late-phase response in humans. Skin biopsies, however, could not detect an effect on the inflammatory skin infiltrate (153). Further evaluation of the newer therapeutic agent, soluble IL-1R type II, is under consideration.

V. Conclusion

There is substantial evidence to indicate that the proinflammatory cytokines IL-1β and TNFα could play a pivotal role in the pathogenesis of allergic disorders. Their potential impact on the severity of the disease is particularly intriguing. Potent specific antagonists are now available for human use. Large-scale studies in patients with RA have demonstrated both their safety and clinical efficacy.

Asthma is a highly prevalent disorder that, especially in the more severe forms, carries significant morbidity and mortality. TNF and/or IL-1 antagonists could prove particularly beneficial for this group of patients.

References

1. Bousquet J, Jeffery PK, Busse WW, Johnson M, Vignola AM. Asthma. From bronchoconstriction to airways inflammation and remodeling. Am J Respir Crit Care Med 2000; 161(5):1720–1745.

2. Konno S, Gonokami Y, Kurokawa M, Kawazu K, Asano K, Okamoto K, Adachi M. Cytokine concentrations in sputum of asthmatic patients. Int Arch Allergy Immunol 1996; 109(1):73–78.
3. Keatings VM, Collins PD, Scott DM, Barnes PJ. Differences in interleukin-8 and tumor necrosis factor-alpha in induced sputum from patients with chronic obstructive pulmonary disease or asthma. Am J Respir Crit Care Med 1996; 153(2):530–534.
4. Broide DH, Lotz M, Cuomo AJ, Coburn DA, Federman EC, Wasserman SI. Cytokines in symptomatic asthma airways. J Allergy Clin Immunol 1992; 89(5):958–967.
5. Cembrzynska-Nowak M, Szklarz E, Inglot AD, Teodorczyk-Injeyan JA. Elevated release of tumor necrosis factor-alpha and interferon-gamma by bronchoalveolar leukocytes from patients with bronchial asthma. Am Rev Respir Dis 1993; 147(2): 291–295.
6. Ying S, Robinson DS, Varney V, Meng Q, Tsicopoulos A, Moqbel R, et al. TNF alpha mRNA expression in allergic inflammation. Clin Exp Allergy 1991; 21(6): 745–750.
7. Ackerman V, Marini M, Vittori E, Bellini A, Vassali G, Mattoli S. Detection of cytokines and their cell sources in bronchial biopsy specimens from asthmatic patients. Relationship to atopic status, symptoms, and level of airway hyperresponsiveness. Chest 1994; 105(3):687–696.
8. Bradding P, Roberts JA, Britten KM, Montefort S, Djukanovic R, Mueller R, et al. Interleukin-4, -5, and -6 and tumor necrosis factor-alpha in normal and asthmatic airways: Evidence for the human mast cell as a source of these cytokines. Am J Respir Cell Mol Biol 1994; 10(5):471–480.
9. Maestrelli P, Di Stefano A, Occari P, Turato G, Milani G, Pivirotto F, et al. Cytokines in the airway mucosa of subjects with asthma induced by toluene diisocyanate. Am J Respir Crit Care Med 1995; 151(3 pt 1):607–612.
10. Sousa AR, Lane SJ, Nakhosteen JA, Lee TH, Poston RN. Expression of interleukin-1 beta (IL-1beta) and interleukin-1 receptor antagonist (IL-1ra) on asthmatic bronchial epithelium. Am J Respir Crit Care Med 1996; 154(4 pt 1):1061–1066.
11. Beutler B, Cerami A. The biology of cachectin/TNF: A primary mediator of the host response. Annu Rev Immunol 1989; 7:625–55:625–655.
12. Jones EY, Stuart DI, Walker NP. Structure of tumour necrosis factor. Nature 1989; 338(6212):225–228.
13. Gearing AJ, Beckett P, Christodoulou M, Churchill M, Clements J, Davidson AH, et al. Processing of tumour necrosis factor-alpha precursor by metalloproteinases. Nature 1994; 370(6490):555–557.
14. Black RA, Rauch CT, Kozlosky CJ, Peschon JJ, Slack JL, Wolfson MF, et al. A metalloproteinase disintegrin that releases tumour-necrosis factor-alpha from cells. Nature 1997; 385(6618):729–733.
15. Moss ML, Jin SL, Milla ME, Bickett DM, Burkhart W, Carter HL, et al. Cloning of a disintegrin metalloproteinase that processes precursor tumour-necrosis factor-alpha. Nature 1997; 385(6618):733–736.
16. Vassalli P. The pathophysiology of tumor necrosis factors. Annu Rev Immunol 1992; 10:411–452.

17. Nedwin GE, Naylor SL, Sakaguchi AY, Smith D, Jarrett-Nedwin J, Pennica D, Goeddel DV, Gray PW. Human lymphotoxin and tumor necrosis factor genes: Structure, homology and chromosomal localization. Nucl Acids Res 1985; 13(17): 6361–6373.
18. Loetscher H, Pan YC, Lahm HW, Gentz R, Brockhaus M, Tabuchi H, Lesslauer W. Molecular cloning and expression of the human 55 kd tumor necrosis factor receptor. Cell 1990; 61(2):351–359.
19. Schall TJ, Lewis M, Koller KJ, Lee A, Rice GC, Wong GH, et al. Molecular cloning and expression of a receptor for human tumor necrosis factor. Cell 1990; 61(2): 361–370.
20. Tartaglia LA, Goeddel DV. Two TNF receptors. Immunol Today 1992; 13(5):151–153.
21. Fiers W. Tumor necrosis factor. Characterization at the molecular, cellular and in vivo level. FEBS Lett 1991; 285(2):199–212.
22. Medvedev AE, Espevik T, Ranges G, Sundan A. Distinct roles of the two tumor necrosis factor (TNF) receptors in modulating TNF and lymphotoxin alpha effects. J Biol Chem 1996; 271(16):9778–9784.
23. Tartaglia LA, Weber RF, Figari IS, Reynolds C, Palladino MA, Goeddel DV. The two different receptors for tumor necrosis factor mediate distinct cellular responses. Proc Natl Acad Sci USA 1991; 88(20):9292–9296.
24. Shalaby MR, Sundan A, Loetscher H, Brockhaus M, Lesslauer W, Espevik T. Binding and regulation of cellular functions by monoclonal antibodies against human tumor necrosis factor receptors. J Exp Med 1990; 172(5):1517–1520.
25. Tartaglia LA, Pennica D, Goeddel DV. Ligand passing: The 75-kDa tumor necrosis factor (TNF) receptor recruits TNF for signaling by the 55-kDa TNF receptor. J Biol Chem 1993; 268(25):18542–18548.
26. Declercq W, Denecker G, Fiers W, Vandenabeele P. Cooperation of both TNF receptors in inducing apoptosis: Involvement of the TNF receptor-associated factor binding domain of the TNF receptor 75. J Immunol 1998; 161(1):390–399.
27. Weiss T, Grell M, Hessabi B, Bourteele S, Muller G, Scheurich P, Wajant H. Enhancement of TNF receptor p60-mediated cytotoxicity by TNF receptor p80: Requirement of the TNF receptor-associated factor-2 binding site. J Immunol 1997; 158(5):2398–2404.
28. Peschon JJ, Torrance DS, Stocking KL, Glaccum MB, Otten C, Willis CR, et al. TNF receptor-deficient mice reveal divergent roles for p55 and p75 in several models of inflammation. J Immunol 1998; 160(2):943–952.
29. Rothe J, Lesslauer W, Lotscher H, Lang Y, Koebel P, Kontgen F, et al. Mice lacking the tumour necrosis factor receptor 1 are resistant to TNF-mediated toxicity but highly susceptible to infection by Listeria monocytogenes. Nature 1993; 364(6440): 798–802.
30. Pfeffer K, Matsuyama T, Kundig TM, Wakeham A, Kishihara K, Shahinian A, et al. Mice deficient for the 55 kd tumor necrosis factor receptor are resistant to endotoxic shock, yet succumb to L. monocytogenes infection. Cell 1993; 73(3):457–467.
31. Sheehan KC, Pinckard JK, Arthur CD, Dehner LP, Goeddel DV, Schreiber RD. Monoclonal antibodies specific for murine p55 and p75 tumor necrosis factor recep-

tors: Identification of a novel in vivo role for p75. J Exp Med 1995; 181(2):607–617.

32. Kaufmann SH. Bacterial and protozoal infections in genetically disrupted mice. Curr Opin Immunol 1994; 6(4):518–525.
33. Erickson SL, de Sauvage FJ, Kikly K, Carver-Moore K, Pitts-Meek S, Gillett N, et al. Decreased sensitivity to tumour-necrosis factor but normal T-cell development in TNF receptor-2-deficient mice. Nature 1994; 372(6506):560–563.
34. Marino MW, Dunn A, Grail D, Inglese M, Noguchi Y, Richards E, et al. Characterization of tumor necrosis factor-deficient mice. Proc Natl Acad Sci USA 1997; 94(15):8093–8098.
35. Carpenter A, Evans TJ, Buurman WA, Bemelmans MH, Moyes D, Cohen J. Differences in the shedding of soluble TNF receptors between endotoxin-sensitive and endotoxin-resistant mice in response to lipopolysaccharide or live bacterial challenge. J Immunol 1995; 155(4):2005–2012.
36. De Togni P, Goellner J, Ruddle NH, Streeter PR, Fick A, Mariathasan S, et al. Abnormal development of peripheral lymphoid organs in mice deficient in lymphotoxin. Science 1994; 264(5159):703–707.
37. Browning JL, Ngam-ek A, Lawton P, DeMarinis J, Tizard R, Chow EP, et al. Lymphotoxin beta, a novel member of the TNF family that forms a heteromeric complex with lymphotoxin on the cell surface. Cell 1993; 72(6):847–856.
38. Crowe PD, VanArsdale TL, Walter BN, Ware CF, Hession C, Ehrenfels B, et al. A lymphotoxin-beta-specific receptor. Science 1994; 264(5159):707–710.
39. Moreland JG, Fuhrman RM, Wohlford-Lenane CL, Quinn TJ, Benda E, Pruessner JA, Schwartz DA. TNF-alpha and IL-1 beta are not essential to the inflammatory response in LPS-induced airway disease. Am J Physiol Lung Cell Mol Physiol 2001; 280(1):L173–L180.
40. Smith S, Skerrett SJ, Chi EY, Jonas M, Mohler K, Wilson CB. The locus of tumor necrosis factor-alpha action in lung inflammation. Am J Respir Cell Mol Biol 1998; 19(6):881–891.
41. Bazzoni F, Beutler B. The tumor necrosis factor ligand and receptor families. N Engl J Med 1996; 334(26):1717–1725.
42. Ledgerwood EC, Pober JS, Bradley JR. Recent advances in the molecular basis of TNF signal transduction. Lab Invest 1999; 79(9):1041–1050.
43. Salvesen GS, Dixit VM. Caspase activation: The induced-proximity model. Proc Natl Acad Sci USA 1999; 96(20):10964–10967.
44. Banchereau J, Steinman RM. Dendritic cells and the control of immunity. Nature 1998; 392(6673):245–252.
45. Roake JA, Rao AS, Morris PJ, Larsen CP, Hankins DF, Austyn JM. Dendritic cell loss from nonlymphoid tissues after systemic administration of lipopolysaccharide, tumor necrosis factor, and interleukin 1. J Exp Med 1995; 181(6):2237–2247.
46. Wang B, Fujisawa H, Zhuang L, Kondo S, Shivji GM, Kim CS, Mak TW, Sauder DN. Depressed Langerhans cell migration and reduced contact hypersensitivity response in mice lacking TNF receptor p75. J Immunol 1997; 159(12):6148–6155.
47. Sallusto F, Lanzavecchia A. Efficient presentation of soluble antigen by cultured human dendritic cells is maintained by granulocyte/macrophage colony-stimulating

factor plus interleukin 4 and downregulated by tumor necrosis factor alpha. J Exp Med 1994; 179(4):1109–1118.

48. Sallusto F, Palermo B, Lenig D, Miettinen M, Matikainen S, Julkunen I, et al. Distinct patterns and kinetics of chemokine production regulate dendritic cell function. Eur J Immunol 1999; 29(5):1617–1625.
49. Rissoan MC, Soumelis V, Kadowaki N, Grouard G, Briere F, de Waal MR, et al. Reciprocal control of T helper cell and dendritic cell differentiation. Science 1999; 283(5405):1183–1186.
50. Becher B, Blain M, Giacomini PS, Antel JP. Inhibition of Th1 polarization by soluble TNF receptor is dependent on antigen-presenting cell-derived IL-12. J Immunol 1999; 162(2):684–688.
51. Shibuya K, Robinson D, Zonin F, Hartley SB, Macatonia SE, Somoza C, et al. IL-1 alpha and TNF-alpha are required for IL-12-induced development of Th1 cells producing high levels of IFN-gamma in BALB/c but not C57BL/6 mice. J Immunol 1998; 160(4):1708–1716.
52. Joseph SB, Miner KT, Croft M. Augmentation of naive, Th1 and Th2 effector CD4 responses by IL-6, IL-1 and TNF. Eur J Immunol 1998; 28(1):277–289.
53. Cope AP, Liblau RS, Yang XD, Congia M, Laudanna C, Schreiber RD, et al. Chronic tumor necrosis factor alters T cell responses by attenuating T cell receptor signaling. J Exp Med 1997; 185(9):1573–1584.
54. Pober JS, Gimbrone MA, Lapierre LA, Mendrick DL, Fiers W, Rothlein R, Springer TA. Overlapping patterns of activation of human endothelial cells by interleukin 1, tumor necrosis factor, and immune interferon. J Immunol 1986; 137(6): 1893–1896.
55. Bevilacqua MP, Pober JS, Mendrick DL, Cotran RS, Gimbrone MA. Identification of an inducible endothelial-leukocyte adhesion molecule. Proc Natl Acad Sci USA 1987; 84(24):9238–9242.
56. Osborn L, Hession C, Tizard R, Vassallo C, Luhowskyj S, Chi-Rosso G, Lobb R. Direct expression cloning of vascular cell adhesion molecule 1, a cytokine-induced endothelial protein that binds to lymphocytes. Cell 1989; 59(6):1203–1211.
57. Striz I, Mio T, Adachi Y, Heires P, Robbins RA, Spurzem JR, et al. IL-4 induces ICAM-1 expression in human bronchial epithelial cells and potentiates TNF-alpha. Am J Physiol 1999; 277(1 pt 1):L58–L64.
58. Pape KA, Khoruts A, Mondino A, Jenkins MK. Inflammatory cytokines enhance the in vivo clonal expansion and differentiation of antigen-activated CD4+ T cells. J Immunol 1997; 159(2):591–598.
59. Ghaffar O, Hamid Q, Renzi PM, Allakhverdi Z, Molet S, Hogg JC, et al. Constitutive and cytokine-stimulated expression of eotaxin by human airway smooth muscle cells. Am J Respir Crit Care Med 1999; 159(6):1933–1942.
60. Blease K, Mehrad B, Lukacs NW, Kunkel SL, Standiford TJ, Hogaboam CM. Antifungal and airway remodeling roles for murine monocyte chemoattractant protein-1/CCL2 during pulmonary exposure to Aspergillus fumigatus conidia. J Immunol 2001; 166(3):1832–1842.
61. Wang JH, Devalia JL, Sapsford RJ, Davies RJ. Effect of corticosteroids on release of RANTES and sICAM-1 from cultured human bronchial epithelial cells, induced by TNF-alpha. Eur Respir J 1997; 10(4):834–840.

62. Pang L, Knox AJ. Regulation of TNF-alpha-induced eotaxin release from cultured human airway smooth muscle cells by beta2-agonists and corticosteroids. FASEB J 2001; 15(1):261–269.
63. Marfaing-Koka A, Devergne O, Gorgone G, Portier A, Schall TJ, Galanaud P, Emilie D. Regulation of the production of the RANTES chemokine by endothelial cells. Synergistic induction by IFN-gamma plus TNF-alpha and inhibition by IL-4 and IL-13. J Immunol 1995; 154(4):1870–1878.
64. Pang L, Knox AJ. Synergistic inhibition by beta(2)-agonists and corticosteroids on tumor necrosis factor-alpha-induced interleukin-8 release from cultured human airway smooth-muscle cells. Am J Respir Cell Mol Biol 2000; 23(1):79–85.
65. Stellato C, Collins P, Ponath PD, Soler D, Newman W, La Rosa G, et al. Production of the novel C-C chemokine MCP-4 by airway cells and comparison of its biological activity to other C-C chemokines. J Clin Invest 1997; 99(5):926–936.
66. Kips J, Pauwels R. Proinflammatory cytokines. In: Barnes PJ, Grunstein MM, Leff AR, Woolley A, eds. Asthma, Vol I. Philadelphia: Lippincott-Raven, 1997:653.
67. Kips JC, Pauwels RA. Airway wall remodelling: Does it occur and what does it mean? Clin Exp Allergy 1999; 29(11):1457–1466.
68. Kume N, Gimbrone MA. Lysophosphatidylcholine transcriptionally induces growth factor gene expression in cultured human endothelial cells. J Clin Invest 1994; 93(2):907–911.
69. Yoshizumi M, Kourembanas S, Temizer DH, Cambria RP, Quertermous T, Lee ME. Tumor necrosis factor increases transcription of the heparin-binding epidermal growth factor-like growth factor gene in vascular endothelial cells. J Biol Chem 1992; 267(14):9467–9469.
70. Takeyama K, Dabbagh K, Lee HM, Agusti C, Lausier JA, Ueki IF, Grattan KM, Nadel JA. Epidermal growth factor system regulates mucin production in airways. Proc Natl Acad Sci USA 1999; 96(6):3081–3086.
71. Holgate ST, Davies DE, Lackie PM, Wilson SJ, Puddicombe SM, Lordan JL. Epithelial-mesenchymal interactions in the pathogenesis of asthma. J Allergy Clin Immunol 2000; 105(2 pt 1):193–204.
72. Shim JJ, Dabbagh K, Ueki IF, Dao-Pick T, Burgel PR, Takeyama K, Tam DC, Nadel JA. IL-13 induces mucin production by stimulating epidermal growth factor receptors and by activating neutrophils. Am J Physiol Lung Cell Mol Physiol 2001; 280(1):L134–L140.
73. Rogalsky V, Todorov G, Den T, Ohnuma T. Increase in protein kinase C activity is associated with human fibroblast growth inhibition. FEBS Lett 1992; 304(2–3): 153–156.
74. Gordon JR, Galli SJ. Promotion of mouse fibroblast collagen gene expression by mast cells stimulated via the Fc epsilon RI. Role for mast cell-derived transforming growth factor beta and tumor necrosis factor alpha. J Exp Med 1994; 180(6):2027–2037.
75. Chou DH, Lee W, McCulloch CA. TNF-alpha inactivation of collagen receptors: Implications for fibroblast function and fibrosis. J Immunol 1996; 156(11):4354–4362.
76. Miyazaki Y, Araki K, Vesin C, Garcia I, Kapanci Y, Whitsett JA, Piguet PF, Vassalli P. Expression of a tumor necrosis factor-alpha transgene in murine lung causes

lymphocytic and fibrosing alveolitis. A mouse model of progressive pulmonary fibrosis. J Clin Invest 1995; 96(1):250–259.

77. Gossart S, Cambon C, Orfila C, Seguelas MH, Lepert JC, Rami J, Carre P, Pipy B. Reactive oxygen intermediates as regulators of TNF-alpha production in rat lung inflammation induced by silica. J Immunol 1996; 156(4):1540–1548.
78. Piguet PF, Collart MA, Grau GE, Sappino AP, Vassalli P. Requirement of tumour necrosis factor for development of silica-induced pulmonary fibrosis. Nature 1990; 344(6263):245–247.
79. Ortiz LA, Lasky J, Lungarella G, Cavarra E, Martorana P, Banks WA, et al. Upregulation of the p75 but not the p55 TNF-alpha receptor mRNA after silica and bleomycin exposure and protection from lung injury in double receptor knockout mice. Am J Respir Cell Mol Biol 1999; 20(4):825–833.
80. Amrani Y, Panettieri RA, Frossard N, Bronner C. Activation of the TNF alpha-p55 receptor induces myocyte proliferation and modulates agonist-evoked calcium transients in cultured human tracheal smooth muscle cells. Am J Respir Cell Mol Biol 1996; 15(1):55–63.
81. Stewart AG, Tomlinson PR, Fernandes DJ, Wilson JW, Harris T. Tumor necrosis factor alpha modulates mitogenic responses of human cultured airway smooth muscle. Am J Respir Cell Mol Biol 1995; 12(1):110–119.
82. Yang CM, Luo SF, Wang CC, Chiu CT, Chien CS, Lin CC, Hsaio LD. Tumour necrosis factor-alpha- and interleukin-1beta-stimulated cell proliferation through activation of mitogen-activated protein kinase in canine tracheal smooth muscle cells. Br J Pharmacol 2000; 130(4):891–899.
83. Panettieri RA, Lazaar AL, Pure E, Albelda SM. Activation of cAMP-dependent pathways in human airway smooth muscle cells inhibits TNF-alpha-induced ICAM-1 and VCAM-1 expression and T lymphocyte adhesion. J Immunol 1995; 154(5):2358–2365.
84. Lazaar AL, Albelda SM, Pilewski JM, Brennan B, Pure E, Panettieri RA. T lymphocytes adhere to airway smooth muscle cells via integrins and CD44 and induce smooth muscle cell DNA synthesis. J Exp Med 1994; 180(3):807–816.
85. Hotta K, Emala CW, Hirshman CA. TNF-alpha upregulates Gialpha and Gqalpha protein expression and function in human airway smooth muscle cells. Am J Physiol 1999; 276(3 pt 1):L405–L411.
86. Kips JC, Tavernier J, Pauwels RA. Tumor necrosis factor causes bronchial hyperresponsiveness in rats. Am Rev Respir Dis 1992; 145(2 Pt 1):332–336.
87. Wheeler AP, Jesmok G, Brigham KL. Tumor necrosis factor's effects on lung mechanics, gas exchange, and airway reactivity in sheep. J Appl Physiol 1990; 68(6): 2542–2549.
88. Thomas PS, Yates DH, Barnes PJ. Tumor necrosis factor-alpha increases airway responsiveness and sputum neutrophilia in normal human subjects. Am J Respir Crit Care Med 1995; 152(1):76–80.
89. Kips JC, Tournoy KG, Pauwels RA. Gene knockout models of asthma. Am J Respir Crit Care Med 2000; 162(3 pt 2):S66–S70.
90. Rudmann DG, Moore MW, Tepper JS, Aldrich MC, Pfeiffer JW, Hogenesch H, et al. Modulation of allergic inflammation in mice deficient in TNF receptors. Am J Physiol Lung Cell Mol Physiol 2000; 279(6):L1047–L1057.

91. Hessel EM, Van Oosterhout AJ, Van A, I, Van Esch B, Hofman G, Van Loveren H, Savelkoul HF, Nijkamp FP. Development of airway hyperresponsiveness is dependent on interferon-gamma and independent of eosinophil infiltration. Am J Respir Cell Mol Biol 1997; 16(3):325–334.
92. Lukacs NW, Strieter RM, Chensue SW, Widmer M, Kunkel SL. TNF-alpha mediates recruitment of neutrophils and eosinophils during airway inflammation. J Immunol 1995; 154(10):5411–5417.
93. Renzetti LM, Paciorek PM, Tannu SA, Rinaldi NC, Tocker JE, Wasserman MA, Gater PR. Pharmacological evidence for tumor necrosis factor as a mediator of allergic inflammation in the airways. J Pharmacol Exp Ther 1996; 278(2):847–853.
94. Zuany-Amorim C, Haile S, Leduc D, Dumarey C, Huerre M, Vargaftig BB, et al. Interleukin-10 inhibits antigen-induced cellular recruitment into the airways of sensitized mice. J Clin Invest 1995; 95(6):2644–2651.
95. Jatakanon A, Uasuf C, Maziak W, Lim S, Chung KF, Barnes PJ. Neutrophilic inflammation in severe persistent asthma. Am J Respir Crit Care Med 1999; 160(5 pt 1):1532–1539.
96. Wenzel SE, Schwartz LB, Langmack EL, Halliday JL, Trudeau JB, Gibbs RL, Chu HW. Evidence that severe asthma can be divided pathologically into two inflammatory subtypes with distinct physiologic and clinical characteristics. Am J Respir Crit Care Med 1999; 160(3):1001–1008.
97. Kips J. Cellular composition of induced sputum and peripheral blood in severe persistent asthma. Eur Respir J 1999; 14:2248.
98. Michel O, Ginanni R, Duchateau J, Vertongen F, Le Bon B, Sergysels R. Domestic endotoxin exposure and clinical severity of asthma. Clin Exp Allergy 1991; 21(4): 441–448.
99. Michel O, Kips J, Duchateau J, Vertongen F, Robert L, Collet H, Pauwels R, Sergysels R. Severity of asthma is related to endotoxin in house dust. Am J Respir Crit Care Med 1996; 154(6 pt 1):1641–1646.
100. Michel O, Duchateau J, Sergysels R. Effect of inhaled endotoxin on bronchial reactivity in asthmatic and normal subjects. J Appl Physiol 1989; 66(3):1059–1064.
101. Sandstrom T, Bjermer L, Rylander R. Lipopolysaccharide (LPS) inhalation in healthy subjects increases neutrophils, lymphocytes and fibronectin levels in bronchoalveolar lavage fluid. Eur Respir J 1992; 5(8):992–996.
102. Michel O, Nagy AM, Schroeven M, Duchateau J, Neve J, Fondu P, Sergysels R. Dose-response relationship to inhaled endotoxin in normal subjects. Am J Respir Crit Care Med 1997; 156(4 pt 1):1157–1164.
103. Lefort J, Singer M, Leduc D, Renesto P, Nahori MA, Huerre M, et al. Systemic administration of endotoxin induces bronchopulmonary hyperreactivity dissociated from TNF-alpha formation and neutrophil sequestration into the murine lungs. J Immunol 1998; 161(1):474–480.
104. Tulic MK, Wale JL, Holt PG, Sly PD. Modification of the inflammatory response to allergen challenge after exposure to bacterial lipopolysaccharide. Am J Respir Cell Mol Biol 2000; 22(5):604–612.
105. Peden DB, Tucker K, Murphy P, Newlin-Clapp L, Boehlecke B, Hazucha M, et al. Eosinophil influx to the nasal airway after local, low-level LPS challenge in humans. J Allergy Clin Immunol 1999; 104(2 pt 1):388–394.

106. Macari DM, Teixeira MM, Ansari T, Jeffery PK, Hellewell PG. Priming and induction of eosinophil trafficking in guinea-pig cutaneous inflammation by tumour necrosis factor alpha. Br J Pharmacol 1998; 125(6):1228–1235.
107. Eldridge MW, Peden DB. Allergen provocation augments endotoxin-induced nasal inflammation in subjects with atopic asthma. J Allergy Clin Immunol 2000; 105(3): 475–481.
108. Dubin W, Martin TR, Swoveland P, Leturcq DJ, Moriarty AM, Tobias PS, et al. Asthma and endotoxin: Lipopolysaccharide-binding protein and soluble CD14 in bronchoalveolar compartment. Am J Physiol 1996; 270(5 pt 1):L736–L744.
109. Kline JN, Cowden JD, Hunninghake GW, Schutte BC, Watt JL, Wohlford-Lenane CL, et al. Variable airway responsiveness to inhaled lipopolysaccharide. Am J Respir Crit Care Med 1999; 160(1):297–303.
110. Arbour NC, Lorenz E, Schutte BC, Zabner J, Kline JN, Jones M, et al. TLR4 mutations are associated with endotoxin hyporesponsiveness in humans. Nat Genet 2000; 25(2):187–191.
111. Wilson AG, Symons JA, McDowell TL, McDevitt HO, Duff GW. Effects of a polymorphism in the human tumor necrosis factor alpha promoter on transcriptional activation. Proc Natl Acad Sci USA 1997; 94(7):3195–3199.
112. Louis R, Leyder E, Malaise M, Bartsch P, Louis E. Lack of association between adult asthma and the tumour necrosis factor alpha-308 polymorphism gene. Eur Respir J 2000; 16(4):604–608.
113. Chagani T, Pare PD, Zhu S, Weir TD, Bai TR, Behbehani NA, et al. Prevalence of tumor necrosis factor-alpha and angiotensin converting enzyme polymorphisms in mild/moderate and fatal/near-fatal asthma. Am J Respir Crit Care Med 1999; 160(1):278–282.
114. Li Kam Wa TC, Mansur AH, Britton J, Williams G, Pavord I, Richards K, et al. Association between −308 tumour necrosis factor promoter polymorphism and bronchial hyperreactivity in asthma. Clin Exp Allergy 1999; 29(9):1204–1208.
115. Albuquerque RV, Hayden CM, Palmer LJ, Laing IA, Rye PJ, Gibson NA, et al. Association of polymorphisms within the tumour necrosis factor (TNF) genes and childhood asthma. Clin Exp Allergy 1998; 28(5):578–584.
116. Fahy JV, Kim KW, Liu J, Boushey HA. Prominent neutrophilic inflammation in sputum from subjects with asthma exacerbation. J Allergy Clin Immunol 1995; 95(4):843–852.
117. Lamblin C, Gosset P, Tillie-Leblond I, Saulnier F, Marquette CH, Wallaert B, Tonnel AB. Bronchial neutrophilia in patients with noninfectious status asthmaticus. Am J Respir Crit Care Med 1998; 157(2):394–402.
118. Tillie L, I, Pugin J, Marquette CH, Lamblin C, Saulnier F, Brichet A, et al. Balance between proinflammatory cytokines and their inhibitors in bronchial lavage from patients with status asthmaticus. Am J Respir Crit Care Med 1999; 159(2):487–494.
119. Dinarello CA. Biologic basis for interleukin-1 in disease. Blood 1996; 87(6):2095–2147.
120. Colotta F, Re F, Muzio M, Bertini R, Polentarutti N, Sironi M, et al. Interleukin-1 type II receptor: A decoy target for IL-1 that is regulated by IL-4. Science 1993; 261(5120):472–475.
121. Re F, Sironi M, Muzio M, Matteucci C, Introna M, Orlando S, et al. Inhibition of

interleukin-1 responsiveness by type II receptor gene transfer: A surface "receptor" with anti-interleukin-1 function. J Exp Med 1996; 183(4):1841–1850.

122. Satoskar AR, Okano M, Connaughton S, Raisanen-Sokolwski A, David JR, Labow M. Enhanced Th2-like responses in IL-1 type 1 receptor-deficient mice. Eur J Immunol 1998; 28(7):2066–2074.
123. Brennan FM, Chantry D, Jackson A, Maini R, Feldmann M. Inhibitory effect of TNF alpha antibodies on synovial cell interleukin-1 production in rheumatoid arthritis. Lancet 1989; 2(8657):244–247.
124. Movat HZ, Burrowes CE, Cybulsky MI, Dinarello CA. Acute inflammation and a Shwartzman-like reaction induced by interleukin-1 and tumor necrosis factor. Synergistic action of the cytokines in the induction of inflammation and microvascular injury. Am J Pathol 1987; 129(3):463–476.
125. Kline JN, Fisher PA, Monick MM, Hunninghake GW. Regulation of interleukin-1 receptor antagonist by Th1 and Th2 cytokines. Am J Physiol 1995; 269(1 pt 1): L92–L98.
126. Symons JA, Young PR, Duff GW. Soluble type II interleukin 1 (IL-1) receptor binds and blocks processing of IL-1 beta precursor and loses affinity for IL-1 receptor antagonist. Proc Natl Acad Sci USA 1995; 92(5):1714–1718.
127. Burger D, Chicheportiche R, Giri JG, Dayer JM. The inhibitory activity of human interleukin-1 receptor antagonist is enhanced by type II interleukin-1 soluble receptor and hindered by type I interleukin-1 soluble receptor. J Clin Invest 1995; 96(1): 38–41.
128. Van Zee KJ, Kohno T, Fischer E, Rock CS, Moldawer LL, Lowry SF. Tumor necrosis factor soluble receptors circulate during experimental and clinical inflammation and can protect against excessive tumor necrosis factor alpha in vitro and in vivo. Proc Natl Acad Sci USA 1992; 89(11):4845–4849.
129. Engelmann H, Aderka D, Rubinstein M, Rotman D, Wallach D. A tumor necrosis factor-binding protein purified to homogeneity from human urine protects cells from tumor necrosis factor toxicity. J Biol Chem 1989; 264(20):11974–11980.
130. Olsson I, Lantz M, Nilsson E, Peetre C, Thysell H, Grubb A, Adolf G. Isolation and characterization of a tumor necrosis factor binding protein from urine. Eur J Haematol 1989; 42(3):270–275.
131. Mohler KM, Torrance DS, Smith CA, Goodwin RG, Stremler KE, Fung VP, et al. Soluble tumor necrosis factor (TNF) receptors are effective therapeutic agents in lethal endotoxemia and function simultaneously as both TNF carriers and TNF antagonists. J Immunol 1993; 151(3):1548–1561.
132. Aderka D, Engelmann H, Maor Y, Brakebusch C, Wallach D. Stabilization of the bioactivity of tumor necrosis factor by its soluble receptors. J Exp Med 1992; 175(2):323–329.
133. Edwards CK. PEGylated recombinant human soluble tumour necrosis factor receptor type I (r-Hu-sTNF-RI): Novel high affinity TNF receptor designed for chronic inflammatory diseases. Ann Rheum Dis 1999; 58(suppl 1):I73–I81.
134. Fisher CJ, Agosti JM, Opal SM, Lowry SF, Balk RA, Sadoff JC, Abraham E. Treatment of septic shock with the tumor necrosis factor receptor:Fc fusion protein. The Soluble TNF Receptor Sepsis Study Group. N Engl J Med 1996; 334(26): 1697–1702.

135. D'haens G, Van Deventer S, Van Hogezand R, Chalmers D, Kothe C, Baert F, et al. Endoscopic and histological healing with infliximab anti-tumor necrosis factor antibodies in Crohn's disease: A European multicenter trial. Gastroenterology 1999; 116(5):1029–1034.
136. Targan SR, Hanauer SB, van Deventer SJ, Mayer L, Present DH, Braakman T, et al. A short-term study of chimeric monoclonal antibody cA2 to tumor necrosis factor alpha for Crohn's disease. Crohn's disease cA2 Study Group. N Engl J Med 1997; 337(15):1029–1035.
137. Mease PJ, Goffe BS, Metz J, VanderStoep A, Finck B, Burge DJ. Etanercept in the treatment of psoriatic arthritis and psoriasis: A randomised trial. Lancet 2000; 356(9227):385–390.
138. Moreland LW, Baumgartner SW, Schiff MH, Tindall EA, Fleischmann RM, Weaver AL, et al. Treatment of rheumatoid arthritis with a recombinant human tumor necrosis factor receptor (p75)-Fc fusion protein [see comments]. N Engl J Med 1997; 337(3):141–147.
139. Moreland LW, Schiff MH, Baumgartner SW, Tindall EA, Fleischmann RM, Bulpitt KJ, et al. Etanercept therapy in rheumatoid arthritis. A randomized, controlled trial. Ann Intern Med 1999; 130(6):478–486.
140. Elliott MJ, Maini RN, Feldmann M, Long-Fox A, Charles P, Bijl H, Woody JN. Repeated therapy with monoclonal antibody to tumour necrosis factor alpha (cA2) in patients with rheumatoid arthritis. Lancet 1994; 344(8930):1125–1127.
141. Elliott MJ, Maini RN, Feldmann M, Kalden JR, Antoni C, Smolen JS, et al. Randomised double-blind comparison of chimeric monoclonal antibody to tumour necrosis factor alpha (cA2) versus placebo in rheumatoid arthritis. Lancet 1994; 344(8930):1105–1110.
142. Weinblatt ME, Kremer JM, Bankhurst AD, Bulpitt KJ, Fleischmann RM, Fox RI, et al. A trial of etanercept, a recombinant tumor necrosis factor receptor:Fc fusion protein, in patients with rheumatoid arthritis receiving methotrexate. N Engl J Med 1999; 340(4):253–259.
143. Warris A, Bjorneklett A, Gaustad P. Invasive pulmonary aspergillosis associated with infliximab therapy. N Engl J Med 2001; 344(14):1099–1100.
144. Luong BT, Chong BS, Lowder DM. Treatment options for rheumatoid arthritis: Celecoxib, leflunomide, etanercept, and infliximab. Ann Pharmacother 2000; 34(6): 743–760.
145. Fisher CJ, Dhainaut JF, Opal SM, Pribble JP, Balk RA, Slotman GJ, et al. Recombinant human interleukin 1 receptor antagonist in the treatment of patients with sepsis syndrome. Results from a randomized, double-blind, placebo-controlled trial. Phase III rhIL-1ra Sepsis Syndrome Study Group. JAMA 1994; 271(23):1836–1843.
146. Opal SM, Fisher CJ, Dhainaut JF, Vincent JL, Brase R, Lowry SF, et al. Confirmatory interleukin-1 receptor antagonist trial in severe sepsis: A phase III, randomized, double-blind, placebo-controlled, multicenter trial. The Interleukin-1 Receptor Antagonist Sepsis Investigator Group. Crit Care Med 1997; 25(7):1115–1124.
147. Campion GV, Lebsack ME, Lookabaugh J, Gordon G, Catalano M. Dose-range and dose-frequency study of recombinant human interleukin-1 receptor antagonist in patients with rheumatoid arthritis. The IL-1ra Arthritis Study Group. Arthritis Rheum 1996; 39(7):1092–1101.

148. Bresnihan B, Alvaro-Gracia JM, Cobby M, Doherty M, Domljan Z, Emery P, et al. Treatment of rheumatoid arthritis with recombinant human interleukin-1 receptor antagonist. Arthritis Rheum 1998; 41(12):2196–2204.
149. Jiang Y, Genant HK, Watt I, Cobby M, Bresnihan B, Aitchison R, McCabe DA. A multicenter, double-blind, dose-ranging, randomized, placebo-controlled study of recombinant human interleukin-1 receptor antagonist in patients with rheumatoid arthritis: Radiologic progression and correlation of Genant and Larsen scores. Arthritis Rheum 2000; 43(5):1001–1009.
150. Bendele AM, Chlipala ES, Scherrer J, Frazier J, Sennello G, Rich WJ, Edwards CK. Combination benefit of treatment with the cytokine inhibitors interleukin-1 receptor antagonist and PEGylated soluble tumor necrosis factor receptor type I in animal models of rheumatoid arthritis. Arthritis Rheum 2000; 43(12):2648–2659.
151. Okada S, Inoue H, Yamauchi K, Iijima H, Ohkawara Y, Takishima T, Shirato K. Potential role of interleukin-1 in allergen-induced late asthmatic reactions in guinea pigs: Suppressive effect of interleukin-1 receptor antagonist on late asthmatic reaction. J Allergy Clin Immunol 1995; 95(6):1236–1245.
152. Watson ML, Smith D, Bourne AD, Thompson RC, Westwick J. Cytokines contribute to airway dysfunction in antigen-challenged guinea pigs: Inhibition of airway hyperreactivity, pulmonary eosinophil accumulation, and tumor necrosis factor generation by pretreatment with an interleukin-1 receptor antagonist. Am J Respir Cell Mol Biol 1993; 8(4):365–369.
153. Mullarkey MF, Leiferman KM, Peters MS, Caro I, Roux ER, Hanna RK, Rubin AS, Jacobs CA. Human cutaneous allergic late-phase response is inhibited by soluble IL-1 receptor. J Immunol 1994; 152(4):2033–2041.

11

Development and Inhibition of Th2 Responses

Realization of Therapeutic Targets

AZZEDDINE DAKHAMA

National Jewish Medical and Research Center
Denver, Colorado

ERWIN W. GELFAND

National Jewish Medical and Research Center
and University of Colorado Health Sciences Center
Denver, Colorado

I. Introduction

Current thinking traces the development of allergic asthma from initial sensitization of naive T-helper (Th) cells (Th0) to environmental allergens through the expression and expansion of chronic allergen-mediated Th2-driven inflammation in the airway mucosa. Thus, T cells are at the epicenter of these responses, in large part because of their ability to synthesize and secrete an array of cytokines that are essential for acute and chronic allergic inflammation, be it in the airways, skin, nose, eyes, or intestine. $CD4^+$ T cells have been implicated as the principal cell type, and the Th2 cytokines they release include interleukin-4 (IL-4), IL-5, IL-6, IL-9, IL-10, IL-13, and granulocyte-macrophage colony stimulating factor (GM-CSF). There is increasing evidence that $CD8^+$ T cells (Tc2 cells), through release of IL-4 and IL-5, may also be involved in allergic diseases.

If Th2 cells are the primary culprits in the development of atopic diseases, then selective targeting or inhibition of Th2 cell responses provides a rational basis for the development of new therapeutic strategies. To achieve this goal, identification of features that differentiate Th2 and Th1 cells is essential to the development of selective immunomodulating drugs. The counterargument to these strategies is that the atopic diseases are not simply a reflection of a Th2 vs. Th1 imbalance or that simply interfering with Th2 responses by stimulating Th1 responses may exacerbate the underlying disease. Even if this Th2 paradigm is correct, controlling atopic disease by targeting Th2 cells may be very difficult in that long-term exposure to allergen may render these cells relatively resistant to immuno- or pharmacomodulation. In this review we examine the theoretical basis for Th2-mediated atopic diseases with a particular focus on asthma, the regulation of Th2 cell development, and the concepts and reality of strategies that interfere with Th2 cell function.

II. Th2 Responses in Asthma

Early postmortem studies of lungs from patients who died of an acute asthma attack have revealed a prominent bronchial tissue infiltration with lymphocytes and eosinophils suggesting involvement of these cells in the pathophysiology of asthma (1,2). With the introduction of fiber-optic bronchoscopy, these inflammatory cells could be sampled in the bronchoalveolar lavage fluid (BALF) and airway tissue from living patients and analyzed in more detail for cellular phenotype and function. Since then, evidence has accumulated to support the central role of T lymphocytes in the pathogenesis of asthma. Initial studies have described an increased proportion of CD4-positive (helper) T cells expressing surface markers of activation (CD25, HLA-DR, VLA-1) in the peripheral blood of patients with acute exacerbation of asthma (3,4). Subsequent studies documented increased numbers of activated T cells in the bronchoalveolar space and airway tissue of patients with bronchial asthma (5–9). These cells appeared to be of a memory phenotype (CD45RO), and their degree of activation generally correlated with severity of the disease (10). Further analyses revealed a predominant Th2 cytokine pattern in atopic asthmatic lung T cells. Using combined immunocytochemistry and in situ hybridization techniques, Robinson et al. (11) showed an increased proportion of T cells expressing mRNA for IL-2, IL-3, IL-4, IL-5, and GM-CSF in the BALF of subjects with atopic asthma compared to healthy control subjects. In atopic asthma, T cells are the predominant source for IL-4 and IL-5 in vivo, although eosinophils (12–16) and mast cells (17–19) can also produce Th2-type cytokines. This predominant Th2 cytokine pattern has also been confirmed in the bronchial tissue of asthmatic patients (20,21).

In general, T-cell activation and the predominant production of IL-4 and IL-5 correlate with airway tissue eosinophilia, asthma severity, and airway hyperresponsiveness in atopic asthma (22,23). These features are also upregulated after local airway challenge with specific allergen, supporting the primary role that Th2 cells play in orchestrating the pathogenesis of asthma (24–26). Del Prete et al. (27) derived T-cell clones from the bronchial mucosa of individuals with atopic asthma and demonstrated that these cells can proliferate in vitro and produce a predominant Th2 cytokine profile in a major histocompatibility complex–

restricted manner when stimulated with specific allergen, further confirming that allergen inhalation results in the local activation of Th2 cells in the airways of exposed atopic asthma patients. Antigen-responsive (memory-type) T cells are recruited to the lungs from the periphery and regional lymph nodes, and upon specific antigen stimulation they expand and produce cytokines. There is substantial evidence to suggest that these cells may recirculate in the periphery (28). In vitro stimulation of circulating T cells from atopic asthmatic individuals with specific allergen can lead to the release of Th2 cytokines, but only levels of stimulated IL-5 production appear to be associated with asthma symptoms whereas IL-4 production is more closely associated with atopy (29,30). In general, a Th2-dominant condition can be predicted from the usual association of the disease with blood or tissue eosinophilia and high IgE levels, as is the case for many atopic disorders, including atopic (extrinsic) asthma. High IgE levels are normally correlated with an increased ratio of IL-4 or IL-13 to IFN-γ, and blood or tissue eosinophilia usually suggests increased levels of IL-5.

A significant proportion (10–30%) of asthmatic subjects are skin prick test negative to common aeroallergens, and their total serum IgE levels are comparable to those of normal subjects (31,32). These patients are more likely to have the onset of symptoms later in life (33), and, like atopic asthmatics, they also have increased numbers of T cells, eosinophils, and high-affinity IgE receptor-expressing cells in their bronchial tissue (34,35). Dominant Th2 function could not be predicted for nonatopic (intrinsic) asthma until the demonstration of increased proportions of IL-4 and IL-5 mRNA and protein-expressing T cells ($CD4^+$ and $CD8^+$) in the bronchial tissue of these patients, providing evidence against the classification of intrinsic asthma as a distinct immunopathological entity (36,37).

These data suggest that Th2 cells may play a role in the pathogenesis of asthma, even in the absence of (obvious) sensitization to common allergens. However, local IgE production may occur as demonstrated by increased expression of germ-line gene transcripts ($I\varepsilon$) and mRNA for the heavy chain of IgE ($C\varepsilon$) in the airway mucosa of nonatopic asthmatic patients (38). Together, these observations led to the hypothesis that unidentified (possibly viral) antigens could be involved in the immunopathological mechanisms of intrinsic asthma (37). Support for this idea includes the demonstration of virus-specific IgE production (39) and a possible switch to IL-5 production by virus-specific $CD8^+$ T cells (40), thereby contributing to the local eosinophilic inflammation in the airways of nonatopic asthmatic subjects.

III. Development of Th1 and Th2 Responses

The distinctive T-helper 1 (Th1) and Th2 cytokine production patterns were originally described among mouse $CD4^+$ T-cell clones and first reported in 1986 by

Mosmann and collaborators (41,42). Th1 and Th2 cytokine patterns correspond to differentiated functional states of activated T cells that can be isolated only after a period of antigenic stimulation and are often categorized as initially primed "effector" or "memory" T cells. Evidence for the existence of Th1 and Th2 clones in humans has been confirmed in subjects with chronic inflammatory diseases (43,44). Th2 cells are characterized by the production of IL-4, IL-5, IL-6, IL-9, IL-10, and IL-13 but not gamma interferon (IFN-γ) or tumor necrosis factor (TNF)-β (also known as lymphotoxin). Th1 cells produce IL-2, IFN-γ, and TNF-β but not Th2 cytokines. A third subset of $CD4^+$ T cells, termed Th0, expresses cytokines of both patterns and may correspond to a primed but uncommitted naive T-cell phenotype (45,46). In humans, the Th1 and Th2 cytokine patterns are not as restricted to a single T-cell subset as in the mouse (47). In general, Th1 responses are involved in cell-mediated immunity and are highly protective against infections caused by intracellular pathogens. Th1 cytokines activate phagocytic and cytotoxic functions and facilitate the production by B cells of complement-fixing antibodies involved in phagocyte-mediated host defense. Th2 cytokines promote antibody production by B lymphocytes (through IL-4 and IL-13) and the growth of mast cells and basophils (through IL-3, IL-4, IL-9, and IL-10) and induce the terminal differentiation, release from bone marrow, and activation of eosinophils (through IL-5). Th2 responses are commonly found in association with high IgE and eosinophil responses in a variety of allergic disorders, including asthma (48–50).

The development of Th1 or Th2 responses involves many factors including the genetic background (51,52), the dose and nature of the antigenic stimulus (53–56), the affinity and strength of peptide binding to MHC molecules (57,58), the route of immunization (59), the nature of the costimulatory signals, and, more critically, the type of cytokines present in the T-cell microenvironment during antigen priming and initiation of the T-cell response (Fig. 1).

A. Cytokines

In vitro studies have demonstrated that the differentiation and effector functions of Th1 and Th2 clones are mutually cross-regulated by the characteristic cytokine products of the reciprocal phenotype. Thus, IFN-γ from Th1 clones selectively inhibited Th2 cell proliferation and IL-4 production whereas IL-4 and IL-10 from Th2 clones inhibited Th1 cell proliferation and IFN-γ production (60–63).

A variety of immune (inflammatory) and nonimmune (structural) cells can also contribute to the production of Th1- and Th2-type cytokines and may therefore participate in the regulation of Th1 and Th2 responses in vivo (50,64,65). Accordingly, the terminology "type 1 and type 2" instead of "Th1 and Th2" has been proposed to characterize disease-associated immune dysregulation in vivo (66,67).

There is now increasing evidence that human $CD8^+$ T cells (66,68,69) and murine $CD8^+$ T cells (70–73) can also develop into type 1 (Tc1) and type 2 (Tc2) cytokine-producing clones. Other cells producing type 1 and type 2 cytokines include subsets of $\gamma\delta$ T cells (74), B cells (75–77), NK cells (78–80), eosinophils (12–16,81), mast cells (82,83), and basophils (84,85).

Monocytes/macrophages, dendritic cells, and mucosal epithelial cells, which are important sources of the regulatory cytokines IL-10 and IL-12 (and possibly TGF-β), also can participate in the Th1(Tc1)/Th2(Tc2) differentiation decision. Because of the diversity of the cellular sources of type 1 and type 2 cytokines, many of these non-T-cell contributions could be transient only and confined to specific anatomical locations. Careful consideration of the timing, the tissue location, and the amount (extent) of such contributions will provide even more conclusive data regarding the ongoing immune response and may help to better define the important cellular targets for the most successful treatments.

B. Dendritic Cells

Recent data suggest that Th-cell polarization may be considerably influenced by distinct subsets of dendritic cells (DCs). The phenotype and functional properties of these cells were initially defined in the mouse system (86–88). Early data derived from in vitro studies suggested that murine $CD8\alpha^-$ DCs stimulate T-cell proliferation and IL-2 production whereas $CD8\alpha^+$ DCs restrict these T-cell responses (89–91). Murine $CD8\alpha^+$ DCs produce high amounts of IL-12 and promote Th1 development by inducing high concentrations of Th1 cytokines but few if any Th2 cytokines. In contrast, $CD8\alpha^-$ DCs produce limited amounts of IL-12 but can induce large amounts of Th2 cytokines and favor Th2 development (92–94).

Human DCs can be differentiated in culture from two distinct DC precursors, monocytes and plasmacytoid cells; both DCs stimulate the proliferation of allogeneic $CD4^+$ T cells (95,96). Human monocyte-derived DCs (DC1) produce high levels of IL-12 and induce the production of large amounts of IFN-γ (Th1 cytokine) but little IL-4, IL-5, and IL-10 (Th2 cytokines) by cocultured naive $CD4^+CD45RA^+$ T cells. Conversely, T cells cultured with plasmacytoid-derived DCs (DC2) secret little Th1 cytokine but large amounts of Th2 cytokines (97,98). Thus IL-12 produced by DCs appears to be dominant in driving the development of Th1 cells (92,99). Antigen exposure via mucosal surfaces such as the respiratory epithelium has been shown to favor immune responses associated with Th2 development (59,100). Consistent with this idea, other studies have demonstrated that resting respiratory tract DCs producing low levels of IL-12 preferentially promote the development of Th2 cells (101), whereas the generation of Th1 cells in the respiratory tract may require obligatory cytokine signals, most notably IL-12. Collectively, these observations support the hypothesis of an alternative

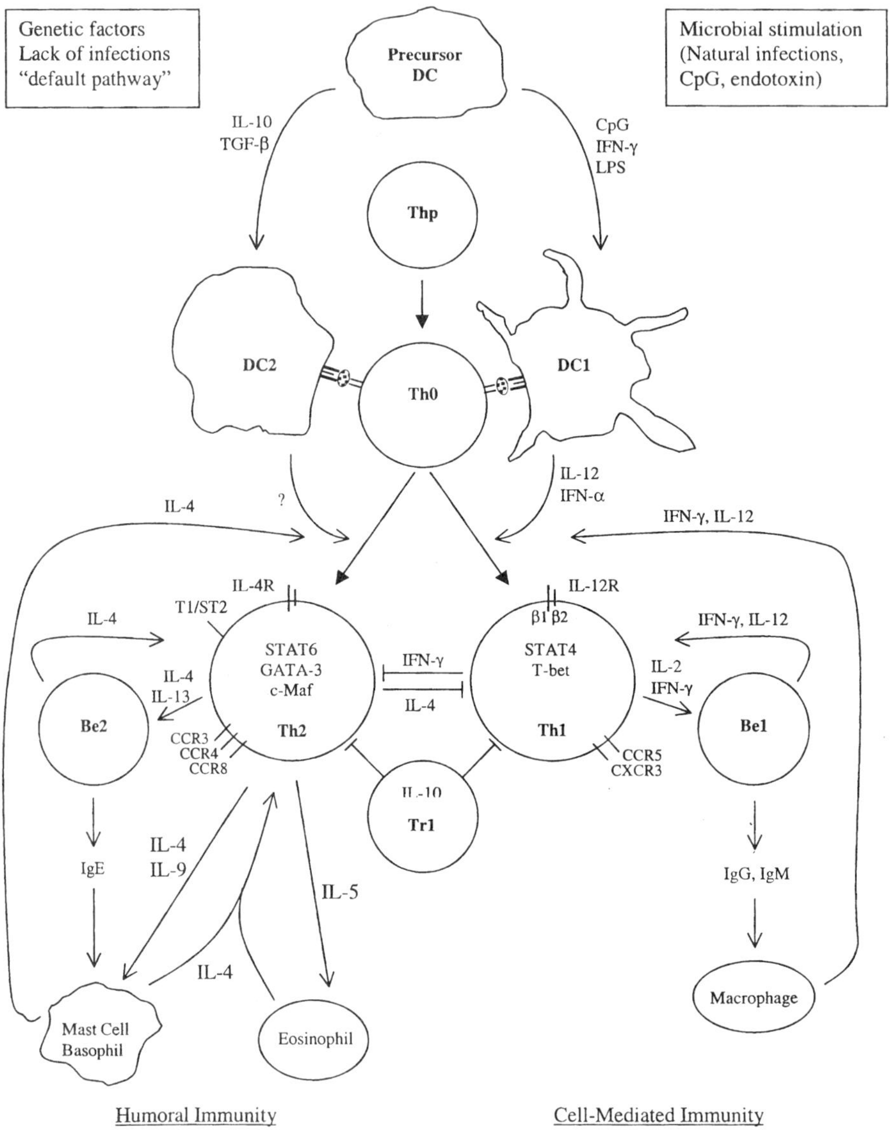
Genetic factors
Lack of infections
"default pathway"
Precursor DC
Microbial stimulation
(Natural infections,
CpG, endotoxin)
IL-10
TGF-β
CpG
IFN-γ
LPS
Thp
DC2
Th0
DC1
?
IL-12
IFN-α
IL-4
IFN-γ, IL-12
IL-4R
T1/ST2
IL-12R
β1 β2
IL-4
STAT6
GATA-3
c-Maf
Th2
IFN-γ
IL-4
STAT4
T-bet
Th1
IFN-γ, IL-12
IL-2
IFN-γ
IL-4
IL-13
Be2
CCR3
CCR4
CCR8
IL-10
Tr1
CCR5
CXCR3
Be1
IgE
IL-4
IL-9
IL-5
IgG, IgM
IL-4
Macrophage
Mast Cell
Basophil
Eosinophil
Humoral Immunity
Cell-Mediated Immunity

''default pathway'' favoring the spontaneous development of Th2 cells in the absence of IL-12 (reviewed in Ref. 102). In the presence of IL-12, the development of Th1 cells would be favored because Th2 cells are usually not responsive to IL-12 owing to a selective downregulation of the IL-12 receptor β2 subunit (IL-12Rβ2) that occurs during the developmental commitment of these cells (103–105). However, it remains possible that other (unknown) molecules or factors expressed by DC2 may direct Th2 development.

C. Costimulatory Signals

Following thymic selection, newly released αβ $CD4^+$ T cells have a naive phenotype and must receive appropriate signals to become effector cells capable of orchestrating inflammatory cell-mediated or humoral responses. When first stimulated with antigen, naive T-helper precursor (Thp) cells become activated and principally produce IL-2 and expand before differentiating into phenotypes that secrete other cytokines. This initial activation step is regulated by engagement of the T-cell receptor (TCR) with selected peptide presented in the context of MHC II molecules and critically requires a number of costimulatory signals (106). In the absence of costimulation, Thp cells become anergic or unresponsive and likely will be depleted. Thus, the fate of Thp cells may be determined by multiple signals that can be delivered by costimulatory molecules of the B7 family expressed on antigen-presenting cells at various stages of the immune response (reviewed in Ref. 107). B7-1 (CD80) and B7-2 (CD86) provide critical signals for T-cell expansion mainly through IL-2 production. The T-cell counterligands

---

Figure 1 Developmental pathways of Th1/Th2 cell differentiation. The differentiation of Th0 cells from naive precursors (Thp) into effector Th1 or Th2 cells is triggered by stimulation with antigen presented by the appropriate antigen-presenting cell (APC). At mucosal sites, the maturation of dendritic cells (DC) is promoted by microbial stimulation. In contrast to immature DC2, mature DC1 produce large amounts of IL-12, which favors Th1 differentiation. In the absence of IL-12 (lack of infections), Th2 differentiation is promoted through a ''default'' pathway by DC2. Once differentiated, Th1 and Th2 cells produce characteristic cytokine patterns and express specific transcription factors and different cytokine and chemokine receptors. Th1 cytokines (IFN-γ, TNF-β) activate phagocytic/cytotoxic functions and promote production of complement-fixing antibodies. Th2 cytokines are involved in allergic responses by promoting IgE production (via IL-4 and IL-13), growth of mast cells/basophils (via IL-4, IL-9, and IL-10), and eosinophilia (through IL-5). Effector Th1 and Th2 cell functions can be downregulated by IL-10-producing regulatory (Tr1) T cells. Th1 and Th2 polarization can be further enhanced by type-1 (IFN-γ) and type-2 (IL-4) cytokines produced by non-T cells (mast cells/basophils, eosinophils, macrophages, and type-1 and type-2 effector B cells (Be1, Be2)), resulting in more chronic responses.

of these molecules are CD28 and CTLA-4. Engagement of CD28 mediates a costimulatory signal that results in T-cell proliferation and prevents the induction of anergy, whereas CTLA-4 delivers a negative regulatory signal to activated T cells (108–111). CD86 appears to be required for initial T-cell activation and dominates during primary responses, whereas CD80 appears to be more critical in sustaining T-cell function during primary and secondary immune responses. Initial studies suggested that CD80 regulates Th1 responses and CD86 regulates Th2 responses (112–114). However, studies of CD80- and CD86-deficient mice showed that CD86, not CD80, was critical for the development of experimental autoimmune encephalomyelitis (EAE), a Th1-mediated inflammatory disease of the central nervous system (115). Other studies suggested that both CD80 and CD86 induce Th1 or Th2 responses (reviewed in Ref. 116).

Another member of the B7 family, called B7-related protein 1 (B7RP-1), has been identified, and its ligand, inducible costimulator (ICOS), was recently discovered (117,118). Unlike CD28, which is expressed on resting T cells, ICOS expression is induced only after T-cell activation and is dramatically reduced by inhibition of B7 signaling (119,120). Recent studies suggest that ICOS–B7RP-1 interaction plays a critical role in the development of humoral responses by promoting isotype switching in both primary and secondary T-cell-dependent B-cell responses (121–123). Other members of the B7 family include programmed death ligands 1 and 2 (PD-L1 and PD-L2) and their receptor PD-1, which contains an inhibitory (ITIM) motif in its cytoplasmic domain (124,125). PD-L1 and PD-L2 are differentially expressed upon activation on monocytes, and their expression can be regulated by IFN-γ and IL-4 or IL-13 (126). Engagement of PD-1 by PD-L1 and PD-L2 may provide negative signals to inhibit Th1 or Th2 responses.

D. Transcription Factors

The signal transducer and activator of transcription (STAT) factors STAT4 and STAT6 play important roles in determining the fate of naive $CD4^+$ T cells, at least during early activation induced by IL-12 and IL-4. STAT4 is essential for IL-12-induced Th1 differentiation (127), and STAT4-deficient mice have defective Th1 development (128). In humans, STAT4 is also activated by type I IFNs, which favor the development of Th1 responses (129–131). Other transcription factors, possibly operating downstream of STAT4, are selectively expressed in Th1 cells. The Ets family member ERM is Th1-specific, and its expression is STAT4-dependent, but its overexpression in STAT4-deficient T cells was not sufficient to restore IFN-γ production (132). The MHC class II transactivator (CIITA) is selectively expressed in Th1 cells and can repress IL-4 (133,134). T-bet, a recently identified Th1-specific transcription factor, is a strong activator of IFN-γ production and can inhibit IL-4 and IL-5 production even when overexpressed in developing Th2 cells (135).

STAT6 is required for IL-4-induced Th2 differentiation (136,137), and early studies reported deficient Th2 responses in STAT6 gene knockout mice (138). However, differentiated Th2 cells can produce IL-4 without the requirement for a continued exogenous IL-4 supply (139). More recently, IL-4-independent and STAT6-independent Th2 development pathways were described (140–143). Downstream of STAT6, the Th2-specific transcription factor GATA-3 plays a critical role in the expression of the Th2 cytokines IL-4, IL-5, and IL-13 (144). STAT6 activation is critical to GATA-3 activation in IL-4-mediated Th2 development (145), and NF-κB appears to be required for the expression of GATA-3 during Th2 development (146). In addition to the conventional IL-4/STAT6 axis, GATA-3 activation can be mediated through CD28 signaling (147). Recent studies suggested that an autoactivation feedback pathway in which GATA-3 activates its own expression would be one mechanism of STAT6-independent Th2 development (148). This may explain why human DC2 can drive Th2 development even in the absence of IL-4 (96). Such "default pathways" would be inhibited by IL-12, which mediates the STAT4 activation signal that can repress GATA-3 expression. The protooncogene c-Maf is another Th2-specific transcription factor with considerable impact on Th2 development (149,150). Unlike GATA-3, which exerts more general effects by regulating the expression of several Th2 cytokines, c-Maf exerts a highly selective effect by promoting the production of IL-4 only and not other Th2 cytokines (151). Both GATA-3 and c-Maf can inhibit Th1 development through an IL-4-independent mechanism (145,150).

E. Recruitment of Th2 Cells

The selective recruitment and trafficking of Th1 and Th2 cells in the lungs involves the coordinated action of chemokines and adhesion molecules. Chemokine receptors are differentially expressed on Th1 and Th2 cells (152–154). Th1 cells preferentially express the chemokine receptors CCR5 and CXCR3 and are selectively attracted by macrophage inflammatory protein-1β (MIP-1β) and interferon-inducible protein 10 (IP-10). Th2 cells preferentially express CCR3, CCR4, and CCR8 and are selectively attracted by eotaxin, I-309, macrophage-derived chemokine (MDC), and thymus and activation-regulated chemokine (TARC). Both CCR3/eotaxin and CCR4/MDC axes have been shown to play a role in the recruitment and retention of Th2 cells within the lung tissue in mouse models of allergic airway inflammation and hyperresponsiveness (155,156). Recent animal studies suggested that Th1 cells, which were recruited to the lungs early during the allergic response, facilitate the recruitment and tissue retention of effector Th2 cells (157,158). This observation may be supported by the ability of TCR-activated Th1 cells to produce Th2-attracting chemokines I-309 and MDC (159). Thus, Th1-derived chemokines may exaggerate Th2 cell-mediated responses, leading to exacerbation of some clinical manifestations of disease, for example virus-mediated exacerbation of asthma attacks.

F. Regulatory T Cells

In addition to the important cytokine-driven effects on T-cell differentiation into Th1- and Th2-like cells, there are regulatory T cells that may impinge on Th-cell differentiation. $CD4^{+}/CD25^{+}$ T cells are potent inhibitors of polyclonal T-cell activation (160). Unlike other regulatory T cells, which produce inhibitory cytokines, these cells suppress immune responses by a contact-dependent mechanism (161–163). TGF-β plays a role in the generation and expansion of these $CD4^{+}/CD25^{+}$ regulatory T cells (164). Another regulatory $CD4^{+}$ T-cell subset, designated T regulatory cells 1 (Tr1), has been isolated among anergic $CD4^{+}$ T cells generated by chronic exposure to alloantigens in the presence of IL-10. These antigen-specific T cells have low proliferative capacity and produce high levels of IL-10, which mediates their immunosuppressive effects (165,166). Anergic T cells suppress other T-cell responses by targeting antigen-presenting cells (167).

IV. Interference with Th2 Function

Because of the predominance of Th2 responses in allergic diseases, asthma in particular, a number of approaches for targeting Th2 responses have been explored. As discussed above and highlighted in Figure 2, a number of cells, receptors, and pathways have theoretical potential for downregulating Th2 responses. Because many of these responses are the result of chronic allergen exposure, they may be relatively resistant to suppression compared to models of primary responses, for example in murine models of allergen-induced inflammation. In addition to the therapeutic strategies to limit Th2 responses, especially taking advantage of features that differentiate Th2 from Th1 cells, some preventive strategies in which induction of Th1 responsiveness is a goal are also reviewed briefly in this section.

A. Corticosteroids

Corticosteroids are currently the most effective treatment in controlling allergic diseases, and if administered early during onset development they may prevent some of the irreversible pathophysiological alterations in asthma (168). Corticosteroids have been proven effective in reducing levels of Th2 cytokines and improving symptoms of asthma (169). Corticosteroids may mediate their anti-

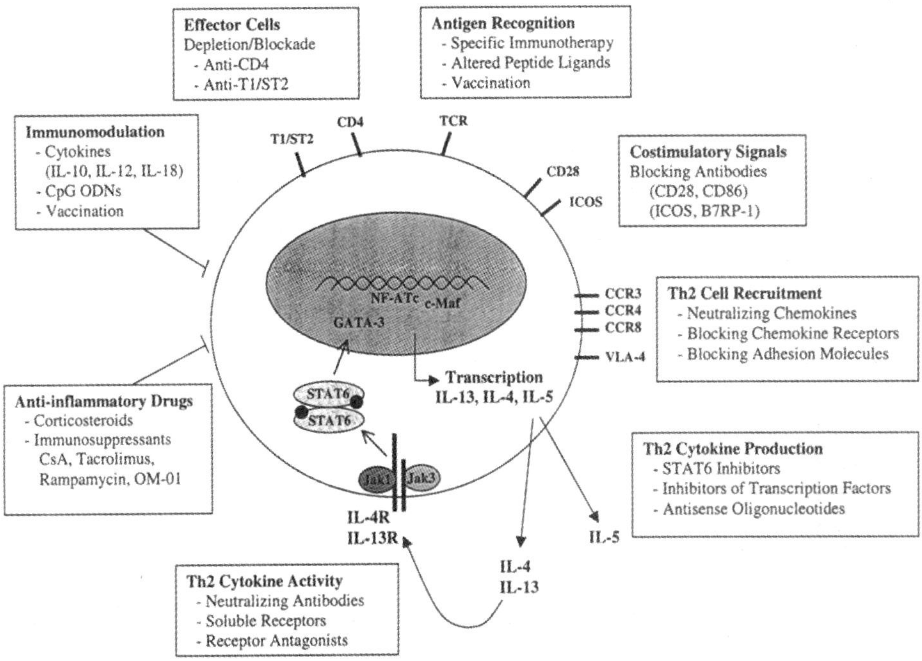

Figure 2 Potential therapeutic targets for inhibition of Th2 responses. Several molecules (cell surface receptors and cytokines) and pathways (Th2-specific transcription factors) are potential therapeutic targets to interfere with Th2 cell differentiation and effector cell function. However, selective targeting of Th2 cells without causing generalized immunosuppression may provide the most successful approach to treatment of Th2-mediated diseases.

inflammatory and immunosuppressive effects principally by inhibiting several transcription factors (e.g., AP-1, NF-κB, NF-AT, STAT) that regulate inflammatory gene expression (170). Corticosteroids interact with cytosolic glucocorticoid (GC) receptors, which dimerize and bind to a specific DNA consensus sequence (GRE), resulting in transactivation (increased activation) of inflammatory genes. Glucocorticoids can also interact with monomeric GC receptors and interfere with the translocation and binding of transcription factors, resulting in transrepression of inflammatory genes. To minimize the undesired side effects of corticosteroids that are mediated largely by transactivation of target genes (through DNA binding), a new generation of corticosteroids (called dissociated steroids) has been generated. Dissociated steroids lack the transactivating properties while maintaining their inhibitory effects on transcription factors (171). Transactivation of certain genes (e.g., β2-adrenergic receptors and IκB) is also part of the beneficial therapeutic effect of corticosteroids in asthma, and whether the use of dissociated steroids will translate to a more effective therapy in patients has not yet been demonstrated. However, there exists a subset of patients whose symptoms are not controlled even by high doses of corticosteroids (172,173), which promoted consideration of other alternative or adjunctive therapies.

B. Immunosuppressants

Clinical studies of cyclosporin A (CsA) suggested its use as a corticosteroid-sparing agent for adjunctive treatment of corticosteroid-dependent asthma (174,175). Treatment of allergic asthmatic patients with CsA attenuated allergen-induced late asthmatic response, but not the early response, an effect that was associated with decreased eosinophilia and eosinophil-associated cytokines and chemokines (176,177). However, the potential side effects of CsA, mainly nephrotoxicity, may limit its clinical use (178,179). A potential alternative to minimize these side effects consists of using inhaled CsA. Repeated inhalation of newly formulated CsA (ADI628) was well tolerated by asthmatic subjects, and no nephrotoxicity or hepatotoxicity was observed after 6 months of treatment (180). CsA and topical tacrolimus (FK506) have also been successfully used for the treatment of severe atopic dermatitis (181–184). These immunosuppressants inhibit T-cell function by interfering with the induction/activation of the nuclear factor of activated T cells (NF-AT), resulting in the suppression of both Th1 and Th2 cytokine production (185). Unlike CsA, FK506, and dexamethasone, which inhibited the production of IL-2, IL-4, and IL-5, the polynactin family member OM-01 appears to be more selective by inhibiting the production of IL-5 but not IL-2 or IL-4 synthesis by allergen-specific human Th clones (186). Thus, drugs that selectively inhibit aspects of T-cell function without causing a generalized immunosuppression may be the most suitable agents for the treatment of severe allergic disorders, including steroid-dependent asthma.

C. Depletion and/or Incapacitation of Effector T Cells

Based on the clear implication of $CD4^+$ T cells in the pathogenesis of asthma, some therapeutic strategies consist of depleting or incapacitating these effectors cells by using monoclonal antibodies (mAbs) to human CD4. The CD4 molecule is involved in MHC class II-dependent recognition of antigen by $CD4^+$ T cells. Initial clinical trials with mouse mAbs to human CD4 provided encouraging data to support the use of these antibodies for the treatment of autoimmune diseases (187,188) or to support organ transplantion (189,190). However, the major side effect of these mouse antibodies is their immunogenicity, which may lead to anaphylaxis in immunocompetent hosts. To overcome this limitation, an IgG1 chimeric human/cynomologus macaque monoclonal antibody to CD4 (keliximab) has been generated (191). The results of clinical trials of keliximab in corticosteroid-dependent asthma patients suggested the use of this antibody as an adjunctive treatment for the management of chronic severe asthma (192). Potential limitation for the long-term use of CD4 mAbs is antibody-mediated depletion of CD4 cells, which may compromise the host's immune response to opportunistic infections. To minimize the CD4 cell depletion, a modified IgG4 derivative of keliximab, clenoliximab, was developed (193). Clenoliximab appears to function as a classical receptor antagonist that blocks the interaction of CD4 with MHC class II and modulates CD4 cells without depleting them.

Th2 cells preferentially express the IL-1 receptor family member T1/ST2 (194,195). T1/ST2 was originally described as a serum-induced late response gene in fibroblasts (196,197). The gene encoding T1/ST2 is closely linked to the IL-1 receptor locus (198). T1/ST2 exists both as a membrane-bound protein with a cytoplasmic domain and as a secreted soluble receptor lacking the transmembrane and cytoplasmic domains (199). A putative T1/ST2 ligand has been identified as a soluble protein, distinct from IL-1, that activates p38MAPK, but its structure and exact biological role have not yet been determined (200). In vivo studies performed in mice suggested an important role for T1/ST2 signaling in Th2-mediated allergic inflammatory responses in the lungs (201). Thus, blockade of T1/ST2 signaling either with a rat mAb to T1/ST2 or with a T1/ST2-Ig fusion protein in allergen-sensitized and airway-challenged mice resulted in considerable decreases in Th2 cytokine production and eosinophilic responses in the lung. T1/ST2 may not be required for the development of Th2 responses (202,203) but appears to play an important role in the activation of Th2 cells, and its expression on Th2 cells polarized in vitro has been shown to be secondary to type 2 cytokine production (204).

Although some effects of these interventions on allergic inflammation can be predicted, further studies and trials are necessary to assess the risk/benefit ratio of these strategies in the management, prevention, and treatment of allergen-induced airway hyperresponsiveness.

D. Inhibition of Th2 Cell Recruitment

Adhesion Molecules

The recruitment of effector Th2 cells into the lung involves specific interactions with adhesion molecules and is critically dependent on the secretion of a subset of chemokines (205,206). The recruitment of T cells is first initiated by a decrease in their rolling through interactions with E-selectin and P-selectin expressed on activated vascular endothelial cells (207). Subsequent interactions with a second family of adhesion molecules, including ICAM-1 (intercellular adhesion molecule-1) and VCAM-1 (vascular cell adhesion molecule-1), result in increased adhesiveness of these cells to the vascular endothelium. Following a gradient of particular chemokines, the T cells are directed to a specific anatomical tissue location. E-selectin, P-selectin, ICAM-1, and VCAM-1 are all upregulated by proinflammatory stimuli. Acute mediators and Th1 cytokines appear to predominantly induce E-selectin, P-selectin, and ICAM-1 (208), whereas Th2 cytokines (IL-4, IL-13) predominantly induce P-selectin and VCAM-1 (209,210). In asthma, the interaction between very late antigen-4 (VLA-4), and VCAM-1 is important for the recruitment of eosinophils and effector T cells, and blockade of VLA-4 has been shown to be effective in abrogating allergic airway responses in animal models (211–214). Small molecule inhibitors of VLA-4 have been developed and shown to be effective in inhibiting allergic airway responses in sensitized sheep (215,216). Recent data suggest that adhesion molecules may also regulate the development and effector function of Th1 and Th2 cells. Blockade of LFA–1/ICAM interaction between dendritic cells and naive T cells enhanced Th2 cytokine production and suppressed the development of Th1 cells (217). Thus, the blocking of adhesion molecules may have an impact at different levels of the immune response, not only on selective adhesion of T cells but also on their differentiation, and may be a helpful strategy in the treatment of allergic responses and asthma if it selectively impairs the recruitment of effector Th2 cells.

Chemokines and Chemokine Receptors

The migration of Th2 cells into inflamed tissue is directed by a subset of CC chemokines that mediate their chemotactic effects through Gi-coupled seven-transmembrane domain receptors differentially expressed on primed Th2 cells. Chemokines also direct the migration of dendritic cells and other leukocytes in tissue and bring T cells and APCs together for closer interactions within the draining lymph nodes. Two functional categories of chemokines are now recognized: inflammatory chemokines and homeostatic chemokines (218,219). Inflammatory chemokines are induced by inflammatory stimuli and are responsible for active recruitment of the appropriate subset of leukocytes, whereas homeostatic chemokines are constitutively expressed in several tissues and regulate basal trafficking of lymphocytes. Certain CC chemokines are particularly involved in the development of allergic airway inflammation and hyperresponsiveness and are preferentially induced by Th2 cytokines (IL-4 and IL-13) but not Th1 cytokines (155,220–226). These include eotaxin, MCP (monocyte chemotactic proteins), RANTES (regulated on activation, normal T cells expressed and secreted), TARC (thymus- and activation-regulated chemokine), and MDC (monocyte-derived chemokine). Interestingly, polarized Th2 cells preferentially express the CC chemokine receptors CCR3 (which binds eotaxin, MCP, and RANTES), CCR4 (which binds MDC and TARC), and CCR8 (which binds I-309). Recent data indicate that certain chemokines and their receptors are involved in a coordinated cooperative manner at different stages of the allergic inflammatory response; whereas the CCR3- eotaxin pathway appears to play a role early during acute responses, the CCR4-MDC subsequently dominates in the recruitment of antigen-specific Th2 cells (156). This selective expression of chemokines and the particular distribution of their receptors on Th2 cells make them potential therapeutic targets for modifying the outcome of allergic airway inflammation and hyperresponsiveness. Thus, an improved understanding of the role of chemokines in regulating T-cell differentiation and trafficking of specialized Th2 cells may lead to the design of novel therapies to correct the defects in many allergic disorders, including asthma.

E. Immunomodulation

Cytokines

Cytokines with immunomodulatory properties such as IL-10 and IL-12 may have some therapeutic potential for the treatment of allergies and asthma. IL-10 is a potent anti-inflammatory cytokine mainly produced by monocytes or macrophages, B cells, and Th2 cells (227). Epithelial cells are another source of IL-10 (228). IL-10 downregulates the expression of MHC class II and the costimulatory molecules CD80 and CD86 (229,230) and inhibits CD28-mediated signaling, resulting in suppression of APC-dependent T-cell effector functions (231). Particularly interesting for its therapeutic use, IL-10 inhibits the synthesis of IL-5 by Th2 cells, decreases the production of eosinophil survival factors (e.g., IL-3 and GM-CSF), and promotes eosinophil death (232). Reduced levels of IL-10 in the BALF and defective IL-10 production by macrophages were measured in patients with asthma in comparison with healthy subjects (226). Inhaled corticosteroids have been shown to increase IL-10 release from alveolar macrophages (233). Thus, administration of exogenous IL-10 to asthmatic patients may restore the balance between pro- and anti-inflammatory cytokines. Repeated administration of recombinant human IL-10 has proved to be safe and effective in controlling inflammatory bowel disease and psoriasis (234,235). Alternatively, increasing the endogenous production of IL-10 may also prove to be beneficial therapeutic strategy. One potential concern is that, at least in murine models of allergen-induced airway hyperresponsiveness, elimination of IL-10 reduces airway hyperresponsiveness, pointing to a role for IL-10 in the development of bronchoconstriction (236,237). Careful investigation of IL-10 receptor function and responsiveness is required for effective IL-10 therapy.

Interleukin-12 is an important endogenous regulator of Th1 cell development. IL-12 is mainly produced by macrophages and APCs and has been shown to promote the differentiation and proliferation of Th1 cells and IFN-γ production by T cells and NK cells. IL-12 can also inhibit Th2 cytokine production and suppress IgE synthesis, suggesting a potential immunomodulatory role in asthma (238–241). IL-12 production by macrophages is reduced in patients with allergic asthma (242), and asthmatic subjects showed lower numbers of IL-12 mRNA-expressing cells in the bronchial tissue than nonasthmatic subjects, but the number of these cells was increased following treatment with corticosteroids (243). Several animal studies suggested a beneficial therapeutic effect of either systemically or locally administered IL-12, which effectively inhibited lung Th2 responses, eosinophilia, and airway hyperresponsiveness (244–247). IL-12 may be ineffective in reversing established Th2 responses, because highly polarized Th2 cells lack the IL-12R β2 subunit, rendering them unresponsive to IL-12 (104,105,248). However, recent data showed that both BAL and peripheral human T cells obtained during allergen-induced late asthmatic responses expressed IL-12R β2 mRNA and were responsive to IL-12 stimulation, which resulted in significant inhibition of antigen-induced IL-5 production and increased IFN-γ production (249). Subcutaneous administration of increasing doses (0.1–0.5 μg/kg) of recombinant human IL-12 to patients with mild allergic asthma resulted in significant decreases in blood and sputum eosinophils but did not inhibit airway hyperresponsiveness to histamine (250). Of the 19 patients studied, four withdrew prematurely because of cardiac arrhythmias, abnormal liver function, or severe flu-like symptoms. Fever, general fatigue, arthralgia, myalgia, and leukopenia are other symptoms reported to be related to IL-12 toxicity, and systemic administration of this cytokine may not be an option for the treatment of airway diseases such as asthma. Alternative options may include local administration of IL-12 to the airways to minimize such side effects.

Interleukin-18 is another cytokine that modulates Th1 and Th2 responses. IL-18 has been recently identified and characterized as an endogenous inducer of IFN-γ production by T cells (251). However, the most remarkable effect of IL-18 is the potentiation of IL-12-driven Th1 responses (252), although IL-18 alone may induce $CD4^+$ T cells to differentiate into Th2 cells when stimulated through the TCR (253). Coadministration of IL-18 and IL-12 has been shown to be effective in inhibiting Th2 responses and airway hyperresponsiveness in mouse models of allergic sensitization (254). Similar results have been described in mice, where IL-18 was overexpressed in the airways using replication-deficient adenovirus vector (255). In other studies, antigen-mediated Th2 responses were deviated toward a Th1-dominated response when IL-18 was administered as an adjuvant with heat-killed *Listeria monocytogenes* (256). An elegant approach consisted of using an allergen–IL-18 fusion DNA vaccine, which not only prevented the development of allergen-mediated Th2 responses but also reversed established airway hyperresponsiveness in mice (257). Thus, IL-18 has interesting potential for clinical use as an adjuvant for antigen (or DNA vaccine)-based immunotherapy. In preliminary trials, IL-18 instillation was not well tolerated in patients with asthma.

In spite of their interesting activities, these cytokines lack some selectivity in their action because they can affect multiple cellular targets that are not involved in the specific immune response, resulting in undesired side effects. Another limitation is their large size and short in vivo half-life, which raise concerns about their delivery and stability and also the cost/effectiveness ratio of their use as a treatment in asthma, which depends on the treatment schedule.

Microbial Products

The increasing prevalence and incidence of allergies and asthma in developed countries are thought to be the result of an unopposed Th2 development due to the lack of natural infections resulting in a defective Th1 response, at least in early life (258). This has led to the concept of immunomodulatory ''anti-allergy'' vaccine strategies consisting of inoculating bacterial products, including bacterial DNA, to favor the development of Th1 responses in early life to counteract the unopposed Th2 development or to restore the Th1/Th2 balance in Th2-dependent diseases such as allergy and asthma. Studies in Japan found an inverse association between the development of atopic disorders and bacillus Calmette-Guérin (BCG) vaccination (259), but this has not been confirmed in other population studies (260–262). BCG inoculation in mice suppressed allergen-induced eosinophilia, reduced IL-4 and IL-5 levels and increased IFN-γ levels in the BAL fluid, and inhibited the development of airway hyperresponsiveness (263,264). Similar results were obtained in mice treated with heat-killed *Mycobacterium vaccae* (265), and clinical trials showed some beneficial immunomodulatory effects with this agent in patients with psoriasis (266,267). However, a recent study found no beneficial effect of using heat-killed (autoclaved) *Mycobacterium vaccae* or a delipidated deglycolipidated preparation in ameliorating symptoms of patients with established asthma (268).

The unmethylated CpG motif-containing oligodeoxynucleotides (CpG ODNs), present at high frequency (1:16) in bacterial DNA, are potent immunostimulatory agents that induce Th1 responses in mice. A number of animal studies suggest that CpG ODNs could have significant therapeutic potential in the treatment of various disorders, including allergy and asthma. CpG ODNs activate B cells and induce T cells to secrete IL-6, IL-12, and IFN-γ (269,270). They induce maturation of immature APCs (271,272), and, through APC-stimulated IL-12 secretion, they activate NK cells to produce large amounts of IFN-γ (273). Studies in mice have shown that CpG ODNs can prevent the development of airway eosinophilia and airway hyperresponsiveness (274–276). Thus, systemic or local (intra-airway) administration of immunostimulatory DNA sequences containing CpG motifs before first allergen exposure may provide a new form of immunotherapy. Another attractive approach in the area of immunotherapy is the use of CpG-rich plasmid DNA constructs containing the coding sequences for the antigen of interest. Conceivably, the inclusion of the CpG motifs in the construct would enhance the resulting immune response to the peptide by inducing larger amounts of IL-12 and type 1 IFNs (277–279). In general, CpG ODNs are well tolerated whether given intravenously, subcutaneously, or intraperitoneally.

However, repeated administration of large doses of CpG ODN may result in splenomegaly due to the expansion of B cells, proliferation of NK cells, and extramedullary hematopoiesis (280). A number of early clinical trials are under way adopting these strategies.

F. Interference with Antigen Recognition

Antigen recognition is a critical step in the development of an allergic response. Upon encounter of specific allergen peptide presented by professional APCs in the context of MHC class II and in conjunction with appropriate costimulatory signals, Th2 cells become activated and secrete a pattern of cytokines that promote the production of antigen-specific IgE responses and further orchestrate other aspects characteristic of the allergic response, including recruitment and activation of effector granulocytes (eosinophils, mast cells, and basophils). Interference with antigen recognition is an attractive approach to prevent the development of allergic responses. Nearly a century ago, immunotherapy was proposed as a preventive method consisting of subcutaneous administration of increasing doses of the putative allergen (281). However, anaphylaxis regularly occurred in patients with high levels of specific IgE. To avoid or minimize this major side effect, it is imperative to develop allergen-derived peptides that can alter T-cell responses without or with very limited (low affinity) binding to IgE (282). Such an approach has been tested in animal models and may ultimately result in the induction of a transient or permanent state of anergy, perhaps involving IL-10-producing regulatory (Tr1) T cells (165,283). Initial approaches using such strategies, using cat dander peptides, for example, have failed to yield consistent results.

Another approach to interfere with antigen recognition involves the generation and use of altered peptide ligands (APLs). APLs are antigen peptide analogs that bear a substitution of a putative T-cell contact residue while retaining similar properties of binding to MHC molecules (284,285). APLs bind to MHC and are recognized by the specific TCR, but unlike the unmodified antigen peptide they do not elicit a specific T-cell response and do not bind IgE. Such TCR antagonism occurs naturally and seems to be involved in thymic selection and development of the T-cell repertoire (286,287), and it may be used by certain viruses to avoid T-cell recognition and escape the immune response (288,289). Altered peptides can also be partial agonists and block only undesirable immune responses (290). APLs have been shown to cause a shift in cytokine production in vitro (291,292) and have been used to inhibit antigen-specific T-cell responses (293,294). The use of APLs may represent an effective approach to preventing or treating allergies without the side effects of conventional immunotherapy. Further studies are still needed to assess the effectiveness and cost/benefit ratio of performing such therapies in humans.

G. Interruption of Costimulatory Signals

The activation of effector T-cell function is critically dependent on the nature of the costimulatory signal delivered to these cells during antigen presentation by professional APCs. Engagement of CD28 and CD80(B7.1)/CD86(B7.2) is essential for initial T-cell activation and expansion (108,109). This response is opposed by binding of CTLA-4 to CD80/CD86, which limits T-cell expansion and cytokine production by recently activated, antigen-experienced T cells (110). Several studies have demonstrated that the prevention of T-cell costimulation in vivo by treatment of sensitized mice with CTLA-4 Ig fusion protein, which interrupts CD28:B7.1/B7.2 interactions, results in marked decreases in Th2 cytokine production, IgE levels, and airway eosinophilia and abrogates airway hyperresponsiveness (295–297). Other studies in mice confirmed these effects and went on to demonstrate that, comparable to the effects obtained with CTLA-4 Ig, airway administration of a monoclonal antibody to B7.2(CD86) inhibited allergen-induced airway eosinophilia, Th2 cytokine secretion, and IgE production and abrogated airway hyperresponsiveness, suggesting the critical involvement of B7.2 in these responses (298). More recent studies suggested that CD28 and ICOS molecules are involved at distinct levels in determining the outcome of the lung immune response, CD28 essentially priming T cells and ICOS regulating effector T-cell responses (299). Accordingly, it is feasible that the interruption of CD28 signaling at the first time of antigen encounter may lead to a state of anergy or antigen-specific unresponsiveness, whereas blocking ICOS signaling may be more effective in inhibiting the effector functions of previously established Th2 responses. Thus, selective targeting of these costimulatory molecules may prove beneficial for the prevention and treatment of Th2-mediated lung mucosal allergic responses. If blockade of T-cell costimulation at the time of antigen presentation may lead to a prolonged state of antigen-specific unresponsiveness, such intervention may have a potential for the treatment of allergic diseases.

H. Inhibition of IL-4 (IL-13)-Mediated Th2 Cell Generation

Although Th2 (and Tc2) cells are considered the predominant source of IL-4 (IL-13) in vivo, other leukocytes such as mast cells and eosinophils may contribute to the production of these cytokines, further perpetuating the chronic inflammation seen in asthma and some allergic disorders. Strategies to inhibit Th2 cytokines include the use of neutralizing antibodies or soluble cytokine receptors that act as blockers, cytokine receptor antagonists, inhibitors of cytokine receptor–mediated signaling pathways, and selective inhibitors of cytokine synthesis.

Interleukin-4 plays a key role in the differentiation and stabilization of the Th2 phenotype (63,300). IL-4 is capable of upregulating its own receptor expression and mediates other effects, including increased expression of CD23 and MHC class II and IgE isotype switch in B cells (301–303). IL-4 also enhances

VCAM-1 and downregulates E-selectin expression on vascular endothelial cells (304,305). In mice, anti-IL-4 antibody was found effective in reducing eosinophil numbers and IgE levels if administered prior to first antigen sensitization (306,307). A recombinant soluble IL-4 receptor (sIL-4R) lacking the transmembrane and cytoplasmic domains has been designed so it can bind secreted IL-4 and block its effects in vitro and in vivo (308,309). In other murine studies, local administration of sIL-4R to the airways was found to be more effective than systemic administration in reducing allergic airway inflammation and IgE responses, but the effects on airway hyperresponsiveness were variable (310,311). Clinical trials of sIL-4R in human asthma suggest its use as a safe medication for management of asthma symptoms (312,313). However, more recent but larger trials with sIL-4R failed to demonstrate significant benefit.

Whereas IL-4 plays a dominant role in the differentiation of Th2 cells, IL-13 also appears to be involved in effector Th2 responses that are mediated through STAT6-dependent pathways and are partially dependent on a common receptor (IL-4Rα) shared with IL-4 (314,315). A soluble form of the high-affinity receptor for IL-13, sIL-13Rα2-Fc fusion protein, which blocks IL-13 binding in vivo (316), was used in a mouse model of *Schistosoma mansoni*–induced pulmonary granuloma and shown to be effective in reducing the size of granuloma and total IgE but did not alter the pattern of Th2 cytokines induced by egg antigens (317). Although the inhibition of either IL-4 or IL-13 is somehow effective, both IL-4 and IL-13 may have to be inhibited to achieve full therapeutic effectiveness. An attractive approach to achieve this is by inhibiting their receptor-mediated effects. In this context, the shared IL-4Rα appears to be the target of choice for interrupting both IL-4- and IL-13-mediated effects.

The IL-4 receptor complex is composed of IL-4Rα and the common gamma (γ_c) chain. Binding of IL-4 to the IL-4R results in the activation of the Janus kinases Jak-1 and Jak-3, which are respectively associated with the IL-4Rα and γ_c chains. This also results in the phosphorylation of the tyrosine residues present in the cytoplasmic domain of the IL-4Rα chain. Phosphorylation of the three conserved tyrosine residues Y575, Y603, and Y631 is critical for the IL-4Rα-mediated signal transduction that leads to the activation of IL-4-induced genes (318,319). These phosphotyrosines serve as docking sites for the Src homology 2 (Sh2) domains of the STAT6 molecules, which are in turn phosphorylated by the activated kinases at the C-terminus tyrosine residue (320). Phosphorylated STAT6 molecules dissociate from the receptor tail and form homodimers, which then translocate to the nucleus and bind to specific DNA motifs with other transcription factors in the promoter regions of IL-4-responsive genes to activate transcription.

The IL-4R also has an ITIM-like motif in its C-terminus, which upon phosphorylation serves as a docking site for the Sh2 domains of the phosphotyrosine phosphatases SHP1/2 or SHIP, but the role of these phosphatases in regulating

IL-4 signaling has not yet been established. In addition, IL-4R activation can be negatively regulated by a series of cytokine-induced suppressors of cytokine signaling (SOCS) such as SOCS-1, which can inhibit the activation of Jak1 and STAT6 in response to IL-4 (321). Because the expression of SOCS (and other functionally related suppressors such as CIS, JAB, and SSI) is dependent on STAT activation and results in the inactivation of the Janus kinases, these suppressor pathways appear to function as a negative loop that modulates the Jak-STAT activation pathway and may therefore terminate IL-4/IL-4R signaling.

Thus, the axis IL-4 (IL-13)–IL-4Rα–Jak1/3–STAT6 is an attractive target for therapeutic intervention of Th2 responses. The importance of this axis is supported by the defective development of Th2 responses seen in IL-4-deficient (322) and STAT6-deficient mice (136–138). Treatment of allergen-sensitized mice with a mutant form of murine IL-4 protein (IL-4R antagonist), which binds IL-4Rα and inhibits both IL-4 and IL-13 signaling, dramatically reduced antigen-induced lung eosinophilia and airway hyperresponsiveness (323). A mutant human IL-13 protein (IL-13E13K) has been recently designed and found to bind IL-13 with higher affinity than unmodified IL-13, but its efficacy in blocking in vivo the effects of IL-13 or both IL-13 and IL-4 has not yet been demonstrated (324).

Downstream of IL-4Rα and associated signaling molecules, the Th2-specific transcription factors c-Maf and GATA-3 also represent specific targets for selective inhibition of Th2 differentiation and cytokine production. The expression of both transcription factors (and STAT6) was shown to be increased in atopic and nonatopic asthma patients compared with healthy control subjects (325,326). In contrast to c-Maf, which transactivates the IL-4 promoter but does not regulate the transcription of other Th2 cytokines (149,151), GATA-3 controls production of the key Th2 cytokines involved in the pathogenesis of allergic airway diseases such as asthma (146,327). Inhibition of GATA-3 using selective pharmacological or antisense oligonucleotide-based strategies may limit the generation of Th2 cells in vivo and possibly attenuate cytokine production by established Th2 cells as suggested by recent data from animal studies (328,329).

V. Conclusions

Atopic or allergic diseases now affect a large percentage of the population of most countries and consume significant proportions of health care spending. As a rule, they are chronic conditions in which therapy is directed toward amelioration of symptoms. For the most part these conditions are incurable, although severity may wax or wane regardless of therapy. The last decade has witnessed an explosion in our understanding of the regulation of the differentiation of precursor T cells into mature Th1 or Th2 cells and the apparent immune deviation from a Th1 to Th2 phenotype that underlies atopy. As a result of this information, numerous targets have been identified to control allergic disease. This has led to the discovery of new classes of drugs as a result of increased understanding of the cellular and molecular events underlying the development of atopy. For many of these targets, development and testing of therapeutic agents is relatively early. A number that have shown potential in animal models have limited or no experience in humans. Results in animal models may or may not carry over to humans. To date, relatively few new drugs have in fact made it to the clinic. Nevertheless, the incredible amount of new knowledge already generated and that is likely to continue to develop should have a major impact on our thinking about and treatment of established allergic disease and on strategies to prevent early sensitization in childhood.

Acknowledgments

This work was supported in part by grants from the NIH (HL-36577, HL-61005) and the Environmental Protection Agency (R825702).

References

1. Dunill MS. The pathology of asthma with special reference to changes in the bronchial mucosa. J Clin Pathol 1968; 13:27–33.
2. Fabbri LM, Danieli D, Crescioli S, Bevilacqua P, Meli S, Saetta M, Mapp CE. Fatal asthma in a subject sensitized to toluene diisocyanate. Am Rev Respir Dis 1988; 137:1494–1498.
3. Corrigan CJ, Hartnell A, Kay AB. T lymphocyte activation in acute severe asthma. Lancet 1988; 1:1129–1132.
4. Corrigan CJ, Kay AB. CD4 T-lymphocyte activation in acute severe asthma. Relationship to disease severity and atopic status. Am Rev Respir Dis 1990; 141:970–977.
5. Azzawi M, Bradley B, Jeffery PK, Frew AJ, Wardlaw AJ, Knowles G, Assoufi B, Collins JV, Durham S, Kay AB. Identification of activated T lymphocytes and eosinophils in bronchial biopsies in stable atopic asthma. Am Rev Respir Dis 1990; 142:1407–1413.
6. Bradley BL, Azzawi M, Jacobson M, Assoufi B, Collins JV, Irani AM, Schwartz LB, Durham SR, Jeffery PK, Kay AB. Eosinophils, T-lymphocytes, mast cells, neutrophils, and macrophages in bronchial biopsy specimens from atopic subjects with asthma: Comparison with biopsy specimens from atopic subjects without asthma and normal control subjects and relationship to bronchial hyperresponsiveness. J Allergy Clin Immunol 1991; 88:661–674.
7. Walker C, Kaegi MK, Braun P, Blaser K. Activated T cells and eosinophilia in bronchoalveolar lavages from subjects with asthma correlated with disease severity. J Allergy Clin Immunol 1991; 88:935–942.

8. Hamid Q, Barkans J, Robinson DS, Durham SR, Kay AB. Co-expression of CD25 and CD3 in atopic allergy and asthma. Immunology 1992; 75:659–663.
9. Wilson JW, Djukanovic R, Howarth PH, Holgate ST. Lymphocyte activation in bronchoalveolar lavage and peripheral blood in atopic asthma. Am Rev Respir Dis 1992; 145:958–960.
10. Robinson DS, Bentley AM, Hartnell A, Kay AB, Durham SR. Activated memory T helper cells in bronchoalveolar lavage fluid from patients with atopic asthma: Relation to asthma symptoms, lung function, and bronchial responsiveness. Thorax 1993; 48:26–32.
11. Robinson DS, Hamid Q, Ying S, Tsicopoulos A, Barkans J, Bentley AM, Corrigan C, Durham SR, Kay AB. Predominant TH2-like bronchoalveolar T-lymphocyte population in atopic asthma. N Engl J Med 1992; 326:298–304.
12. Broide DH, Paine MM, Firestein GS. Eosinophils express interleukin 5 and granulocyte macrophage-colony-stimulating factor mRNA at sites of allergic inflammation in asthmatics. J Clin Invest 1992; 90:1414–1424.
13. Dubucquoi S, Desreumaux P, Janin A, Klein O, Goldman M, Tavernier J, Capron A, Capron M. Interleukin 5 synthesis by eosinophils: Association with granules and immunoglobulin-dependent secretion. J Exp Med 1994; 179:703–708.
14. Moqbel R, Ying S, Barkans J, Newman TM, Kimmitt P, Wakelin M, Taborda-Barata L, Meng Q, Corrigan CJ, Durham SR, Kay AB. Identification of messenger RNA for IL-4 in human eosinophils with granule localization and release of the translated product. J Immunol 1995; 155:4939–4947.
15. Nonaka M, Nonaka R, Woolley K, Adelroth E, Miura K, Okhawara Y, Glibetic M, Nakano K, O'Byrne P, Dolovich J, Jordana M. Distinct immunohistochemical localization of IL-4 in human inflamed airway tissues. IL-4 is localized to eosinophils in vivo and is released by peripheral blood eosinophils. J Immunol 1995; 155: 3234–3244.
16. Moller GM, de Jong TA, Overbeek SE, van der Kwast TH, Postma DS, Hoogsteden HC. Ultrastructural immunogold localization of interleukin 5 to the crystalloid core compartment of eosinophil secondary granules in patients with atopic asthma. J Histochem Cytochem 1996; 44:67–69.
17. Bradding P, Feather IH, Howarth PH, Mueller R, Roberts JA, Britten K, Bews JP, Hunt TC, Okayama Y, Heusser CH, Bullock GR, Church MK, Holgate ST. Interleukin 4 is localized to and released by human mast cells. J Exp Med 1992; 176: 1381–1386.
18. Jaffe JS, Glaum MC, Raible DG, Post TJ, Dimitry E, Govindarao D, Wang Y, Schulman ES. Human lung mast cell IL-5 gene and protein expression: Temporal analysis of upregulation following IgE-mediated activation. Am J Respir Cell Mol Biol 1995; 13:665–675.
19. Jaffe JS, Raible DG, Post TJ, Wang Y, Glaum MC, Butterfield JH, Schulman ES. Human lung mast cell activation leads to IL-13 mRNA expression and protein release. Am J Respir Cell Mol Biol 1996; 15:473–481.
20. Ying S, Durham SR, Corrigan CJ, Hamid Q, Kay AB. Phenotype of cells expressing mRNA for TH2-type (interleukin 4 and interleukin 5) and TH1-type (interleukin 2 and interferon gamma) cytokines in bronchoalveolar lavage and bronchial biopsies from atopic asthmatic and normal control subjects. Am J Respir Cell Mol Biol 1995; 12:477–487.

21. Humbert M, Durham SR, Ying S, Kimmitt P, Barkans J, Assoufi B, Pfister R, Menz G, Robinson DS, Kay AB, Corrigan CJ. IL-4 and IL-5 mRNA and protein in bronchial biopsies from patients with atopic and nonatopic asthma: Evidence against ''intrinsic'' asthma being a distinct immunopathologic entity. Am J Respir Crit Care Med 1996; 154:1497–1504.
22. Robinson DS, Ying S, Bentley AM, Meng Q, North J, Durham SR, Kay AB, Hamid Q. Relationships among numbers of bronchoalveolar lavage cells expressing messenger ribonucleic acid for cytokines, asthma symptoms, and airway methacholine responsiveness in atopic asthma. J Allergy Clin Immunol 1993; 92:397–403.
23. Walker C, Bauer W, Braun RK, Menz G, Braun P, Schwarz F, Hansel TT, Villiger B. Activated T cells and cytokines in bronchoalveolar lavages from patients with various lung diseases associated with eosinophilia. Am J Respir Crit Care Med 1994; 150:1038–1048.
24. Bentley AM, Meng Q, Robinson DS, Hamid Q, Kay AB, Durham SR. Increases in activated T lymphocytes, eosinophils, and cytokine mRNA expression for interleukin-5 and granulocyte/macrophage colony-stimulating factor in bronchial biopsies after allergen inhalation challenge in atopic asthmatics. Am J Respir Cell Mol Biol 1993; 8:35–42.
25. Robinson D, Hamid QA, Bentley A, Ying S, Kay AB, Durham SR. Activation of CD4+ T cells, increased TH2-type cytokine mRNA expression, and eosinophil recruitment in bronchoalveolar lavage after allergen inhalation challenge in patients with atopic asthma. J Allergy Clin Immunol 1993; 92:313–324.
26. Huang SK, Xiao HQ, Kleine-Tebbe J, Paciotti G, Marsh DG, Lichtenstein LM, Liu MC. IL-13 expression at the sites of allergen challenge in patients with asthma. J Immunol 1995; 155:2688–2694.
27. Del Prete GF, De Carli M, D'Elios MM, Maestrelli P, Ricci M, Fabbri L, Romagnani S. Allergen exposure induces the activation of allergen-specific Th2 cells in the airway mucosa of patients with allergic respiratory disorders. Eur J Immunol 1993; 23:1445–1449.
28. Hamid QA, Cameron LA. Recruitment of T cells to the lung in response to antigen challenge. J Allergy Clin Immunol 2000; 106(5 suppl):S227–S234.
29. Tang C, Rolland IM, Ward C, Bish R, Thien F, Walters EH. Seasonal comparison of cytokine profiles in atopic asthmatics and atopic non-asthmatics. Am J Respir Crit Care Med 1996; 154:1615–1622.
30. Till S, Dickason R, Huston D, Humbert M, Robinson D, Larche M, Durham S, Kay AB, Corrigan C. IL-5 secretion by allergen-stimulated CD4+ T cells in primary culture: Relationship to expression of allergic disease. J Allergy Clin Immunol 1997; 99:563–569.
31. Wüthrich B, Schindler C, Leuenberg P, Ackermann-Liebrich U. Prevalence of atopy and pollinosis in the adult population of Switzerland (SAPALDIA study). Swiss Study on Air Pollution and Lung Diseases in Adults. Int Arch Allergy Immunol 1995; 106:149–156.
32. Godard P, Bousquet J, Michel FB. Extrinsinc and intrinsic asthma: Still a matter for debate? Clin Asthma Rev 1997; 1:19–22.
33. Rackemann FM. A working classification of asthma. Am J Med 1947; 3:601–606.
34. Bentley AM, Menz G, Storz C, Robinson DS, Bradley B, Jeffery PK, Durham SR,

Kay AB. Identification of T lymphocytes, macrophages, and activated eosinophils in the bronchial mucosa in intrinsic asthma. Relationship to symptoms and bronchial responsiveness. Am Rev Respir Dis 1992; 146:500–506.

35. Humbert M, Grant JA, Taborda-Barata L, Durham SR, Pfister R, Menz G, Barkans J, Ying S, Kay AB. High-affinity IgE receptor (FcepsilonRI)-bearing cells in bronchial biopsies from atopic and nonatopic asthma. Am J Respir Crit Care Med 1996; 153:1931–1937.
36. Ying S, Humbert M, Barkans J, Corrigan CJ, Pfister R, Menz G, Larche M, Robinson DS, Durham SR, Kay AB. Expression of IL-4 and IL-5 mRNA and protein product by CD4+ and CD8+ T cells, eosinophils, and mast cells in bronchial biopsies obtained from atopic and nonatopic (intrinsic) asthmatics. J Immunol 1997; 158:3539–3544.
37. Humbert M, Menz G, Ying S, Corrigan CJ, Robinson DS, Durham SR, Kay AB. The immunopathology of extrinsic (atopic) and intrinsic (non-atopic) asthma: More similarities than differences. Immunol Today 1999; 20:528–533.
38. Durham SR, Gould HJ, Thienes CP, Jacobson MR, Masuyama K, Rak S, Lowhagen O, Schotman E, Cameron L, Hamid QA. Expression of epsilon germ-line gene transcripts and mRNA for the epsilon heavy chain of IgE in nasal B cells and the effects of topical corticosteroid. Eur J Immunol 1997; 27:2899–2906.
39. Welliver RC, Wong DT, Sun M, Middleton E Jr, Vaughan RS, Ogra PL. The development of respiratory syncytial virus-specific IgE and the release of histamine in nasopharyngeal secretions after infection. N Engl J Med 1981; 305:841–846.
40. Coyle AJ, Erard F, Bertrand C, Walti S, Pircher H, Le Gros G. Virus-specific CD8+ cells can switch to interleukin 5 production and induce airway eosinophilia. J Exp Med 1995; 181:1229–1233.
41. Mosmann TR, Cherwinski H, Bond MW, Giedlin MA, Coffman RL. Two types of murine helper T cell clone. I. Definition according to profiles of lymphokine activities and secreted proteins. J Immunol 1986; 136:2348–2357.
42. Cherwinski HM, Schumacher JH, Brown KD, Mosmann TR. Two types of mouse helper T cell clone. III. Further differences in lymphokine synthesis between Th1 and Th2 clones revealed by RNA hybridization, functionally monospecific bioassays, and monoclonal antibodies. J Exp Med 1987; 166:1229–1244.
43. Del Prete GF, De Carli M, Mastromauro C, Biagiotti R, Macchia D, Falagiani P, Ricci M, Romagnani S. Purified protein derivative of Mycobacterium tuberculosis and excretory-secretory antigen(s) of Toxocara canis expand in vitro human T cells with stable and opposite (type 1 T helper or type 2 T helper) profile of cytokine production. J Clin Invest 1991; 88:346–350.
44. Wierenga EA, Snoek M, Jansen HM, Bos JD, van Lier RA, Kapsenberg ML. Human atopen-specific types 1 and 2 T helper cell clones. J Immunol 1991; 147:2942–2949.
45. Firestein GS, Roeder WD, Laxer JA, Townsend KS, Weaver CT, Hom JT, Linton J, Torbett BE, Glasebrook AL. A new murine CD4+ T cell subset with an unrestricted cytokine profile. J Immunol 1989; 143:518–525.
46. Paliard X, de Waal Malefijt R, Yssel H, Blanchard D, Chretien I, Abrams J, de Vries J, Spits H. Simultaneous production of IL-2, IL-4, and IFN-gamma by activated human CD4+ and CD8+ T cell clones. J Immunol 1988; 141:849–855.

47. Romagnani S. Lymphokine production by human T cells in disease states. Annu Rev Immunol 1994; 12:227–257.
48. Romagnani S. Human TH1 and TH2 subsets: Doubt no more. Immunol Today 1991; 12:256–257.
49. Lucey DR, Clerici M, Shearer GM. Type 1 and type 2 cytokine dysregulation in human infectious, neoplastic, and inflammatory diseases. Clin Microbiol Rev 1996; 9:532–562.
50. Mosmann TR, Sad S. The expanding universe of T-cell subsets: Th1, Th2 and more. Immunol Today 1996; 17:138–146.
51. Barnes KC, Marsh DG. The genetics and complexity of allergy and asthma. Immunol Today 1998; 19:325–332.
52. Barnes KC. Evidence for common genetic elements in allergic disease. J Allergy Clin Immunol 2000; 106(5 suppl):S192–S200.
53. Parish CR, Liew FY. Immune response to chemically modified flagellin. 3. Enhanced cell-mediated immunity during high and low zone antibody tolerance to flagellin. J Exp Med 1972; 135:298–311.
54. Bretscher PA, Wei G, Menon JN, Bielefeldt-Ohmann H. Establishment of stable, cell-mediated immunity that makes ''susceptible'' mice resistant to Leishmania major. Science 1992; 257:539–542.
55. Hosken NA, Shibuya K, Heath AW, Murphy KM, O'Garra A. The effect of antigen dose on CD4+ T helper cell phenotype development in a T cell receptor-alpha beta-transgenic model. J Exp Med 1995; 182:1579–1584.
56. Guery JC, Galbiati F, Smiroldo S, Adorini L. Selective development of T helper (Th)2 cells induced by continuous administration of low dose soluble proteins to normal and beta(2)-microglobulin-deficient BALB/c mice. J Exp Med 1996; 183: 485–497.
57. Murray JS, Pfeiffer C, Madri J, Bottomly K. Major histocompatibility complex (MHC) control of CD4 T cell subset activation. II. A single peptide induces either humoral or cell-mediated responses in mice of distinct MHC genotype. Eur J Immunol 1992; 22:559–565.
58. Pfeiffer C, Stein J, Southwood S, Ketelaar H, Sette A, Bottomly K. Altered peptide ligands can control CD4 T lymphocyte differentiation in vivo. J Exp Med 1995; 181:1569–1574.
59. Constant SL, Lee KS, Bottomly K. Site of antigen delivery can influence T cell priming: Pulmonary environment promotes preferential Th2-type differentiation. Eur J Immunol 2000; 30:840–847.
60. Mosmann TR, Coffman RL. TH1 and TH2 cells: Different patterns of lymphokine secretion lead to different functional properties. Annu Rev Immunol 1989; 7:145–173.
61. Fiorentino DF, Bond MW, Mosmann TR. Two types of mouse T helper cell. IV. Th2 clones secrete a factor that inhibits cytokine production by Th1 clones. J Exp Med 1989; 170:2081–2095.
62. Maggi E, Parronchi P, Manetti R, Simonelli C, Piccinni MP, Rugiu FS, De Carli M, Ricci M, Romagnani S. Reciprocal regulatory effects of IFN-gamma and IL-4 on the in vitro development of human Th1 and Th2 clones. J Immunol 1992; 148: 2142–2147.

63. Seder RA, Paul WE, Davis MM, Fazekas de St Groth B. The presence of interleukin 4 during in vitro priming determines the lymphokine-producing potential of CD4+ T cells from T cell receptor transgenic mice. J Exp Med 1992; 176:1091–1098.
64. Bloom BR, Salgame P, Diamond B. Revisiting and revising suppressor T cells. Immunol Today 1992; 13:131–136.
65. Liles WC, Van Voorhis WC. Review: Nomenclature and biologic significance of cytokines involved in inflammation and the host immune response. J Infect Dis 1995; 172:1573–1580.
66. Salgame P, Abrams JS, Clayberger C, Goldstein H, Convit J, Modlin RL, Bloom BR. Differing lymphokine profiles of functional subsets of human CD4 and CD8 T cell clones. Science 1991; 254:279–282.
67. Clerici M, Shearer GM. A TH1 → TH2 switch is a critical step in the etiology of HIV infection. Immunol Today 1993; 14:107–111.
68. Maggi E, Giudizi MG, Biagiotti R, Annunziato F, Manetti R, Piccinni MP, Parronchi P, Sampognaro S, Giannarini L, Zuccati G, Romagnani S. Th2-like CD8+ T cells showing B cell helper function and reduced cytolytic activity in human immunodeficiency virus type 1 infection. J Exp Med 1994; 180:489–495.
69. Paganelli R, Scala E, Ansotegui IJ, Ausiello CM, Halapi E, Fanales-Belasio E, D'Offizi G, Mezzaroma I, Pandolfi F, Fiorilli M, Cassone A, Aiuti F. CD8+ T lymphocytes provide helper activity for IgE synthesis in human immunodeficiency virus-infected patients with hyper-IgE. J Exp Med 1995; 18:423–428.
70. Seder RA, Boulay JL, Finkelman F, Barbier S, Ben-Sasson SZ, Le Gros G, Paul WE. CD8+ T cells can be primed in vitro to produce IL-4. J Immunol 1992; 148: 1652–1656.
71. Erard F, Wild MT, Garcia-Sanz JA, Le Gros G. Switch of CD8 T cells to noncytolytic CD8−CD4-cells that make TH2 cytokines and help B cells. Science 1993; 260:1802–1805.
72. Croft M, Carter L, Swain SL, Dutton RW. Generation of polarized antigen-specific CD8 effector populations: Reciprocal action of interleukin (IL)-4 and IL-12 in promoting type 2 versus type 1 cytokine profiles. J Exp Med 1994; 180:1715– 1728.
73. Coyle AJ, Erard F, Bertrand C, Walti S, Pircher H, Le Gros G. Virus-specific CD8+ cells can switch to interleukin 5 production and induce airway eosinophilia. J Exp Med 1995; 181:1229–1233.
74. Ferrick DA, Schrenzel MD, Mulvania T, Hsieh B, Ferlin WG, Lepper H. Differential production of interferon-gamma and interleukin-4 in response to Th1- and Th2-stimulating pathogens by gamma delta T cells in vivo. Nature 1995; 373:255–257.
75. O'Garra A, Stapleton G, Dhar V, Pearce M, Schumacher J, Rugo H, Barbis D, Stall A, Cupp J, Moore K, Vieira P, Mosmann T, Whitmore A, Arnold L, Haughton G, Howard M. Production of cytokines by mouse B cells: B lymphomas and normal B cells produce interleukin 10. Int Immunol 1990; 2:821–832.
76. Schultze JL, Michalak S, Lowne J, Wong A, Gilleece MH, Gribben JG, Nadler LM. Human non-germinal center B cell interleukin (IL)-12 production is primarily regulated by T cell signals CD40 ligand, interferon gamma, and IL-10: Role of B cells in the maintenance of T cell responses. J Exp Med 1999; 189:1–12.
77. Harris DP, Haynes L, Sayles PC, Duso DK, Eaton SM, Lepak NM, Johnson LL,

Swain SL, Lund FE. Reciprocal regulation of polarized cytokine production by effector B and T cells. Nat Immunol 2000; 1:475–482.
78. Trinchieri G. Biology of natural killer cells. Adv Immunol 1989; 47:187–376.
79. Walker C, Checkel J, Cammisuli S, Leibson PJ, Gleich GJ. IL-5 production by NK cells contributes to eosinophil infiltration in a mouse model of allergic inflammation. J Immunol 1998; 161:1962–1969.
80. Bendelac A, Hunziker RD, Lantz O. Increased interleukin 4 and immunoglobulin E production in transgenic mice overexpressing NK1 T cells. J Exp Med 1996; 184:1285–1293.
81. Woerly G, Roger N, Loiseau S, Capron M. Expression of Th1 and Th2 immunoregulatory cytokines by human eosinophils. Int Arch Allergy Immunol 1999; 118:95–97.
82. Plaut M, Pierce JH, Watson CJ, Hanley-Hyde J, Nordan RP, Paul WE. Mast cell lines produce lymphokines in response to cross-linkage of Fc epsilon RI or to calcium ionophores. Nature 1989; 339:64–67.
83. Bradding P, Feather IH, Wilson S, Bardin PG, Heusser CH, Holgate ST, Howarth PH. Immunolocalization of cytokines in the nasal mucosa of normal and perennial rhinitic subjects. The mast cell as a source of IL-4, IL-5, and IL-6 in human allergic mucosal inflammation. J Immunol 1993; 151:3853–3865.
84. Seder RA, Paul WE, Dvorak AM, Sharkis SJ, Kagey-Sobotka A, Niv Y, Finkelman FD, Barbieri SA, Galli SJ, Plaut M. Mouse splenic and bone marrow cell populations that express high-affinity Fc epsilon receptors and produce interleukin 4 are highly enriched in basophils. Proc Natl Acad Sci USA 1991; 88:2835–2839.
85. MacGlashan D Jr, White JM, Huang SK, Ono SJ, Schroeder JT, Lichtenstein LM. Secretion of IL-4 from human basophils. The relationship between IL-4 mRNA and protein in resting and stimulated basophils. J Immunol 1994; 152:3006–3016.
86. Vremec D, Zorbas M, Scollay R, Saunders DJ, Ardavin CF, Wu L, Shortman K. The surface phenotype of dendritic cells purified from mouse thymus and spleen: Investigation of the CD8 expression by a subpopulation of dendritic cells. J Exp Med 1992; 176:47–58.
87. Inaba K, Pack M, Inaba M, Sakuta H, Isdell F, Steinman RM. High levels of a major histocompatibility complex II-self peptide complex on dendritic cells from the T cell areas of lymph nodes. J Exp Med 1997; 186:665–672.
88. Salomon B, Cohen JL, Masurier C, Klatzmann D. Three populations of mouse lymph node dendritic cells with different origins and dynamics. J Immunol 1998; 160:708–717.
89. Kronin V, Winkel K, Suss G, Kelso A, Heath W, Kirberg J, von Boehmer H, Shortman K. A subclass of dendritic cells regulates the response of naive CD8 T cells by limiting their IL-2 production. J Immunol 1996; 157:3819–3827.
90. Suss G, Shortman K. A subclass of dendritic cells kills CD4 T cells via Fas/Fas-ligand-induced apoptosis. J Exp Med 1996; 183:1789–1796.
91. Vremec D, Pooley J, Hochrein H, Wu L, Shortman K. CD4 and CD8 expression by dendritic cell subtypes in mouse thymus and spleen. J Immunol 2000; 164:2978–2986.
92. Maldonado-Lopez R, De Smedt T, Michel P, Godfroid J, Pajak B, Heirman C, Thielemans K, Leo O, Urbain J, Moser M. CD8alpha+ and CD8alpha− subclasses

of dendritic cells direct the development of distinct T helper cells in vivo. J Exp Med 1999; 189:587–592.

93. Maldonado-Lopez R, De Smedt T, Pajak B, Heirman C, Thielemans K, Leo O, Urbain J, Maliszewski CR, Moser M. Role of CD8alpha+ and CD8alpha− dendritic cells in the induction of primary immune responses in vivo. J Leukoc Biol 1999; 66:242–246.
94. Pulendran B, Smith JL, Caspary G, Brasel K, Pettit D, Maraskovsky E, Maliszewski CR. Distinct dendritic cell subsets differentially regulate the class of immune response in vivo. Proc Natl Acad Sci USA 1999; 96:1036–1041.
95. Grouard G, Rissoan MC, Filgueira L, Durand I, Banchereau J, Liu YJ. The enigmatic plasmacytoid T cells develop into dendritic cells with interleukin (IL)-3 and CD40-ligand. J Exp Med 1997; 185:1101–1111.
96. Rissoan MC, Soumelis V, Kadowaki N, Grouard G, Briere F, de Waal Malefyt R, Liu YJ. Reciprocal control of T helper cell and dendritic cell differentiation. Science 1999; 283:1183–1186.
97. Kapsenberg ML, Hilkens CM, Wierenga EA, Kalinski P. The role of antigen-presenting cells in the regulation of allergen-specific T cell responses. Curr Opin Immunol 1998; 10:607–613.
98. Kalinski P, Hilkens CM, Wierenga EA, Kapsenberg ML. T-cell priming by type-1 and type-2 polarized dendritic cells: The concept of a third signal. Immunol Today 1999; 20:561–567.
99. O'Garra A. Cytokines induce the development of functionally heterogeneous T helper cell subsets. Immunity 1998; 8:275–283.
100. Bochner BS, Undem BJ, Lichtenstein LM. Immunological aspects of allergic asthma. Annu Rev Immunol 1994; 12:295–335.
101. Stumbles PA, Thomas JA, Pimm CL, Lee PT, Venaille TJ, Proksch S, Holt PG. Resting respiratory tract dendritic cells preferentially stimulate T helper cell type 2 (Th2) responses and require obligatory cytokine signals for induction of Th1 immunity. J Exp Med 1998; 188:2019–2031.
102. Moser M, Murphy KM. Dendritic cell regulation of TH1-TH2 development. Nat Immunol 2000; 1:199–205.
103. Szabo SJ, Jacobson NG, Dighe AS, Gubler U, Murphy KM. Developmental commitment to the Th2 lineage by extinction of IL-12 signaling. Immunity 1995; 2: 665–675.
104. Szabo SJ, Dighe AS, Gubler U, Murphy KM. Regulation of the interleukin (IL)-12R beta 2 subunit expression in developing T helper 1 (Th1) and Th2 cells. J Exp Med 1997; 185:817–824.
105. Rogge L, Papi A, Presky DH, Biffi M, Minetti LJ, Miotto D, Agostini C, Semenzato G, Fabbri LM, Sinigaglia F. Antibodies to the IL-12 receptor beta 2 chain mark human Th1 but not Th2 cells in vitro and in vivo. J Immunol 1999; 162:3926–3932.
106. Schwartz RH. A cell culture model for T lymphocyte clonal anergy. Science 1990; 248:1349–1356.
107. Coyle AJ, Gutierrez-Ramos JC. The expanding B7 superfamily: Increasing complexity in costimulatory signals regulating T cell function. Nat Immunol 2001; 2: 203–209.

108. Jenkins MK, Taylor PS, Norton SD, Urdahl KB. CD28 delivers a costimulatory signal involved in antigen-specific IL-2 production by human T cells. J Immunol 1991; 147:2461–2466.
109. Harding FA, McArthur JG, Gross JA, Raulet DH, Allison JP. CD28-mediated signalling co-stimulates murine T cells and prevents induction of anergy in T-cell clones. Nature 1992; 356:607–609.
110. Walunas TL, Lenschow DJ, Bakker CY, Linsley PS, Freeman GJ, Green JM, Thompson CB, Bluestone JA. CTLA-4 can function as a negative regulator of T cell activation. Immunity 1994; 1:405–413.
111. Tivol EA, Borriello F, Schweitzer AN, Lynch WP, Bluestone JA, Sharpe AH. Loss of CTLA-4 leads to massive lymphoproliferation and fatal multiorgan tissue destruction, revealing a critical negative regulatory role of CTLA-4. Immunity 1995; 3:541–547.
112. Corry DB, Reiner SL, Linsley PS, Locksley RM. Differential effects of blockade of CD28-B7 on the development of Th1 or Th2 effector cells in experimental leishmaniasis. J Immunol 1994; 153:4142–4148.
113. Freeman GJ, Boussiotis VA, Anumanthan A, Bernstein GM, Ke XY, Rennert PD, Gray GS, Gribben JG, Nadler LM. B7-1 and B7-2 do not deliver identical costimulatory signals, since B7-2 but not B7-1 preferentially costimulates the initial production of IL-4. Immunity 1995; 2:523–532.
114. Kuchroo VK, Das MP, Brown JA, Ranger AM, Zamvil SS, Sobel RA, Weiner HL, Nabavi N, Glimcher LH. B7-1 and B7-2 costimulatory molecules activate differentially the Th1/Th2 developmental pathways: Application to autoimmune disease therapy. Cell 1995; 80:707–718.
115. Girvin AM, Dal Canto MC, Rhee L, Salomon B, Sharpe A, Bluestone JA, Miller SD. A critical role for B7/CD28 costimulation in experimental autoimmune encephalomyelitis: A comparative study using costimulatory molecule-deficient mice and monoclonal antibody blockade. J Immunol 2000; 164:136–143.
116. Thompson CB. Distinct roles for the costimulatory ligands B7-1 and B7-2 in T helper cell differentiation? Cell 1995; 81:979–982.
117. Hutloff A, Dittrich AM, Beier KC, Eljaschewitsch B, Kraft R, Anagnostopoulos I, Kroczek RA. ICOS is an inducible T-cell co-stimulator structurally and functionally related to CD28. Nature 1999; 397:263–266.
118. Yoshinaga SK, Whoriskey JS, Khare SD, Sarmiento U, Guo J, Horan T, Shih G, Zhang M, Coccia MA, Kohno T, Tafuri-Bladt A, Brankow D, Campbell P, Chang D, Chiu L, Dai T, Duncan G, Elliott GS, Hui A, McCabe SM, Scully S, Shahinian A, Shaklee CL, Van G, Mak TW, Senaldi G. T-cell co-stimulation through B7RP-1 and ICOS. Nature 1999; 402:827–832.
119. Coyle AJ, Lehar S, Lloyd C, Tian J, Delaney T, Manning S, Nguyen T, Burwell T, Schneider H, Gonzalo JA, Gosselin M, Owen LR, Rudd CE, Gutierrez-Ramos JC. The CD28-related molecule ICOS is required for effective T cell-dependent immune responses. Immunity 2000; 13:95–105.
120. McAdam AJ, Chang TT, Lumelsky AE, Greenfield EA, Boussiotis VA, Duke-Cohan JS, Chernova T, Malenkovich N, Jabs C, Kuchroo VK, Ling V, Collins M, Sharpe AH, Freeman GJ. Mouse inducible costimulatory molecule (ICOS) expres-

sion is enhanced by CD28 costimulation and regulates differentiation of CD4+ T cells. J Immunol 2000; 165:5035–5040.

121. Dong C, Juedes AE, Temann UA, Shresta S, Allison JP, Ruddle NH, Flavell RA. ICOS co-stimulatory receptor is essential for T-cell activation and function. Nature 2001; 409:97–101.
122. McAdam AJ, Greenwald RJ, Levin MA, Chernova T, Malenkovich N, Ling V, Freeman GJ, Sharpe AH. ICOS is critical for CD40-mediated antibody class switching. Nature 2001; 409:102–105.
123. Tafuri A, Shahinian A, Bladt F, Yoshinaga SK, Jordana M, Wakeham A, Boucher LM, Bouchard D, Chan VS, Duncan G, Odermatt B, Ho A, Itie A, Horan T, Whorisky JS, Pawson T, Penninger JM, Ohashi PS, Mak TW. ICOS is essential for effective T-helper-cell responses. Nature 2001; 409:105–109.
124. Ishida Y, Agata Y, Shibahara K, Honjo T. Induced expression of PD-1, a novel member of the immunoglobulin gene superfamily, upon programmed cell death. EMBO J 1992; 11:3887–3895.
125. Freeman GJ, Long AJ, Iwai Y, Bourque K, Chernova T, Nishimura H, Fitz LJ, Malenkovich N, Okazaki T, Byrne MC, Horton HF, Fouser L, Carter L, Ling V, Bowman MR, Carreno BM, Collins M, Wood CR, Honjo T. Engagement of the PD-1 immunoinhibitory receptor by a novel B7 family member leads to negative regulation of lymphocyte activation. J Exp Med 2000; 192:1027–1034.
126. Latchman Y, Wood CR, Chernova T, Chaudhary D, Borde M, Chernova I, Iwai Y, Long AJ, Brown JA, Nunes R, Greenfield EA, Bourque K, Boussiotis VA, Carter LL, Carreno BM, Malenkovich N, Nishimura H, Okazaki T, Honjo T, Sharpe AH, Freeman GJ. PD-L2 is a second ligand for PD-I and inhibits T cell activation. Nat Immunol 2001; 2:261–268.
127. Kaplan MH, Sun YL, Hoey T, Grusby MJ. Impaired IL-12 responses and enhanced development of Th2 cells in Stat4-deficient mice. Nature 1996; 382:174–177.
128. Jacobson NG, Szabo SJ, Weber-Nordt RM, Zhong Z, Schreiber RD, Darnell JE Jr, Murphy KM. Interleukin 12 signaling in T helper type 1 (Th1) cells involves tyrosine phosphorylation of signal transducer and activator of transcription (Stat)3 and Stat4. J Exp Med 1995; 181:1755–1762.
129. Parronchi P, De Carli M, Manetti R, Simonelli C, Sampognaro S, Piccinni MP, Macchia D, Maggi E, Del Prete G, Romagnani S. IL-4 and IFN (alpha and gamma) exert opposite regulatory effects on the development of cytolytic potential by Th1 or Th2 human T cell clones. J Immunol 1992; 149:2977–2983.
130. Wenner CA, Guler ML, Macatonia SE, O'Garra A, Murphy KM. Roles of IFN-gamma and IFN-alpha in IL-12-induced T helper cell-1 development. J Immunol 1996; 156:1442–1447.
131. Cho SS, Bacon CM, Sudarshan C, Rees RC, Finbloom D, Pine R, O'Shea JJ. Activation of STAT4 by IL-12 and IFN-alpha: Evidence for the involvement of ligand-induced tyrosine and serine phosphorylation. J Immunol 1996; 157:4781–4789.
132. Ouyang W, Jacobson NG, Bhattacharya D, Gorham JD, Fenoglio D, Sha WC, Murphy TL, Murphy KM. Thc Ets transcription factor ERM is Th1-specific and induced by IL-12 through a Stat4-dependent pathway. Proc Natl Acad Sci USA 1999; 96: 3888–3893.

133. Gourley T, Roys S, Lukacs NW, Kunkel SL, Flavell RA, Chang CH. A novel role for the major histocompatibility complex class I transactivator CIITA in the repression of IL-4 production. Immunity 1999; 10:377–386.
134. Sisk TJ, Gourley T, Roys S, Chang CH. MHC class II transactivator inhibits IL-4 gene transcription by competing with NF-AT to bind the coactivator CREB binding protein (CBP)/p300. J Immunol 2000; 165:2511–2517.
135. Szabo SJ, Kim ST, Costa GL, Zhang X, Fathman CG, Glimcher LH. A novel transcription factor, T-bet, directs Th1 lineage commitment. Cell 2000; 100:655–669.
136. Kaplan MH, Schindler U, Smiley ST, Grusby MJ. Stat6 is required for mediating responses to IL-4 and for development of Th2 cells. Immunity 1996; 4:313–319.
137. Takeda K, Tanaka T, Shi W, Matsumoto M, Minami M, Kashiwamura S, Nakanishi K, Yoshida N, Kishimoto T, Akira S. Essential role of Stat6 in IL-4 signalling. Nature 1996; 380:627–630.
138. Shimoda K, van Deursen J, Sangster MY, Sarawar SR, Carson RT, Tripp RA, Chu C, Quelle FW, Nosaka T, Vignali DA, Doherty PC, Grosveld G, Paul WE, Ihle JN. Lack of IL-4-induced Th2 response and IgE class switching in mice with disrupted Stat6 gene. Nature 1996; 380:630–633.
139. Huang H, Hu-Li J, Chen H, Ben-Sasson SZ, Paul WE. IL-4 and IL-13 production in differentiated T helper type 2 cells is not IL-4 dependent. J Immunol 1997; 159: 3731–3738.
140. Noben-Trauth N, Shultz LD, Brombacher F, Urban JF Jr, Gu H, Paul WE. An interleukin 4 (IL-4)-independent pathway for CD4+ T cell IL-4 production is revealed in IL-4 receptor-deficient mice. Proc Natl Acad Sci USA 1997; 94:10838–10843.
141. Dent AL, Hu-Li J, Paul WE, Staudt LM. T helper type 2 inflammatory disease in the absence of interleukin 4 and transcription factor STAT6. Proc Natl Acad Sci USA 1998; 95:13823–13828.
142. Kaplan MH, Wurster AL, Smiley ST, Grusby MJ. Stat6-dependent and-independent pathways for IL-4 production. J Immunol 1999; 163:6536–6540.
143. Jankovic D, Kullberg MC, Noben-Trauth N, Caspar P, Paul WE, Sher A. Single cell analysis reveals that IL-4 receptor/Stat6 signaling is not required for the in vivo or in vitro development of CD4+ lymphocytes with a Th2 cytokine profile. J Immunol 2000; 164:3047–3055.
144. Zheng W, Flavell RA. The transcription factor GATA-3 is necessary and sufficient for Th2 cytokine gene expression in CD4 T cells. Cell 1997; 89:587–596.
145. Ouyang W, Ranganath SH, Weindel K, Bhattacharya D, Murphy TL, Sha WC, Murphy KM. Inhibition of Th1 development mediated by GATA-3 through an IL-4-independent mechanism. Immunity 1998; 9:745–755.
146. Das J, Chen CH, Yang L, Cohn L, Ray P, Ray A. A critical role for NF-kappa B in GATA3 expression and TH2 differentiation in allergic airway inflammation. Nat Immunol 2001; 2:45–50.
147. Rodriguez-Palmero M, Hara T, Thumbs A, Hunig T. Triggering of T cell proliferation through CD28 induces GATA-3 and promotes T helper type 2 differentiation in vitro and in vivo. Eur J Immunol 1999; 29:3914–3924.
148. Ouyang W, Lohning M, Gao Z, Assenmacher M, Ranganath S, Radbruch A, Mur-

phy KM. Stat6-independent GATA-3 autoactivation directs IL-4-independent Th2 development and commitment. Immunity 2000; 12:27–37.
149. Ho IC, Hodge MR, Rooney JW, Glimcher LH. The proto-oncogene c-maf is responsible for tissue-specific expression of interleukin-4. Cell 1996; 85:973–983.
150. Ho IC, Lo D, Glimcher LH. c-maf promotes T helper cell type 2 (Th2) and attenuates Th1 differentiation by both interleukin 4-dependent and -independent mechanisms. J Exp Med 1998; 188:1859–1866.
151. Kim JI, Ho IC, Grusby MJ, Glimcher LH. The transcription factor c-Maf controls the production of interleukin-4 but not other Th2 cytokines. Immunity 1999; 10: 745–751.
152. Sallusto F, Mackay CR, Lanzavecchia A. Selective expression of the eotaxin receptor CCR3 by human T helper 2 cells. Science 1997; 277:2005–2007.
153. Bonecchi R, Bianchi G, Bordignon PP, D'Ambrosio D, Lang R, Borsatti A, Sozzani S, Allavena P, Gray PA, Mantovani A, Sinigaglia F. Differential expression of chemokine receptors and chemotactic responsiveness of type 1 T helper cells (Th1s) and Th2s. J Exp Med 1998; 187:129–134.
154. Zingoni A, Soto H, Hedrick JA, Stoppacciaro A, Storlazzi CT, Sinigaglia F, D'Ambrosio D, O'Garra A, Robinson D, Rocchi M, Santoni A, Zlotnik A, Napolitano M. The chemokine receptor CCR8 is preferentially expressed in Th2 but not Th1 cells. J Immunol 1998; 161:547–551.
155. Gonzalo JA, Pan Y, Lloyd CM, Jia GQ, Yu G, Dussault B, Powers CA, Proudfoot AE, Coyle AJ, Gearing D, Gutierrez-Ramos JC. Mouse monocyte-derived chemokine is involved in airway hyperreactivity and lung inflammation. J Immunol 1999; 163:403–411.
156. Lloyd CM, Delaney T, Nguyen T, Tian J, Martinez-A C, Coyle AJ, Gutierrez-Ramos JC. CC chemokine receptor (CCR)3/eotaxin is followed by CCR4/monocyte-derived chemokine in mediating pulmonary T helper lymphocyte type 2 recruitment after serial antigen challenge in vivo. J Exp Med 2000; 191:265–274.
157. Randolph DA, Stephens R, Carruthers CJ, Chaplin DD. Cooperation between Th1 and Th2 cells in a murine model of eosinophilic airway inflammation. J Clin Invest 1999; 104:1021–1029.
158. Randolph DA, Carruthers CJ, Szabo SJ, Murphy KM, Chaplin DD. Modulation of airway inflammation by passive transfer of allergen-specific Th1 and Th2 cells in a mouse model of asthma. J Immunol 1999; 162:2375–2383.
159. Iellem A, Colantonio L, Bhakta S, Sozzani S, Mantovani A, Sinigaglia F, D'Ambrosio D. Inhibition by IL-12 and IFN-alpha of I-309 and macrophage-derived chemokine production upon TCR triggering of human Th1 cells. Eur J Immunol 2000; 30:1030–1039.
160. Suri-Payer E, Amar AZ, Thornton AM, Shevach EM. CD4+CD25+ T cells inhibit both the induction and effector function of autoreactive T cells and represent a unique lineage of immunoregulatory cells. J Immunol 1998; 160:1212–1218.
161. Thornton AM, Shevach EM. Suppressor effector function of CD4+CD25+ immunoregulatory T cells is antigen nonspecific. J Immunol 2000; 164:183–190.
162. Cederbom L, Hall H, Ivars F. CD4+CD25+ regulatory T cells down-regulate costimulatory molecules on antigen-presenting cells. Eur J Immunol 2000; 30:1538–1543.

163. Kuniyasu Y, Takahashi T, Itoh M, Shimizu J, Toda G, Sakaguchi S. Naturally anergic and suppressive CD25+CD4+ T cells as a functionally and phenotypically distinct immunoregulatory T cell subpopulation. Int Immunol 2000; 12:1145–1155.
164. Yamagiwa S, Gray JD, Hashimoto S, Horwitz DA. A role for TGF-beta in the generation and expansion of CD4+CD25+ regulatory T cells from human peripheral blood. J Immunol 2001; 166:7282–7289.
165. Groux H, O'Garra A, Bigler M, Rouleau M, Antonenko S, de Vries JE, Roncarolo MG. A CD4+ T-cell subset inhibits antigen-specific T-cell responses and prevents colitis. Nature 1997; 389:737–742.
166. Cottrez F, Hurst SD, Coffman RL, Groux H. T regulatory cells 1 inhibit a Th2-specific response in vivo. J Immunol 2000; 165:4848–4853.
167. Vendetti S, Chai JG, Dyson J, Simpson E, Lombardi G, Lechler R. Anergic T cells inhibit the antigen-presenting function of dendritic cells. J Immunol 2000; 165: 1175–1181.
168. Barnes PJ, Pedersen S, Busse WW. Efficacy and safety of inhaled corticosteroids. New developments. Am J Respir Crit Care Med 1998; 157(3 pt 2):S1–S53.
169. Robinson D, Hamid Q, Ying S, Bentley A, Assoufi B, Durham S, Kay AB. Prednisolone treatment in asthma is associated with modulation of bronchoalveolar lavage cell interleukin-4, interleukin-5, and interferon-gamma cytokine gene expression. Am Rev Respir Dis 1993; 148:401–406.
170. Barnes PJ. Anti-inflammatory actions of glucocorticoids: Molecular mechanisms. Clin Sci (Lond) 1998; 94:557–572.
171. Vayssiere BM, Dupont S, Choquart A, Petit F, Garcia T, Marchandeau C, Gronemeyer H, Resche-Rigon M. Synthetic glucocorticoids that dissociate transactivation and AP-1 transrepression exhibit antiinflammatory activity in vivo. Mol Endocrinol 1997; 11:1245–1255.
172. Carmichael J, Paterson IC, Diaz P, Crompton GK, Kay AB, Grant IW. Corticosteroid resistance in chronic asthma. Br Med J 1981; 282:1419–1422.
173. Alvarez J, Surs W, Leung DY, Ikle D, Gelfand EW, Szefler SJ. Steroid-resistant asthma: Immunologic and pharmacologic features. J Allergy Clin Immunol 1992; 89:714–721.
174. Alexander AG, Barnes NC, Kay AB. Trial of cyclosporin in corticosteroid-dependent chronic severe asthma. Lancet 1992; 339:324–328.
175. Lock SH, Kay AB, Barnes NC. Double-blind, placebo-controlled study of cyclosporin A as a corticosteroid-sparing agent in corticosteroid-dependent asthma. Am J Respir Crit Care Med 1996; 153:509–514.
176. Sihra BS, Kon OM, Durham SR, Walker S, Barnes NC, Kay AB. Effect of cyclosporin A on the allergen-induced late asthmatic reaction. Thorax 1997; 52:447–452.
177. Khan LN, Kon OM, Macfarlane AJ, Meng Q, Ying S, Barnes NC, Kay AB. Attenuation of the allergen-induced late asthmatic reaction by cyclosporin A is associated with inhibition of bronchial eosinophils, interleukin-5, granulocyte macrophage colony-stimulating factor, and eotaxin. Am J Respir Crit Care Med 2000; 162(4 pt 1):1377–1382.
178. Kay AB. Immunosuppressive agents in chronic severe asthma. Allergy Proc 1994; 15:147–150.

179. Nizankowska E, Soja J, Pinis G, Bochenek G, Sladek K, Domagala B, Pajak A, Szczeklik A. Treatment of steroid-dependent bronchial asthma with cyclosporin. Eur Respir J 1995; 8:1091–1099.
180. Rohatagi S, Calic F, Harding N, Ozoux ML, Bouriot JP, Kirkesseli S, DeLeij L, Jensen BK. Pharmacokinetics, pharmacodynamics, and safety of inhaled cyclosporin A (ADI628) after single and repeated administration in healthy male and female subjects and asthmatic patients. J Clin Pharmacol 2000; 40:1211–1226.
181. Mizoguchi M, Kawaguchi K, Ohsuga Y, Ikari Y, Yanagawa A, Mizushima Y. Cyclosporin ointment for psoriasis and atopic dermatitis. Lancet 1992; 339:1120.
182. Nakagawa H, Etoh T, Ishibashi Y, Higaki Y, Kawashima M, Torii H, Harada S. Tacrolimus ointment for atopic dermatitis. Lancet 1994; 344:883.
183. Bieber T. Topical tacrolimus (FK 506): A new milestone in the management of atopic dermatitis. J Allergy Clin Immunol 1998; 102(4 pt 1):555–557.
184. Bottari V, Frezzolini A, Ruffelli M, Puddu P, Fontana L, De Pita O. Cyclosporin A (CyA) reduces sCD30 serum levels in atopic dermatitis: A possible new immune intervention. Allergy 1999; 54:507–510.
185. Schreiber SL, Crabtree GR. The mechanism of action of cyclosporin A and FK506, Immunol Today 1992; 13:136–142.
186. Mori A, Kaminuma O, Ogawa K, Nakata A, Egan RW, Akiyama K, Okudaira H. Control of IL-5 production by human helper T cells as a treatment for eosinophilic inflammation: Comparison of in vitro and in vivo effects between selective and nonselective cytokine synthesis inhibitors. J Allergy Clin Immunol 2000; 106(1 pt 2):S58–S64.
187. Herzog C, Walker C, Pichler W, Aeschlimann A, Wassmer P, Stockinger H, Knapp W, Rieber P, Muller W. Monoclonal anti-CD4 in arthritis. Lancet 1987; 2:1461–1462.
188. Hafler DA, Ritz J, Schlossman SF, Weiner HL. Anti-CD4 and anti-CD2 monoclonal antibody infusions in subjects with multiple sclerosis. Immunosuppressive effects and human anti-mouse responses. J Immunol 1988; 141:131–138.
189. Morel P, Vincent C, Cordier G, Panaye G, Carosella E, Revillard JP. Anti-CD4 monoclonal antibody administration in renal transplanted patients. Clin Immunol Immunopathol 1990; 56:311–322.
190. Reinke P, Volk HD, Miller H, Neuhaus K, Fietze E, Herberger J, Herberger D, von Baehr R, Emmrich F. Anti-CD4 therapy of acute rejection in long-term renal allograft recipients. Lancet 1991; 338:702–703.
191. Newman R, Alberts J, Anderson D, Carner K, Heard C, Norton F, Raab R, Reff M, Shuey S, Hanna N. ''Primatization'' of recombinant antibodies for immunotherapy of human diseases: A macaque/human chimeric antibody against human CD4. Biotechnology 1992; 10:1455–1460.
192. Kon OM, Sihra BS, Compton CH, Leonard TB, Kay AB, Barnes NC. Randomised, dose-ranging, placebo-controlled study of chimeric antibody to CD4 (keliximab) in chronic severe asthma. Lancet 1998; 352:1109–1113.
193. Newman R, Hariharan K, Reff M, Anderson DR, Braslawsky G, Santoro D, Hanna N, Bugelski PJ, Brigham-Burke M, Crysler C, Gagnon RC, Dal Monte P, Doyle ML, Hensley PC, Reddy MP, Sweet RW, Truneh A. Modification of the Fc region of a primatized IgG antibody to human CD4 retains its ability to modulate CD4

receptors but does not deplete CD4(+) T cells in chimpanzees. Clin Immunol 2001; 98:164–174.

194. Lohning M, Stroehmann A, Coyle AJ, Grogan JL, Lin S, Gutierrez-Ramos JC, Levinson D, Radbruch A, Kamradt T. T1/ST2 is preferentially expressed on murine Th2 cells, independent of interleukin 4, interleukin 5, and interleukin 10, and important for Th2 effector function. Proc Natl Acad Sci USA 1998; 95:6930–6935.
195. Xu D, Chan WL, Leung BP, Huang Fp, Wheeler R, Piedrafita D, Robinson JH, Liew FY. Selective expression of a stable cell surface molecule on type 2 but not type 1 helper T cells. J Exp Med 1998; 187:787–794.
196. Klemenz R, Hoffmann S, Werenskiold AK. Serum- and oncoprotein-mediated induction of a gene with sequence similarity to the gene encoding carcinoembryonic antigen. Proc Natl Acad Sci USA 1989; 86:5708–5712.
197. Tominaga S. A putative protein of a growth specific cDNA from BALB/c-3T3 cells is highly similar to the extracellular portion of mouse interleukin 1 receptor. FEBS Lett 1989; 258:301–304.
198. Tominaga S, Jenkins NA, Gilbert DJ, Copeland NG, Tetsuka T. Molecular cloning of the murine ST2 gene. Characterization and chromosomal mapping. Biochim Biophys Acta 1991; 1090:1–8.
199. Yanagisawa K, Takagi T, Tsukamoto T, Tetsuka T, Tominaga S. Presence of a novel primary response gene ST2L, encoding a product highly similar to the interleukin 1 receptor type 1. FEBS Lett 1993; 318:83–87.
200. Kumar S, Minnich MD, Young PR. ST2/T1 protein functionally binds to two secreted proteins from Balb/c 3T3 and human umbilical vein endothelial cells but does not bind interleukin 1. J Biol Chem 1995; 270:27905–27913.
201. Coyle AJ, Lloyd C, Tian J, Nguyen T, Erikkson C, Wang L, Ottoson P, Persson P, Delaney T, Lehar S, Lin S, Poisson L, Meisel C, Kamradt T, Bjerke T, Levinson D, Gutierrez-Ramos JC. Crucial role of the interleukin 1 receptor family member T1/ST2 in T helper cell type 2-mediated lung mucosal immune responses. J Exp Med 1999; 190:895–902.
202. Hoshino K, Kashiwamura S, Kuribayashi K, Kodama T, Tsujimura T, Nakanishi K, Matsuyama T, Takeda K, Akira S. The absence of interleukin 1 receptor-related T1/ST2 does not affect T helper cell type 2 development and its effector function. J Exp Med 1999; 190:1541–1548.
203. Senn KA, McCoy KD, Maloy KJ, Stark G, Frohli E, Rulicke T, Klemenz R. T1-deficient and T1-Fc-transgenic mice develop a normal protective Th2-type immune response following infection with Nippostrongylus brasiliensis. Eur J Immunol 2000; 30:1929–1938.
204. Meisel C, Bonhagen K, Lohning M, Coyle AJ, Gutierrez-Ramos JC, Radbruch A, Kamradt T. Regulation and function of T1/ST2 expression on CD4+ T cells: Induction of type 2 cytokine production by T1/ST2 cross-linking. J Immunol 2001; 166:3143–3150.
205. Springer TA. Traffic signals for lymphocyte recirculation and leukocyte emigration: The multistep paradigm. Cell 1994; 76:301–314.
206. Moser B, Loetscher P. Lymphocyte traffic control by chemokines. Nat Immunol 2001; 2:123–128.

207. Butcher EC. Leukocyte-endothelial cell recognition: Three (or more) steps to specificity and diversity. Cell 1991; 67:1033–1036.
208. Bevilacqua MP. Endothelial-leukocyte adhesion molecules. Annu Rev Immunol 1993; 11:767–804.
209. Schleimer RP, Sterbinsky SA, Kaiser J, Bickel CA, Klunk DA, Tomioka K, Newman W, Luscinskas FW, Gimbrone MA Jr, McIntyre BW, Bochner BS. IL-4 induces adherence of human eosinophils and basophils but not neutrophils to endothelium. Association with expression of VCAM-1. J Immunol 1992; 148:1086–1092.
210. Bochner BS, Klunk DA, Sterbinsky SA, Coffman RL, Schleimer RP. IL-13 selectively induces vascular cell adhesion molecule-1 expression in human endothelial cells. J Immunol 1995; 154:799–803.
211. Abraham WM, Sielczak MW, Ahmed A, Cortes A, Lauredo IT, Kim J, Pepinsky B, Benjamin CD, Leone DR, Lobb RR, Weller PF. Alpha 4-integrins mediate antigen-induced late bronchial responses and prolonged airway hyperresponsiveness in sheep. J Clin Invest 1994; 93:776–787.
212. Pretolani M, Ruffie C, Lapa e Silva JR, Joseph D, Lobb RR, Vargaftig BB. Antibody to very late activation antigen 4 prevents antigen-induced bronchial hyperreactivity and cellular infiltration in the guinea pig airways. J Exp Med 1994; 180: 795–805.
213. Henderson WR Jr, Chi EY, Albert RK, Chu SJ, Lamm WJ, Rochon Y, Jonas M, Christie PE, Harlan JM. Blockade of CD49d (alpha4 integrin) on intrapulmonary but not circulating leukocytes inhibits airway inflammation and hyperresponsiveness in a mouse model of asthma. J Clin Invest 1997; 100:3083–3092.
214. Kanehiro A, Takeda K, Joetham A, Tomkinson A, Ikemura T, Irvin CG, Gelfand EW. Timing of administration of anti- VLA-4 differentiates airway hyperresponsiveness in the central and peripheral airways in mice. Am J Respir Crit Care Med 2000; 162:1132–1139.
215. Abraham WM, Ahmed A, Sielczak MW, Narita M, Arrhenius T, Elices MJ. Blockade of late-phase airway responses and airway hyperresponsiveness in allergic sheep with a small-molecule peptide inhibitor of VLA-4. Am J Respir Crit Care Med 1997; 156:696–703.
216. Abraham WM, Gill A, Ahmed A, Sielczak MW, Lauredo IT, Botinnikova Y, Lin KC, Pepinsky B, Leone DR, Lobb RR, Adams SP. A small-molecule, tight-binding inhibitor of the integrin alpha(4)beta(1) blocks antigen-induced airway responses and inflammation in experimental asthma in sheep. Am J Respir Crit Care Med 2000; 162:603–611.
217. Salomon B, Bluestone JA. LFA-1 interaction with ICAM-1 and ICAM-2 regulates Th2 cytokine production. J Immunol 1998; 161:5138–5142.
218. Baggiolini M. Chemokines and leukocyte traffic. Nature 1998; 392:565–568.
219. Sallusto F, Lanzavecchia A, Mackay CR. Chemokines and chemokine receptors in T-cell priming and Th1/Th2-mediated responses. Immunol Today 1998; 19:568–574.
220. Lukacs NW, Strieter RM, Warmington K, Lincoln P, Chensue SW, Kunkel SL. Differential recruitment of leukocyte populations and alteration of airway hyper-

reactivity by C-C family chemokines in allergic airway inflammation. J Immunol 1997; 158:4398–4404.

221. Rothenberg ME, MacLean JA, Pearlman E, Luster AD, Leder P. Targeted disruption of the chemokine eotaxin partially reduces antigen-induced tissue eosinophilia. J Exp Med 1997; 185:785–970.
222. Ying S, Robinson DS, Meng Q, Rottman J, Kennedy R, Ringler DJ, Mackay CR, Daugherty BL, Springer MS, Durham SR, Williams TJ, Kay AB. Enhanced expression of eotaxin and CCR3 mRNA and protein in atopic asthma. Association with airway hyperresponsiveness and predominant co-localization of eotaxin mRNA to bronchial epithelial and endothelial cells. Eur J Immunol 1997; 27:3507–3516.
223. Campbell EM, Kunkel SL, Strieter RM, Lukacs NW. Temporal role of chemokines in a murine model of cockroach allergen-induced airway hyperreactivity and eosinophilia. J Immunol 1998; 161:7047–7053.
224. Gonzalo JA, Lloyd CM, Wen D, Albar JP, Wells TN, Proudfoot A, Martinez-A C, Dorf M, Bjerke T, Coyle AJ, Gutierrez-Ramos JC. The coordinated action of CC chemokines in the lung orchestrates allergic inflammation and airway hyperresponsiveness. J Exp Med 1998; 188:157–167.
225. Conti P, DiGioacchino M. MCP-1 and RANTES are mediators of acute and chronic inflammation. Allergy Asthma Proc 2001; 22:133–137.
226. Kawasaki S, Takizawa H, Yoneyama H, Nakayama T, Fujisawa R, Izumizaki M, Imai T, Yoshie O, Homma I, Yamamoto K, Matsushima K. Intervention of thymus and activation-regulated chemokine attenuates the development of allergic airway inflammation and hyperresponsiveness in mice. J Immunol 2001; 166:2055–2062.
227. Borish L. IL-10: Evolving concepts. J Allergy Clin Immunol 1998; 101:293–297.
228. Bonfield TL, Konstan MW, Burfeind P, Panuska JR, Hilliard JB, Berger M. Normal bronchial epithelial cells constitutively produce the anti-inflammatory cytokine interleukin-10, which is downregulated in cystic fibrosis. Am J Respir Cell Mol Biol 1995; 13:257–261.
229. Flores Villanueva PO, Reiser H, Stadecker MJ. Regulation of T helper cell responses in experimental murine schistosomiasis by IL-10. Effect on expression of B7 and B7-2 costimulatory molecules by macrophages. J Immunol 1994; 153: 5190–5199.
230. Buelens C, Willems F, Delvaux A, Pierard G, Delville JP, Velu T, Goldman M. Interleukin-10 differentially regulates B7-1 (CD80) and B7-2 (CD86) expression on human peripheral blood dendritic cells. Eur J Immunol 1995; 25:2668–2672.
231. Akdis CA, Joss A, Akdis M, Blaser K. Mechanism of IL-10-induced T cell inactivation in allergic inflammation and normal response to allergens. Int Arch Allergy Immunol 2001; 124:180–182.
232. Pretolani M, Goldman M. IL-10: A potential therapy for allergic inflammation? Immunol Today 1997; 18:277–280.
233. John M, Lim S, Seybold J, Jose P, Robichaud A, O'Connor B, Barnes PJ, Chung KF. Inhaled corticosteroids increase interleukin-10 but reduce macrophage inflammatory protein-1 alpha, granulocyte-macrophage colony-stimulating factor, and interferon-gamma release from alveolar macrophages in asthma. Am J Respir Crit Care Med 1998; 157:256–262.
234. van Deventer SJ, Elson CO, Fedorak RN. Multiple doses of intravenous interleukin

10 in steroid-refractory Crohn's disease. Crohn's Disease Study Group. Gastroenterology 1997; 113:383–389.
235. Asadullah K, Docke WD, Ebeling M, Friedrich M, Belbe G, Audring H, Volk HD, Sterry W. Interleukin 10 treatment of psoriasis: Clinical results of a phase 2 trial. Arch Dermatol 1999; 135:187–192.
236. Makela MJ, Kanehiro A, Borish L, Dakhama A, Loader J, Joetham A, Xing Z, Jordana M, Larsen GL, Gelfand EW. IL-10 is necessary for the expression of airway hyperresponsiveness but not pulmonary inflammation after allergic sensitization. Proc Natl Acad Sci USA 2000; 97:6007–6012.
237. van Scott MR, Justice JP, Bradfield JF, Enright E, Sigounas A, Sur S. IL-10 reduces Th2 cytokine production and eosinophilia but augments airway reactivity in allergic mice. Am J Physiol Lung Cell Mol Physiol 2000; 278:L667–L674.
238. Lamont AG, Adorini L. IL-12: A key cytokine in immune regulation. Immunol Today 1996; 17:214–217.
239. Gately MK, Renzetti LM, Magram J, Stern AS, Adorini L, Gubler U, Presky DH. The interleukin-12/interleukin-12-receptor system: Role in normal and pathologic immune responses. Annu Rev Immunol 1998; 16:495–521.
240. McDyer JF, Wu CY, Seder RA. The regulation of IL-12: Its role in infectious, autoimmune, and allergic diseases. J Allergy Clin Immunol 1998; 102:11–15.
241. Wills-Karp M. Interleukin-12 as a target for modulation of the inflammatory response in asthma. Allergy 1998; 53:113–119.
242. van der Pouw Kraan TC, Boeije LC, de Groot ER, Stapel SO, Snijders A, Kapsenberg ML, van der Zee JS, Aarden LA. Reduced production of IL-12 and IL-12-dependent IFN-gamma release in patients with allergic asthma. J Immunol 1997; 158:5560–5565.
243. Naseer T, Minshall EM, Leung DY, Laberge S, Ernst P, Martin RJ, Hamid Q. Expression of IL-12 and IL-13 mRNA in asthma and their modulation in response to steroid therapy. Am J Respir Crit Care Med 1997; 155:845–851.
244. Iwamoto I, Kumano K, Kasai M, Kurasawa K, Nakao A. Interleukin-12 prevents antigen-induced eosinophil recruitment into mouse airways. Am J Respir Crit Care Med 1996; 154:1257–1260.
245. Kips JC, Brusselle GJ, Joos GF, Peleman RA, Tavernier JH, Devos RR, Pauwels RA. Interleukin-12 inhibits antigen-induced airway hyperresponsiveness in mice. Am J Respir Crit Care Med 1996; 153:535–539.
246. Sur S, Lam J, Bouchard P, Sigounas A, Holbert D, Metzger WJ. Immunomodulatory effects of IL-12 on allergic lung inflammation depend on timing of doses. J Immunol 1996; 157:4173–4180.
247. Schwarze J, Hamelmann E, Cieslewicz G, Tomkinson A, Joetham A, Bradley K, Gelfand EW. Local treatment with IL-12 is an effective inhibitor of airway hyperresponsiveness and lung eosinophilia after airway challenge in sensitized mice. J Allergy Clin Immunol 1998; 102:86–93.
248. Rogge L, Barberis-Maino L, Biffi M, Passini N, Presky DH, Gubler U, Sinigaglia F. Selective expression of an interleukin-12 rcccptor component by human T helper 1 cells. J Exp Med 1997; 185:825–831.
249. Varga EM, Wachholz P, Nouri-Aria KT, Verhoef A, Corrigan CJ, Till SJ, Durham SR. T cells from human allergen-induced late asthmatic responses express IL-12

receptor beta 2 subunit mRNA and respond to IL-12 in vitro. J Immunol 2000; 165:2877–2885.
250. Bryan SA, O'Connor BJ, Matti S, Leckie MJ, Kanabar V, Khan J, Warrington SJ, Renzetti L, Rames A, Bock JA, Boyce MJ, Hansel TT, Holgate ST, Barnes PJ. Effects of recombinant human interleukin-12 on eosinophils, airway hyper-responsiveness, and the late asthmatic response. Lancet 2000; 356:2149–2153.
251. Okamura H, Tsutsi H, Komatsu T, Yutsudo M, Hakura A, Tanimoto T, Torigoe K, Okura T, Nukada Y, Hattori K, Akita K, Namba M, Tanabe F, Konishi K, Fukuda S, Kurimoto M. Cloning of a new cytokine that induces IFN-gamma production by T cells. Nature 1995; 378:88–91.
252. Yoshimoto T, Okamura H, Tagawa YI, Iwakura Y, Nakanishi K. Interleukin 18 together with interleukin 12 inhibits IgE production by induction of interferon-gamma production from activated B cells. Proc Natl Acad Sci USA 1997; 94:3948–3953.
253. Xu D, Trajkovic V, Hunter D, Leung BP, Schulz K, Gracie JA, McInnes IB, Liew FY. IL-18 induces the differentiation of Th1 or Th2 cells depending upon cytokine milieu and genetic background. Eur J Immunol 2000; 30:3147–3156.
254. Hofstra CL, Van Ark I, Hofman G, Kool M, Nijkamp FP, Van Oosterhout AJ. Prevention of Th2-like cell responses by coadministration of IL-12 and IL-18 is associated with inhibition of antigen-induced airway hyperresponsiveness, eosinophilia, and serum IgE levels. J Immunol 1998; 161:5054–5060.
255. Walter DM, Wong CP, DeKruyff RH, Berry GJ, Levy S, Umetsu DT. IL-18 gene transfer by adenovirus prevents the development of and reverses established allergen-induced airway hyperreactivity. J Immunol 2001; 166:6392–6398.
256. Hansen G, Yeung VP, Berry G, Umetsu DT, DeKruyff RH. Vaccination with heat-killed Listeria as adjuvant reverses established allergen-induced airway hyperreactivity and inflammation: Role of CD8+ T cells and IL-18. J Immunol 2000; 164: 223–230.
257. Maecker HT, Hansen G, Walter DM, DeKruyff RH, Levy S, Umetsu DT. Vaccination with allergen-IL-18 fusion DNA protects against, and reverses established, airway hyperreactivity in a murine asthma model. J Immunol 2001; 166:959–965.
258. Erb KJ. Atopic disorders: A default pathway in the absence of infection? Immunol Today 1999; 20:317–322.
259. Shirakawa T, Enomoto T, Shimazu S, Hopkin JM. The inverse association between tuberculin responses and atopic disorder. Science 1997; 275:77–79.
260. Strannegard IL, Larsson LO, Wennergren G, Strannegard O. Prevalence of allergy in children in relation to prior BCG vaccination and infection with atypical mycobacteria. Allergy 1998; 53:249–254.
261. Omenaas E, Jentoft HF, Vollmer WM, Buist AS, Gulsvik A. Absence of relationship between tuberculin reactivity and atopy in BCG vaccinated young adults. Thorax 2000; 55:454–458.
262. Suzuki N, Kudo K, Sano Y, Ito K. Can Mycobacterium tuberculosis infection prevent asthma and other allergic disorders? Int Arch Allergy Immunol 2001; 124: 113–116.
263. Erb KJ, Holloway JW, Sobeck A, Moll H, Le Gros G. Infection of mice with Myco-

bacterium bovis-Bacillus Calmette-Guerin (BCG) suppresses allergen-induced airway eosinophilia. J Exp Med 1998; 187:561–569.

264. Herz U, Gerhold K, Gruber C, Braun A, Wahn U, Renz H, Paul K. BCG infection suppresses allergic sensitization and development of increased airway reactivity in an animal model. J Allergy Clin Immunol 1998; 102:867–874.

265. Wang CC, Rook GA. Inhibition of an established allergic response to ovalbumin in BALB/c mice by killed Mycobacterium vaccae. Immunology 1998; 93:307–313.

266. Lehrer A, Bressanelli A, Wachsmann V, Bottasso O, Bay ML, Singh M, Stanford C, Stanford J. Immunotherapy with Mycobacterium vaccae in the treatment of psoriasis. FEMS Immunol Med Microbiol 1998; 21:71–77.

267. Balagon MV, Walsh DS, Tan PL, Cellona RV, Abalos RM, Tan EV, Fajardo TT, Watson JD, Walsh GP. Improvement in psoriasis after intradermal administration of heat-killed Mycobacterium vaccae. Int J Dermatol 2000; 39:51–58.

268. Shirtcliffe PM, Easthope SE, Cheng S, Weatherall M, Tan PL, Le Gros G, Beasley R. The effect of delipidated deglycolipidated (DDMV) and heat-killed Mycobacterium vaccae in asthma. Am J Respir Crit Care Med 2001; 163:1410–1414.

269. Krieg AM, Yi AK, Matson S, Waldschmidt TJ, Bishop GA, Teasdale R, Koretzky GA, Klinman DM. CpG motifs in bacterial DNA trigger direct B-cell activation. Nature 1995; 374:546–549.

270. Klinman DM, Yi AK, Beaucage SL, Conover J, Krieg AM. CpG motifs present in bacteria DNA rapidly induce lymphocytes to secrete interleukin 6, interleukin 12, and interferon gamma. Proc Natl Acad Sci USA 1996; 93:2879–2883.

271. Jakob T, Walker PS, Krieg AM, Udey MC, Vogel JC. Activation of cutaneous dendritic cells by CpG-containing oligodeoxynucleotides: A role for dendritic cells in the augmentation of Th1 responses by immunostimulatory DNA. J Immunol 1998; 161:3042–3049.

272. Sparwasser T, Koch ES, Vabulas RM, Heeg K, Lipford GB, Ellwart JW, Wagner H. Bacterial DNA and immunostimulatory CpG oligonucleotides trigger maturation and activation of murine dendritic cells. Eur J Immunol 1998; 28:2045–2054.

273. Chace JH, Hooker NA, Mildenstein KL, Krieg AM, Cowdery JS. Bacterial DNA-induced NK cell IFN-gamma production is dependent on macrophage secretion of IL-12. Clin Immunol Immunopathol 1997; 84:185–193.

274. Broide D, Schwarze J, Tighe H, Gifford T, Nguyen MD, Malek S, Van Uden J, Martin-Orozco E, Gelfand EW, Raz E. Immunostimulatory DNA sequences inhibit IL-5, eosinophilic inflammation, and airway hyperresponsiveness in mice. J Immunol 1998; 161:7054–7062.

275. Kline JN, Waldschmidt TJ, Businga TR, Lemish JE, Weinstock JV, Thorne PS, Krieg AM. Modulation of airway inflammation by CpG oligodeoxynucleotides in a murine model of asthma. J Immunol 1998; 160:2555–2559.

276. Sur S, Wild JS, Choudhury BK, Sur N, Alam R, Klinman DM. Long term prevention of allergic lung inflammation in a mouse model of asthma by CpG oligodeoxynucleotides. J Immunol 1999; 162:6284–6293.

277. Sato Y, Roman M, Tighe H, Lee D, Corr M, Nguyen MD, Silverman GJ, Lotz M, Carson DA, Raz E. Immunostimulatory DNA sequences necessary for effective intradermal gene immunization. Science 1996; 273:352–354.

278. Klinman DM, Yamshchikov G, Ishigatsubo Y. Contribution of CpG motifs to the immunogenicity of DNA vaccines. J Immunol 1997; 158:3635–3639.
279. Tighe H, Takabayashi K, Schwartz D, Van Nest G, Tuck S, Eiden JJ, Kagey-Sobotka A, Creticos PS, Lichtenstein LM, Spiegelberg HL, Raz E. Conjugation of immunostimulatory DNA to the short ragweed allergen amb a 1 enhances its immunogenicity and reduces its allergenicity. J Allergy Clin Immunol 2000; 106: 124–134.
280. Lipford GB, Sparwasser T. Hematopoietic remodeling triggered by CpG DNA. Curr Top Microbiol Immunol 2000; 247:119–129.
281. Noon L. Prophylactic inoculation against hay fever. Lancet 1911; I:1572–1573.
282. Takai T, Yokota T, Yasue M, Nishiyama C, Yuuki T, Mori A, Okudaira H, Okumura Y. Engineering of the major house dust mite allergen Der f 2 for allergen-specific immunotherapy. Nat Biotechnol 1997; 15:754–758.
283. Akdis CA, Blaser K. IL-10-induced anergy in peripheral T cell and reactivation by microenvironmental cytokines: Two key steps in specific immunotherapy. FASEB J 1999; 13:603–609.
284. De Magistris MT, Alexander J, Coggeshall M, Altman A, Gaeta FC, Grey HM, Sette A. Antigen analog-major histocompatibility complexes act as antagonists of the T cell receptor. Cell 1992; 68:625–634.
285. Sette A, Alexander J, Ruppert J, Snoke K, Franco A, Ishioka G, Grey HM. Antigen analogs/MHC complexes as specific T cell receptor antagonists. Annu Rev Immunol 1994; 12:413–431.
286. Page DM, Alexander J, Snoke K, Appella E, Sette A, Hedrick SM, Grey HM. Negative selection of CD4+ CD8+ thymocytes by T-cell receptor peptide antagonists. Proc Natl Acad Sci USA 1994; 91:4057–4061.
287. Robey E, Fowlkes BJ. Selective events in T cell development. Annu Rev Immunol 1994; 12:675–705.
288. Bertoletti A, Sette A, Chisari FV, Penna A, Levrero M, De Carli M, Fiaccadori F, Ferrari C. Natural variants of cytotoxic epitopes are T-cell receptor antagonists for antiviral cytotoxic T cells. Nature 1994; 369:407–410.
289. Klenerman P, Meier UC, Phillips RE, McMichael AJ. The effects of natural altered peptide ligands on the whole blood cytotoxic T lymphocyte response to human immunodeficiency virus. Eur J Immunol 1995; 25:1927–1931.
290. Jameson SC, Bevan MJ. T cell receptor antagonists and partial agonists. Immunity 1995; 2:1–11.
291. Kumar V, Bhardwaj V, Soares L, Alexander J, Sette A, Sercarz E. Major histocompatibility complex binding affinity of an antigenic determinant is crucial for the differential secretion of interleukin 4/5 or interferon gamma by T cells. Proc Natl Acad Sci USA 1995; 92:9510–9514.
292. Windhagen A, Scholz C, Hollsberg P, Fukaura H, Sette A, Hafler DA. Modulation of cytokine patterns of human autoreactive T cell clones by a single amino acid substitution of their peptide ligand. Immunity 1995; 2:373–380.
293. Ikagawa S, Matsushita S, Chen YZ, Ishikawa T, Nishimura Y. Single amino acid substitutions on a Japanese cedar pollen allergen (Cry j 1)-derived peptide induced alterations in human T cell responses and T cell receptor antagonism. J Allergy Clin Immunol 1996; 97:53–64.

294. De Palma R, Wu S, Sallusto F, Di Felice G, Martucci P, Geraci D, Colombo P, Troise C, Sacerdoti G, Nocera A, Gorski J. Use of antagonist peptides to inhibit in vitro T cell responses to Par j 1, the major allergen of Parietaria judaica pollen. J Immunol 1999; 162:1982–1987.
295. Krinzman SJ, De Sanctis GT, Cernadas M, Mark D, Wang Y, Listman J, Kobzik L, Donovan C, Nassr K, Katona I, Christiani DC, Perkins DL, Finn PW. Inhibition of T cell costimulation abrogates airway hyperresponsiveness in a murine model. J Clin Invest 1996; 98:2693–2699.
296. Van Oosterhout AJ, Hofstra CL, Shields R, Chan B, Van Ark I, Jardieu PM, Nijkamp FP. Murine CTLA4-IgG treatment inhibits airway eosinophilia and hyperresponsiveness and attenuates IgE upregulation in a murine model of allergic asthma. Am J Respir Cell Mol Biol 1997; 17:386–392.
297. Padrid PA, Mathur M, Li X, Herrmann K, Qin Y, Cattamanchi A, Weinstock J, Elliott D, Sperling AI, Bluestone JA. CTLA4Ig inhibits airway eosinophilia and hyperresponsiveness by regulating the development of Th1/Th2 subsets in a murine model of asthma. Am J Respir Cell Mol Biol 1998; 18:453–462.
298. Tsuyuki S, Tsuyuki J, Einsle K, Kopf M, Coyle AJ. Costimulation through B7-2 (CD86) is required for the induction of a lung mucosal T helper cell 2 (TH2) immune response and altered airway responsiveness. J Exp Med 1997; 185:1671–1679.
299. Gonzalo JA, Tian J, Delaney T, Corcoran J, Rottman JB, Lora J, Al-Garawi A, Kroczek R, Gutierrez-Ramos JC, Coyle AJ. ICOS is critical for T helper cell-mediated lung mucosal inflammatory responses. Nat Immunol 2001; 2:597–604.
300. Hsieh CS, Heimberger AB, Gold JS, O'Garra A, Murphy KM. Differential regulation of T helper phenotype development by interleukins 4 and 10 in an alpha beta T-cell-receptor transgenic system. Proc Natl Acad Sci USA 1992; 89:6065–6069.
301. Ohara J, Paul WE. Up-regulation of interleukin 4/B-cell stimulatory factor 1 receptor expression. Proc Natl Acad Sci USA 1988; 85:8221–8225.
302. Noelle R, Krammer PH, Ohara J, Uhr JW, Vitetta ES. Increased expression of Ia antigens on resting B cells: An additional role for B-cell growth factor. Proc Natl Acad Sci USA 1984; 81:6149–6153.
303. Defrance T, Aubry JP, Rousset F, Vanbervliet B, Bonnefoy JY, Arai N, Takebe Y, Yokota T, Lee F, Arai K, De Vries J, Banchereau J. Human recombinant interleukin 4 induces Fc epsilon receptors (CD23) on normal human B lymphocytes. J Exp Med 1987; 165:1459–1467.
304. Thornhill MH, Wellicome SM, Mahiouz DL, Lanchbury JS, Kyan-Aung U, Haskard DO. Tumor necrosis factor combines with IL-4 or IFN-gamma to selectively enhance endothelial cell adhesiveness for T cells. The contribution of vascular cell adhesion molecule-1-dependent and -independent binding mechanisms. J Immunol 1991; 146:592–598.
305. Bennett BL, Cruz R, Lacson RG, Manning AM. Interleukin-4 suppression of tumor necrosis factor alpha-stimulated E-selectin gene transcription is mediated by STAT6 antagonism of NF-kappaB. J Biol Chem 1997; 272:10212–10219.
306. Lukacs NW, Strieter RM, Chensue SW, Kunkel SL. Interleukin-4-dependent pulmonary eosinophil infiltration in a murine model of asthma. Am J Respir Cell Mol Biol 1994; 10:526–532.

307. Zhou CY, Crocker IC, Koenig G, Romero FA, Townley RG. Anti-interleukin-4 inhibits immunoglobulin E production in a murine model of atopic asthma. J Asthma 1997; 34:195–201.
308. Maliszewski CR, Sato TA, Vanden Bos T, Waugh S, Dower SK, Slack J, Beckmann MP, Grabstein KH. Cytokine receptors and B cell functions. I. Recombinant soluble receptors specifically inhibit IL-1- and IL-4-induced B cell activities in vitro. J Immunol 1990; 144:3028–3033.
309. Sato TA, Widmer MB, Finkelman FD, Madani H, Jacobs CA, Grabstein KH, Maliszewski CR. Recombinant soluble murine IL-4 receptor can inhibit or enhance IgE responses in vivo. J Immunol 1993; 150:2717–2723.
310. Renz H, Bradley K, Enssle K, Loader JE, Larsen GL, Gelfand EW. Prevention of the development of immediate hypersensitivity and airway hyperresponsiveness following in vivo treatment with soluble IL-4 receptor. Int Arch Allergy Immunol 1996; 109:167–176.
311. Henderson WR Jr, Chi EY, Maliszewski CR. Soluble IL-4 receptor inhibits airway inflammation following allergen challenge in a mouse model of asthma. J Immunol 2000; 164:1086–1095.
312. Borish LC, Nelson HS, Lanz MJ, Claussen L, Whitmore JB, Agosti JM, Garrison L. Interleukin-4 receptor in moderate atopic asthma. A phase I/II randomized, placebo-controlled trial. Am J Respir Crit Care Med 1999; 160:1816–1823.
313. Borish LC, Nelson HS, Corren J, Bensch G, Busse WW, Whitmore JB, Agosti JM. Efficacy of soluble IL-4 receptor for the treatment of adults with asthma. J Allergy Clin Immunol 2001; 107:963–970.
314. Urban JF Jr, Noben-Trauth N, Donaldson DD, Madden KB, Morris SC, Collins M, Finkelman FD. IL-13, IL-4Ralpha, and Stat6 are required for the expulsion of the gastrointestinal nematode parasite Nippostrongylus brasiliensis. Immunity 1998; 8:255–264.
315. McKenzie GJ, Emson CL, Bell SE, Anderson S, Fallon P, Zurawski G, Murray R, Grencis R, McKenzie AN. Impaired development of Th2 cells in IL-13-deficient mice. Immunity 1998; 9:423–432.
316. Donaldson DD, Whitters MJ, Fitz LJ, Neben TY, Finnerty H, Henderson SL, O'Hara RM Jr, Beier DR, Turner KJ, Wood CR, Collins M. The murine IL-13 receptor alpha 2: Molecular cloning, characterization, and comparison with murine IL-13 receptor alpha 1. J Immunol 1998; 161:2317–2324.
317. Chiaramonte MG, Schopf LR, Neben TY, Cheever AW, Donaldson DD, Wynn TA. IL-13 is a key regulatory cytokine for Th2 cell-mediated pulmonary granuloma formation and IgE responses induced by Schistosoma mansoni eggs. J Immunol 1999; 162:920–930.
318. Ryan JJ, McReynolds LJ, Keegan A, Wang LH, Garfein E, Rothman P, Nelms K, Paul WE. Growth and gene expression are predominantly controlled by distinct regions of the human IL-4 receptor. Immunity 1996; 4:123–132.
319. Reichel M, Nelson BH, Greenberg PD, Rothman PB. The IL-4 receptor alpha-chain cytoplasmic domain is sufficient for activation of JAK-1 and STAT6 and the induction of IL-4-specific gene expression. J Immunol 1997; 158:5860–5867.
320. Darnell JE Jr. STATs and gene regulation. Science 1997; 277:1630–1635.

321. Losman JA, Chen XP, Hilton D, Rothman P. Cutting edge: SOCS-1 is a potent inhibitor of IL-4 signal transduction. J Immunol 1999; 162:3770–3774.
322. Kopf M, Le Gros G, Bachmann M, Lamers MC, Bluethmann H, Kohler G. Disruption of the murine IL-4 gene blocks Th2 cytokine responses. Nature 1993; 362: 245–248.
323. Tomkinson A, Duez C, Cieslewicz G, Pratt JC, Joetham A, Shanafelt MC, Gundel R, Gelfand EW. A murine IL-4 receptor antagonist that inhibits IL-4- and IL-13-induced responses prevents antigen-induced airway eosinophilia and airway hyperresponsiveness. J Immunol 2001; 166:5792–5800.
324. Oshima Y, Puri RK. Characterization of a powerful high affinity antagonist that inhibits biological activities of human interleukin-13. J Biol Chem 2001; 276: 15185–15191.
325. Nakamura Y, Ghaffar O, Olivenstein R, Taha RA, Soussi-Gounni A, Zhang DH, Ray A, Hamid Q. Gene expression of the GATA-3 transcription factor is increased in atopic asthma. J Allergy Clin Immunol 1999; 103:215–222.
326. Christodoulopoulos P, Cameron L, Nakamura Y, Lemiere C, Muro S, Dugas M, Boulet LP, Laviolette M, Olivenstein R, Hamid Q. Th2 cytokine-associated transcription factors in atopic and nonatopic asthma: Evidence for differential signal transducer and activator of transcription 6 expression. J Allergy Clin Immunol 2001; 107:586–591.
327. Ray A, Cohn L. Th2 cells and GATA-3 in asthma: New insights into the regulation of airway inflammation. J Clin Invest 1999; 104:985–993.
328. Zhang DH, Yang L, Cohn L, Parkyn L, Homer R, Ray P, Ray A. Inhibition of allergic inflammation in a murine model of asthma by expression of a dominant-negative mutant of GATA-3. Immunity 1999; 11:473–482.
329. Finotto S, De Sanctis GT, Lehr HA, Herz U, Buerke M, Schipp M, Bartsch B, Atreya R, Schmitt E, Galle PR, Renz H, Neurath MF. Treatment of allergic airway inflammation and hyperresponsiveness by antisense-induced local blockade of GATA-3 expression. J Exp Med 2001; 193:1247–1260.

12

Cell Adhesion Molecule Blockers and/or Modulators

Potential Therapeutic Tools in Asthma

THEODORE F. REISS and S. BALACHANDRA DASS

Merck Research Laboratories
Rahway, New Jersey

I. Introduction

Asthma is an inflammatory disease characterized by infiltration and distribution of inflammatory cells in the airway wall and mucosa (1–3). The model for the expression of the asthmatic phenotype currently includes complex interactions among the structural elements of the airways, inflammatory leukocytes and other types of cells, cytokines and chemokines, adhesion molecules, and various other activating and/or stimulating factors. This biological model suggests that there are numerous potential targets for novel therapies in asthma; however, the relative importance of these pathways is unknown. Therefore, the development of compounds that disrupt specific pathways not only offers the potential for new therapy but also helps define the important biological pathways and refine the model of asthma.

This review summarizes our current knowledge of a pathway believed to be important in the asthmatic process. The presence of inflammatory cells in the airways is associated with and thought to require the activity of cell adhesion molecules. We describe the form and function of these molecules and their ligands, their involvement in the recruitment and migration of leukocytes, and their presence and expression in asthmatic patients. A number of strategies that have been employed to block and/or modulate their function are discussed; in addition, we report some previously unpublished data from clinical studies on a specific cell adhesion blocker.

II. Cell Adhesion Molecules

The adhesion molecules are glycoproteins that mediate interactions between cells and between cells and the extracellular matrix. They are believed to play a significant role in the cellular activation and trafficking of eosinophils, lymphocytes, and other inflammatory cells from the vascular compartment to the airways tissue (extensively reviewed in Refs. 4–8). In addition to their involvement in immune functions, they participate in a variety of other processes, such as tissue and organ development during embryogenesis, tumor metastasis, angiogenesis, nerve cell functions, atherosclerosis, hematopoiesis and stem cell development, signal transduction, and cellular apoptosis. Three families of adhesion molecules that are associated with the inflammatory process in asthma have been described: selectins, integrins, and the immunoglobulin superfamily (Table 1).

Selectins consist of three differentially expressed proteins: E-selectin is expressed on cytokine-activated endothelial cells, P-selectin is expressed on acti-

Table 1 Principal Cell Adhesion Molecules, Their Ligands, and Cellular Localization

Cell adhesion molecule	Ligand
Selectins	
E-selectin[a]	**ESL-1, L-selectin**
L-selectin[b]	*MadCAM-1, GlyCAM-1, P-selectin, E-selectin*
P-selectin	**PSGL-1, L-selectin**
Integrins	
VLA-4	*VCAM-1*
LFA-1	*ICAM-1, ICAM-2*
Mac-1	*ICAM-1*
$\boldsymbol{\alpha_4\beta_7}$	*MadCAM-1, VCAM-1*
Immunoglobulin family	
ICAM-1	**LFA-1, Mac-1**
VCAM-1	**VLA-4**
PECAM-1[c]	PECAM-1, $\alpha_v\beta_3$

[a] Endothelial receptors are shown in italics.
[b] Leukocyte receptors are in bold font.
[c] PECAM-1 is found on both the leukocytes and the endothelium. See text for further details.

vated platelets and endothelial cells, and L-selectin is constitutively expressed on circulating leukocytes. The N-terminal lectin domain in their structure allows for binding of carbohydrate ligands. Ligands that bind the selectins are glycosylated proteins and glycolipids that have in common a sialyl Lewis^x moiety and other fucose-containing carbohydrate determinants. P-selectin glycoprotein ligand-1 (PSGL-1) is found on all leukocytes and is recognized by all three selectins. A number of cell-surface molecules have been proposed to bind E-selectin, including E-selectin ligand-1 (ESL-1), which has been shown to express the sialyl Lewis^x moiety. Other selectin ligands belonging to the sialomucin family are the L-selectin ligands MadCAM-1 (mucosal addressin cell adhesion molecule-1) and GlyCAM-1 (glycosylated cell adhesion molecule-1), found on high endothelial venules in mucosal or peripheral lymph nodes, and possibly CD34, found on endothelial microvilli.

Integrins are structurally related heterodimeric glycoproteins composed of an α chain and a β chain that bind endothelial cells and matrix proteins. Some important members of the integrin family are the β_2 (CD18) and α_4 (CD49d) integrins. The β_2 integrin subfamily is expressed on all leukocytes and consists of a β_2 subunit linked to one of the following four α subunits: CD11a (α_L), CD11b (α_M), CD11c (α_X), or CD11d (α_D). Lymphocytes produce primarily CD11a/CD18 (LFA-1 or lymphocyte function associated antigen-1), whereas eosinophils, neutrophils, and monocytes produce all four β_2 integrins. The β_2 integrins bind to various members of the immunoglobulin supergene family, such as intercellular cell adhesion molecule-1 (ICAM-1), ICAM-2, or ICAM-3. Of particular relevance in allergic disease is the constitutively produced $\alpha_4\beta_1$ integrin (CD49d/CD29, VLA-4 or very late activation antigen-4), expressed on lymphocytes, monocytes, and eosinophils. VLA-4 mediates the binding of lymphocytes, eosinophils, and basophils to vascular cell adhesion molecule-1 (VCAM-1) and fibronectin. The integrin $\alpha_4\beta_7$ (CD49d/CD$^-$), expressed on eosinophils and some lymphocytes, mediates the binding of eosinophils to VCAM-1, MadCAM-1, and fibronectin and requires activation for this purpose.

The immunoglobulin (Ig) superfamily consists of a series of cell-surface proteins that mediate antigen recognition, complement binding, and activation, proliferation, and trafficking of lymphocytes. ICAM-1 and ICAM-2 are constitutively expressed on endothelial cells; the former molecule is further transcriptionally upregulated following cellular activation by various cytokines. ICAM-1 binds the integrins LFA-1 and Mac-1 ($\alpha_M\beta_2$), and ICAM-2 is recognized by LFA-1. ICAM-3, expressed constitutively on leukocytes (but not so on endothelial cells), is recognized by LFA-1 and mediates interactions between leukocytes. VCAM-1 is a cytokine-inducible molecule that is expressed on endothelial cells and is recognized by the integrins VLA-4 and $\alpha_4\beta_7$. The platelet endothelial cell adhesion molecule-1 (PECAM-1) is expressed constitutively on endothelial cells, leukocytes, and platelets and may be involved in leukocyte adhesion and migration between endothelial cells.

The adhesion molecules that are relevant to the asthmatic process are produced not only by the endothelial cells and leukocytes but also by other cells, such as mast cells in the lungs that express β_1 integrins; lung macrophages that produce ICAM-1, VLA-4, PSGL-1, L-selectin, and CD11b; lung dendritic cells that produce VLA-4 and PSGL-1; and bronchial epithelial cells that, unlike microvascular endothelial cells, express only ICAM-1 (4).

III. Recruitment and Migration of Leukocytes

The recruitment and migration of leukocytes from the vascular compartments into tissue sites is a complex process that involves the participation of a number of adhesion molecules (5,7,9,10). The adhesion process is a sequence of events that begins with leukocyte tethering and rolling along the endothelium of mesenteric venules. These weak interactions between the endothelium and the migrating cell are mediated by the selectins and their counterligands (11) and by members of the integrin family such as VLA-4 (12,13). The next step is firm leukocyte adhesion to endothelial cells; this requires activation of leukocytes by contact with endothelial adhesion molecules or by signals from cytokines (interleukins) and/or chemokines (eotaxins) (14–16). Associated with this process is an increased avidity and expression of β_1 and β_2 integrins on the leukocytes, which then enter into adhesion complexes with ICAM-1, ICAM-2, and VCAM-1 on cytokine-activated endothelium. The final phase is transendothelial migration of the leukocytes (diapedesis) from the apical to the basolateral surface. This process is primarily mediated by the β_2 integrins (17,18), VLA-4 (18,19), L-selectin (17), and various cytokines (interleukins, granulocyte-macrophage colony stimulating factor), chemokines (eotaxin, RANTES, MCP, MIP), and other chemotactic factors (14,15,20). Following diapedesis, leukocytes migrate up a gradient of chemotactic stimulus.

IV. Presence and Expression of Cell Adhesion Molecules in Asthmatic Patients

There is a considerable literature on cell adhesion molecule expression in allergic diseases, particularly asthma. Because of limitations in identifying significant differences in expression following immunostaining techniques, a number of these studies have provided conflicting findings; nevertheless, a general picture pointing to a significant role for these molecules in the inflammatory process has emerged. For instance, Montefort et al. (21) did not demonstrate any significant difference in expression of endothelial and epithelial ICAM-1 or endothelial E-selectin in the bronchial mucosa between normal subjects and symptomatic atopic asthmatic individuals. However, following segmental allergen challenge in atopic asthmatic subjects, an increase in leukocyte infiltration that was associated with increased expression of E-selectin and endothelial ICAM-1, but not VCAM-1, was shown by using bronchial biopsies (22). Bentley et al. (23) showed an increase in endothelial ICAM-1 and E-selectin levels in intrinsic asthmatic patients compared with nonasthmatic control individuals; epithelial expression of ICAM-1 was also more frequent in asthmatic patients than in the controls. In a study of allergic and nonallergic asthmatic patients and control subjects, Gosset et al. (24) demonstrated a significant increase in epithelial and endothelial ICAM-1 and in endothelial E-selectin and VCAM-1 that was correlated with eosinophil and total leukocyte infiltration in allergic asthma. Ohkawara et al. (25) examined the expression of adhesion molecules in the bronchial tissues of asthmatic patients with airflow limitation. Their studies using in situ hybridization and immunoelectron microscopy suggested that ICAM-1, VCAM-1, and E-selectin are newly synthesized prior to spontaneous asthma attacks. Endothelial cells in capillaries and venules were strongly positive for VCAM-1 in these asthmatic subjects, pointing to a key role for this molecule in the recruitment of eosinophils.

It is not clear if soluble forms of cell adhesion molecules serve as markers that reflect airways inflammation. Montefort et al. (26) detected increased levels of soluble ICAM-1 and E-selectin (but not VCAM-1) in the sera from patients suffering acute asthma, compared to samples from stable asthmatic patients and normal patients. In addition, following segmental antigen challenge, increased levels of soluble ICAM-1 (which correlated with increased leukocyte counts) were detected in the bronchoalveolar lavage (BAL) fluid of patients with asthma (27). Zangrilli et al. (28) reported a marked increase in soluble VCAM-I levels in BAL fluid following segmental challenge that correlated with increased numbers of eosinophils and concentrations of IL-4 and IL-5. Fukuda et al. (29) showed an increase in VCAM-1 expression (but not endothelial E-selectin and ICAM-1) in allergic asthmatic patients that correlated with eosinophil counts (but not with neutrophils), but only in patients with detectable IL-4 in BAL fluid.

Other studies demonstrated an association between increased endothelial VCAM-1 expression and eosinophil infiltration in nonallergic chronic hyperplastic sinusitis with nasal polyposis (30) and an increase in ICAM-1 on nasal epithelial cells in allergic subjects (31).

V. Cell Adhesion Molecule Blockers and/or Modulators

Novel pharmaceutical approaches have been employed to block and/or modulate the functioning of cell adhesion molecules in an attempt to prevent the activation and recruitment of inflammatory cells from the vascular space and their migration to the airways (4–6,9,32). Numerous studies have used the specificity of monoclonal antibodies (mAb) to block cell adhesion molecule functions. An mAb to ICAM-1 was shown to reduce airway hyperresponsiveness and eosinophilia in a monkey model of asthma (33). Certain mAbs to the α_4 chain of $\alpha_4\beta_1$ (VLA-4) and $\alpha_4\beta_7$ when used in lung antigen challenge models in several species can block the late-phase response and airways hyperresponsiveness. In particular, mAb HP1/2 was efficacious in a sheep model of allergic airways challenge whether given intravenously or as an aerosol (34,35). In a mouse model of late-phase allergic pulmonary inflammation, intrapulmonary blockage of the α_4 integrin using an mAb (administered intranasally) resulted in an amelioration of lung inflammation and hyperresponsiveness to methacholine (36).

Monoclonal antibodies to selectins have also been effective in ameliorating asthma in model systems (37). For instance, allergic sheep treated with an L-selectin-specific mAb (DU1-29, in aerosol form) before antigen challenge showed a reduction in both early and late airway responses and did not develop post-challenge airway hyperresponsiveness (38).

Soluble adhesion molecule–IgG constructs (immunoadhesins) have been shown to be effective as inhibitors of leukocyte trafficking in animal models of lung inflammation (4). Jackson et al. (39) described novel, highly potent, cyclic peptides that used functional groups similar to the binding epitope of VCAM-1 that competitively inhibited VLA-4 binding to VCAM-1 and fibronectin and inhibited lymphocyte migration in vivo. A small-molecule inhibitor of VLA-4 (that prevents VLA-4-mediated binding to fibronectin) administered by aerosol to allergic sheep resulted in a significant decrease in the early antigen-induced bronchial response and almost complete inhibition of the late-phase airway response (40). The inhibitor prevented an increase in lymphocyte and eosinophil numbers (as measured in biopsy specimens) and blocked macrophage adherence to fibronectin. Pretreatment of allergic sheep with a nebulized dose of BIO-1211, a high affinity, selective, small-molecule inhibitor of VLA-4, inhibited early and late airway responses following antigen challenge (41). Similarly, Abraham et al. (42) showed that single doses of BIO-1211 (whether given by aerosol or intravenously), either before or after antigen challenge, blocked allergen-induced late responses and post-antigen-induced airway hyperresponsiveness in allergic sheep. This chemical also provided dose-dependent inhibition of the early airway response to antigen. Sheep treated with BIO-1211 before challenge showed significantly reduced numbers of eosinophils in BAL fluid and inflammatory cells (eosinophils, lymphocytes, metachromatic-staining cells, and neutrophils) in bronchial biopsies obtained after challenge (42).

Dimeric and trimeric biphenyl-based compounds such as TBC-1269, consisting of simple nonoligosaccharide selectin antagonists, inhibited the binding of sialyl Lewis^x-bearing HL-60 cells to selectin fusion proteins (43). TBC-1269 also inhibited early airway responses and reduced the number of neutrophils recovered in BAL fluid in allergic sheep (38). Treatment with sialyl Lewis^x (known to inhibit the binding of leukocytes to E-selectin in vitro) or its mimetic CGP69669A led to a disruption of E-selectin-dependent leukocyte rolling in the mouse postcapillary venules (44). In this regard, it must be noted that inhibition of α-1,3-fucosyltransferase VII, an enzyme that regulates selectin function, is another possible approach to asthma therapy (32).

Neutrophil inhibitory factor, a β_2 integrin antagonist, inhibited neutrophil adhesion to endothelial cells in vitro and prevented lipopolysaccharide-induced lung neutrophil infiltration and injury in the mouse (45). Agusti et al. (46) showed that the compound Leumedin NPC 15669 and an antibody to ICAM-1 both prevented neutrophil recruitment and goblet cell degranulation in guinea pigs, implicating leukocytes in the response. Eosinophil count, sICAM-1, and fibronectin binding to eosinophils in BAL fluid from atopic asthmatic patients significantly decreased after the administration of Y-24180, a potent and long-acting antagonist to platelet-activating factor receptor (47). Tyrphostin AG-490, a specific Janus kinase 2 inhibitor, inhibited β_1 integrin adhesiveness of eosinophils in vitro; the in vivo administration of this chemical prevented antigen-induced eosinophil infiltration in the airways of sensitized mice in a dose-dependent manner (48).

Other available agents that may have some effect on the cell adhesion molecule pathways include cetirizine, an antihistamine (49,50); the phosphodiesterase inhibitors theophylline and ibudilast (51,52); and the cytokine inhibitor rooperol (53). Additional approaches include the use of antisense technology; an antisense oligonucleotide ISIS 2302 was shown to inhibit ICAM-1 expression in the treatment of Crohn's disease and was well tolerated in patients (54). Cytokines that induce adhesion molecule expression and metalloproteinases that are involved in L-selectin shedding are other possible (but nonspecific) targets (5).

VI. Clinical Experience

The available evidence from in vivo animal studies strongly suggests that the adhesion molecule pathways play a critical role in human disease—hence the hypothesis that compounds that disrupt the action of cell adhesion molecules and the activation and migration of inflammatory cells will show utility in a wide range of diseases believed to be inflammatory in origin. However, as previously described, adhesion molecules are required for many other biological processes; as a result, there are significant potential liabilities associated with the use of adhesion molecule antagonists. For instance, these molecules seem to be required for embryo implantation and development (55,56) and may have effects on the functioning of the bone marrow or vascular marginated pool of cells. It is clear that such mechanism-based effects must be managed effectively before these agents can serve as potential therapeutic tools in diseases like asthma.

Table 2 Baseline Characteristics of Patients

Age (years, mean ± SD)	34.9 ± 10.0
Gender (% female)	22.9
Duration of asthma (years, mean ± SD)	20.6 ± 12.2
β-Agonist use (puffs/day)	4.7 ± 2.8
FEV_1 (% predicted)	66.8 ± 11.1

To date there have been no published efficacy trials of adhesion molecule antagonists in the treatment of asthma, although there are a number of compounds in early development. Recently, the first prototype VLA-4 antagonist was tested. This compound, which demonstrated activity in the sheep model of asthma (41,42), was administered by inhalation to adult asthmatic patients in a randomized, double-blind, placebo-controlled study of 3 weeks duration, at a nebulized dose of 25 mg. In this trial, patients had moderate asthma (Table 2); patients on inhaled corticosteroids were excluded from the study. The results showed that there was no significant difference between the placebo group and the test compound group in the measured parameters of forced expiratory volume in 1 s (FEV_1), peak expiratory flow rate (PEFR), daytime symptoms score, and daily β-agonist use. The safety profile of this potential therapy was similar to that seen with placebo, and there were no important clinical or laboratory adverse events. Although this compound was active in the sheep model of the early and late-phase antigen challenge and was used in humans at a similar concentration, subsequent data (not shown) suggest that it may not have been a sufficiently potent adhesion molecule antagonist in the human lung to test the hypothesis of an effect in asthma.

New adhesion molecule antagonists are keenly anticipated. These could not only serve as potential therapies but also provide useful insight into the still evolving pathophysiological model of asthma and other inflammatory diseases of the airway.

References

1. Sterk PJ. Pathophysiology of asthma. In: Yeadon M, Diamant Z, eds. New and Exploratory Therapeutic Agents for Asthma. New York: Marcel Dekker, 2000:27–56.
2. Lordan JL, Djukanovic R. Anti-inflammatory drugs in asthma: The pathophysiology of asthma. In: Sampson AP, Church MK, eds. Anti-Inflammatory Drugs in Asthma. Basel: Birkhauser Verlag, 1999:1–33.
3. Jeffery KP. Airway pathology in asthma. In: Barnes PJ, Rodger IW, Thomson NC, eds. Asthma: Basic Mechanisms and Clinical Management. San Diego: Academic Press, 1998:47–64.

4. Hellewell PG. Adhesion molecule strategies. Pulm Pharmacol Ther 1999; 12:137–141.
5. Schleimer RP, Bochner BS. The role of adhesion molecules in allergic inflammation and their suitability as targets of antiallergic therapy. Clin Exp Allergy 1998; 28(suppl 3):15–23.
6. Wardlaw A. Adhesion molecules. In: Barnes PJ, Rodger IW, Thomson NC, eds. Asthma: Basic Mechanisms and Clinical Management. San Diego: Academic Press, 1988:239–251.
7. Nourshargh S. Adhesion molecules and asthma. J Pharm Pharmacol 1997;49(suppl 3):33–38.
8. Henricks PA, Bloemen PG, Nijkamp FP. Adhesion molecules and the recruitment of eosinophils to the airways. Res Immunol 1997; 148:18–28.
9. Foster PS, Hogan SP. Cytokine and adhesion molecule antagonists. In: Sampson AP, Church MK, eds. Anti-Inflammatory Drugs in Asthma. Basel: Birkhauser Verlag, 1999:251–272.
10. Bloemen PG, Henricks PA, Nijkamp FP. Cell adhesion molecules and asthma. Clin Exp Allergy 1997; 27:128–141.
11. Sriramarao P, von Andrian UH, Butcher EC, Bourdon MA, Broide DH. L-selectin and very late antigen-4 integrin promote eosinophil rolling at physiological shear rates in vivo. J Immunol 1994; 153:4238–4246.
12. Berlin C, Bargatze RF, Campbell JJ, von Andrian UH, Szabo MC, Hasslen SR, Nelson RD, Berg EL, Erlandsen SL, Butcher EC. Alpha 4 integrins mediate lymphocyte attachment and rolling under physiologic flow. Cell 1995; 80:413–422.
13. Alon R, Kassner PD, Carr MW, Finger EB, Hemler ME, Springer TA. The integrin VLA-4 supports tethering and rolling in flow on VCAM-1. J Cell Biol 1995; 128: 1243–1253.
14. Simson L, Foster PS. Chemokine and cytokine cooperativity: Eosinophil migration in the asthmatic response. Immunol Cell Biol 2000; 78:415–422.
15. Carlos AG, Carlos ML, Conceicao SM, Alcinda M. Cytokines and asthma. J Invest Allergol Clin Immunol 1997; 7:270–273.
16. Hogan SP, Foster PS. Cellular and molecular mechanisms involved in the regulation of eosinophil trafficking in vivo. Med Res Rev 1996; 16:407–432.
17. Ebisawa M, Bochner BS, Georas SN, Schleimer RP. Eosinophil transendothelial migration induced by cytokines. I. Role of endothelial and eosinophil adhesion molecules in IL-1 beta-induced transendothelial migration. J Immunol 1992; 149:4021–4028.
18. Moser R, Fehr J, Bruijnzeel PL. IL-4 controls the selective endothelium-driven transmigration of eosinophils from allergic individuals. J Immunol 1992; 149:1432–1438.
19. Weg VB, Williams TJ, Lobb RR, Nourshargh S. A monoclonal antibody recognizing very late activation antigen-4 inhibits eosinophil accumulation in vivo. J Exp Med 1993; 177:561–566.
20. Ebisawa M, Liu MC, Yamada T, Kato M, Lichtenstein LM, Bochner BS, Schleimer RP. Eosinophil transendothelial migration induced by cytokines. II. Potentiation of eosinophil transendothelial migration by eosinophil-active cytokines. J Immunol 1994; 152:4590–4596.

21. Montefort S, Roche WR, Howarth PH, Djukanovic R, Gratziou C, Carroll M, Smith L, Britten KM, Haskard D, Lee TH, et al. Intercellular adhesion molecule-1 (ICAM-1) and endothelial leucocyte adhesion molecule-1 (ELAM-1) expression in the bronchial mucosa of normal and asthmatic subjects. Eur Respir J 1992; 5:815–823.
22. Montefort S, Gratziou C, Goulding D, Polosa R, Haskard DO, Howarth PH, Holgate ST, Carroll MP. Bronchial biopsy evidence for leukocyte infiltration and upregulation of leukocyte-endothelial cell adhesion molecules 6 hours after local allergen challenge of sensitized asthmatic airways. J Clin Invest 1994; 93:1411–1421.
23. Bentley AM, Durham SR, Robinson DS, Menz G, Storz C, Cromwell O, Kay AB, Wardlaw AJ. Expression of endothelial and leukocyte adhesion molecules intercellular adhesion molecule-1, E-selectin, and vascular cell adhesion molecule-1 in the bronchial mucosa in steady-state and allergen-induced asthma. J Allergy Clin Immunol 1993; 92:857–868.
24. Gosset P, Tillie-Leblond I, Janin A, Marquette CH, Copin MC, Wallaert B, Tonnel AB. Expression of E-selectin, ICAM-1 and VCAM-1 on bronchial biopsies from allergic and non-allergic asthmatic patients. Int Arch Allergy Immunol 1995; 106: 69–77.
25. Ohkawara Y, Yamauchi K, Maruyama N, Hoshi H, Ohno I, Honma M, Tanno Y, Tamura G, Shirato K, Ohtani H. In situ expression of the cell adhesion molecules in bronchial tissues from asthmatics with air flow limitation: In vivo evidence of VCAM-1/VLA-4 interaction in selective eosinophil infiltration. Am J Respir Cell Mol Biol 1995; 12:4–12.
26. Montefort S, Lai CK, Kapahi P, Leung J, Lai KN, Chan HS, Haskard DO, Howarth PH, Holgate ST. Circulating adhesion molecules in asthma. Am J Respir Crit Care Med 1994; 149:1149–1152.
27. Takahashi N, Liu MC, Proud D, Yu XY, Hasegawa S, Spannhake EW. Soluble intercellular adhesion molecule 1 in bronchoalveolar lavage fluid of allergic subjects following segmental antigen challenge. Am J Respir Crit Care Med 1994; 150:704–709.
28. Zangrilli JG, Shaver JR, Cirelli RA, Cho SK, Garlisi CG, Falcone A, Cuss FM, Fish JE, Peters SP. sVCAM-1 levels after segmental antigen challenge correlate with eosinophil influx, IL-4 and IL-5 production, and the late phase response. Am J Respir Crit Care Med 1995; 151:1346–1353.
29. Fukuda T, Fukushima Y, Numao T, Ando N, Arima M, Nakajima H, Sagara H, Adachi T, Motojima S, Makino S. Role of interleukin-4 and vascular cell adhesion molecule-1 in selective eosinophil migration into the airways in allergic asthma. Am J Respir Cell Mol Biol 1996; 14:84–94.
30. Hamilos DL, Leung DY, Wood R, Bean DK, Song YL, Schotman E, Hamid Q. Eosinophil infiltration in nonallergic chronic hyperplastic sinusitis with nasal polyposis (CHS/NP) is associated with endothelial VCAM-1 upregulation and expression of TNF-alpha. Am J Respir Cell Mol Biol 1996; 15:443–450.
31. Ciprandi G, Pronzato C, Ricca V, Passalacqua G, Bagnasco M, Canonica GW. Allergen-specific challenge induces intercellular adhesion molecule 1 (ICAM-1 or CD54) on nasal epithelial cells in allergic subjects. Relationships with early and late inflammatory phenomena. Am J Respir Crit Care Med 1994; 150:1653–1659.

32. Rogers DF, Giembycz MA. Asthma therapy for the 21st century. Trends Pharmacol Sci 1998; 19:160–164.
33. Wegner CD, Gundel RH, Reilly P, Haynes N, Letts LG, Rothlein R. Intercellular adhesion molecule-1 (ICAM-1) in the pathogenesis of asthma. Science 1990; 247: 456–459.
34. Lobb RR, Abraham WM, Burkly LC, Gill A, Ma W, Knight JA, Leone DR, Antognetti G, Pepinsky RB. Pathophysiologic role of alpha 4 integrins in the lung. Ann NY Acad Sci 1996; 796:113–123.
35. Lobb RR, Pepinsky B, Leone DR, Abraham WM. The role of alpha 4 integrins in lung pathophysiology. Eur Respir J Suppl 1996; 22:104–108.
36. Henderson WR, Chi EY, Albert RK, Chu SJ, Lamm WJ, Rochon Y, Jonas M, Christie PE, Harlan JM. Blockade of CD49d (alpha4 integrin) on intrapulmonary but not circulating leukocytes inhibits airway inflammation and hyperresponsiveness in a mouse model of asthma. J Clin Invest 1997; 100:3083–3092.
37. Symon FA, Wardlaw AJ. Selectins and their counter receptors: A bitter sweet attraction. Thorax 1996; 51:1155–1157.
38. Abraham WM, Ahmed A, Sabater JR, Leuredo IT, Botvinnikova Y, Bjercke RJ, Hu X, Revelle BM, Kogan TP, Scott IL, Dixon RA, Yeh ET, Beck PJ. Selectin blockade prevents antigen-induced late bronchial responses and airway hyperresponsiveness in allergic sheep. Am J Respir Crit Care Med 1999; 159:1205–1214.
39. Jackson DY, Quan C, Artis DR, Rawson T, Blackburn B, Struble M, Fitzgerald G, Chan K, Mullins S, Burnier JP, Fairbrother WJ, Clark K, Berisini M, Chui H, Renz M, Jones S, Fong S. Potent alpha 4 beta 1 peptide antagonists as potential anti-inflammatory agents. J Med Chem 1997; 40:3359–3368.
40. Abraham WM, Ahmed A, Sielczak MW, Narita M, Arrhenius T, Elices MJ. Blockade of late-phase airway responses and airway hyperresponsiveness in allergic sheep with a small-molecule peptide inhibitor of VLA-4. Am J Respir Crit Care Med 1997; 156:696–703.
41. Lin KC, Ateeq HS, Hsiung SH, Chong LT, Zimmerman CN, Castro A, Lee WC, Hammond CE, Kalkunte S, Chen LL, Pepinsky RB, Leone DR, Sprague AG, Abraham WM, Gill A, Lobb RR, Adams SP. Selective, tight-binding inhibitors of integrin alpha4betal that inhibit allergic airway responses. J Med Chem 1999; 42:920–934.
42. Abraham WM, Gill A, Ahmed A, Sielczak MW, Lauredo IT, Botinnikova Y, Lin KC, Pepinsky B, Leone DR, Lobb RR, Adams SP. A small-molecule, tight-binding inhibitor of the integrin alpha(4)beta(1) blocks antigen-induced airway responses and inflammation in experimental asthma in sheep. Am J Respir Crit Care Med 2000; 162:603–611.
43. Kogan TP, Dupre B, Bui H, McAbee KL, Kassir JM, Scott IL, Hu X, Vanderslice P, Beck PJ, Dixon RA. Novel synthetic inhibitors of selectin-mediated cell adhesion: Synthesis of 1,6-bis[3-(3-carboxymethylphenyl)-4-(2-alpha-D-mannopyranosyloxy) phenyl]hexane (TBC1269). J Med Chem 1998; 41:1099–1111.
44. Norman KE, Anderson GP, Kolb HC, Ley K, Ernst B. Sialyl Lewis(x) (sLe(x)) and an sLe(x) mimetic, CGP69669A, disrupt E-selectin-dependent leukocyte rolling in vivo. Blood 1998; 91:475–483.
45. Zhou MY, Lo SK, Bergenfeldt M, Tiruppathi C, Jaffe A, Xu N, Malik AB. In vivo

expression of neutrophil inhibitory factor via gene transfer prevents lipopolysaccharide-induced lung neutrophil infiltration and injury by a beta2 integrin-dependent mechanism. J Clin Invest 1998; 101:2427–2437.

46. Agusti C, Takeyama K, Cardell LO, Ueki I, Lausier J, Lou YP, Nadel JA. Goblet cell degranulation after antigen challenge in sensitized guinea pigs. Role of neutrophils. Am J Respir Crit Care Med 1998; 158:1253–1258.
47. Mizuki M, Komatsu H, Akiyama Y, Iwane S, Tsuda T. Inhibition of eosinophil activation in bronchoalveolar lavage fluid from atopic asthmatics by Y-24180, an antagonist to platelet-activating factor. Life Sci 1999; 65:2031–2039.
48. Kumano K, Nakao A, Nakajima H, Miike S, Kurasawa K, Saito Y, Iwamoto I. Blockade of JAK2 by tyrphostin AG-490 inhibits antigen-induced eosinophil recruitment into the mouse airways. Biochem Biophys Res Commun 2000; 270:209–214.
49. Sedgwick JB, Busse WW. Inhibitory effect of cetirizine on cytokine-enhanced in vitro eosinophil survival. Ann Allergy Asthma Immunol 1997; 78:581–585.
50. Mincarini M, Cagnoni F, Canonica GW, Cordone G, Sismondini A, Semino C, Pietra G, Melioli G. Quantitative flow cytometric analysis of the effects of cetirizine on the expression of ICAM-1/CD54 on primary cultured nasal cells. Allergy 2000; 55: 226–231.
51. Spoelstra FM, Berends C, Dijkhuizen B, de Monchy JG, Kauffman HF. Effect of theophylline on CD11b and L-selectin expression and density of eosinophils and neutrophils in vitro. Eur Respir J 1998; 12:585–591.
52. Chihara J, Urayama O, Kayaba H, Honda K, Saito N, Hayashi N, Kurachi D, Yamamoto T. Inhibitory effect of ibudilast (KC-404) on the expression of the beta2 integrin family on an eosinophilic cell line (EoL-1). Ann Allergy Asthma Immunol 1998; 81:448–450.
53. Bereta J, Bereta M, Allison AC, Kruger PB, Koj A. Inhibitory effect of di-catechol rooperol on VCAM-1 and iNOS expression in cytokine-stimulated endothelium. Life Sci 1997; 60:325–334.
54. Yacyshyn BR, Bowen-Yacyshyn MB, Jewell L, Tami JA, Bennett CF, Kisner DL, Shanahan WR. A placebo-controlled trial of ICAM-1 antisense oligonucleotide in the treatment of Crohn's disease. Gastroenterology 1998; 114:1133–1142.
55. Crossin KL. Cell adhesion molecules in embryogenesis and disease. Ann NY Acad Sci 1991; 615:172–186.
56. Campbell S, Swann HR, Seif MW, Kimber SJ, Aplin JD. Cell adhesion molecules on the oocyte and preimplantation human embryo. Hum Reprod 1995; 10:1571–1578.

13

Allergen-Specific Immunotherapy

A. BARRY KAY and MARK LARCHÉ

National Heart and Lung Institute
Imperial College
London, England

I. Introduction

The prevalence of atopic allergic disease increased substantially toward the end of the twentieth century and is set to rise further. This group of diseases now constitutes the most common cause of chronic ill health in the developed world. Despite considerable attention from the pharmaceutical industry, little progress has been made in the development of disease-modifying therapies. In contrast, recent activity has focused almost exclusively on treatment of symptoms (palliation) rather than cause. The failure of palliative approaches to address the issue of increasing incidence of disease is in evidence in the case of allergic diseases and is a continuing focus of concern. At present, the most frequently employed nonpalliative form of disease-modifying therapy is specific allergen immunotherapy (SIT) in which increasing doses of whole allergen extract are administered in order to desensitize the allergic subject.

II. Specific Allergen Immunotherapy

Desensitizing immunotherapy was initially described by Noon and Freeman working at St. Mary's Hospital in London at the beginning of the last century (1,2). The technique involved administering increasing doses of crudely prepared whole allergen extract to sensitized subjects until symptoms were ameliorated. The first controlled trial of specific allergen immunotherapy was performed by Frankland and Augustin (also at St. Mary's Hospital) in 1954 (3). Since that time, SIT has been widely evaluated and modified and has been shown to be efficacious in venom hypersensitivity, seasonal or perennial allergic rhinitis, and mild allergic asthma. The role of allergen immunotherapy in the treatment of allergic disease, together with guidelines for its use, was summarized in a WHO position paper (4). Double-blind studies have shown that SIT with allergen extracts for grass pollen- and cat dander-induced rhinitis/asthma can be highly efficacious (3–5). However, questions continue to be raised about safety, particularly in relation to immediate IgE-mediated anaphylactic reactions. Although widely practiced in mainland Europe and in the United States, SIT is given in the United Kingdom on a routine basis only to patients with seasonal allergic rhinitis due to grass pollen (hayfever) who have failed to respond adequately to antiallergy drugs and in patients with anaphylaxis due to wasp or bee venom hypersensitivity. Only high quality standardized allergen extracts licensed under the provision of the U.K. Medicines Act and associated European directives are recommended (6).

III. Immune Response to Allergen

Allergen challenge in the clinical laboratory, in both the skin and the lung, has provided a useful model for investigating allergic inflammation. We have employed allergen inhalation challenge in asthmatic subjects in order to study the cellular mechanisms underlying allergic asthma. Allergen inhalation challenge of atopic asthmatic individuals results in an early asthmatic reaction (EAR) followed by a late asthmatic reaction (LAR). The EAR is rapid, peaking at 15 min, and is dependent on the IgE-mediated release of mast cell–derived mediators such as histamine and leukotrienes (7–9). In contrast, the LAR reaches a maximum at 6–9 h and is believed to represent, at least in part, the cellular inflammatory component of the asthmatic response. In this sense it has served as a useful model of chronic asthma. The LAR is characterized by infiltration of the airway by activated eosinophils and CD4 T cells, with increased numbers of T cells expressing mRNA for the Th2-type (IL-4 and IL-5) and eosinophil-active cytokines (IL-3, IL-5, and GM-CSF), (10,11). The ability of diverse agents such as antihistamines, anti-IgE monoclonal antibodies, leukotriene receptor antagonists, and cyclosporin A to partially inhibit the decreased airway function that characterizes the LAR suggests that a number of mechanisms may contribute to late-phase allergic inflammation.

IV. Effects of SIT

Evidence suggests that SIT may exert effects on several aspects of the immune system including modulation of the allergen-specific antibody response and modification of T-cell function. SIT may induce a form of ''immune deviation'' from a Th2 to a Th1 phenotype by downregulation of IL-4 and/or upregulation of IFN-γ. Alternatively, induction of tolerance, anergy, activation-induced cell death or hyporesponsiveness, and/or the production of cells with active suppressor function may have a role in the efficacy attributed to this form of therapy.

V. Modulation of the IgE-Dependent Early-Phase Response to Allergen

Atopic allergic disorders are diagnosed on the basis of elevated allergen-specific IgE and an accompanying history of relevant symptomatology. Interleukin-4 (IL-4) and IL-13 are required for isotype switch to Cε and Cγ4 in addition to contact-dependent signaling through CD40 and CD40 ligand (12). Furthermore, at later stages antigen-specific IgE antibody production by memory B cells also depends on IL-4 and IL-13.

Successful immunotherapy is accompanied by a variety of changes in the quality of the allergen-specific immune response (Fig. 1). One of the most notable is the increase in the specific IgG4/IgE ratio. It has been proposed that specific IgG4 may compete with IgE for allergen, thus preventing interaction of the latter with mast cells and basophils. Recent studies demonstrated that the majority of IgG4 in multiply sensitized allergic individuals is bispecific as a result of recombination of individual IgG4 chains (13). The monospecific molecules generated may be important in the mode of action of IgG4 in successful immunotherapy. Although there is an initial elevation in serum IgE concentrations during conventional immunotherapy with a gradual decrease to normal over a period of months, target organ sensitivity may decrease in the face of these elevations in serum IgE as a result of the more rapid increase in IgG4. Thus, although serum levels of both isotypes increase during the early phase of treatment, the ratio of specific IgE to IgG4 decreased by 10- to 100-fold (14). The presence of high levels of bee venom phospholipase A2-specific IgG4 in hyperimmune, nonallergic beekeepers has been linked to high levels of expression of IL-10 (15).

Interleukin-10 (IL-10) has been shown to play a key role in the regulation of allergen-specific IgG4 and IgE. IL-10 was shown to decrease epsilon transcripts induced by IL-4 in B-cell cultures in vitro when added during the first 3 days of

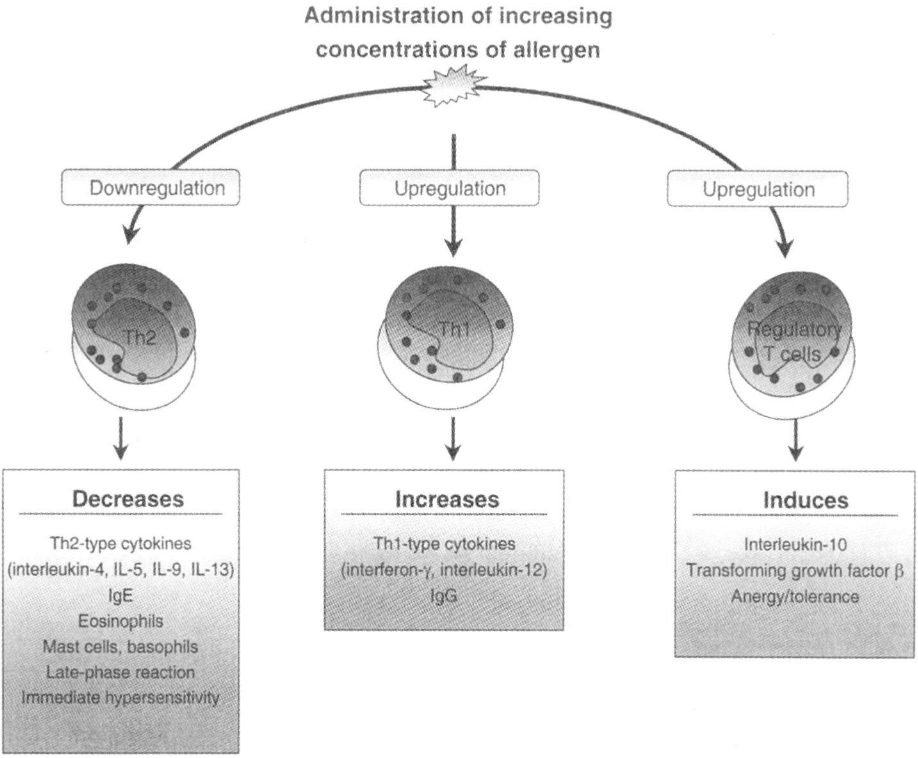

Figure 1 Proposed mechanisms of specific immunotherapy (hyposensitization or desensitization). Specific immunotherapy is associated with a downregulation of Th2 cells, immune deviation to Th1 cells, and the induction of regulatory T cells (e.g., Tr1/Th3). This in turn leads to inhibition of allergic inflammation and increases in cytokines that control IgE production (IFN-γ, IL-12), blocking antibodies (IgG), and cytokines involved in anergy or tolerance (i.e., IL-10 and TGF-β). Other immunological tricks such as linked suppression, bystander tolerance, and infectious tolerance may also be involved.

culture. Paradoxically, when added later, IL-10 enhanced IgE production. Interestingly, independently of the time of addition to cultures, IL-10 enhanced IgG4 production, probably by increasing IL-4-dependent class switching to gamma 4 (16). In bee venom hypersensitivity, IL-10 was a potent suppressor of both total and phospholipase A (PLA)-specific IgE while simultaneously increasing IgG4 formation (14). The issue of whether or not intact B-cell epitopes are required for the induction of allergen-specific IgG4 has been raised with regard to peptide immunotherapy. Data from Muller et al. (17) suggest that peptides alone, perhaps through the induction of IL-10, are capable of inducing IgG4. Increases in serum allergen-specific IgG concentrations after immunotherapy may be related to increases in IL-10 and IL-12, both of which are increased after SIT. Thus, suggested mechanisms by which IgG may downregulate the allergic response include (1) competition with IgE for allergen binding (classical blocking antibody theory), (2) prevention of aggregation of FcεRI-bound IgE through steric hindrance, and (3) interference with antigen trapping and focusing by IgE bound to antigen-presenting cells (18).

Successful immunotherapy reduces both the early- and late-phase responses to allergen. The decrease in the magnitude of the immediate response is likely to be due, at least partially, to a reduction in the numbers of tissue mast cells (19) and the previously described alteration in the ratio of IgG4 to IgE. Additionally, SIT characteristically inhibits, often dramatically, the late-phase reaction (LPR), and this in turn is associated with decreases in the numbers of mast cells, basophils, and eosinophils in both blood and target organs (19–22).

VI. Modulation of T-Cell Responses Following SIT

T lymphocytes are present in increased numbers at the site of allergic inflammation, and their numbers increase further following allergen challenge. In vitro experiments have shown that immunotherapy inhibited IL-4-dependent proliferation and production of IFN-γ by peripheral blood T cells but that addition of IL-2 or IL-15 to cultures restored proliferation and IFN-γ production but not IL-4 production (23). These data suggest that T-cell anergy was induced in this model.

Data from a number of studies suggest that immunotherapy is associated with profound modulation of T-cell function with either immune deviation from a Th1 to Th2 phenotype, induction of anergy, or both. There is some evidence, mostly from experimental animals, that $CD8^+$ T cells with suppressor activity may also be induced by SIT (24). SIT results in a decrease in antigen-induced recruitment to tissues of $CD4^+$ T cells and eosinophils with concomitant increases in cells expressing HLA-DR and CD25 (21). This may be the result of augmentation of HLA-DR and CD25 by interferon-gamma (IFN-γ) derived from Th1 cells. Thus immunotherapy is associated with a decrease in recruitment of CD4 cells, possible enhancement of $CD8^+$ cell function, downregulation of IL-4 and IL-5, and increases in IL-10 and IL-12.

It has been proposed that SIT, like other forms of immune modulation, involves immunological tricks in which nonresponsiveness induced to one epitope of a molecule either confers "tolerance" to the whole molecule (linked suppression) or adjacent molecules (bystander tolerance) or is passed to the next generation of regulatory T cells (infectious tolerance).

In addition to its role in the regulation of IgG4 and IgE synthesis, IL-10 has been demonstrated to exert a variety of effects on T cells and effector leukocytes in the late-phase allergic response. IL-10 inhibits T-cell proliferation and cytokine responses of both Th1 and Th2 cells and also blocks costimulatory pathways in T cells. In vitro, IL-10 induces a long-term antigen-specific anergic state in human $CD4^+$ T cells and can give rise to a regulatory, IL-10-producing population termed Tr1 cells (25). IL-10 may play a critical role in decreasing mast cell numbers and reactivity as well as in downregulating eosinophil function (15,26). Furthermore, IL-10 inhibits GM-CSF production and CD40 expression by activated eosinophils (27).

VII. Novel Forms of Immunotherapy

Antigen dose has been demonstrated to be an important factor in the commitment of T cells to produce cytokines of a Th1 or Th2 phenotype in murine models (28,29) and also in the induction of T-cell nonresponsiveness. Thus increasing antigen concentrations favor a Th1 phenotype whereas IL-4 was decreased at high antigen doses. This indicates that in certain situations Th1 and Th2 cells do not represent stable phenotypes but may be modulated by the dose of antigen. Therefore, in specific immunotherapy the concentration of antigen may be critical in determining the formation of IgE or IgG, resulting in either hypersensitivity or immunity.

An important feature of the efficacy associated with SIT is the delivery of relatively high doses of allergen (compared to natural exposure), which may exert its effect through the mechanism described above such as the induction of a Th1 cytokine phenotype. Indeed, the common monthly maintenance dose for aeroallergen immunotherapy is between 5 and 20 μg, a figure several orders of magnitude higher than those encountered during natural exposure.

Delivery of high doses of allergen carries with it the risk of IgE-mediated events including systemic anaphylaxis, resulting from widespread mast cell degranulation, which may be life-threatening. A variety of approaches have been initiated by which the ability of material used for immunotherapy to interact with IgE has been reduced. A further feature of these approaches is that attempts are also made to retain regions of the molecule, particularly linear epitopes, that interact with T-cell receptors. Some of these strategies, such as the generation of allergoids, have been clinically evaluated and shown to be efficacious. Others, such as recombinant allergens, naturally occurring allergen isoforms, and allergen-derived peptides, are currently at an earlier stage of development and require further analysis in controlled trials.

VIII. Allergoids

Modification of antibody-binding epitopes on the outer surface of native allergen molecules to generate ''allergoids'' has most frequently been achieved with formaldehyde, which modifies lysine residues and results in cross-linking of amino acid side chains, destroying three-dimensional epitopes in the process (30). A variety of allergoid preparations, including ragweed (31,32), grass pollen (33–37), *Parietaria* (38), and mite allergens (39,40), have been evaluated. Routes of administration and treatment regimens have varied in line with unmodified allergen immunotherapy and have included protocols (33–36) and sublingual/oral administration (40).

IX. Naturally Occurring Allergen Isoforms

Isolation, by purification or recombinant expression, of allergens derived from plants and trees has identified naturally occurring isoforms of allergens that have a reduced capacity to bind IgE (41). The relative lack of interaction with IgE generally results from amino acid substitutions or deletions within the IgE binding site or at sites that induce conformational changes in the molecule, preventing or substantially reducing IgE binding. These observations have led to suggestions that immunotherapy performed with hypoallergenic isoforms may allow higher doses to be used for immunotherapy, thereby providing a more effective method of modulating the T-cell response to allergens. Induction of IgE responses in previously naive individuals has, however, been observed during SIT with allergen isoforms (42,43), which may limit their effectiveness in immunotherapy.

X. Recombinant Allergens

A number of groups have employed recombinant DNA technology to clone, sequence, and express allergen proteins in the laboratory. Detailed analysis of IgE-binding epitopes has resulted in the mapping of IgE binding sites for a number of the major allergens. More recently, these findings together with the prior observations concerning the relative lack of immunogenicity associated with some allergen isoforms have been exploited by the use of in vitro mutagenesis to create allergen proteins in which single amino acids have been modified, or deletions introduced, to produce molecules with substantially reduced IgE-binding capacity (44–48).

Allergen engineering and the identification of low-IgE-binding allergen isoforms offer the prospect of purified, standardized allergen reagents for the diagnosis and therapy of allergic diseases. However, the large numbers of isoforms occurring naturally, particularly for plant and tree allergens, may make such approaches unfeasible.

XI. DNA Vaccines

In contrast to strategies that employ whole proteins or peptides to modify the immune response to allergens, recent interest has focused on direct immunization with DNA encoding allergen proteins. A number of variations on the theme of

DNA vaccination have been investigated. Unmethylated CpG motifs (ACGT) have been used to induce Th1 immune responses either alone or in combination with allergen proteins. Additionally, plasmid vectors encoding whole protein allergen genes have been injected directly into animals either before or after allergen challenge (49).

Palindromic nucleotide sequences containing the motif ACGT are found in microbial DNA and have previously been shown to induce the production of interferons in human peripheral blood mononuclear cells (50), activate B cells (51), and stimulate the production of Th1-enhancing cytokines such as IL-12, IFN-γ, and TNF-α in mice (52,53).

Recently, oligonucleotides containing CpG motifs were evaluated in murine models of asthma. Inhibition of IL-5 resulted in failure to release eosinophils from the bone marrow and was characterized by an inhibition of airways eosinophilia accompanied by modulation of airways inflammation and hyperresponsiveness (54,55). Mice were sensitized with recombinant Der p 5 following immunization with plasmid DNA encoding the allergen under the control of a CMV promoter (or empty vector control). Allergen-specific IgE levels were found to be 90% lower in mice immunized with the Der p 5 construct. In addition, Der p 5–specific CD8 T cells were shown to produce high levels of IFN-γ and could adoptively transfer suppression of IgE responses (56). In a rat model of asthma, immunization with plasmid constructs encoding a house dust mite allergen prevented IgE synthesis, histamine release in the lung, and airways hyperresponsiveness induced by allergen challenge (57). In addition to immunization with plasmid vectors encoding allergen proteins, inhibition of mucosal Th2-type immune responses has also been achieved following cytokine gene transfer. Li et al. (58) expressed IFN-γ in the airway epithelium of mice following gene transfer and observed inhibition of both allergen- and T-cell-induced airways eosinophilia.

Thus, strategies to abrogate Th2-type cytokine production via immunization with DNA motifs or plasmids encoding allergen and cytokine genes hold promise for therapy of allergic disease including asthma (Fig. 2). However, the majority of data collected in this area to date have come from murine models of disease. A cautionary note has been sounded by Li and colleagues (59), who demonstrate distinct, strain-dependent antibody isotype responses to plasmid-encoded Ara h 2. On the basis of their findings the authors highlight the importance of selecting appropriate animal strains for investigation of DNA vaccines ultimately intended for human use.

XII. Peptide Immunotherapy

A. Anergy and/or Tolerance

Activation of $CD4^+$ T cells is dependent upon the presentation of peptide fragments of processed antigen by MHC class II on antigen-presenting cells to spe-

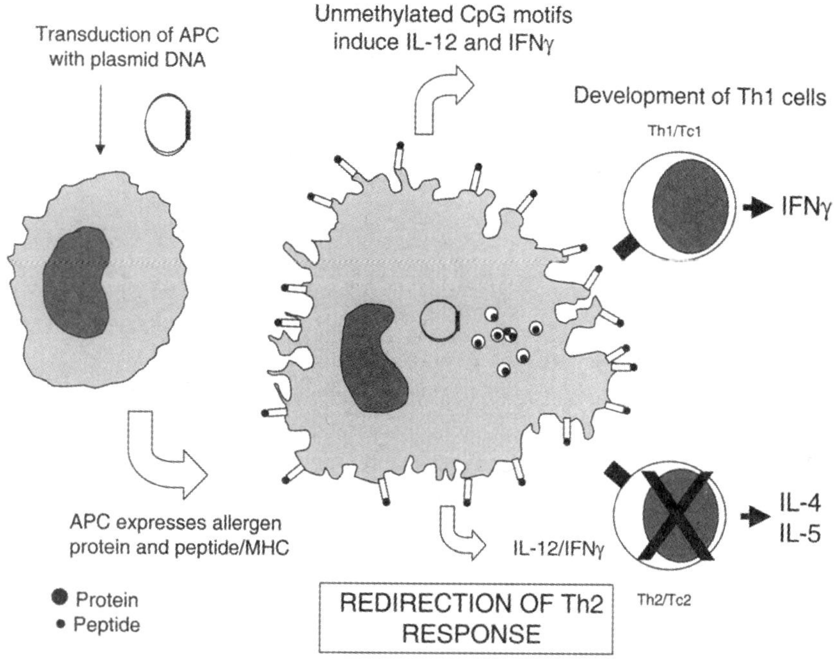

Figure 2 Mechanisms of immune deviation by plasmid DNA vaccination. Following intradermal or subcutaneous administration of plasmid DNA containing unmethylated CpG motifs (immunostimulatory sequences; ISS) and encoding an antigen or antigen peptide (or in certain cases, cytokine), antigen-presenting cells (APCs) are transduced. APCs become activated and produce IL-12, IL-18, IFN-α, and IFN-γ in response to ISS sequences. Proteins (peptides or cytokines) encoded by the plasmid insert are transcribed and translated. Peptide fragments bind to MHC molecules and are presented to specific T cells at the APC surface. Cytokines induced by ISS encourage Th1/Tc1 development and antagonize Th2/Tc2 development and effector function.

cific T-cell receptors (TcRs) (60). Productive T-cell responses also require costimulation through such pathways as CD28-CD80/CD86 (61,62). Much attention has focused on functional inactivation of such T-cell responses leading to ''tolerance.'' Presentation of antigen to high affinity TcR during thymic maturation leads to cell death by thymic deletion or central tolerance. Peripheral T-cell tolerance may result from deletion following activation-induced cell death (AICD) or, equally, failure to receive TcR-mediated stimulation, inhibition of migration, and active suppression. The absence of costimulation leads to T-cell unresponsiveness (''anergy'') to rechallenge (63,64). In murine models the injection of peptides produces T-cell anergy or nonresponsiveness through as yet unexplained mechanisms (65). For example, production of IgG and IL-2 by lymphocytes from

Fel d 1–primed mice was decreased after multiple injections of a peptide fragment of the priming allergen (65), and intranasal administration of peptides from Der p 1 could prevent sensitization and could also inhibit lymphocyte responses in previously sensitized mice (66). There is good evidence for peptide-induced nonresponsiveness of human CD4 cells in vitro (67,68).

B. Clinical Trials

Despite reservations regarding the use of peptides to treat allergic diseases in outbred human populations, peptide-based immunotherapy has recently been evaluated in subjects with allergic disease induced by either cat or ragweed allergens. Two relatively large peptides from the major cat allergen Fel d 1, termed IPC-1 and IPC-2, were evaluated by Norman et al. (69). Following four injections of peptide in three dose groups, clinical efficacy was observed only at the highest dose of peptide (4×750 μg). Both nasal and lung symptom scores improved in response to peptide therapy, although treatment was associated with a significant incidence of adverse events that occurred a few minutes to several hours after peptide injection. Further studies from the same group (70) demonstrated reduced IL-4 production in IPC-1/IPC-2-specific T-cell lines following therapy. A similar reduction in IL-4 production was reported by Pène et al. (71). Peripheral blood mononuclear cells were stimulated with cat dander extract before and after treatment with IPC-1/IPC-2. A significant reduction (compared to background levels) of IL-4 production was observed in the high-dose group (1500–4500 μg) but not in the lower dose groups. A reduction in allergen PD_{20} was also observed in response to both high- and medium-dose (150–450 μg) regimens compared to baseline but not compared to placebo. Simons et al. (72) also observed late-onset symptoms of rhinitis, asthma, and pruritis following treatment of cat allergic subjects with four weekly doses of 250 μg of IPC-1/IPC-2. In this placebo-controlled study of 42 individuals, the authors found no change in cytokine secretion patterns of PBMC before and after therapy. Furthermore, no change in early- and late-phase skin responses to whole allergen were observed at several time points after treatment. In a multicenter study of 133 patients, Maguire et al. (73) reported an improvement in pulmonary function in subjects receiving eight injections of 750 μg IPC-1/IPC-2 who had diminished baseline FEV_1 but only at a single time point (3 weeks) following therapy. A large number of adverse events were reported in this study, including some that required the use of adrenaline. In keeping with other studies evaluating IPC-1/IPC-2, late-onset adverse reactions diminished with successive doses of peptide, suggesting the induction of hyporesponsiveness. Thus, a relatively modest improvement in symptom scores combined with frequent adverse reactions resulted in cat and ragweed vaccines being withdrawn from clinical trials.

More recently, Muller et al. (74) identified three T-cell peptide epitopes in the bee venom phospholipase A_2 (PLA2) molecule and used these peptides to desensitize five allergic subjects. Peptides were well tolerated and, despite the differing MHC backgrounds of the subjects, T-cell responses to all three peptides were observed, suggesting that the problems of using peptide immunotherapy in an outbred population such as humans may not present as much of a problem as has been envisaged in the past.

C. T-Cell Tolerance is Preceded by T-Cell Activation

In addition to rapid onset reactions, Norman et al. (69) also observed asthma-like symptoms commencing several hours after administration of IPC-1/IPC-2. We hypothesized that these reactions were the result of direct MHC-restricted activation of allergen-specific T cells. To determine whether T-cell peptides, which do not cross-link IgE, can induce an isolated LAR, we designed three Fel d 1 chain 1–derived peptides (FC1Ps) of 16 or 17 residues and administered them by intradermal injection into cat-allergic asthmatic subjects. Furthermore, by repeated administration of peptides, we tested the hypothesis that specific hyporesponsiveness could be induced.

Haselden et al. established that the peptides, by virtue of their small size, did not release histamine from basophil-enriched mononuclear cells (75). Following intradermal injection of 80 μg of FC1P, nine of 40 cat-allergic asthmatic subjects experienced a fall in FEV_1 that started at 3–4 h and reached a plateau by 6 h (75). In none of the 40 subjects were immediate lung reactions observed. We hypothesized that these responses represented isolated Th2 cell–dependent LARs. Recognition of antigenic peptides by T cells requires that the peptide be presented to the T cell in the context of an appropriate MHC molecule or "restriction element." Because not all individuals developed a response, the HLA DRB1 haplotype of all subjects was determined (75). Using allergen-specific T-cell lines derived from the study subjects prior to peptide injection and L cells (transformed fibroblasts) transfected with appropriate HLA-DR alleles, it was determined that peptide FC1P3 could be presented to T cells by both HLA-DRB1*0101 and two microvariants of DR13 (HLA-DRB1*1301 and HLA-DRB1*1302) (75), leading to proliferation and secretion of IL-5. Additionally, another of the three peptides (FC1P2) could be presented by HLA-DRB1*0405 to T cells derived from an autologous (HLA-DRB1*0405) subject and, interestingly, to an individual expressing HLA-DRB1*0408.

D. MHC-Based Allergen Peptide Vaccine

The recognition of the two peptides in the context of more than one MHC molecule suggests that these peptides are capable of promiscuous binding. This observation may be of some significance, because one argument against the use of peptides for disease-modulating immunotherapy in humans is that since humans differ widely in their MHC haplotypes, a very large (and therefore impractical) number of peptides will have to be employed in any therapeutic preparation. In fact, what our findings suggest is not only that individual peptides are capable of binding promiscuously to more than one MHC molecule but also that there is a degree of plasticity at the level of the T-cell receptor, because a T-cell receptor from an HLA-DRB1*0408 individual can recognize FC1P2 when it is presented in the context of HLA-DRB1*0405. Based on these early observations, therefore, it appears that a relatively small number of carefully selected peptides from an allergen may be efficacious in the treatment of allergic disease. This concept has been supported by data from Texier et al. (76).

Thus, it was possible to account for FC1P-mediated induction of LAR by virtue of the nine individuals expressing a DR1, DR4, or DR13 allele. These findings strongly support the hypothesis that direct, MHC-restricted activation of Th2 lymphocytes by allergen-derived peptides leads to the development of the LAR, suggesting that both the Th2 component of asthma and strategies to downregulate this response are founded firmly in MHC-restricted Th2-cell recognition of allergen epitopes.

During the course of these investigations, three subjects displaying an isolated LAR were given a further dose of peptide, and this was followed by a markedly reduced or absent response (75), suggesting that T-cell hyporesponsiveness had been induced by the initial injection, strongly supporting the hypothesis. Interestingly, following a further peptide injection more than 1 year after the first, LARs of similar magnitude to the initial response were observed (75). These findings suggested that hyporesponsiveness lasted for more than several weeks but less than 1 year. Collectively, these observations were further investigated with a larger mixture of overlapping peptides from the same allergen.

Data obtained with FC1P indicated that in order to elicit peptide LAR and subsequent nonresponsiveness in the majority of cat-allergic asthmatic subjects, administration of synthetic peptides covering the entire sequence of the Fel d 1 molecule would be required, because recognition of individual regions of the molecule was restricted by MHC haplotype. Thus 16 overlapping peptides were designed spanning both chains of the Fel d 1 molecule. Four of the 16 proved to be poorly soluble in aqueous solution and were therefore excluded from the mixture of peptides, termed MOPs (multiple overlapping peptides), that were subsequently administered to cat-allergic asthmatic subjects.

Initially, dose–response experiments were undertaken to establish the relationship between peptide dose and both the magnitude and frequency of isolated LARs. Isolated LARs in cat-allergic asthmatic volunteers could be induced at doses as low as 1 μg of each of the 12 peptides as a mixture. Furthermore, at 1 μg of peptide, one out of eight individuals experienced an isolated LAR. At a dose of 2.5 μg, two out of eight individuals developed reactions that were of greater magnitude than at 1 μg. Finally, at a dose of 5 μg, 50% of individuals

(4/8) developed LARs that were generally of greater magnitude than the reactions observed with lower doses. In common with the earlier FC1P peptide preparation, a second injection of cat allergen (Fel d 1)-derived T-cell peptides was associated with a marked reduction, or absence, of the late asthmatic reaction (Fig. 3) and that up to 40 weeks was required to return to baseline values (Fig. 4). The cutaneous late-phase reaction to whole cat dander was also inhibited, even in subjects who did not experience an initial late asthmatic reaction (Fig. 5). These observations were associated with a significant decrease in peptide- and whole allergen-induced proliferation of peripheral blood mononuclear cells and the production of interleukin-4, interleukin-13, and interferon-gamma in cultures (Fig. 6). Thus, allergen-derived peptides induce tolerance to subsequent peptide injection in the target organ (the lung), reduce late-phase cutaneous responsiveness to whole allergen, and alter in vitro T-cell reactivity.

The cellular mechanisms that underlie the peptide-induced, MHC-restricted reactions and subsequent hyporesponsiveness described in this review remain to be elucidated. Recently much attention has focused on T cells that may regulate the immune response. A number of such regulatory T-cell populations have been described in animal studies (25,77–79). The mechanisms by which these cells modulate Th1 or Th2 responses require further clarification, but cytokines such as

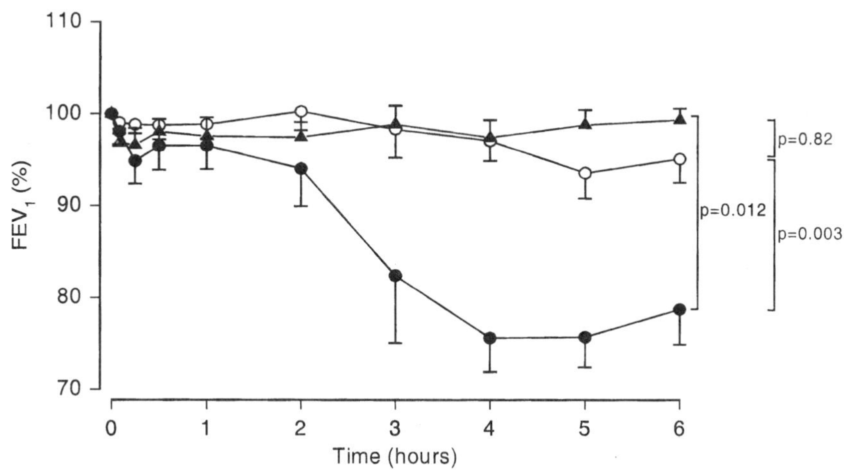

Figure 3 The effect on FEV_1 of readministering Fel d 1 peptides to cat-allergic asthmatic individuals who previously developed a late asthmatic reaction following the first injection. Seven subjects who developed an LAR following intradermal challenge of Fel d 1 peptides (filled circles) were challenged on a second occasion 2–14 weeks later (open circles), and the pooled results were compared with the control day (filled triangles). The points represent the mean (±SEM).

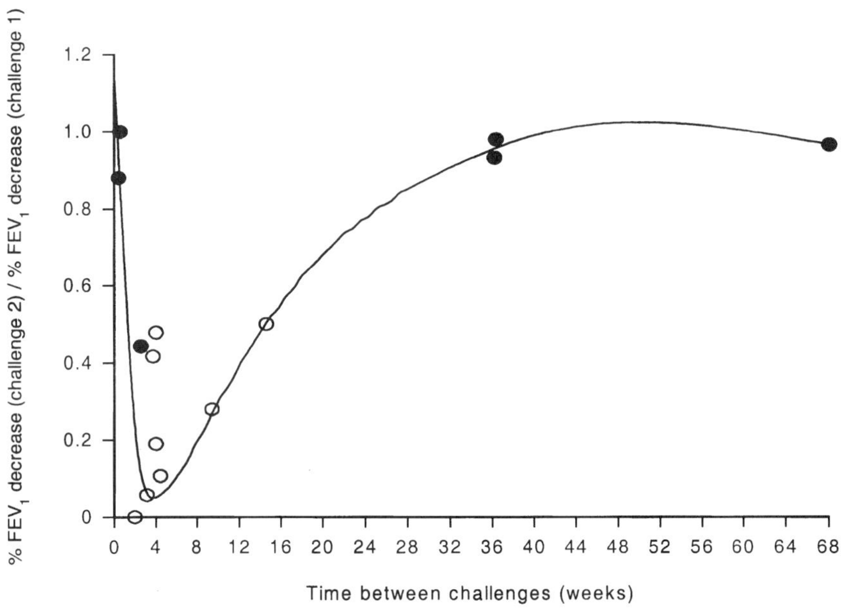

Figure 4 A comparison over time of the percentage decrease in the FEV_1 on the first and second challenge in cat-allergic subjects who developed an LAR following intradermal challenge with Fel d 1 peptides (5.0 μg). In the subjects studied the time interval between the two challenges varied from a few days to 68 weeks. Asthmatic subjects (open circles) had a percentage decrease in FEV_1 of <20% on the second challenge and remained asymptomatic. Those depicted by the filled circles had an LAR (i.e., a decrease in FEV_1 of >20%) on the second occasion and experienced wheezy breathlessness (as all subjects did on the first challenge).

IL-10 and TGF-β are likely to be important factors in this ''regulation.'' Linked suppression is a phenomenon, demonstrated in animal models, in which the administration of a single epitope from a protein modifies the responses of nontolerant T cells specific for other epitopes within the same protein and, in some models, epitopes derived from other proteins (''bystander suppression'') (80). The mechanism(s) of linked suppression vary from model to model (81,82). Induction of nonresponsiveness to whole proteins following administration of a single peptide epitope has been demonstrated in a number of models (65,83–87). Hoyne et al. (88) demonstrated linked suppression in T-cell responses to epitopes within the same allergen protein after inhalation challenge of a single immunodominant epitope. The phenomenon of linked suppression has not been demonstrated in vivo in a human model. However, because neither the FC1P nor MOP preparation spans the entire Fel d 1 molecule, it will be possible within this model to investi-

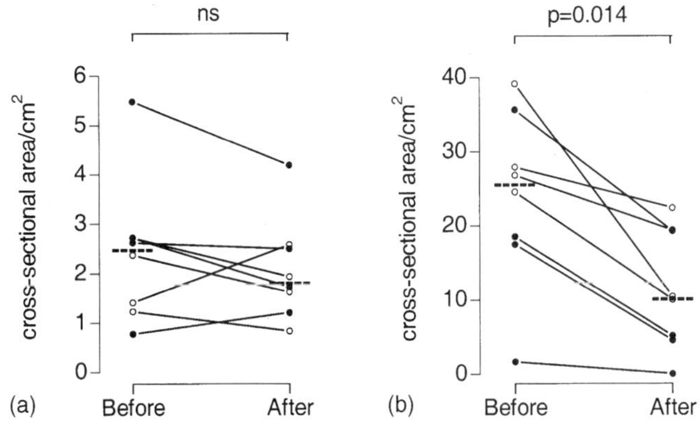

Figure 5 The effect of a single injection of Fel d 1 peptides (5.0 μg) on the (a) early-phase (15 min) and (b) late-phase (6 h) cutaneous reaction to whole cat dander. Subjects who had an LAR on the first injection are represented by the filled circles, and those who did not, by the open circles. The interval between the injection of Fel d 1 peptides and the reassessment of cutaneous reactivity to whole cat dander was 2 weeks.

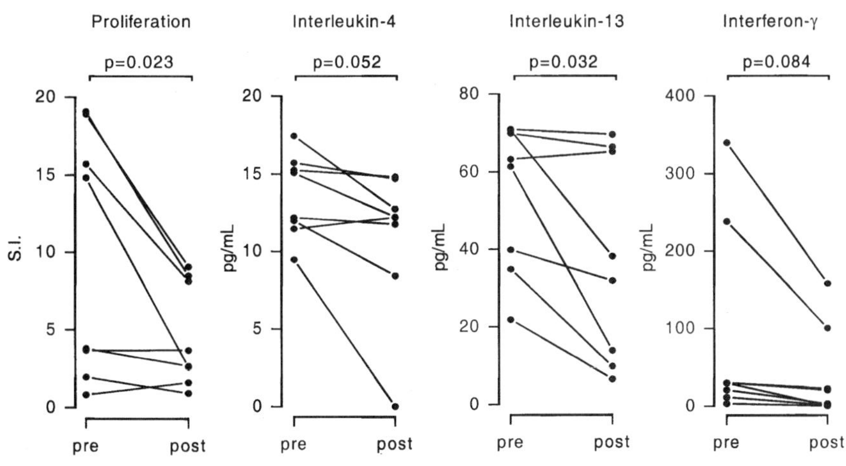

Figure 6 The effect of a single injection of Fel d 1 peptides (5 μg) on the PBMC responses (proliferation and IFN-γ, IL-4, and IL-13 production) to whole cat dander. Proliferative responses are expressed as median with interquartile range and cytokine responses as mean ± standard error.

gate whether T-cell responses (in vitro) to peptides not injected into patients are downregulated at the same time as those to injected peptides. If this can be demonstrated, it will be the first demonstration of linked suppression in a human in vivo situation.

XIII. Conclusions

Specific immunotherapy has been successfully performed on sensitized individuals for 90 years. Although efficacious, this form of therapy is associated with the risk of adverse IgE-mediated events including systemic anaphylaxis. The mechanisms underlying successful SIT include modulation of the specific immune response to allergen that are manifested by a relative decrease in Th2-type responses and a concomitant increase in Th1-type parameters. Additionally, increases in the allergen-specific IgG4/IgE ratio have been consistently observed, which may be dependent upon cytokines such as IL-10 from T cells, B cells, and monocytes.

Attempts to reduce the interaction between allergen preparations and IgE have led to the development of effective therapies such as allergoids and also, more recently, to experimental strategies including naturally occurring hypoallergenic allergen isoforms, engineered allergens with reduced IgE-binding capacity, and the use of T-cell peptide epitopes.

Experience in our own laboratory with peptides derived from the major cat allergen Fel d 1 suggests that peptides can be used to induce profound and long-lasting hyporesponsiveness in vivo, in the absence of adverse events. This provides an exciting opportunity to effectively modify existing disease and to go some way toward redressing the continuing increase in the prevalence of allergic diseases.

Acknowledgments

We thank our colleagues Drs. B.M. Haselden, W. Oldfield, D.S. Robinson, S. Ying, and Ms. K. Shirley for their important contributions to this work. We also thank the following collaborators: Dr. Meinir Jones, Professor Robert Lechler, Dr. Giovanna Lombardi, Professor Jonathan Lamb, Dr. Carolyn Katovich-Hurley, Dr. John Richert, Dr. Amanda Bennett, and Professor Martin Church.

References

1. Noon L. Prophylactic inoculation against hay fever. Lancet 1911; 1:1572.
2. Freeman J. Vaccination against hay fever: Report of results during the first three years. Lancet 1914; 1:1178.

3. Frankland AW, Augustin R. Prophylaxis of summer hayfever and asthma. A controlled trial comparing crude grass pollen extracts with the isolated main protein component. Lancet 1954; i:1055–1057.
4. WHO. Allergen immunotherapy: Therapeutic vaccines for allergic diseases. WHO Position Paper. Allergy 1998; suppl 53:1–42.
5. Durham SR, Till SJ. Immunologic changes associated with allergen immunotherapy. J Allergy Clin Immunol 1998; 102:157–164.
6. Kay AB, Frew AJ, Coleman JW, et al. Position Paper on Allergen Immunotherapy. Report of a BSACI Working Party. Clin Exp Allergy 1993; suppl 3:1–44.
7. Metzger WJ, Zavala D, Richerson HB, Moseley P, Iwamota P, Monick M, Sjoerdsma K, Hunninghake GW. Local allergen challenge and bronchoalveolar lavage of allergic asthmatic lungs. Description of the model and local airway inflammation. Am Rev Respir Dis 1987; 135:433–440.
8. Sedgwick JB, Calhoun WJ, Gleich GJ, Kita H, Abrams JS, Schwartz LB, Volovitz B, Ben-Yaakov-M, Busse WW. Immediate and late airway response of allergic rhinitis patients to segmental antigen challenge. Characterization of eosinophil and mast cell mediators. Am Rev Respir Dis 1991; 144:1274–1281.
9. Liu MC, Hubbard WC, Proud D, Stealey BA, Galli SJ, Kagey-Sobotka A, Bleecker ER, Lichtenstein LM. Immediate and late inflammatory responses to ragweed antigen challenge of the peripheral airways in allergic asthmatics. Cellular, mediator, and permeability changes. Am Rev Respir Dis 1991; 144:51–58.
10. Bentley AM, Meng Q, Robinson DS, Hamid Q, Kay AB, Durham SR. Increases in activated T lymphocytes, eosinophils, and cytokine mRNA expression for interleukin-5 and granulocyte/macrophage colony-stimulating factor in bronchial biopsies after allergen inhalation challenge in atopic asthmatics. Am J Respir Cell Mol Biol 1993; 8:35–42.
11. Ying S, Humbert M, Barkans J, Corrigan CJ, Pfister R, Menz G, Robinson DS, Larché M, Durham SR, Kay AB. Expression of IL-4 and IL-5 mRNA and protein product by CD4+ and CD8+ T cells, eosinophils, and mast cells in bronchial biopsies obtained from atopic and nonatopic (intrinsic) asthmatics. J Immunol 1997; 158: 3539–3544.
12. Vercelli D. Molecular regulation of the IgE immune response. Clin Exp Allergy 1995; 25(suppl 2):43–45.
13. Schuurman J, Van Ree R, Perdok GJ, Van Doorn HR, Tan KY, Aalberse RC. Normal human immunoglobulin G4 is bispecific: It has two different antigen-combining sites. Immunology 1999; 97:693–698.
14. Akdis CA, Blesken T, Akdis M, Alkan SS, Wüthrich B, Heusser CH, Blaser K. Induction and differential regulation of bee venom phospholipase A_2-specific human IgE and IgG4 antibodies in vitro requires allergen-specific and nonspecific activation of T and B cells. J Allergy Clin Immunol 1997; 99:345–353.
15. Akdis CA, Blesken T, Akdis M, Wüthrich B, Blaser K. Role of interleukin 10 in specific immunotherapy. J Clin Invest 1998; 102:98–106.
16. Jeannin P, Lecoanet S, Delneste Y, Gauchat JF, Bonnefoy JY. IgE versus IgG4 production can be differentially regulated by IL-10. J Immunol 1998; 160:3555–3561.
17. Muller U, Akdis CA, Fricker M, Akdis M, Blesken T, Bettens F, Blaser K. Success-

ful immunotherapy with T-cell epitope peptides of bee venom phospholipase A_2 induces specific T-cell anergy in patients allergic to bee venom. J Allergy Clin Immunol 1998; 101:747–754.

18. Stingl G, Maurer D. IgE-mediated allergen presentation via Fc epsilon RI on antigen-presenting cells. Int Arch Allergy Immunol 1997; 113:24–29.
19. Durham SR, Varney VA, Gaga M, Jacobson MR, Varga EM, Frew AJ, Kay AB. Grass pollen immunotherapy decreases the number of mast cells in the skin. Clin Exp Allergy 1999; 29:1490–1496.
20. Nish WA, Charlesworth EN, Davis TL, Whisman BA, Valtier S, Charlesworth MG, Leiferman KM. The effect of immunotherapy on the cutaneous late phase response to antigen. J Allergy Clin Immunol 1994; 93:484–493.
21. Varney VA, Hamid QA, Gaga M, Ying S, Jacobson M, Frew AJ, Kay AB, Durham SR. Influence of grass pollen immunotherapy on cellular infiltration and cytokine mRNA expression during allergen-induced late-phase cutaneous responses. J Clin Invest 1993; 92:644–651.
22. Furin MJ, Norman PS, Creticos PS, Proud D, Kagey-Sobotka A, Lichtenstein LM, et al. Immunotherapy decreases antigen-induced eosinophil cell migration into the nasal cavity. J Allergy Clin Immunol 1991; 88:27–32.
23. Akdis CA, Akdis M, Blesken T, Wymann D, Alkan SS, Müller U, Blaser K. Epitope-specific T cell tolerance to phospholipase A_2 in bee venom immunotherapy and recovery by IL-2 and IL-15 in vitro. J Clin Invest 1996; 98:1676–1683.
24. Renz H, Lack G, Saloga J, Schwinzer R, Bradley K, Loader J, Kupfer A, Larson GL, Gelfand EW. Inhibition of IgE production and normalization of airways responsiveness by sensitized CD8 T cells in a mouse model of allergen-induced sensitization. J Immunol 1994; 152:351–360.
25. Groux H, O'Garra A, Bigler M, Rouleau M, Antonenko S, de Vries JE, Roncarolo MG. A CD4+ T-cell subset inhibits antigen-specific T-cell responses and prevents colitis. Nature 1997; 389:737–742.
26. Akdis CA, Blaser K. IL-10-induced anergy in peripheral T cell and reactivation by microenvironmental cytokines: Two key steps in specific immunotherapy. FASEB J 1999; 13:603–609.
27. Borish L. IL-10: Evolving concepts. J Allergy Clin Immunol 1998; 101:293–297.
28. Hosken NA, Shibuya K, Heath AW, Murphy KM, O'Garra A. The effect of antigen dose on CD4+ T helper cell phenotype development in a T cell receptor-alpha beta-transgenic model. J Exp Med 1995; 182:1579–1584.
29. Constant SL, Bottomly K. Induction of Th1 and Th2 CD4+ T cell responses: The alternative approaches. Annu Rev Immunol 1997; 15:297–322.
30. Marsh DG, Lichtenstein LM, Campbell DH. Studies on "allergoids" prepared from naturally occurring allergens. I. Assay of allergenicity and antigenicity of formalinized rye group component. Immunology 1970; 18:705–722.
31. Norman PS, Lichtenstein LM, Marsh DG. Studies on allergoids from naturally occurring allergens. IV. Efficacy and safety of long-term allergoid treatment of ragweed hay fever. J Allergy Clin Immunol 1981; 68:460–470.
32. Norman PS, Lichtenstein LM, Kagey-Sobotka A, Marsh DG. Controlled evaluation of allergoid in the immunotherapy of ragweed hay fever. J Allergy Clin Immunol 1982; 70:248–260.

33. Bousquet J, Hejjaoui A, Skassa-Brociek W, Guerin B, Maasch HJ, Dhivert H, Michel FB. Double-blind, placebo-controlled immunotherapy with mixed grass-pollen allergoids. I. Rush immunotherapy with allergoids and standardized orchard grass-pollen extract. J Allergy Clin Immunol 1987; 80:591–598.
34. Bousquet J, Maasch H, Martinot B, Hejjaoui A, Wahl R, Michel FB. Double-blind, placebo-controlled immunotherapy with mixed grass-pollen allergoids. II. Comparison between parameters assessing the efficacy of immunotherapy. J Allergy Clin Immunol 1988; 82:439–446.
35. Bousquet J, Maasch HJ, Hejjaoui A, Skassa-Brociek W, Wahl R, Dhivert H, Michel FB. Double-blind, placebo-controlled immunotherapy with mixed grass-pollen allergoids. III. Efficacy and safety of unfractionated and high-molecular-weight preparations in rhinoconjunctivitis and asthma. J Allergy Clin Immunol 1989; 84:546–556.
36. Bousquet J, Hejjaoui A, Soussana M, Michel FB. Double-blind, placebo-controlled immunotherapy with mixed grass-pollen allergoids. IV. Comparison of the safety and efficacy of two dosages of a high-molecular-weight allergoid. J Allergy Clin Immunol 1990; 85:490–497.
37. Pastorello EA, Pravettoni V, Incorvaia C, Mambretti M, Franck E, Wahl R, Zanussi C. Clinical and immunological effects of immunotherapy with alum-absorbed grass allergoid in grass-pollen-induced hay fever. Allergy 1992; 47:281–290.
38. Tari MG, Mancino M, Ghezzi E, Frank E, Cromwell O. Immunotherapy with an alum-adsorbed Parietaria-pollen allergoid: A 2-year, double-blind, placebo-controlled study. Allergy 1997; 52:65–74.
39. Pecoud A, Nicod L, Badan M, Agrell B, Dreborg S, Kolly M. Effects of one-year hyposensitization in allergic rhinitis. Comparison of two house dust mite extracts. Allergy 1990; 45:386–392.
40. Passalacqua G, Albano M, Fregonese L, Riccio A, Pronzato C, Mela GS, Canonica GW. Randomised controlled trial of local allergoid immunotherapy on allergic inflammation in mite-induced rhinoconjunctivitis. Lancet 1998; 351:629–632.
41. Ferreira F, Hirtenlehner K, Jilek A, Godnik-Cvar J, Breiteneder H, Grimm R, Hoffmann-Sommergruber K, Scheiner O, Kraft D, Breitenbach M, Rheinberger HJ, Ebner C. Dissection of immunoglobulin E and T lymphocyte reactivity of isoforms of the major birch pollen allergen Bet v 1: Potential use of hypoallergenic isoforms for immunotherapy. J Exp Med 1996; 183:599–609.
42. Breiteneder H, Ferreira F, Hoffmann-Sommergruber K, Ebner C, Breitenbach M, Rumpold H, Kraft D, Scheiner O. Four recombinant isoforms of Cor a I, the major allergen of hazel pollen, show different IgE-binding properties. Eur J Biochem 1993; 212:355–362.
43. Schenk S, Hoffmann-Sommergruber K, Breiteneder H, Ferreira F, Fischer G, Scheiner O, Kraft D, Ebner C. Four recombinant isoforms of Cor a 1, the major allergen of hazel pollen, show different reactivities with allergen-specific T-lymphocyte clones. Eur J Biochem 1994; 224:717–722.
44. Ferreira F, Ebner C, Kramer B, Casari G, Briza P, Kungl AJ, Grimm R, Jahn-Schmid B, Breiteneder H, Kraft D, Breitenbach M, Rheinberger HJ, Scheiner O. Modulation of IgE reactivity of allergens by site-directed mutagenesis: Potential use of hypoallergenic variants for immunotherapy. FASEB J 1998; 2:231–242.
45. Stanley JS, King N, Burks AW, Huang SK, Sampson H, Cockrell G, Helm RM, West

CM, Bannon GA. Identification and mutational analysis of the immunodominant IgE binding epitopes of the major peanut allergen Ara h 2. Arch Biochem Biophys 1997; 342:244–253.

46. Smith AM, Chapman MD. Reduction in IgE binding to allergen variants generated by site-directed mutagenesis: Contribution of disulfide bonds to the antigenic structure of the major house dust mite allergen Der p 2. Mol Immunol 1996; 33:399–405.
47. Takai T, Yokota T, Yasue M, Nishiyama C, Yuuki T, Mori A, Okudaira H, Okumura Y. Engineering of the major house dust mite allergen Der f 2 for allergen-specific immunotherapy. Nat Biotechnol 1997; 15:754–758.
48. Schramm G, Kahlert H, Suck R, Weber B, Stuwe HT, Muller WD, Bufe A, Becker MW, Schlaak MW, Jager L, Cromwell O, Fiebig H. ''Allergen engineering'': Variants of the timothy grass pollen allergen Phl p 5b with reduced IgE-binding capacity but conserved T cell reactivity. Immunology 1999; 162:2406–2414.
49. Tighe H, Corr M, Roman M, Raz E. Gene vaccination: Plasmid DNA is more than just a blueprint. Immunol Today 1998; 19:89–97.
50. Yamamoto T, Yamamoto S, Katakota T, Komura K, Kohase M, Tokungaga T. Synthetic oligonucleotides with certain palindromic sequences stimulate interferon production of human peripheral blood lymphocytes in vitro. Jpn J Cancer Res 1994; 85:775–779.
51. Krieg AM, Yi AM, Matson S, Waldschmidt TJ, Bishop GA, Teasdale R, Koretsky GA, Klinsman DM. CpG motifs in bacterial DNA trigger direct B cell activation. Nature 1995; 374:546–549.
52. Halpern MD, Kurlander RJ, Pisetsky DS. Bacterial DNA induces murine interferon-gamma production by stimulation of interleukin-12 and tumor necrosis factor-alpha. Cell Immunol 1996; 167:72–78.
53. Klinsman DM, Yi AK, Beaucage SL, Conover J, Krieg AM. CpG motifs present in bacterial DNA rapidly induce lymphocytes to secrete interleukin 6, interleukin 12 and interferon-γ. Proc Natl Acad Sci USA 1996; 93:2879–2883.
54. Kline JN, Waldschmidt TJ Businga TR, Lemish JE, Weinstock JV, Thorne PS, Krieg AM. Modulation of airway inflammation by CpG oligodeoxynucleotides in a murine model of asthma. J Immunol 1998; 160:2555–2559.
55. Broide D, Schwarze J, Tighe H, Gifford T, Nguyen M-D, Malek S, van Uden J, Gelfand E, Raz E. Immunostimulatory DNA sequences inhibit IL-5, eosinophilic inflammation and airway hyperresponsiveness in mice. J Immunol 1998; 161:7054–7062.
56. Hsu CH, Chua KY, Tao MH, Huang SK, Hsieh KH. Inhibition of specific IgE response in vivo by allergen-gene transfer. Int Immunol 1996; 8:1405–1411.
57. Hsu CH, Chua KY, Tao MH, Lai YL, Wu HD, Huang SK, Hsieh KH. Immunoprophylaxis of allergen-induced immunoglobulin E synthesis and airway hyperresponsiveness in vivo by genetic immunization. Nat Med 1996; 2:540–544.
58. Li XM, Chopra RK, Chou TY, Schofield BH, Wills-Karp M, Huang SK. Mucosal IFN-gamma gene transfer inhibits pulmonary allergic responses in mice. J Immunol 1996; 157:3216–3219.
59. Li X, Huang CK, Schofield BH, Burks AW, Bannon GA, Kim KH, Huang SK,

Sampson HA. Strain-dependent induction of allergic sensitization caused by peanut allergen DNA immunization in mice. J Immunol 1999; 162:3045–3052.

60. Jorgensen JL, Reay PA, Ehrich EW, Davis MM. Molecular components of T-cell recognition. Annu Rev Immunol 1992; 10:835–873.
61. Schwartz RH. Costimulation of T lymphocytes: The role of CD28, CTLA-4, and B7/BB1 in interleukin-2 production and immunotherapy. Cell 1992; 71:1065–1068.
62. Larché M, Till SJ, Haselden B-M, North J, Barkans J, Kay AB, Robinson DS. Costimulation through CD86 is involved in airway presenting cell and T cell responses to allergen in atopic asthmatics. J Immunol 1998; 161:6375–6382.
63. Schwartz RH. T cell clonal anergy. Curr Opin Immunol 1997; 9:351–357.
64. Lamb JR, Skidmore BJ, Green N, Chiller JM, Feldmann M. Induction of tolerance in influenza virus-immune T lymphocyte clones with synthetic peptides of influenza hemagglutinin. J Exp Med 1983; 157:1434–1447.
65. Briner TJ, Kuo MC, Keating KM, Rogers BL, Greenstein JL. Peripheral T-cell tolerance induced in naive and primed mice by subcutaneous injection of peptides from the major cat allergen Fel d I. Proc Natl Acad Sci USA 1993; 90:7608–7612.
66. Hoyne GF, O'Hehir RE, Wraith DC, Thomas WR, Lamb JR. Inhibition of T cell and antibody responses to house dust mite allergen by inhalation of the dominant T cell epitope in naive and sensitized mice. J Exp Med 1993; 178:1783–1788.
67. O'Hehir RE, Garman RD, Greenstein JL, Lamb JR. The specificity and regulation of T-cell responsiveness to allergens. Annu Rev Immunol 1991; 9:67–95.
68. Higgins JA, Lamb JR, Marsh SG, Tonks S, Hayball JD, Rosen-Bronson S, Bodmer JG, O'Hehir RE. Peptide-induced nonresponsiveness of HLA-DP restricted human T cells reactive with Dermatophagoides spp. (house dust mite). J Allergy Clin Immunol 1992; 90:749–756.
69. Norman PS, Ohman JL Jr, Long AA, Creticos PS, Gefter MA, Shaked Z, Wood RA, Eggleston PA, Hafner KB, Rao P, Lichtenstein LM, Jones NH, Nicodemus CF. Treatment of cat allergy with T-cell reactive peptides. Am J Respir Crit Care Med 1996; 154:1623–1628.
70. Marcotte GV, Braun CM, Norman PS, Nicodemus CF, Kagey-Sobotka A, Lichtenstein LM, Essayan DM. Effects of peptide therapy on ex vivo T-cell responses. J Allergy Clin Immunol 1998; 101:506–513.
71. Pène J, Desroches A, Paradis L, Lebel B, Farce M, Nicodemus CF, Yssel H, Bousquet J. Immunotherapy with Fel d 1 peptides decreases IL-4 release by peripheral blood T cells of patients allergic to cats. J Allergy Clin Immunol 1998; 102:571–578.
72. Simons FE, Imada M, Li Y, Watson WT, HayGlass KT. Fel d 1 peptides: Effect on skin tests and cytokine synthesis in cat-allergic human subjects. Int Immunol 1996; 8:1937–1945.
73. Maguire P, Nicodemus C, Robinson D, Aaronson D, Umetsu DT. The safety and efficacy of ALLER VAX CAT in cat allergic patients. Clin Immunol 1999; 93:222–231.
74. Muller U, Akdis CA, Fricker M, Akdis M, Blesken T, Bettens F, Blaser K. Successful immunotherapy with T-cell epitope peptides of bee venom phospholipase A2

induces specific T-cell anergy in patients allergic to bee venom. J Allergy Clin Immunol 1998; 101:747–754.

75. Haselden BM, Kay AB, Larché M. IgE-independent MHC-restricted T cell peptide epitope-induced late asthmatic reactions. J Exp Med 1999; 189:1885–1894.
76. Texier C, Pouvelle S, Busson M, Herve M, Charron D, Menez A, Maillere B. HLA-DR restricted peptide candidates for bee venom immunotherapy. J Immunol 2000; 164:3177–3184.
77. Weiner HL, Inobe J, Kuchroo V, Chen Y. Induction and characterisation of TGFβ secreting Th3 cells. FASEB J 1996; 10:A1444.
78. Powrie F, Carlino J, Leach MW, Mauze S, Coffman RL. A critical role for transforming growth factor-β but not IL-4 in the suppression of T helper type 1-mediated colitis by CD45RB(low) CD4+ T cells. J Exp Med 1996; 183:2669–2674.
79. Bridoux F, Badou A, Saoudi A, Bernard I, Druet E, Pasquier R, Druet P, Pelletier L. Transforming growth factor beta (TGF-beta)-dependent inhibition of T helper cell 2 (Th2)-induced autoimmunity by self-major histocompatibility complex (MHC) class II-specific, regulatory CD4(+) T cell lines. J Exp Med 1997; 185: 1769–1775.
80. Davies JD, Leong LYW, Mellor A, Cobbold SP, Waldmann H. T cell suppression in transplantation tolerance through linked suppression. J Immunol 1996; 156:3602–3607.
81. Lombardi G, Sidhu S, Batchelor R, Lechler R. Anergic T cells as suppressor cells in vitro. Science 1994; 264:1587–1589.
82. Chen Y, Kuchroo VK, Inobe J, Hafler DA, Weiner HL. Regulatory T cell clones induced by oral tolerance: Suppression of autoimmune encephalomyelitis. Science 1994; 265:1237–1240.
83. Gaur A, Wiers B, Liu A, Rothbard J, Fathman GC. Amelioration of experimental autoimmune encephalomyelitis by myelin basic protein synthetic peptide-induced anergy. Science 1992; 258:1491–1494.
84. Ku G, Kronenberg M, Peacock DJ, Banquerigo ML, Braun BS, Reeve JR, Brahn E. Prevention of experimental autoimmune arthritis with a peptide fragment of type II collagen. Eur J Immunol 1993; 23:591–599.
85. Vaysburd M, Lock C, McDevitt H. Prevention of insulin-dependent diabetes mellitus in non-obese diabetic mice by immunogenic but not tolerated peptides. J Exp Med 1995; 182:897–902.
86. Staines NA, Harper N, Ward FJ, Malmstrom V, Holmdahl R, Bansal S. Mucosal tolerance and suppression of collagen-induced arthritis (CIA) induced by nasal inhalation of synthetic peptide 184–198 of bovine type II collagen (CII) expressing a dominant T cell epitope. Clin Exp Immunol 1996; 103:368–375.
87. Clayton JP, Gammon GM, Ando DG, Kono DH, Hood L, Sercarz EE. Peptide-specific prevention of experimental allergic encephalomyelitis. J Exp Med 1989; 169:1681–1691.
88. Hoyne GF, Jarnicki AG, Thomas WR, Lamb JR. Characterization of the specificity and duration of T cell tolerance to intranasally administered peptides in mice: A role for intramolecular epitope suppression. Int Immunol 1997; 9:1165–1173.

14

Glucocorticoid Effects on Mediator Modulation

T. K. LOKE, C. J. CORRIGAN, and TAK H. LEE

Guy's, King's and St. Thomas' School of Medicine
London, England

I. Introduction

Glucocorticoids play a vital role in the cellular functions and homeostatic mechanisms that govern normal physiological function. Synthetic analogs, which act via the glucocorticoid receptor, are able to mimic the actions of endogenous cortisol in controlling activation of genes that are important in inflammation. By understanding how glucocorticoids work to modulate the expression of inflammatory mediators known to be implicated in the asthmatic airway, it may be possible to provide more efficacious drugs to broaden the pharmacological options currently available for asthma and other allergic conditions.

II. Overview of Glucocorticoid Effects

Glucocorticoids are the most effective treatment currently available for reducing airway inflammation, bronchial hyperresponsiveness, and airway obstruction that occurs in asthma. The pluripotent effects of glucocorticoid therapy have been extensively studied and reviewed in the past decade (1–3). Nevertheless, the anti-inflammatory actions of glucocorticoids are still not fully understood. Glucocorticoids have long been known to increase the synthesis of anti-inflammatory proteins found in asthmatic airways. For instance, glucocorticoids upregulate the expression of lipocortin-1 in rat and human leukocytes (4). Lipocortin-1, an inhibitor of phospholipase A_2, has acute anti-inflammatory properties and has been shown to inhibit the production of lipid mediators such as leukotrienes, prostaglandins, and platelet-activating factor (PAF). Originally thought to be the predominant mode by which glucocorticoids exert their anti-inflammatory action, the importance of lipocortin-1 has since been superseded by other proteins due to its rather nonspecific effects as well as to doubts about the ability of glucocorticoids to induce lipoprotein-1 expression in some cells. Glucocorticoids are also capable of inducing other anti-inflammatory mediators, such as secretory leukocyte protease inhibitor (SLPI), macrophage migratory inhibitory factor (MIF), and interleukin-1 (IL-1) type II ''decoy'' receptor, the roles of which have been discussed elsewhere (5–7). These effects are often cell-specific and, in the case of MIF, are dependent on the concentrations of steroids within the relevant cell and tissue type. Nevertheless, these findings are not sufficient to explain the ability of glucocorticoids to reduce inflammation in a wide range of cells studied to date.

Most of the anti-inflammatory effects of glucocorticoids in asthma may be due to inhibition of inflammatory mediators elaborated by cells resident in and recruited to the bronchial mucosa and lumen. These mediators, known as cytokines, are produced by many types of cells and act on target cells to cause a wide array of cellular functions, including activation, proliferation, differentiation, and apoptosis (8,9). These proteins are characterized by a wide pleiotropy and redundancy of functions in that each cytokine has many overlapping functions, with each function potentially mediated by more than one cytokine. Some cytokines (e.g., IL-1, IL-2, IL-4) can promote and regulate their own expression as well as the expression of other proinflammatory mediators. Other cytokines known as chemokines have chemoattractant properties and are important for the recruitment of specific inflammatory cells to the sites where these chemokines are preferentially expressed. Thus cytokines and chemokines, by acting via their specific cellular receptors, can convey a variety of extracellular signals to neighboring cells and tissue, which makes them key messengers in orchestrating the inflammatory process within the bronchial mucosa and lumen.

Our current understanding of how glucocorticoids modulate the expression and concentrations of asthma-relevant cytokines and chemokines is mostly derived from in vitro experiments as well as from studies utilizing bronchial biopsies and bronchoalveolar lavage. Numerous studies have confirmed the ability of glucocorticoids to reduce the inflammatory infiltrate within the bronchial mucosa, local T-cell activation, and associated cytokine expression that is known to be upregulated in the asthmatic airway (10–14). Recently, the technique of sputum induction has provided a further tool to study noninvasively changes in mediator expression in subjects with mild to moderate asthma following glucocorticoid therapy (15). Glucocorticoids have also been shown to inhibit mediator release from alveolar macrophages and peripheral blood monocytes (16,17), eosinophils (18–20), and T lymphocytes in vitro. Elevated percentages of peripheral blood CD4-positive T lymphocytes from asthmatic patients expressed cytokine mRNA encoding IL-3, IL-5, and GM-CSF, which were downregulated following glucocorticoid therapy (21–23). The transcription of genes for IL-1β, TNF-α, GM-CSF, IL-2, IL-3, IL-4, IL-5, IL-6, and chemokines IL-8, RANTES, MCP-1, and MIP-1α is amenable to glucocorticoid inhibition, and mechanisms for these inhibitory effects are discussed below.

The epithelium is increasingly recognized as an important source of asthma-relevant cytokines and chemokines. In addition, epithelial cells express inducible nitric oxide synthase (iNOS), endothelin-1, prostaglandins (PGE_2 and $PGF_{2\alpha}$), growth factors such as transforming growth factor α (TGF-α), platelet-derived growth factor (PDGF), and insulin-like growth factor (IGF), which may contribute to airway inflammation. By altering the cellular response to normal growth and repair mechanisms these factors may also play a role in the process of airway remodeling. As glucocorticoids reduce local production of many of these mediators, it is tempting to speculate on the long-term effects of glucocorticoids in halting the decline in lung function. The data available on this, however, are controversial. Trigg et al. (24) demonstrated a significant reduction in type 3 collagen deposition in the subepithelial layer following short-term inhaled corticosteroid therapy. In contrast, Minshall et al. (25) could not show any improvement in the epithelial thickness and integrity in the upper airways of patients with allergic rhinitis following 1 year of treatment with topical steroids. This is despite evidence from in vitro studies for the inhibition of epithelial proinflammatory mediators by steroids (2,26).

The response of different types of cells to glucocorticoids with regard to production of cytokines and inflammatory mediators is diverse and is often determined by critical factors in the cellular environment. As a result, data from cell culture work and stimulation assays have not consistently reflected in vivo observations, which may, in part, be due to the different experimental conditions employed and the type of stimulus used as well as complex cell–cell interactions that are not present in these experimental models. These in vitro studies have nevertheless provided important insights into mechanisms by which glucocorticoids exert their anti-inflammatory action. The effects of glucocorticoids on cellular function, as applied to asthma and allergic conditions, are summarized below.

A. Glucocorticoid Effects on Monocytes and Macrophages

Macrophages are numerically the most abundant cells in the bronchial lumen of asthmatic and healthy individuals. They release a wide variety of inflammatory mediators, including enzymes (PAF, lysozyme, collagenase, and elastase), eicosanoids (leukotrienes LTB_4 and LTC_4), and growth factors. Release of such factors can be initiated by the cross-linking of surface IgE to both high- and low-affinity IgE Fc receptors on the surface of monocytes and macrophages, the numbers of which are increased in atopic asthmatic patients (27,28). Circumstantially, monocytes and alveolar macrophages would appear to be particularly suitable targets for glucocorticoid action. Indeed, glucocorticoids have been shown to reduce the production of arachidonic acid metabolites by alveolar macrophages (29) as well as the release of cytokines IL-1, TNF-α, and GM-CSF (30) and enzymes (collagenase and elastase) (31) in vitro. Glucocorticoids are also important in modulating the antigen-presenting activity of macrophages and monocytes. The enhanced capacity of alveolar macrophages, cultured in GM-CSF, to present antigen and thereby activate T lymphocytes is dependent on physiological levels of glucocorticoids being present in vitro (32). Glucocorticoids are also able to diminish markedly the number of circulating monocytes, especially those bearing IgE receptor (FCεRII) in blood.

B. Glucocorticoid Effects on Eosinophils

Eosinophil infiltration is a prominent feature of asthmatic airways. Allergen inhalation results in a marked increase in eosinophils in bronchoalveolar lavage (BAL) fluid at the time of the late reaction, and there is a relationship between peripheral blood eosinophilia and bronchial hyperresponsiveness. Eosinophils release a variety of membrane-derived mediators, including LTC_4 and PAF, and granule-associated proteins such as major basic protein and eosinophil cationic protein, which are toxic to airway epithelium. These mediators are suppressed by glucocorticoids in vivo (33–35). Eosinophils synthesize chemokines such as IL-8, MIP-1α (macrophage inflammatory protein), RANTES (regulated upon activation, normal T cell expressed and secreted), and MCP-1 (monocyte chemoattractant protein), which are inhibited by glucocorticoids (36). Eosinophils may also play a role in airway remodeling by producing fibrogenic cytokines such as IL-6, IL-11, and TGF-β (transforming growth factor beta).

Eosinophil production, differentiation, and survival are processes dependent on cytokines such as IL-3, IL-5, and GM-CSF. These cytokines, in particular IL-5, induce release of the eosinophils into the circulation in collaboration with eosinophil-active chemokines such as eotaxin. The production of eosinophils in the bone marrow and their subsequent migration to tissues are processes that are exquisitely sensitive to glucocorticoid suppression. These effects are presumably mediated by cytokines and chemokines, because eosinophil progenitor cells are not responsive to glucocorticoids directly (37). Treatment of asthmatic subjects with 2 weeks of prednisolone significantly reduced the number of activated eosinophils in the bronchial mucosa compared to placebo-treated patients. This effect was associated with inhibition of IL-3, IL-5, and GM-CSF production (14,38–40). IL-5 is the main cytokine involved in the development of eosinophilia in vivo (41,42). It is responsible for the terminal stages of eosinophil maturation and can also prolong eosinophil survival (43–45). IL-5 mRNA levels, as determined by in situ hybridization techniques, have been shown to be upregulated in the bronchial mucosa of asthmatic subjects, and the amounts of IL-5 mRNA have broadly correlated with the numbers of activated T cells and eosinophils in bronchial biopsy specimens from the same individuals (46). The ability of glucocorticoids to directly inhibit IL-5 synthesis (47) and suppress production of other eosinophil-active chemokines such as RANTES, MCP-3, MCP-4, and eotaxin (26,48) serves, in part, to explain the efficacy by which glucocorticoids inhibit eosinophil chemotaxis, activation, and release of eosinophil products (49).

C. Glucocorticoid Effects on Mast Cells and Basophils

Mast cells and basophils are the principal histamine-producing cells in atopic rhinitis and asthma. Histamine is stored in preformed granules, and its release is triggered by cross-linking of IgE to high-affinity FcεR1 receptors found on the surface of these cells. Mast cells and basophils also produce arachidonic acid metabolites such as LTC_4 in response to allergens and pharmacological and neurogenic stimuli. IL-4 production by these cells is thought to mediate IgE production by B cells and consequently the recruitment of eosinophils and lymphocytes to sites of its release. These cells therefore play a crucial role in initiating and perpetuating allergic inflammation and are therefore particularly relevant targets for mediator modulation.

The effects of glucocorticoids on mast cells and basophils appear to be heterogeneous. Several studies have shown that oral or inhaled glucocorticoids may reduce the numbers of mast cells in bronchial biopsies or BAL of asthmatic patients (50,51). Studies of allergic rhinitis, however, have not shown any effects on mast cell numbers in nasal biopsies even after 4 weeks of treatment (52,53). There is no evidence for the direct effect of glucocorticoids on the release of mediators by skin and airway mast cells in response to physiological stimuli in vitro, despite the fact that mast cells are a potential source of many cytokines (e.g., IL-4, IL-5, IL-6, TNF-α), proteases (chymase, tryptase), and other proinflammatory mediators (kinins, prostaglandins, leukotrienes). In contrast to this, basophils appear to be sensitive to glucocorticoid inhibition, and the number of circulating basophils is also reduced by glucocorticoid treatment (54,55).

D. Glucocorticoid Effects on T Lymphocytes

T lymphocytes are the main cells involved in orchestrating the inflammatory process in asthma (56). Activated $CD4^+$ T-cell subsets are characterized by their ability to produce specific cytokine profiles, which are crucial for the initiation and propagation of distinct immune effector mechanisms (57). At least two subsets have been described: Th1 cells, which produce IL-2 and IFN-γ, and Th2 cells, which produce IL-4 and IL-5. Both subsets produce IL-3 and GM-CSF. These two T-cell subsets are believed to be derived from a common precursor subtype (Th0), which produces both patterns of cytokines. The development of either a Th1 or Th2 pattern of cytokine synthesis by both murine and human T cells expanded in vitro is enhanced by IFN-γ or IL-4 in culture medium, respectively (58–61). These cells elaborate a whole host of cytokines and chemokines that are susceptible to glucocorticoid inhibition. Glucocorticoids are also effective at inhibiting T-cell proliferation, mainly by suppression of IL-2 synthesis (62,63). By altering the cytokine profile produced by Th1 and Th2 cell subsets through mechanisms that will be discussed later, glucocorticoids are able to attenuate and alter the nature of the ensuing inflammatory response. For example, treatment of asthmatic patients with glucocorticoids has been shown to downregulate expression of mRNA encoding Th2-derived cytokines (e.g., IL-5) but to upregulate expression of Th1-derived cytokines (e.g., IL-12 and IFNγ), which are themselves inhibitory to further Th2 T-cell functional differentiation.

E. Glucocorticoid Effects on Neutrophils

Contrary to the effects seen in other inflammatory cells, the number of neutrophils circulating in the peripheral circulation is increased following administration of exogenous glucocorticoids. This is partly due to decreased margination of neutrophils in the peripheral circulation but also to increased recruitment of neutrophils from the bone marrow. In vitro glucocorticoid treatment is known to enhance the formation of neutrophil colonies (64). Whether neutrophils contribute directly to airway pathology in asthma is still rather unclear. Nevertheless, neutrophils are known to produce proteases, cytokines, lipid mediators, and reactive oxygen species that promote airway inflammation. Increased neutrophil numbers have been observed in the airways of patients with severe asthma, and concentrations of LTB_4, a potent neutrophil chemoattractant, have also been found to be increased in the BAL of patients with occupational asthma (65). Neutrophils are not particularly susceptible to the anti-inflammatory actions of glucocorticoids in vitro. GRβ (the transcriptionally inactive isoform of the glucocorticoid receptor), whose expression is increased in neutrophils, is postulated to play a role in this (66).

F. Glucocorticoid Effects on Epithelial Cells

The role of epithelial cells in promoting airway inflammation and contributing to structural changes in the airway lumen has become a topic of rigorous study in recent years. The epithelium is the first point of contact with the external environment and is therefore a particularly suitable target for modulation by pharmacological agents with anti-inflammatory and bronchodilating properties. Apart from providing a structural barrier to entry by external antigens, airway epithelial cells also produce a wide array of mediators, the homeostatic function of which is somehow disrupted in asthma, leading to a cascade of inflammatory events thought to contribute to airways remodeling.

In this regard, epithelial cells are the source of inducible cyclooxygenase and may produce the prostanoids PGE_2 and prostaglandin F2α ($PGF_{2\alpha}$) with opposing effects on bronchial smooth muscle tone. They also produce endothelin-1, a potent bronchoconstrictor, in response to stimulation by several cytokines including IL-1, IL-2, IL-6, and TNF-α (67). In addition, they produce inducible nitric oxide synthase (iNOS) in response to a variety of cytokines (68). Glucocorticoids have wide-ranging inhibitory effects on epithelial cells and reduce production by these cells of endothelin-1, metabolites of inducible cyclooxygenase, and nitric oxide.

In addition to these mediators, epithelial cells are capable of proinflammatory effects through the secretion of a broad representation of chemokines and growth factors. They are a potential source of a wide range of both CXC and CC chemokines, such as IL-8 and GROα (CXC chemokines) and MCP-4, RANTES, and eotaxin (CC chemokines). Potentially fibrogenic growth factors produced by the cells include TGF-β, platelet-derived growth factor (PDGF), and insulin growth factor (IGF). Glucocorticoids have been shown to inhibit the production of many of these mediators, including IL-1, IL-6, IL-8, TNF-α, GM-CSF, and RANTES. Finally, glucocorticoids reduce the expression of a variety of leukocyte adhesion molecules on epithelial cells, such as intracellular adhesion molecule-1 (ICAM-1) and vascular adhesion molecule-1 (VCAM-1) (69), which are important for the migration of neutrophils and eosinophils into the lumen of the airway (70). Further work on airway epithelial cells is required to ascertain whether glucocorticoids are capable of producing similar effects in vivo, based on current experimental observations.

G. Other Effects

Glucocorticoids may enhance cellular responses to β2 agonists in a number of ways. Glucocorticoids increase transcription of β2-adrenergic receptors in vitro (71) and prevent downregulation of β2-receptor transcription in response to chronic β2-agonist exposure (72). Glucocorticoids also reduce plasma exudation and increases in vascular permeability by inhibiting local production of vasoactive peptides, such as histamine, bradykinin, and prostaglandins. The half-life of these peptides is reduced due to increased degradation by neutral endopeptidases and angiotensin-converting enzyme. These enzymes are known to be induced by glucocorticoids (73).

III. The Glucocorticoid Receptor

The glucocorticoid receptor (GR) is a member of a superfamily of ligand-associated nuclear receptors, which includes the vitamin D3, thyroid hormone, and retinoid hormone receptors (74). The GR and other hormone receptors in this family are structurally organized into five homologous domains (see Fig. 1), each responsible for certain functions and each with different degrees of conservation within this family. These are

1. N-terminal/transactivation domain
2. DNA-binding domain
3. C-terminal/ligand-binding domain
4. GR dimerization region
5. Nuclear localization regions

The N-terminal domain is responsible for most of the transactivating activity and is the least conserved of all the domains. It is the immunogenetic site of the receptor and also possesses marked cell-type and promoter specificity. In contrast, the DNA-binding domain is the most highly conserved region of the receptor. This is a cysteine-rich 70 amino acid sequence that folds into two zinc finger motifs, each of them with a zinc atom tetrahedrally coordinated to four cysteine residues. The zinc finger structures confer high affinity of the GR to glucocorticoid response elements (GREs) on DNA promoter regions. The ligand-binding domain is located at the C-terminal end of the GR and is the next most conserved region of the receptor. This region binds the ligand in a hydrophobic pocket and participates in several other functions, including dimerization and hormone-dependent transcriptional activation. It is also the binding site of heat shock protein (HSP90), which is responsible in part for maintaining a GR conformation that facilitates glucocorticoid binding (75).

Cloning of the human GR has identified two isoforms, GRα and GRβ, that are generated as a result of alternative splicing of the GR primary transcript (76,77). The two isoforms are identical through to amino acid 727 but then diverge, with GRα having an additional 50 amino acids and GRβ having an addi-

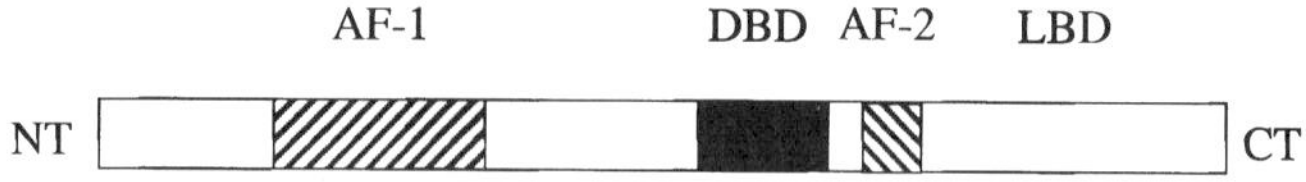

Figure 1 Functional domains of the glucocorticoid receptor. AF-1 and AF-2 = activating domains; CT = carboxy terminal; DBD = DNA-binding domain; LBD = ligand = binding domain; NT = amino terminal.

tional 15 nonhomologous amino acids. GRα is transcriptionally active, in contrast to GRβ, which is not capable of binding ligand or activating gene transcription. Although positive immunoreactivity for GRβ has been detected in various tissues and cell types, its functional significance is still unknown (77–81). Both isoforms are subjected to transcriptional regulation by glucocorticoids in vitro (82). Following incubation with dexamethasone (10^{-6} M), expression of mRNA for GRα and GRβ in human respiratory epithelial cells was decreased to 55% of control, and this effect was not abolished in the presence of cycloheximide, an inhibitor of protein synthesis.

In the absence of ligand, GR exists as oligomers in the cytoplasmic compartment, closely associated to a variety of coregulatory proteins such as HSP90, p60, p23 immunophilins, and calreticulin. These receptor chaperones, whose functions have only recently been appreciated, serve to regulate the steroid-binding and DNA-binding activities of GR (83). Upon associating with steroids, GR undergoes phosphorylation, dissociates from HSP90 molecules, and forms homodimers. Translocation to the nucleus where it interacts with DNA at GRE sites proceeds in a temperature-dependent fashion (84).

The stability of the GR complexes is affected by various factors. Activation and degradation of GR in vitro is inhibited by molybdate (85) and stabilized by phosphorylated sugars. GR levels vary throughout the cell cycle and are dependent on the presence and absence of glucocorticoids (82) and heat shock proteins (86). Like other steroid hormone receptors, GR undergoes cell cycle-dependent and hormone-dependent phosphorylation (87). Phosphorylation sites occur exclusively in the N-terminal domain and mainly within the transactivation region corresponding to AF-1 (see Fig. 1). GR phosphorylation is thought to play an important role in altering cellular responsiveness to glucocorticoids during the cell cycle. Cell cycle changes have long been known to affect cell sensitivity to glucocorticoids. For example, HeLa cells, mitogen- and antigen-stimulated human peripheral lymphocytes, and rat lymph node cells exhibit a substantial increase in GR hormone binding sites per cell during the S phase compared to the G1 phase (88–90). In addition, transcription of endogenous metallothionein-1 gene is resistant to induction by glucocorticoids in murine L cell fibroblasts arrested in G2 phase (91). Work on other cell lines has shown that GR exists in a hyperphosphorylated state during the G2/M phase, in contrast to the hypophosphorylated stage in the S phase (87,92). Hormone-induced hyperphosphorylation, which normally occurs in the S phase, fails to occur in the G2/M phase, suggesting that variations in the basal phosphorylated states of GR regulate GR sensitivity to glucocorticoids. Moreover, changes in the basal phosphorylated state of GR as cells progress from the S to G2/M phase may be responsible for determining the differential effects of glucocorticoids during different stages of the cell cycle.

IV. The Effects of Glucocorticoids on Gene Transcription

The glucocorticoid receptor regulates the transcription of target genes by binding to specific elements of DNA following ligand-activated nuclear translocation. Glucocorticoid response elements (GREs) have been found in the promoter regions in many genes implicated in asthma (93). Most GREs comprise palindromic sequences, composed of 6 bp half-sites separated by a 3 bp spacer. Binding of GR dimers to this sequence usually results in promoter enhancement. Although this prototypical model of GR action is well established, accumulating evidence in the past decade regarding the interactions of GR with other transcription factors (94) and coactivators (95) has questioned the necessity of DNA binding for its transcriptional regulation and served to highlight the complexity of interplay between transcription factors at the DNA level in modulating mediator expression. In this section we summarize the current models by which glucocorticoids, through interaction with their receptor GR, control expression of asthma-relevant cytokines and chemokines.

The transcription factors activator protein-1 (AP-1) and nuclear factor kappa B (NFκB) upregulate a whole host of inflammatory genes implicated in asthma (see Fig. 2). Activation of gene transcription usually follows binding of these transcription factors to their DNA consensus sites upstream to the transcription initiation sites. Glucocorticoids are known to downregulate expression of asthma-relevant cytokines and chemokines by interfering with binding of these transcription factors to cognate DNA binding sites. An "nGRE" model has been proposed to account for transcriptional hindrance of these nuclear factors mediated by GR, which can occur without binding of GR to DNA. This is believed to involve protein–protein interactions that may induce conformational changes in DNA binding sites. Alternatively, binding of GR and other coregulatory molecules recruited to the transcriptional machinery may result in critical alterations in the DNA binding affinities of the GR complex and of other nuclear factors. The overall effect can be either transcriptional inhibition (or transrepression) of the gene involved, i.e., if GR is able to outcompete other nuclear factors for DNA binding, or transactivation, if the opposite is true. Such a "competitive nGRE" model may explain the mutuality of effect that is seen in GR-mediated repression of both AP-1- and NFκB-dependent transcription. Not only is GR capable of repressing AP-1- and NFκB-dependent transcription, but AP-1 and NFκB may also repress GR-dependent transcription (96–98). Direct interactions between GR and AP-1 (98) as well as between GR and NFκB (99,100) have been observed and support the hypothesis that GR-mediated transrepression of genes induced by various stimuli proceeds via steric interactions with other nuclear factors. The strength of DNA binding for each of these transcription factors, including GR, may be regulated by the local environment in the transcription complex and the presence and absence of coregulatory molecules that either stabilize or destabilize

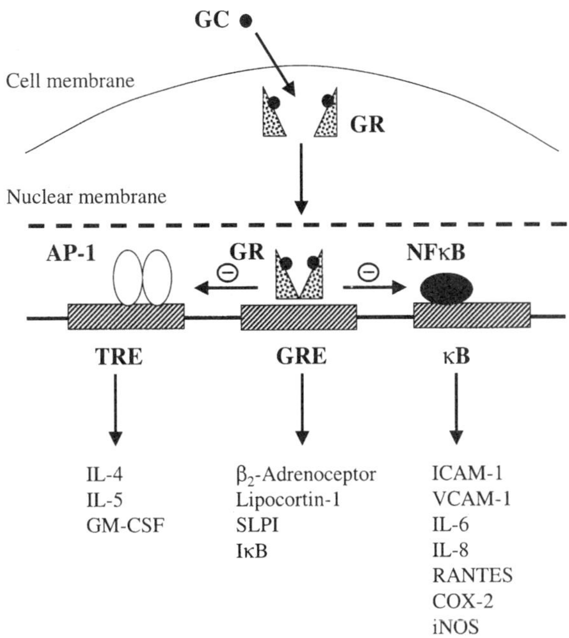

Figure 2 Schematic diagram of the molecular interactions of GR with other transcription factors (AP-1 and NFκB). GRE = glucocorticoid response element; κB = κB motifs for NFκB DNA binding; TRE = TPA response element.

DNA contacts in this environment as well as the extent of chromatin packing that can determine the accessibility of relevant transcription factors to cognate DNA sites. In any given case, it is likely that a combination of these mechanisms will be involved in determining the levels of gene expression of asthmatic mediators, at least at a transcriptional level.

The ability of GR to inhibit transcription of inflammatory genes is also influenced by other regulatory nuclear proteins. Of these, CREB binding protein (CBP) and its functional analog (p300) have attracted much attention (101). These proteins are capable of binding to and coactivating with many activators, including CREB, AP-1, NFκB, and STATs as well as GR and other steroid hormone receptors (100,102,103). CBP and p300 also possess histone acetyl transferase (HAT) activity, which facilitates chromatin unfolding and allows greater access of RNA polymerase II to transcription sites. CBP and other GR-associated coactivators (95) interact with GR in a ligand-dependent manner and are able to enhance transcriptional activity by the receptor through histone acetylation. Histone deacetylase (HDAC) activity also appears to be an intrinsic property of GR and other nuclear hormone receptors. Recruitment of histone deacetylases to the promoters of inflammatory genes may result in loss of acetyl groups from core histone proteins, leading to transcriptional silencing. The balance of HAT/HDAC activity associated with the multimeric GR complex may therefore dictate the overall effect of GR on gene transcription. In other words, high HAT/HDAC activity can be expected to result in increased transcriptional activity; conversely, low HAT/HDAC activity would lead to enhanced repression of the gene. Manipulation of HAT/HDAC activity associated with GR may thus provide a novel mechanism for regulating the transcriptional effects of glucocorticoids.

Transcription interference through interactions of GR with other transcription factors and activators has only partly explained some of the in vitro and in vivo effects associated with downregulation of proinflammatory genes. For example, IL-1β-induced upregulation of COX-2 protein in A549 epithelial cells is downregulated by dexamethasone, despite high mRNA levels of COX-2 at relevant time points (104). Similar dexamethasone-dependent effects have been reported for IL-1β, GM-CSF, IL-6, IL-8, IFN-γ, and iNOS in various other types of cells. Activation of GM-CSF promoter constructs in human T cells is not inhibited by dexamethasone, despite clear downregulation of GM-CSF protein expression in these cells. A possible mechanism for this effect may involve GR-mediated induction of mediators that sequester or inactivate transcription factors. One such example involves upregulation of the cytoplasmic NFκB inhibitor IκBα that prevents nuclear translocation and DNA binding by retention of NFκB heterodimers in the cytoplasm. Glucocorticoids also enhance phosphorylation of JUN N-terminal kinase (JNK), a crucial step in the phosphorylation of c-jun, which is important for constitutive AP-1 activity. Post-transcriptional mechanisms may also contribute to GR-mediated inhibition of cytokine production. In the case of GM-CSF, this may involve destabilization of newly transcribed mRNA. It has been demonstrated that the 3[1]-untranslated region of GM-CSF mRNA contains a number of repeated AU-rich motives that play a part in mRNA destabilizing and translational blockage (105,106). Protein binding to these regions can mediate selective mRNA degradation, providing another possible method by which levels of mRNA in cells can be regulated.

Finally, glucocorticoid-induced cell apoptosis is believed to be mediated by transcriptional control. Inhibition of T-cell proliferation by glucocorticoids involves blocking cell cycle progression at G0/G1, possibly by induction of cell cycle genes such as G1 progressive factor and cyclin D3 (107). Activation-induced cell death (AICD), however, may require new protein synthesis, regulated at the transcription level. It is interesting to note that transgenic mice with defects in GR dimerization are able to survive to full term and are apparently healthy, implicating functions that are independent of GR DNA binding in normal physiological processes. However, thymocytes from these $GR_{DIM\text{-}DIM}$ mice display resistance to dexamethasone-induced apoptosis, which suggests a crucial role for glucocorticoids in regulating cellular proliferation in the context of the inflammatory process (108,109).

V. Mechanisms of Glucocorticoid Resistance in Asthma

Although the majority of asthma sufferers show improvement in lung function indices following treatment with glucocorticoids, a subgroup of patients do not respond despite being treated with high-dose systemic steroids. These patients, whose asthma tends to be severe, provide a valuable insight into the mechanisms of glucocorticoid action. Glucocorticoid (GC) resistance is not limited to asthma and is a feature of other inflammatory diseases such as Crohn's disease, rheumatoid arthritis, and other autoimmune disorders (110–113). GC resistance has also been described in several species of New World primates (114). These animals have high plasma-free cortisol concentrations with low-affinity glucocorticoid receptors despite being apparently healthy. Thus, GC resistance represents a heterogeneous syndrome with different etiologies, the causes of which have important implications for biology and medicine in a wider sense.

Glucocorticoid responsiveness is probably a continuous spectrum, with individuals who demonstrate GC resistance falling at one end of the unimodal distribution. We have defined GC resistance as failure of an asthmatic patient to improve the forced expiratory volume at 1 second (FEV_1) by 15% after an adequate course of steroids (40 mg/day oral prednisolone for 2 weeks) despite showing clear reversibility (>15%) to β2 agonists. This is in contrast to GC-sensitive individuals, who show an improvement of >30% in FEV_1 measurements after an equivalent course of steroids. These definitions reflect polar extremes of the dose–response curve but are important to allow valid comparisons of both subgroups to be made for research purposes.

The mechanism of GC resistance is poorly understood. Studies in our department have shown that GC-resistant asthmatic patients show no abnormalities of GC metabolism or the hypothalmic-pituitary-adrenal (HPA) axis (115) and no molecular abnormalities of the glucocorticoid receptor (116–118). Freshly isolated peripheral blood mononuclear cells (PBMCs) from GC-resistant and GC-sensitive asthmatic individuals showed no significant differences in the proportion of T-cell subsets, monocytes, and B lymphocytes (119). GC resistance, however, is associated with impaired in vitro and in vivo responsiveness of PBMCs to the suppressive effect of glucocorticoids (115,120–124). This phenomenon of "proinflammatory" GC resistance is phenotypically and biochemically distinct from the rare syndrome of primary cortisol resistance, which results in end organ glucocorticoid resistance secondary to sequence abnormalities of the GR. In particular, peripheral T lymphocytes from GC-resistant individuals show an increased activation status as measured by elevated expression of CD25

(IL-2 receptor) and HLA-DR activation antigens on these cells. Leung et al. (125) also examined bronchoalveolar lavage (BAL) airway cells from GC-sensitive and GC-resistant asthmatic subjects. They found that baseline BAL cells from GC-resistant patients had significantly higher numbers of cells expressing mRNA for IL-2 and IL-4 compared to BAL cells from GC-sensitive patients. However, no significant differences were observed in the expression of IL-5 mRNA between these two patient populations. Following a 1 week course of prednisolone (40 mg/day), there was a significant decrease in cells expressing IL-4 mRNA and IL-5 mRNA in BAL cells from GC-sensitive patients, an effect that was not observed in GC-resistant patients. These findings suggest that GC resistance may be a primary phenomenon or a phenomenon associated with increased immune activation of immunoregulatory cells in the airways and blood of GC-resistant individuals. Kam et al. (126) found that incubation of PBMCs from normal subjects with a combination of IL-2 and IL-4 was able to reduce glucocorticoid responsiveness of T cells, an effect that was reversible upon incubating in medium alone, and not a result of changes in the proportion of CD4:CD8 lymphocyte subsets.

Glucocorticoid resistance is not cell-specific. Wilkinson et al. (123) showed that monocyte-primed supernatants from asthmatic subjects secrete a 3 kDa peptide that is proinflammatory in vitro for neutrophils and eosinophils. This activity is inhibited in a dose–response and rank-order fashion by hydrocortisone, methylprednisolone, and dexamethasone in GC-sensitive asthmatic subjects but to a lesser extent in GC-resistant asthmatic subjects (117). Sousa et al. (127) provided evidence for an in vivo defect in the responsiveness of the macrophage–T cell interaction to the suppressive effects of glucocorticoids in GC-resistant asthma. We used the classical tuberculin cutaneous delayed hypersensitivity immune response to investigate in vivo defects in mononuclear cell function in nine GC-resistant and six GC-sensitive asthmatic subjects who demonstrated sensitivity to intradermal purified protein derivative (PPD) of *Mycobacterium tuberculosis*. In a double-blind, crossover, placebo-controlled study, patients were given oral prednisolone or placebo starting on day 0 and a predetermined intradermal dose of PPD on day 7, and on day 9 the site of the induration was measured and biopsied for immunohistochemical analysis. There was no difference in skin induration between the GC-sensitive and GC-resistant groups during the placebo limb of the study ($p = 0.38$). Prednisolone significantly suppressed the cutaneous induration ($p < 0.003$) in the GC-sensitive group but not in the GC-resistant group. Compared to placebo, there was suppression by prednisolone of the number of macrophages ($p = 0.018$), eosinophils ($p = 0.009$), and T memory cells ($p = 0.009$) in the GC-sensitive group but not in the GC-resistant group. There was no significant suppression by prednisolone in the number of neutrophils or monocytes or immature macrophages in either group. There was no difference in intercellular adhesion molecule-1 (ICAM-1), vascular cell adhesion molecule-

1 (VCAM-1), or endothelial leukocyte adhesion molecule-1 (ELAM-1) expression in blood vessels or epidermis between the GC-sensitive and GC-resistant groups, with no suppression by prednisolone in either group. These findings suggest a generalized in vivo defect in the responsiveness of cellular immune mechanisms to the suppressive effects of glucocorticoids in GC-resistant asthma. The differential suppressive effects of glucocorticoids on cellular recruitment in the PPD response between the GC-sensitive and GC-resistant individuals are not due to modulation of expression of endothelial adhesion molecules. More recently, we also showed that the GRβ isoform of the glucocorticoid receptor is significantly elevated in PPD indurated skin biopsies from these GC-resistant patients, compared to GC-sensitive patients, and that prednisolone treatment resulted in a significant alteration in the proportion of GRα:GRβ isoforms colocalized to the same cells in GC-sensitive patients, which was unaltered in the GC-resistant subgroup (128). Expression of GRβ in neutrophils, known to be relatively unresponsive to glucocorticoids, was found to be significantly higher than in PBMCs, and this was increased following stimulation with IL-8 (66,129,130). Brown et al. (131) also showed that the cutaneous vasoconstrictor responses in asthmatic subjects correlated with the airways response to oral glucocorticoids, further emphasizing the possibility that GC resistance may be a more generalized phenomenon.

VI. Molecular Basis of Glucocorticoid-Resistant Asthma

Although our understanding of glucocorticoid receptor interactions with DNA has increased significantly in recent years, the mechanisms by which glucocorticoids fail to inhibit cellular activation and cytokine production are still far from clear. We have implicated abnormal regulation of the AP-1 in the molecular mechanism of GC resistance, a phenomenon that may be confined to T cells and monocytes (see Fig. 3). Previous studies in our department showed that glucocorticoid-exposed PBMCs from GC-resistant asthmatic individuals have fewer activated glucocorticoid receptors available for DNA binding than those from GC-sensitive asthmatic subjects (132) but elevated DNA binding of AP-1 following phorbol ester stimulation (133). These cells also demonstrate significantly elevated basal, as well as phorbol ester-stimulated, transcription and translation of c-fos. Furthermore, phorbol ester stimulation of cells from GC-sensitive patients induced a GC-resistant phenotype that was associated with direct interaction between the activated glucocorticoid receptor (GR) and c-fos, detected by coimmunoprecipitation (134). Binding of GR to other transcription factors activated in inflammation (e.g., CREB and NFκB) was unaffected. Our interpretation of these data is that mononuclear cells from GC-resistant asthmatic patients inappropriately overexpress AP-1, which sequesters and neutralizes activated GR, thus causing refractoriness to glucocorticoid-induced inhibitory responses.

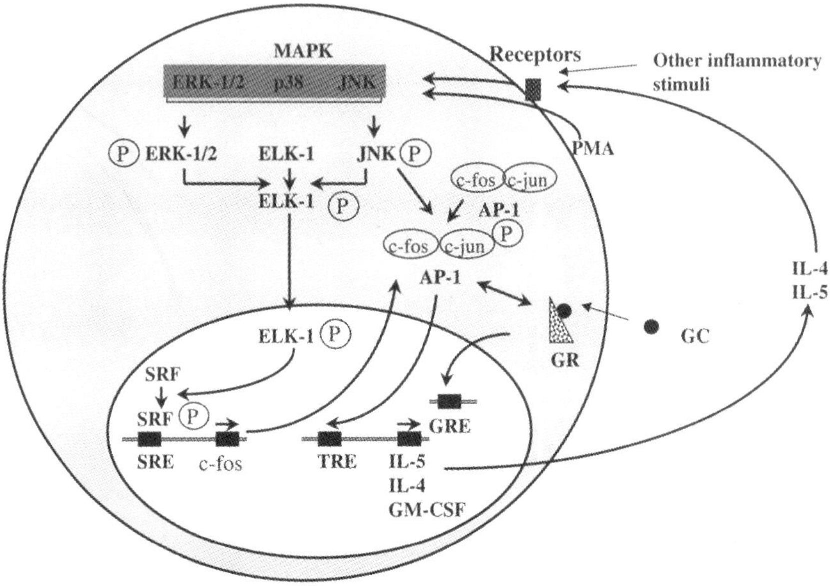

Figure 3 Pathways for activation of AP-1. ERK = extracellular signal-regulated kinases; JNK = Jun amino-terminal kinases; MAPK = mitogen-activated protein kinases; P = phosphate moiety; PMA = phorbol 12-myristate 13-acetate; SRE = serum response element; SRF = serum response factor.

Higher protein levels of GRβ have been found in other GC-resistant states (128,135), which supports a role for GRβ in GC resistance. It is possible that GRα-mediated transactivation of glucocorticoid target genes may be inhibited by GRβ via several mechanisms. These may involve competitive interactions between GRα and GRβ for GRE-binding sites. Another possibility is that GRβ may attenuate GRα-mediated gene transrepression by mechanisms that may not require DNA binding (squelching). Alternatively, interaction of GRβ with other coregulatory proteins that are normally associated with GRα may result in loss of transactivating functions for the latter. Further work directed at GRα–GRβ interactions will need to be done before these issues can be resolved.

VII. Summary

Despite the development of more selective anti-inflammatory therapies for asthma, glucocorticoids (GCs) remain the most effective treatment for this condition. The ability of GCs to act at many levels in preventing cellular activation and expression of important mediators underscores its effectiveness as an anti-inflammatory agent.

In the past decade, our understanding of interactions between GR and other nuclear factors (such as AP-1 and NFκB) as well as coregulatory molecules that modulate expression of proinflammatory genes has increased dramatically. Enhanced immune activation, as reflected by overexpression of AP-1 in GC-resistant asthmatic subjects, may explain the poor response of these individuals to the therapeutic effects of GCs. Further work targeting transcriptional regulation of these genes, using specific transcription inhibitors, may provide novel pharmacological options for modulating the immune processes that occur in asthma and other inflammatory conditions.

References

1. Lane SJ, Lee TH. Corticosteroids: Chemistry and mode of action. In: Leff AR, Hefta J, McCurdy, Stanley C, eds. Pulmonary Pharmacology and Therapeutics. New York: McGraw-Hill, 1996:553–560.
2. Schwiebert LM, Beck LA, Stellato C, Bickel CA, Bochner BS, Schleimer RP, Schwiebert LA. Glucocorticosteroid inhibition of cytokine production: Relevance to antiallergic actions. J Allergy Clin Immunol 1996; 97(1 pt 2):143–152.
3. Barnes PJ. Inhaled glucocorticoids for asthma. N Engl J Med 1995; 332(13):868–875.
4. Flower RJ, Rothwell NJ. Lipocortin-1: Cellular mechanisms and clinical relevance. Trends Pharmacol Sci 1994; 15(3):71–76.
5. Abbinante-Nissen JM, Simpson LG, Leikauf GD. Corticosteroids increase secretory leukocyte protease inhibitor transcript levels in airway epithelial cells. Am J Physiol 1995; 268(4 pt 1):L601–L606.
6. Calandra T, Bernhagen J, Metz CN, Spiegel LA, Bacher M, Donnelly T, Cerami A, Bucala R. MIF as a glucocorticoid-induced modulator of cytokine production. Nature 1995; 377(6544):68–71.
7. Re F, Muzio M, De Rossi M, Polentarutti N, Giri JG, Mantovani A, Colotta F. The type II "receptor" as a decoy target for interleukin 1 in polymorphonuclear leukocytes: Characterization of induction by dexamethasone and ligand binding properties of the released decoy receptor. J Exp Med 1994; 179(2):739–743.
8. Chung KF, Barnes PJ. Cytokines in asthma. Thorax 1999; 54(9):825–857.
9. Lane SJ, Sousa AR, Cousins DJ, Staynov DZ, Lee TH. Topical Glucocorticoids in Asthma: Mechanisms and Clinical Actions. Longboat Key, FL: Marcel Dekker, 1994:309–347.
10. Robinson DS, Ying S, Bentley AM, Meng Q, North J, Durham SR, Kay AB, Hamid Q. Relationships among numbers of bronchoalveolar lavage cells expressing messenger ribonucleic acid for cytokines, asthma symptoms, and airway methacholine responsiveness in atopic asthma. J Allergy Clin Immunol 1993; 92(3):397–403.

11. Lundgren R, Soderberg M, Horstedt P, Stenling R. Morphological studies of bronchial mucosal biopsies from asthmatics before and after ten years of treatment with inhaled steroids. Eur Respir J 1988; 1(10):883–889.
12. Duddridge M, Ward C, Hendrick DJ, Walters EH. Changes in bronchoalveolar lavage inflammatory cells in asthmatic patients treated with high dose inhaled beclomethasone dipropionate. Eur Respir J 1993; 6(4):489–497.
13. Djukanovic R, Wilson JW, Britten KM, Wilson SJ, Walls AF, Roche WR, Howarth PH, Holgate ST. Effect of an inhaled corticosteroid on airway inflammation and symptoms in asthma. Am Rev Respir Dis 1992; 145(3):669–674.
14. Bentley AM, Hamid Q, Robinson DS, Schotman E, Meng Q, Assoufi B, Kay AB, Durham SR. Prednisolone treatment in asthma. Reduction in the numbers of eosinophils, T cells, tryptase-only positive mast cells, and modulation of IL-4, IL-5, and interferon-gamma cytokine gene expression within the bronchial mucosa. Am J Respir Crit Care Med 1996; 153(2):551–556.
15. Hargreave FE. Induced sputum and response to glucocorticoids. J Allergy Clin Immunol 1998; 102(5):S102–S105.
16. Berkman N, Jose PJ, Williams TJ, Schall TJ, Barnes PJ, Chung KF. Corticosteroid inhibition of macrophage inflammatory protein-1 alpha in human monocytes and alveolar macrophages. Am J Physiol 1995; 269(4 pt 1):L443–L452.
17. Linden M, Brattsand R. Effects of a corticosteroid, budesonide, on alveolar macrophage and blood monocyte secretion of cytokines: Differential sensitivity of GM-CSF, IL-1 beta, and IL-6. Pulm Pharmacol 1994; 7(1):43–47.
18. Sano A, Munoz NM, Sano H, Choi J, Zhu X, Jacobs B, Leff AR. Inhibition of cPLA2 translocation and leukotriene C4 secretion by fluticasone propionate in exogenously activated human eosinophils. Am J Respir Crit Care Med 1999; 159(6): 1903–1909.
19. Juan M, Mullol J, Roca-Ferrer J, Fuentes M, Perez M, Vilardell C, Yague J, Picado C. Regulation of ICAM-3 and other adhesion molecule expressions on eosinophils in vitro. Effects of dexamethasone. Allergy 1999; 54(12):1293–1298.
20. Miyamasu M, Misaki Y, Izumi S, Takaishi T, Morita Y, Nakamura H, Matsushima K, Kasahara T, Hirai K. Glucocorticoids inhibit chemokine generation by human eosinophils. J Allergy Clin Immunol 1998; 101(1 pt 1):75–83.
21. Corrigan CJ, Hamid Q, North J, Barkans J, Moqbel R, Durham S, Gemou-Engesaeth V, Kay AB. Peripheral blood CD4 but not CD8 T-lymphocytes in patients with exacerbation of asthma transcribe and translate messenger RNA encoding cytokines which prolong eosinophil survival in the context of a Th2-type pattern: Effect of glucocorticoid therapy. Am J Respir Cell Mol Biol 1995; 12(5):567–578.
22. Doi S, Gemou-Engesaeth V, Kay AB, Corrigan CJ. Polymerase chain reaction quantification of cytokine messenger RNA expression in peripheral blood mononuclear cells of patients with acute exacerbations of asthma: Effect of glucocorticoid therapy. Clin Exp Allergy 1994; 24(9):854–867.
23. Gemou-Engesaeth V, Bush A, Kay AB, Hamid Q, Corrigan CJ. Inhaled glucocorticoid therapy of childhood asthma is associated with reduced peripheral blood T cell activation and 'Th2-type' cytokine mRNA expression. Pediatrics 1997; 99(5): 695–703.

24. Trigg CJ, Manolitsas ND, Wang J, Calderon MA, McAulay A, Jordan SE, Herdman MJ, Jhalli N, Duddle JM, Hamilton SA. Placebo-controlled immunopathologic study of four months of inhaled corticosteroids in asthma. Am J Respir Crit Care Med 1994; 150(1):17–22.
25. Minshall E, Ghaffar O, Cameron L, O'Brien F, Quinn H, Rowe-Jones J, Davies RJ, Prior A, Lund VJ, Mackay IS, Nolop K, Lutsky B, Durham SR, Hamid Q. Assessment by nasal biopsy of long-term use of mometasone furoate aqueous nasal spray (Nasonex) in the treatment of perennial rhinitis. Otolaryngol Head Neck Surg 1998; 118(5):648–654.
26. Stellato C, Beck LA, Gorgone GA, Proud D, Schall TJ, Ono SJ, Lichtenstein LM, Schleimer RP. Expression of the chemokine RANTES by a human bronchial epithelial cell line. Modulation by cytokines and glucocorticoids. J Immunol 1995; 155(1):410–418.
27. Borish L, Mascali JJ, Rosenwasser LJ. IgE-dependent cytokine production by human peripheral blood mononuclear phagocytes. J Immunol 1991; 146(1):63–67.
28. Humbert M, Grant JA, Taborda-Barata L, Durham SR, Pfister R, Menz G, Barkans J, Ying S, Kay AB. High-affinity IgE receptor (FcepsilonRI)-bearing cells in bronchial biopsies from atopic and nonatopic asthma. Am J Respir Crit Care Med 1996; 153(6 pt 1):1931–1937.
29. Yoss EB, Spannhake EW, Flynn JT, Fish JE, Peters SP. Arachidonic acid metabolism in normal human alveolar macrophages: Stimulus specificity for mediator release and phospholipid metabolism, and pharmacologic modulation in vitro and in vivo. Am J Respir Cell Mol Biol 1990; 2(1):69–80.
30. Snyder DS, Unanue ER. Corticosteroids inhibit murine macrophage Ia expression and interleukin 1 production. J Immunol 1982; 129(5):1803–1805.
31. Werb Z. Biochemical actions of glucocorticoids on macrophages in culture. Specific inhibition of elastase, collagenase, and plasminogen activator secretion and effects on other metabolic functions. J Exp Med 1978; 147(6):1695–1712.
32. Caulfield JJ, Fernandez MH, Sousa AR, Lane SJ, Lee TH, Hawrylowicz CM. Regulation of major histocompatibility complex class II antigens on human alveolar macrophages by granulocyte-macrophage colony-stimulating factor in the presence of glucocorticoids. Immunology 1999; 98(1):104–110.
33. Robin JL, Seldin DC, Austen KF, Lewis RA. Regulation of mediator release from mouse bone marrow-derived mast cells by glucocorticoids. J Immunol 1985; 135(4):2719–2726.
34. Charlesworth EN, Kagey-Sobotka A, Schleimer RP, Norman PS, Lichtenstein LM. Prednisone inhibits the appearance of inflammatory mediators and the influx of eosinophils and basophils associated with the cutaneous late-phase response to allergen. J Immunol 1991; 146(2):671–676.
35. Scadding GK, Darby YC, Austin CE. Effect of short-term treatment with fluticasone propionate nasal spray on the response to nasal allergen challenge. Br J Clin Pharmacol 1994; 38(5):447–451.
36. Weller PF. Human eosinophils. J Allergy Clin Immunol 1997; 100(3):283–287.
37. Gleich GJ, Hunt LW, Bochner BS. Glucocorticoid effects on human eosinophils. In:

Schleimer RP, Busse WW, O'Byrne PM, eds. Topical Glucocorticoids in Asthma: Mechanisms and Clinical Actions. New York: Marcel Dekker, 1997:279.

38. Corrigan CJ, Hamid Q, North J, Barkans J, Moqbel R, Durham S, Gemou-Engesaeth V, Kay AB. Peripheral blood CD4 but not CD8 T-lymphocytes in patients with exacerbation of asthma transcribe and translate messenger RNA encoding cytokines which prolong eosinophil survival in the context of a Th2-type pattern: Effect of glucocorticoid therapy. Am J Respir Cell Mol Biol 1995; 12(5): 567–578.
39. Hallsworth MP, Litchfield TM, Lee TH. Glucocorticoids inhibit granulocyte-macrophage colony-stimulating factor-1 and interleukin-5 enhanced in vitro survival of human eosinophils. Immunology 1992; 75(2):382–385.
40. Lamas AM, Leon OG, Schleimer RP. Glucocorticoids inhibit eosinophil responses to granulocyte-macrophage colony-stimulating factor. J Immunol 1991; 147(1): 254–259.
41. Shi HZ, Xiao CQ, Zhong D, Qin SM, Liu Y, Liang GR, Xu H, Chen YQ, Long XM, Xie ZF. Effect of inhaled interleukin-5 on airway hyperreactivity and eosinophilia in asthmatics. Am J Respir Crit Care Med 1998; 157(1):204–209.
42. Venge J, Lampinen M, Hakansson L, Rak S, Venge P. Identification of IL-5 and RANTES as the major eosinophil chemoattractants in the asthmatic lung. J Allergy Clin Immunol 1996; 97(5):1110–1115.
43. Lopez AF, Sanderson CJ, Gamble JR, Campbell HD, Young IG, Vadas MA. Recombinant human interleukin 5 is a selective activator of human eosinophil function. J Exp Med 1988; 167(1):219–224.
44. Yamaguchi Y, Hayashi Y, Sugama Y, Miura Y, Kasahara T, Kitamura S, Torisu M, Mita S, Tominaga A, Takatsu K. Highly purified murine interleukin 5 (IL-5) stimulates eosinophil function and prolongs in vitro survival. IL-5 as an eosinophil chemotactic factor. J Exp Med 1988; 167(5):1737–1742.
45. Clutterbuck EJ, Hirst EM, Sanderson CJ. Human interleukin-5 (IL-5) regulates the production of eosinophils in human bone marrow cultures: Comparison and interaction with IL-1, IL-3, IL-6, and GMCSF. Blood 1989; 73(6):1504–1512.
46. Ying S, Humbert M, Barkans J, Corrigan CJ, Pfister R, Menz G, Larche M, Robinson DS, Durham SR, Kay AB. Expression of IL-4 and IL-5 mRNA and protein product by CD4+ and CD8+ T cells, eosinophils, and mast cells in bronchial biopsies obtained from atopic and nonatopic (intrinsic) asthmatics. J Immunol 1997; 158(7):3539–3544.
47. Mori A, Kaminuma O, Suko M, Inoue S, Ohmura T, Hoshino A, Asakura Y, Miyazawa K, Yokota T, Okumura Y, Ito K, Okudaira H. Two distinct pathways of interleukin-5 synthesis in allergen-specific human T-cell clones are suppressed by glucocorticoids. Blood 1997; 89(8):2891–2900.
48. Jahnsen FL, Haye R, Gran E, Brandtzaeg P, Johansen FE. Glucocorticosteroids inhibit mRNA expression for eotaxin, eotaxin-2, and monocyte-chemotactic protein-4 in human airway inflammation with eosinophilia. J Immunol 1999; 163(3):1545–1551.
49. Schleimer RP, Bochner BS. The effects of glucocorticoids on human eosinophils. J Allergy Clin Immunol 1994; 94(6 pt 2):1202–1213.
50. Adelroth E, Rosenhall L, Johansson SA. Inflammatory cells and eosinophilic activ-

ity in asthmatics investigated by bronchoalveolar lavage. The effects of antiasthmatic treatment with budesonide or terbutaline. Am Rev Respir Dis 1990; 142(1):91–99.

51. Laitinen LA, Laitinen A. A comparative study of the effects of an inhaled corticosteroid, budesonide, and a β2-agonist, terbutaline, on airway inflammation in newly diagnosed asthma: A randomised, double-blind, parallel-group controlled trial. J Allergy Clin Immunol 1992; 90(1):32–42.
52. Pipkorn U, Andersson P. Budesonide and nasal mucosal histamine content and anti-IgE induced histamine release. Allergy 1982; 37(8):591–595.
53. Spector SL, English G, Jones L. Clinical and nasal biopsy response to treatment of perennial rhinitis. J Allergy Clin Immunol 1980; 66(2):129–137.
54. Schleimer RP. Inhibition of basophil histamine release by anti-inflammatory steroids. Nature 1981; 292(5822):454–455.
55. Schleimer RP. The effects of glucocorticoids on mast cells and basophils. In: Schleimer RP, Claman HN, Oronsky A, eds. Anti-inflammatory Steroid Action: Basic and Clinical Aspects. San Diego: Academic Press, 1989:226.
56. Corrigan CJ. T and B lymphocytes and the development of allergic reactions. In: Kay AB, ed. Allergy and Allergic Diseases. Oxford, England: Blackwell Scientific, 1997:36–57.
57. Mosmann TR, Coffman RL. Th1 and Th2 cells: Different patterns of lymphokine secretion lead to different functional properties. Annu Rev Immunol 1989; 7:145–173.
58. Coffman RL, Varkila K, Scott P, Chatelain R. Role of cytokines in the differentiation of CD4+ T-cell subsets in vivo. Immunol Rev 1991; 123:189–207.
59. Swain SL, Weinberg AD, English M, Huston G. IL-4 directs the development of Th2-like helper effectors. J Immunol 1990; 145(11):3796–3806.
60. Gajewski TF, Goldwasser E, Fitch FW. Anti-proliferative effect of IFN-gamma in immune regulation. II. IFN-gamma inhibits the proliferation of murine bone marrow cells stimulated with IL-3, IL-4, or granulocyte-macrophage colony-stimulating factor. J Immunol 1988; 141(8):2635–2642.
61. Maggi E, Parronchi P, Manetti R, Simonelli C, Piccinni MP, Rugiu FS, De Carli M, Ricci M, Romagnani S. Reciprocal regulatory effects of IFN-gamma and IL-4 on the in vitro development of human Th1 and Th2 clones. J Immunol 1992; 148(7):2142–2147.
62. Gillis S, Crabtree GR, Smith KA. Glucocorticoid-induced inhibition of T cell growth factor production. I. The effect on mitogen-induced lymphocyte proliferation. J Immunol 1979; 123(4):1624–1631.
63. Larsson EL. Cyclosporin A and dexamethasone suppress T cell responses by selectively acting at distinct sites of the triggering process. J Immunol 1980; 124(6):2828–2833.
64. Bjornson BH, Harvey JM, Rose L. Differential effect of hydrocortisone on eosinophil and neutrophil proliferation. J Clin Invest 1985; 76(3):924–929.
65. Wenzel SE, Schwartz LB, Langmack EL, Halliday JL, Trudeau JB, Gibbs RL, Chu HW. Evidence that severe asthma can be divided pathologically into two inflammatory subtypes with distinct physiologic and clinical characteristics. Am J Respir Crit Care Med 1999; 160(3):1001–1008.

66. Strickland I, Kisich K, Hauk PJ, Vottero A, Chrousos GP, Klemm DJ, Leung DY. High constitutive glucocorticoid receptor beta in human neutrophils enables them to reduce their spontaneous rate of cell death in response to corticosteroids. J Exp Med 2001; 193(5):585–594.
67. Nakano J, Takizawa H, Ohtoshi T, Shoji S, Yamaguchi M, Ishii A, Yanagisawa M, Ito K. Endotoxin and pro-inflammatory cytokines stimulate endothelin-1 expression and release by airway epithelial cells. Clin Exp Allergy 1994; 24(4):330–336.
68. Guo FH, De Raeve HR, Rice TW, Stuehr DJ, Thunnissen FB, Erzurum SC. Continuous nitric oxide synthesis by inducible nitric oxide synthase in normal human airway epithelium in vivo. Proc Natl Acad Sci USA 1995; 92(17):7809–7813.
69. Atsuta J, Sterbinsky SA, Schwiebert LA, Bochner BS, Schleimer RP. Regulation of ICAM-1 and VCAM-1 expression in the human bronchial epithelial cell line BEAS-2B and involvement in eosinophil adhesion. J Allergy Clin Immunol 1997; 91(1 pt 2):S386.
70. Albelda SM. Endothelial and epithelial cell adhesion molecules. Am J Respir Cell Mol Biol 1991; 4(3):195–203.
71. Mak JC, Nishikawa M, Barnes PJ. Glucocorticosteroids increase beta 2-adrenergic receptor transcription in human lung. Am J Physiol 1995; 268(1 pt 1):L41–L46.
72. Mak JC, Nishikawa M, Shirasaki H, Miyayasu K, Barnes PJ. Protective effects of a glucocorticoid on downregulation of pulmonary beta 2-adrenergic receptors in vivo. J Clin Invest 1995; 96(1):99–106.
73. Borson DB, Gruenert DC. Glucocorticoids induce neutral endopeptidase in transformed human tracheal epithelial cells. Am J Physiol 1991; 260(2 pt 1):L83–L89.
74. Evans RM. The steroid and thyroid hormone receptor superfamily. Science 1988; 240(4854):889–895.
75. Pratt WB. The role of heat shock proteins in regulating the function, folding, and trafficking of the glucocorticoid receptor. J Biol Chem 1993; 268(29):21455–21458.
76. Hollenberg SM, Weinberger C, Ong ES, Cerelli G, Oro A, Lebo R, Thompson EB, Rosenfeld MG, Evans RM. Primary structure and expression of a functional human glucocorticoid receptor cDNA. Nature 1985; 318(6047):635–641.
77. Oakley RH, Sar M, Cidlowski JA. The human glucocorticoid receptor beta isoform. Expression, biochemical properties, and putative function. J Biol Chem 1996; 271(16):9550–9559.
78. Bamberger CM, Bamberger AM, de Castro M, Chrousos GP. Glucocorticoid receptor beta, a potential endogenous inhibitor of glucocorticoid action in humans. J Clin Invest 1995; 95(6):2435–2441.
79. Hecht K, Carlstedt-Duke J, Stierna P, Gustafsson J, Bronnegard M, Wikstrom AC. Evidence that the beta-isoform of the human glucocorticoid receptor does not act as a physiologically significant repressor. J Biol Chem 1997; 272(42):26659–26664.
80. Dahia PL, Honegger J, Reincke M, Jacobs RA, Mirtella A, Fahlbusch R, Besser GM, Chew SL, Grossman AB. Expression of glucocorticoid receptor gene isoforms in corticotropin-secreting tumors. J Clin Endocrinol Metab 1997; 82(4):1088–1093.
81. Korn SH, Wouters EF, Wesseling G, Arends JW, Thunnissen FB. In vitro and in vivo modulation of alpha- and beta-glucocorticoid-receptor mRNA in human bronchial epithelium. Am J Respir Crit Care Med 1997; 155(3):1117–1122.

82. Pujols L, Mullol J, Perez M, Roca-Ferrer J, Juan M, Xaubet A, Cidlowski JA, Picado C. Expression of the human glucocorticoid receptor alpha and beta isoforms in human respiratory epithelial cells and their regulation by dexamethasone. Am J Respir Cell Mol Biol 2001; 24(1):49–57.
83. Pratt WB, Toft DO. Steroid receptor interactions with heat shock protein and immunophilin chaperones. Endocr Rev 1997; 18(3):306–360.
84. Miesfeld RL. The structure and function of steroid receptor proteins. Crit Rev Biochem Mol Biol 1989; 24(2):101–117.
85. Leach KL, Dahmer MK, Hammond ND, Sando JJ, Pratt WB. Molybdate inhibition of glucocorticoid receptor inactivation and transformation. J Biol Chem 1979; 254(23):11884–11890.
86. Vedeckis WV, Ali M, Allen HR. Regulation of glucocorticoid receptor protein and mRNA levels. Cancer Res 1989; 49(8 suppl):2295s–2302s.
87. Hu JM, Bodwell JE, Munck A. Cell cycle-dependent glucocorticoid receptor phosphorylation and activity. Mol Endocrinol 1994; 8(12):1709–1713.
88. Cidlowski JA, Michaels GA. Alteration in glucocorticoid binding site number during the cell cycle in HeLa cells. Nature 1977; 266(5603):643–645.
89. Smith KA, Crabtree GR, Kennedy SJ, Munck AU. Glucocorticoid receptors and glucocorticoid sensitivity of mitogen stimulated and unstimulated human lymphocytes. Nature 1977; 267(5611):523–526.
90. Crabtree GR, Munck A, Smith KA. Glucocorticoids and lymphocytes. II. Cell cycle-dependent changes in glucocorticoid receptor content. J Immunol 1980; 125(1):13–17.
91. Hsu SC, Qi M, DeFranco DB. Cell cycle regulation of glucocorticoid receptor function. EMBO J 1992; 11(9):3457–3468.
92. Orti E, Hu LM, Munck A. Kinetics of glucocorticoid receptor phosphorylation in intact cells. Evidence for hormone-induced hyperphosphorylation after activation and recycling of hyperphosphorylated receptors. J Biol Chem 1993; 268(11):7779–7784.
93. Newton R. Molecular mechanisms of glucocorticoid action: What is important? Thorax 2000; 55(7):603–613.
94. Barnes PJ, Adcock IM. Transcription factors and asthma. Eur Respir J 1998; 12(1): 221–234.
95. Leo C, Chen JD. The SRC family of nuclear receptor coactivators. Gene 2000; 245(1):1–11.
96. Schule R, Rangarajan P, Kliewer S, Ransone LJ, Bolado J, Yang N, Verma IM, Evans RM. Functional antagonism between oncoprotein c-Jun and the glucocorticoid receptor. Cell 1990; 62(6):1217–1226.
97. Jonat C, Rahmsdorf HJ, Park KK, Cato AC, Gebel S, Ponta H, Herrlich P. Antitumor promotion and antiinflammation: Down-modulation of AP-1 (Fos/Jun) activity by glucocorticoid hormone. Cell 1990; 62(6):1189–1204.
98. Yang-Yen HF, Chambard JC, Sun YL, Smeal T, Schmidt TJ, Drouin J, Karin M. Transcriptional interference between c-Jun and the glucocorticoid receptor: Mutual inhibition of DNA binding due to direct protein–protein interaction. Cell 1990; 62(6):1205–1215.
99. Ray A, Prefontaine KE. Physical association and functional antagonism between

the p65 subunit of transcription factor NF-kappa B and the glucocorticoid receptor. Proc Natl Acad Sci USA 1994; 91(2):752–756.

100. McKay LI, Cidlowski JA. CBP (CREB binding protein) integrates NF-kappaB (nuclear factor-kappaB) and glucocorticoid receptor physical interactions and antagonism. Mol Endocrinol 2000; 14(8):1222–1234.

101. Giordano A, Avantaggiati ML. p300 and CBP: Partners for life and death. J Cell Physiol 1999; 181(2):218–230.

102. Kamei Y, Xu L, Heinzel T, Torchia J, Kurokawa R, Gloss B, Lin SC, Heyman RA, Rose DW, Glass CK, Rosenfeld MG. A CBP integrator complex mediates transcriptional activation and AP-1 inhibition by nuclear receptors. Cell 1996; 85(3):403–414.

103. Sheppard KA, Phelps KM, Williams AJ, Thanos D, Glass CK, Rosenfeld MG, Gerritsen ME, Collins T. Nuclear integration of glucocorticoid receptor and nuclear factor-kappaB signaling by CREB-binding protein and steroid receptor coactivator-1. J Biol Chem 1998; 273(45):29291–29294.

104. Newton R, Seybold J, Kuitert LM, Bergmann M, Barnes PJ. Repression of cyclooxygenase-2 and prostaglandin E2 release by dexamethasone occurs by transcriptional and post-transcriptional mechanisms involving loss of polyadenylated mRNA. J Biol Chem 1998; 273(48):32312–32321.

105. Huarte J, Stutz A, O'Connell ML, Gubler P, Belin D, Darrow AL, Strickland S, Vassalli JD. Transient translational silencing by reversible mRNA deadenylation. Cell 1992; 69(6):1021–1030.

106. Kruys V, Marinx O, Shaw G, Deschamps J, Huez G. Translational blockade imposed by cytokine-derived UA-rich sequences. Science 1989; 245(4920):852–855.

107. Reisman D, Thompson EA. Glucocorticoid regulation of cyclin D3 gene transcription and mRNA stability in lymphoid cells. Mol Endocrinol 1995; 9(11):1500–1509.

108. Cole TJ, Blendy JA, Monaghan AP, Krieglstein K, Schmid W, Aguzzi A, Fantuzzi G, Hummler E, Unsicker K, Schutz G. Targeted disruption of the glucocorticoid receptor gene blocks adrenergic chromaffin cell development and severely retards lung maturation. Genes Dev 1995; 9(13):1608–1621.

109. Reichardt HM, Kaestner KH, Tuckermann J, Kretz O, Wessely O, Bock R, Gass P, Schmid W, Herrlich P, Angel P, Schutz G. DNA binding of the glucocorticoid receptor is not essential for survival. Cell 1998; 93(4):531–541.

110. Chikanza LC, Panayi GS. The effects of hydrocortisone on in vitro lymphocyte proliferation and interleukin-2 and -4 production in corticosteroid sensitive and resistant subjects. Eur J Clin Invest 1993; 23(12):845–850.

111. Curley RK, Holden CA. Steroid-resistant bullous pemphigoid treated with cyclosporin A. Clin Exp Dermatol 1991; 16(1):68–69.

112. Coman E, Reinus JF. Cyclosporin use in steroid-resistant Crohn's disease: Grasping at new straws? Am J Gastroenterol 1990; 85(6):758–759.

113. Dundar S, Ozdemir O, Ozcebe O. Cyclosporin in steroid-resistant auto-immune haemolytic anaemia. Acta Haematol 1991; 86(4):200–202.

114. Chrousos GP, Renquist D, Brandon D, Eil C, Pugeat M, Vigersky R, Cutler GB Jr, Loriaux DL, Lipsett MB. Glucocorticoid hormone resistance during primate

evolution: Receptor-mediated mechanisms. Proc Natl Acad Sci USA 1982; 79(6): 2036–2040.

115. Corrigan CJ, Brown PH, Barnes NC, Szefler SJ, Tsai JJ, Frew AJ, Kay AB. Glucocorticoid resistance in chronic asthma. Glucocorticoid pharmacokinetics, glucocorticoid receptor characteristics, and inhibition of peripheral blood T cell proliferation by glucocorticoids in vitro. Am Rev Respir Dis 1991; 144(5):1016–1025.
116. Corrigan CJ. Glucocorticoid-resistant asthma. T-lymphocyte defects. Am J Respir Crit Care Med 1996; 154(2 pt 2):S53–S55.
117. Lane SJ, Lee TH. Glucocorticoid receptor characteristics in monocytes of patients with corticosteroid-resistant bronchial asthma. Am Rev Respir Dis 1991; 143(5 pt 1):1020–1024.
118. Lane SJ, Arm JP, Staynov DZ, Lee TH. Chemical mutational analysis of the human glucocorticoid receptor cDNA in glucocorticoid-resistant bronchial asthma. Am J Respir Cell Mol Biol 1994; 11(1):42–48.
119. Poznansky MC, Gordon AC, Douglas JG, Krajewski AS, Wyllie AH, Grant IW. Resistance to methylprednisolone in cultures of blood mononuclear cells from glucocorticoid-resistant asthmatic patients. Clin Sci (Colch) 1984; 67(6):639–645.
120. Kay AB, Diaz P, Carmicheal J, Grant IW. Corticosteroid-resistant chronic asthma and monocyte complement receptors. Clin Exp Immunol 1981; 44(3):576–580.
121. Wilkinson JR, Crea AE, Clark TJ, Lee TH. Identification and characterization of a monocyte-derived neutrophil-activating factor in corticosteroid-resistant bronchial asthma. J Clin Invest 1989; 84(6):1930–1941.
122. Lane SJ, Wilkinson JR, Cochrane GM, Lee TH, Arm JP. Differential in vitro regulation by glucocorticoids of monocyte-derived cytokine generation in glucocorticoid-resistant bronchial asthma. Am Rev Respir Dis 1993; 147(3):690–696.
123. Wilkinson JR, Lane SJ, Lee TH. Effects of corticosteroids on cytokine generation and expression of activation antigens by monocytes in bronchial asthma. Int Arch Allergy Appl Immunol 1991; 94(1–4):220–221.
124. Corrigan CJ, Brown PH, Barnes NC, Tsai JJ, Frew AJ, Kay AB. Glucocorticoid resistance in chronic asthma. Peripheral blood T lymphocyte activation and comparison of the T lymphocyte inhibitory effects of glucocorticoids and cyclosporin A. Am Rev Respir Dis 1991; 144(5):1026–1032.
125. Leung DY, Martin RJ, Szefler SJ, Sher ER, Ying S, Kay AB, Hamid Q. Dysregulation of interleukin 4, interleukin 5, and interferon gamma gene expression in steroid-resistant asthma. J Exp Med 1995; 181(1):33–40.
126. Kam JC, Szefler SJ, Surs W, Sher ER, Leung DY. Combination IL-2 and IL-4 reduces glucocorticoid receptor-binding affinity and T cell response to glucocorticoids. J Immunol 1993; 151(7):3460–3466.
127. Sousa AR, Lane SJ, Atkinson BA, Poston RN, Lee TH. The effects of prednisolone on the cutaneous tuberculin response in patients with corticosteroid-resistant bronchial asthma. J Allergy Clin Immunol 1996; 97(2):698–706.
128. Sousa AR, Lane SJ, Cidlowski JA, Staynov DZ, Lee TH. Glucocorticoid resistance in asthma is associated with elevated in vivo expression of the glucocorticoid receptor beta-isoform. J Allergy Clin Immunol 2000; 105(5):943–950.
129. Schleimer RP, Freeland HS, Peters SP, Brown KE, Derse CP. An assessment of the effects of glucocorticoids on degranulation, chemotaxis, binding to vascular

endothelium and formation of leukotriene B4 by purified human neutrophils. J Pharmacol Exp Ther 1989; 250(2):598–605.

130. Cox G. Glucocorticoid treatment inhibits apoptosis in human neutrophils. Separation of survival and activation outcomes. J Immunol 1995; 154(9):4719–4725.
131. Brown PH, Teelucksingh S, Matusiewicz SP, Greening AP, Crompton GK, Edwards CR. Cutaneous vasoconstrictor response to glucocorticoids in asthma. Lancet 1991; 337(8741):576–580.
132. Adcock IM, Lane SJ, Brown CR, Peters MJ, Lee TH, Barnes PJ. Differences in binding of glucocorticoid receptor to DNA in steroid-resistant asthma. J Immunol 1995; 154(7):3500–3505.
133. Adcock IM, Lane SJ, Brown CR, Lee TH, Barnes PJ. Abnormal glucocorticoid receptor-activator protein 1 interaction in steroid-resistant asthma. J Exp Med 1995; 182(6):1951–1958.
134. Lane SJ, Adcock IM, Richards D, Hawrylowicz C, Barnes PJ, Lee TH. Corticosteroid-resistant bronchial asthma is associated with increased c-fos expression in monocytes and T lymphocytes. J Clin Invest 1998; 102(12):2156–2164.
135. Shahidi H, Vottero A, Stratakis CA, Taymans SE, Karl M, Longui CA, Chrousos GP, Daughaday WH, Gregory SA, Plate JM. Imbalanced expression of the glucocorticoid receptor isoforms in cultured lymphocytes from a patient with systemic glucocorticoid resistance and chronic lymphocytic leukemia. Biochem Biophys Res Commun 1999; 254(3):559–565.

15

Future Therapies for Asthma

PETER J. BARNES

Imperial College
National Heart and Lung Institute
London, England

I. Introduction

Current therapies for asthma are highly effective in the majority of patients. To improve upon existing inhaled therapies, which are not only effective but also very safe and without significant adverse effects, is a major challenge for the pharmaceutical industry. New drugs therefore need to answer clinical needs that are unmet by currently used therapy. Many novel classes of drugs are considered in this book, and although some of these drugs have shown promise in animal models and small clinical studies, none of them so far reaches the efficacy of existing treatments.

Asthma is a highly complex inflammatory disease process that involves multiple inflammatory and structural cells, all of which release a multitude of inflammatory mediators (1,2). This implies that highly selective therapies are unlikely to have good efficacy, because they will deal with only one specific aspect of the complex disease process. For example, histamine mimics many features of the pathophysiology of asthma, and histamine is released from mast cells in patients with asthma, particularly during exacerbations, but antihistamines such as loratadine, cetirizine, and fexofenadine, which are potent histamine H_1-receptor antagonists, are ineffective in clinical asthma. This is almost certainly because blocking a single mediator does not inhibit the actions of the many other mediators that produce the same effects as histamine. This means that there is a trade-off between efficacy and specificity. It is hoped that more specific drugs would have fewer side effects than drugs that block many different mechanisms. Oral corticosteroids are highly effective in the treatment of asthma and would be efficacious in almost every patient, but of course the side effects preclude their regular use in all but the most severely asthmatic patients. This led to the introduction of topically acting inhaled corticosteroids, which have become the mainstay of modern asthma management.

II. The Future of Existing Therapies

A relatively small number of drug classes have been found useful in asthma therapy. It is likely that some will continue to be used, but others will be less used.

A. Bronchodilators

There are three classes of bronchodilator treatment currently used in asthma management.

β_2-Agonists

β_2-Agonists are by far the most effective bronchodilators in asthma, giving rapid relief of symptoms when taken by inhalation. Their efficacy in asthma is related to the fact that they act as functional antagonists, blocking the bronchoconstrictor action of all bronchoconstrictor mediators. The long-acting inhaled β_2-agonists are effective and long-lasting bronchodilators that give an important clinical improvement when added to any dose of inhaled corticosteroids in patients with mild, moderate, or even severe asthma (3,4). They provide sustained bronchodilation and bronchoprotection when given twice daily. Pharmaceutical companies are now searching for once-daily inhaled β_2-agonists. Anticholinergic drugs are much less effective as bronchodilators in asthma, which is not surprising, because they inhibit only the bronchoconstriction due to acetylcholine and have no effect on the multiple other bronchoconstrictors released in asthma.

Theophylline

Theophylline is also less effective than β_2-agonists as a bronchodilator because the dose is limited by side effects. However, it is becoming apparent that may of the clinical benefits of theophylline are due to some anti-inflammatory action and that this can be achieved at lower doses than are needed for bronchodilation (5). In the future it is likely that inhaled β_2-agonists will remain the bronchodilators of choice.

New Bronchodilators

Novel classes of bronchodilators have been explored, including potassium channel openers, phosphodiesterase 3 inhibitors, nitrovasodilators, and vasoactive intestinal peptide (6). All of these drugs relax human airways in vitro, but unfortunately they have turned out to be more potent in vascular smooth muscle, resulting in vasodilator side effects that have limited the dose of drug that can be given. These new classes of drugs are therefore no longer in development as bronchodilators for asthma, and bronchodilators are not considered further in this chapter.

B. Controller Drugs

Corticosteroids

Corticosteroids are by far the most effective drugs in long-term control of chronic asthma, and inhaled corticosteroids are the mainstay of therapy (7,8). Inhaled corticosteroids provide good control of asthma, give marked protection against exacerbations, are highly cost-effective, and are virtually free of side effects at the doses most patients need (9). At high doses there is a risk of systemic side effects, but patients who require such big doses would have previously needed oral steroids, which have a much greater risk of systemic side effects. Inhaled corticosteroids have a relatively flat dose–response curve in most patients with asthma, so for most patients high doses are unnecessary. If asthma is not controlled on a low dose of inhaled steroids another class of drugs is preferable, particularly long-acting inhaled β_2-agonists, but also low-dose theophylline and antileukotrienes.

Cromones

The cromones (cromolyn sodium and nedocromil sodium) are much less effective in the control of asthma than inhaled corticosteroids but continue to be used, particularly in children, because of their safety. However, although effective in acute challenges, these drugs are not very effective in long-term control, and they have a very short duration of action, making them inconvenient to use. Indeed, a recent meta-analysis concluded that cromolyn sodium was virtually ineffective in childhood asthma (10). Furthermore, the very low doses of inhaled corticosteroids that are equivalent to the effects of cromones have no side effects. This has made the use of cromones obsolete.

Antileukotrienes

Antileukotrienes, which include the cysteinyl-leukotriene receptor-1 antagonists zafirlukast and montelukast, and 5′-lipoxygenase inhibitors, of which zileuton is the only available drug, are the only new classes of treatment introduced as asthma therapy in over 30 years. They have significant effects on measurements of asthma control, have weak anti-inflammatory effects, and have the advantage that they are effective by oral administration and are without significant class-related side effects (11). However, it is becoming apparent that they are far less effective than low does of inhaled corticosteroids in every parameter that has so far been measured (12–14). This means that they are not an adequate substitute for inhaled corticosteroids in the treatment of mild asthma. However, they may have add-on benefit in patients already treated with inhaled corticosteroids, although they are less effective in this respect than long-acting inhaled β_2-agonists (15). Antileukotrienes do not appear to provide benefit when added to other treatments in patients with severe asthma who are still symptomatic (16). Antileukotrienes are a much more specific type of therapy than corticosteroids, so it is not surprising that they should be less effective. It is possible that some patients may do well on this treatment if leukotrienes play an important role in their asthma pathophysiology, and it is possible that these good responders might be recognized through the presence of certain polymorphisms in the leukotriene pathways (see later).

Theophylline

Theophylline is now considered more an anti-inflammatory drug than a bronchodilator when low doses are used (giving plasma concentrations of 5–10 mg/L). Low-dose theophylline inhibits the inflammatory process in patients with severe asthma already treated with maximal doses of inhaled corticosteroids, as demonstrated by clinical deterioration and increased inflammatory cells after theophylline withdrawal (17). Theophylline also has anti-inflammatory effects in mild asthma (18) and is a useful add-on therapy in patients on low to high doses of inhaled corticosteroids (19–21). It is likely that theophylline will continue to be used clinically in patients with more severe asthma because it has some effects that may not be achieved by corticosteroids.

Steroid-Sparing Therapies

Various immunomodulatory drugs have been introduced to reduce the need for oral steroid maintenance therapy in patients with severe disease (22). These treatments include methotrexate, cyclosporin A, intravenous immunoglobulin, and oral gold. None of these treatments is very effective, and all have a high risk of troublesome effects, so they are little used (23).

Fixed Steroid–β-Agonist Combination Inhalers

Inhaled corticosteroids together with inhaled long-acting β2-agonists provide by far the most effect way of controlling asthma, in terms of symptom control and reduction in exacerbations. There is a positive interaction between β_2-agonists and corticosteroids, with corticosteroids increasing expression of β_2-adrenergic receptors and β_2-agonists enhancing the anti-inflammatory action of corticosteroids under certain conditions. The development of fixed combination inhalers is therefore a logical development, particularly because the duration of action of current inhaled corticosteroids and that of long-acting β_2-agonists are similar. Two fixed combination inhalers are now available: fluticasone/salmeterol (Seretide, Advair) and budesonide/formoterol [Symbicort (in Europe)] (15,24). Fixed combination inhalers are more convenient to patients and should improve compliance with long-term therapy, because delivering a bronchodilator with the inhaled corticosteroids should ensure that the use of inhaled corticosteroids continues. It is likely that these fixed combination inhalers will become the main therapeutic approach for the majority of asthmatic patients over the next 15 years.

III. The Need for New Treatments for Asthma

Despite the fact that effective and safe treatments for asthma are already available, there is a need for new treatments in the future.

Inhaled corticosteroids are highly effective in controlling asthma, but compliance with regular treatment is very poor (25). Many patients are worried about systemic side effects of steroids, and there has been particular concern about stunting of growth in children. An alternative anti-inflammatory drug would therefore have a potential advantage.

Inhaled therapies are the most effective treatments for asthma and reduce the risk of systemic side effects that are due to the nonspecific systemic actions of the drugs. There would be major advantages to an oral therapy for asthma. This would be easier to develop and might improve compliance. Drugs that inhibit the underlying allergic inflammatory process might also treat associated allergic symptoms, such as rhinitis and eczema. Because 85% of patients with asthma also have rhinitis and rhinitis exacerbates asthma, this could be an important advance in therapy (26). However, the risk of oral therapy is that there will be systemic adverse effects, so any treatment will need to be specific for the pathophysiology of asthma or atopy.

A small proportion of patients with asthma are not well controlled on current therapy, although they may improve on high doses of oral steroids. These patients appear to be relatively steroid-resistant; patients who are completely resistant to steroids are rarely seen (27,28). These patients require some other form of treatment that overcomes the poor response to steroids.

It is not certain whether current therapies alter the progression of the disease or can reverse and prevent the structural changes (remodeling) that occur in the airway wall in some patients with chronic disease. There is circumstantial evidence that inhaled corticosteroids used early in the course of asthma may reduce the impairment in lung function found in some patients, but definitive evidence is lacking because of the difficulty in serially monitoring structural changes in the airways. Drugs that prevent disease progression would be of particular value in patients susceptible to these changes.

None of the existing treatments is obviously disease-modifying, that is, a treatment that will maintain control even when withdrawn. This concept is well established in the management of other inflammatory diseases such as rheumatoid arthritis but has not yet been fully explored in asthma.

None of the currently available treatments are curative. Even when asthma is completely controlled by inhaled corticosteroids, stopping steroids results in loss of asthma control, showing that although corticosteroids are effective in suppressing the airway inflammation, they do not deal with the underlying causal mechanisms. The prospects of a cure become greater as the molecular and genetic mechanisms of asthma are unraveled.

A. Strategies for New Drug Development

There are several approaches to the development of new treatments for asthma (29,30).

New therapies have been developed by improving existing classes of drugs though extending the duration of action (for example, long-acting inhaled β_2-agonists), by improving pharmacokinetics (for example, fluticasone and budesonide), or by improving drug selectivity for the target (such as the more selective muscarinic antagonist tiotropium bromide).

A second approach is through logical development, because disease targets are discovered through research and a better understanding of the disease process. Examples are antileukotrienes, anti-interleukin-5 antibodies, and CCR3 antagonists, which are obvious approaches and usually undertaken by several pharmaceutical companies in parallel.

The most difficult approach is to develop completely novel drugs by serendipity. These may be discovered in other therapeutic areas or may target a novel mechanism discovered through research.

IV. New Corticosteroids

Corticosteroids are the most effective currently available treatment for atopic diseases, and high doses of oral corticosteroids control virtually every patient with asthma. However, systemic side effects limit the dose that can be given over long periods, and in the early 1970s this led to the development of topical steroids, which have local anti-inflammatory effects. Inhaled corticosteroids have dramatically improved the treatment of asthma and are now first-line treatment for persistent asthma in all patients (9,31). Concern about systemic absorption of inhaled steroid led to the development of corticosteroids that are metabolized locally.

However, these "soft steroids," such as butixicort 21-propionate and tipredane, proved to have poor efficacy in clinical studies, because they are metabolized before they exert any anti-inflammatory action. Ciclesonide is a prodrug that is inactive, but the active steroid is released by esterases in the lung. This steroid is effective and may have a good safety profile (32).

Advances in understanding the molecular mechanisms whereby corticosteroids suppress inflammation at a molecular level may lead to the development of safer steroids or drugs that mimic their key anti-inflammatory actions (see Sec. VIII). Corticosteroids bind to a cytosolic glucocorticoid receptor that translocates to the nucleus and binds as a homodimer to DNA to activate genes, including anti-inflammatory genes. However, the major anti-inflammatory effect of corticosteroids is suppression of multiple inflammatory genes, including cytokines, inflammatory enzymes, adhesion molecules, and inflammatory mediator receptors; this is why corticosteroids are so effective in complex inflammatory conditions such as atopic diseases. Most of the anti-inflammatory actions of corticosteroids can be accounted for by inhibiting transcription factors, such as activator protein-1 (AP-1), nuclear factor-κB (NF-κB), and nuclear factor of activated T-cells (NF-AT), that regulate inflammatory gene expression (33). These effects are mediated, at least in part, by deacetylation of core histones that have been acetylated via activation of these transcription factors (34). This provides new targets for the discovery of nonsteroidal anti-inflammatory agents.

A. Dissociated Corticosteroids

Systemic side effects of corticosteroids are largely mediated via DNA binding and histone acetylation, whereas anti-inflammatory effects are mediated largely independently of DNA binding and via histone deacetylation (35). It may therefore be possible to dissociate the side effects from the anti-inflammatory effects and develop oral steroids without adverse effects. Several dissociated corticosteroids have now been synthesized, and a separation between *trans*-activation (DNA binding) and *trans*-repression (transcription factor inhibition) has been demonstrated in gene reporter systems and in intact cells in vitro (36). Whether this will translate to in vivo differences is less certain (37), and because all corticosteroids have to bind to a single class of glucocorticoid receptor a clear separation of effects may never be possible. Identification of the major targets for corticosteroid action, such as NF-κB, or deacetylation of core histones may be a more promising approach for the future.

V. Mediator Antagonists

Many inflammatory mediators are involved in atopic diseases, and in asthma over 80 different mediators have been identified (2). Several of these antagonists are discussed in the preceding chapters. Because of the multiplicity and the duplication of effects of these mediators, it is very unlikely that a single mediator antagonist could be as effective as corticosteroids, although they may be expected to have fewer side effects than systemic steroids. It is difficult to predict which antagonists will be most useful until potent and selective drugs are tested in patients with asthma. Unfortunately, animal models have proved to be particularly misleading in this area, because mediators play different roles in different species. For example, serotonin is a potent bronchoconstrictor in rats but has no effect on human airways. Histamine and substance P are potent constrictors of human airways but are bronchodilators in sheep and mice, respectively! Platelet-activating factor (PAF) is a mediator that mimics closely the pathophysiology of asthma and induces airway hyperresponsiveness in normal humans. PAF receptor antagonists are effective in most animal models of asthma, but even potent PAF antagonists have proved to be of no value in symptomatic human asthma (38). Yet some mediator antagonists may be more useful, because some mediators may play a more dominant role or may be upstream of a complex mediator cascade. A good example is the use of tumor necrosis factor-α (TNF-α) inhibitors in severe rheumatoid arthritis, a situation where many other mediators are also involved (39).

One approach to overcoming the relatively weak effects of single mediator antagonists is to combine antagonists. For example, antihistamine and antileukotrienes together are apparently more effective than either drug alone (40).

A. Cytokine Modulators

Multiple cytokines have been implicated in the pathophysiology of atopic diseases, although some cytokines play a more critical role in atopic inflammation (41). There are several possible approaches to inhibiting specific cytokines (42). These range from drugs that inhibit cytokine synthesis (corticosteroids, cyclosporin A, tacrolimus), humanized blocking antibodies, to cytokines or their receptors, soluble receptors to mop up secreted cytokines, receptor antagonists, or drugs that block the signal transduction pathways activated by cytokines (Fig. 1). There are some cytokines that suppress the allergic inflammatory process, and these may also have therapeutic potential.

Anti-IL-5

Interleukin-5 plays a key role in orchestrating the eosinophilic inflammation of asthma (see Chap. 7). Blocking antibodies to IL-5 inhibit eosinophilic inflammation and airway hyperresponsiveness (AHR) in animal models of asthma, including primates (43). This blocking effect may last for over 3 months after a single injection, making the treatment of chronic asthma with such a therapy a feasible proposition. Humanized monoclonal antibodies to IL-5 have been developed, and a single injection reduces blood eosinophils for over 3 months and prevents eosinophil recruitment into the airways after allergen challenge (44). However, this

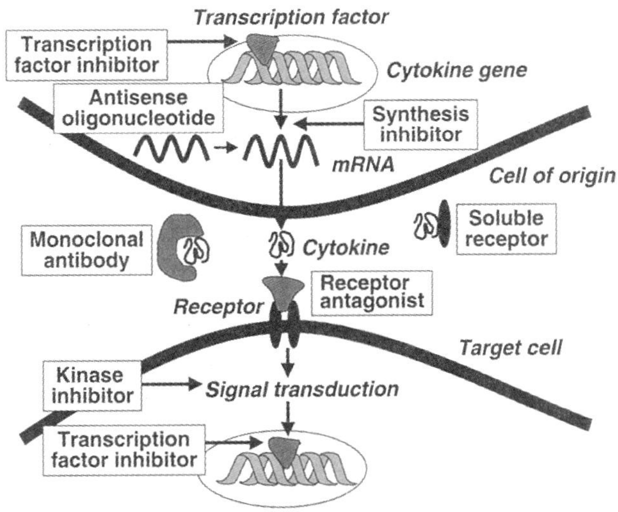

Figure 1 Inhibition of cytokine synthesis. Several strategies are available to inhibit the production or effects of cytokines.

treatment has no effect on the early or late response to allergen challenge or on AHR, suggesting that eosinophils may be less important for these responses than was previously believed. A clinical study showed no effect on asthma control in symptomatic patients who were treated with steroids (45). The lack of effect of anti-IL-5 on airway responsiveness despite a profound reduction in circulating eosinophils must cast some doubt on the role of eosinophils in human asthma and also on the strategy to develop other anti-eosinophil drugs, such as CCR3 antagonists and VLA-4 inhibitors as novel antiasthma drugs.

Anti-IL-4

Interleukin-4 is a more upstream target than IL-5, because it plays a critical role in the formation of IgE and has a unique role in the differentiation of Th2 cells (46). There are several strategies for inhibiting IL-4, including soluble receptors, mutated IL-4 blocking protein, monoclonal antibodies, and inhibitors of the transcription factor STAT-6 (see Chap. 6). Preliminary studies suggest that this approach appears to be more effective than anti-IL-5 (47).

Anti-IL-13

There is increasing evidence that IL-13 in mice mimics many of the features of asthma, including AHR, increased IgE, and mucus hypersecretion (48) and may be a good target because it is produced in much larger amounts in asthmatic airways than the related cytokine IL-4. A soluble IL-13Rα2-Fc fusion protein, which blocks the effects of IL-13 but not IL-4, has been used successfully to neutralize IL-13 in mice (49).

Anti-IL-9

Interleukin-9 is produced by Th2 cells and appears to have an amplifying effect on the expression of IL-4 and IL-5 (49,50). This suggests that IL-9 may be a useful upstream target in asthma, and humanized monoclonal IL-9 antibodies are now in clinical development (as discussed in Chap. 7).

Anti-TNF

Tumor necrosis factor-α (TNF-α) is expressed in asthmatic airways and may play a key role in amplifying atopic inflammation, through the activation of NF-κB, AP-1 and other transcription factors (51). In rheumatoid arthritis inhibitors of TNF-α have produced remarkable clinical responses, even in patients who are relatively unresponsive to steroids (52). TNF antibodies (such as infliximab) or soluble TNF receptors (such as entanercept) are a logical approach to asthma therapy, particularly in patients with severe disease. There is also a search for small-molecule inhibitors of TNF, of which the most promising are inhibitors of TNF-α-converting enzyme, because these could be given orally. Other new anti-inflammatory treatments, including phosphodiesterase-4 inhibitors and p38 mitogen-activated protein (MAP) kinase inhibitors, are also effective in inhibiting TNF-α release from inflammatory cells.

B. Chemokine Inhibitors

Over 50 chemokines are involved in the recruitment of inflammatory cells, and they activate over 20 surface receptors (53). Because these are in the G-protein coupled receptor superfamily of receptors it is feasible to develop small-molecule inhibitors (54). In asthma there has been particular interest in CCR3 that are expressed predominantly on eosinophils and also on basophils, mast cells, and some Th2 cells. Blocking CCR3 is a logical approach to the treatment of asthma (discussed in Chap. 8), and several small-molecule inhibitors are now in clinical development. They have the advantage of oral absorption and should be safe, but the lack of effect of reducing eosinophils in asthmatic patients raises some doubts about their potential.

In murine models of asthma other chemokine receptors have been implicated in the recruitment of inflammatory cells, including CCR2 and CCR4. There is particular interest in the potential for CCR4 inhibitors, because CCR4 is important in the recruitment of Th2 cells (55). In more severe asthma there is a predominance of neutrophils, and this has suggested that chemokines involved in neutrophil recruitment should be targeted. IL-8 is increased in the induced sputum of these patients (56) and recruits neutrophils via activation of CXCR2. Small molecule inhibitors of these receptors are now in clinical development (57).

VI. Anti-Inflammatory Cytokines

Some cytokines have anti-inflammatory effects in allergic inflammation and therefore have therapeutic potential (58). Although it may not be feasible or cost-effective to administer these proteins as long-term therapy, it may be possible to develop drugs that increase the release of these endogenous cytokines or activate their receptors and specific signal transduction pathways.

A. Interleukin-1 Receptor Antagonist

Interleukin-1 receptor antagonist binds to IL-1 receptors and blocks the action of IL-1β. In experimental animals it reduces AHR (59), but clinical studies have been disappointing (60).

B. Interleukin-10

Interleukin-10 is a potent anti-inflammatory cytokine that inhibits the synthesis of many inflammatory proteins, including cytokines (TNF-α, GM-CSF, IL-5, chemokines) and inflammatory enzymes (iNOS), that are overexpressed in asthma (61). Indeed, there may be a defect in IL-10 transcription and secretion from macrophages in asthma that may increase the intensity and duration of the inflammatory response (62). In sensitized animals IL-10 is effective in suppressing the inflammatory response to allergen (63), suggesting that IL-10 might be effective in the treatment of asthma. Specific allergen immunotherapy results in increased production of IL-10 by T-helper cells, and this may contribute to the beneficial effects of immunotherapy (64).

Recombinant human IL-10 has shown to have some benefit in controlling inflammatory bowel disease, where similar cytokines are expressed, and is given as a weekly injection (65). In the future, drugs that activate the unique signal transduction pathways activated by the IL-10 receptor or drugs that increase endogenous production of IL-10 may be developed. In mice, drugs that elevate cyclic AMP increase IL-10 production, but this does not appear to be the case in human cells (66). Specific allergen immunotherapy may increase local IL-10 production (64).

C. Interferons

Interferon-γ (IFN-γ) inhibits Th2 cells and should therefore reduce atopic inflammation. In sensitized animals nebulized IFN-γ inhibits eosinophilic inflammation induced by allergen exposure (67). Administration of IFN-γ by nebulization to asthmatic patients did not significantly reduce eosinophilic inflammation, however, possibly due to the difficulty in obtaining a high enough concentration locally in the airways (68). Interestingly, allergen immunotherapy increases IFN-γ production by circulating T cells in patients with clinical benefit (69) and increases the numbers of IFN-γ-expressing cells in nasal biopsies of patients with allergic rhinitis (70). A preliminary report suggests that IFN-γ may be useful in the treatment of patients with severe asthma who have reduced responsiveness to corticosteroids (71).

D. Interleukin-12

Interleukin-12 is the endogenous regulator of Th1 cell development and regulates the balance of Th1 and Th2 cells (72). The administration of IL-12 to rats inhibits allergen-induced inflammation (73) and inhibits sensitization to allergens. IL-12 releases IFN-γ but has additional effects on T-cell differentiation. Recombinant human IL-12 has been administered to humans and has several toxic effects that are diminished by slow escalation of the dose (74). In asthmatic patients, IL-12 reduces circulating eosinophils but does not inhibit allergen responses or reduce AHR (75). In addition, side effects such as malaise are common, thus precluding the use of systemic IL-12 for treatment of atopic diseases. In mice, administration of an IL-12-allergen fusion protein results in the development of a specific Th1 response to allergens with an increase in specific IgG2 rather than the normal Th2 response with specific IgE formation (76). This suggests the possibility of using IL-12 to provide a more specific immunotherapy.

E. Interleukin-18

Interleukin-18 was originally described as IFN-γ releasing factor but has a different mechanism of action than IL-12 (77). IL-12 and IL-18 appear to have a synergistic effect on inducing IFN-γ release and inhibiting IL-4-dependent IgE production and airway hyperresponsiveness. Adenovirus transfer of IL-18 in mice effectively blocks allergen-induced inflammation and airway hyperresponsiveness, indicating the therapeutic potential for IL-18 (78).

VII. New Anti-Inflammatory Drugs

There has been an intensive search for anti-inflammatory treatments that are as effective as corticosteroids in asthma but with fewer side effects.

A. Phosphodiesterase-4 Inhibitors

Phosphodiesterases (PDEs) break down cyclic nucleotides that inhibit cell activation, and at least nine families of enzymes have now been characterized. Theophylline has been used for a long time in asthma therapy and is a weak nonselective

PDE inhibitor. PDE4 is the predominant family of PDEs in inflammatory cells, including mast cells, eosinophils, T lymphocytes, macrophages, and structural cells such as sensory nerves and epithelial cells (79). This has suggested that PDE4 inhibitors would be useful as an anti-inflammatory treatment in atopic disease, particularly as there is some evidence for overexpression of PDE4 in cells of atopic patients (80). In animal models of asthma, PDE4 inhibitors reduce eosinophil infiltration and AHR responses to allergen (81). Several PDE4 inhibitors have been now tested in asthma, but with disappointing results. Most of the PDE4 inhibitors so far tested clinically have had unacceptable side effects, particularly nausea and vomiting. Several approaches might overcome these problems. It is possible that vomiting is due to inhibition of a particular subtype of PDE4. At least four human PDE4 genes have been identified, and each has several splice variants (79,81). This raises the possibility that subtype-selective inhibitors may be developed that may preserve the anti-inflammatory effect while having less likelihood of side effects. PDE4D appears to be of particular importance in inflammatory cells, such as T lymphocytes and eosinophils, and may be a more specific target (82), and subtype-selective PDE4 inhibitors are in development. There has recently been interest in PDE7 as a therapeutic target, because antisense oligonucleotides that reduce PDE7 expression inhibit the activation of T lymphocytes (83). No selective PDE7 inhibitors have so far been reported, but high throughput screening is under way.

B. Transcription Factor Inhibitors

Transcription factors, such as NF-κB and AP-1, play an important role in the orchestration of asthmatic inflammation (84,85), and this has prompted a search for specific blockers of these transcription factors. There are several possible approaches to inhibition of NF-κB, including gene transfer of the inhibitor of NF-κB (IκB), inhibitors of IκB kinases (IKKs), NF-κB-inducing kinase (NIK), and IκB ubiquitin ligase, which regulate the activity of NF-κB, and the development of drugs that inhibit the degradation of IκB (86). One concern about this approach is that effective inhibitors of NF-κB may result in immune suppression and impair host defenses, because knockout mice that lack NF-κB proteins succumb to septicemia. However, there are alternative pathways of NF-κB activation that might be more important in inflammatory disease (87).

Cyclosporin A and tacrolimus inhibit T-lymphocyte function by blocking the transcription factor NF-AT (nuclear factor of activated T-cells) by blocking activation of calcineurin (88). This results in suppression of IL-2, IL-4, IL-5, and GM-CSF and therefore is of therapeutic potential in asthma.

C. MAP Kinase Inhibitors

There are three major MAP kinase cascades and increasing recognition that these pathways are involved in chronic inflammation and the expression of multiple inflammatory genes (89). There has been particular interest in the p38 MAP kinase pathway that is blocked by a novel class of drugs, the cytokine suppressant anti-inflammatory drugs (CSAIDs), such as SB203580 and RWJ67657 (90). These drugs inhibit the synthesis of many inflammatory cytokines, chemokines, and inflammatory enzymes. Interestingly, they appear to have a preferential inhibitory effect on synthesis of Th2 compared to Th1 cytokines, indicating their potential application in the treatment of atopic diseases (91). Furthermore, p38 MAPK inhibitors decrease eosinophil survival by activating apoptotic pathways (92). Whether this new class of anti-inflammatory drugs will prove to be safe in long-term studies remains to be established. However, as with corticosteroids, topical application is a possibility to limit toxicity. Inhibitors of the other major MAP kinase pathways (ERK and JNK) have also been developed.

D. Tyrosine Kinase Inhibitors

A pivotal role in signaling the high-affinity IgE receptor (FcεRI) in mast cells is played by the protein tyrosine kinase *syk* kinase, and in *syk*-deficient mice mast cell degranulation is inhibited. This suggests that *syk* might be an important potential target for the development of mast cell stabilizing drugs (93). *syk* is also involved in antigen receptor signaling of B and T lymphocytes and in eosinophil survival in response to IL-5 and GM-CSF (94), so *syk* inhibitors might have several useful beneficial effects in atopic diseases. Another tyrosine kinase, *lyn*, is upstream of *syk*, and an inhibitor of *lyn* kinase, PP1, has an inhibitory effect on eosinophil and mast cell activation (95–97). Because *lyn* and *syk* are widely distributed in the immune system, however, there must be concerns about the long-term safety of selective inhibitors that may necessitate topical administration.

E. Cell Adhesion Blockers

Infiltration of inflammatory cells into tissues depends upon adhesion of circulating inflammatory cells to endothelial cells prior to migration to the inflammatory site (98). This depends upon specific glycoprotein adhesion molecules, including integrins and selectins, on both leukocytes and endothelial cells, which may be upregulated or show increased binding affinity in response to various inflammatory stimuli such as cytokines or lipid mediators. Blocking adhesion molecules using monoclonal antibodies or small-molecule inhibitors is a potential therapeutic approach (see Chap. 13). The interaction between VLA-4 and VCAM-1 is important for eosinophil inflammation, and humanized antibodies to VLA-4 (α4β1) have been developed (99). Small-molecule peptide inhibitors of VLA-4 have been developed that are effective in inhibiting allergen-induced responses in sensitized sheep (100). Whereas the blocking of adhesion molecules is an attractive new approach to the treatment of inflammatory disease, there may be potential danger in inhibiting immune responses leading to more frequent infection or risk of neoplasia.

VIII. Immunomodulators

T lymphocytes may play a critical role in initiating and maintaining the inflammatory process in asthma via the release of cytokines that result in eosinophilic inflammation, suggesting that T-cell inhibitors may be useful in controlling inflammation. Many new drugs for asthma have targeted eosinophilic inflammation (Fig. 2).

A. Nonselective Immunosuppressants

The nonspecific immunomodulator cyclosporin A reduces the dose of oral steroids needed to control asthma in patients with severe asthma (101), but its effi-

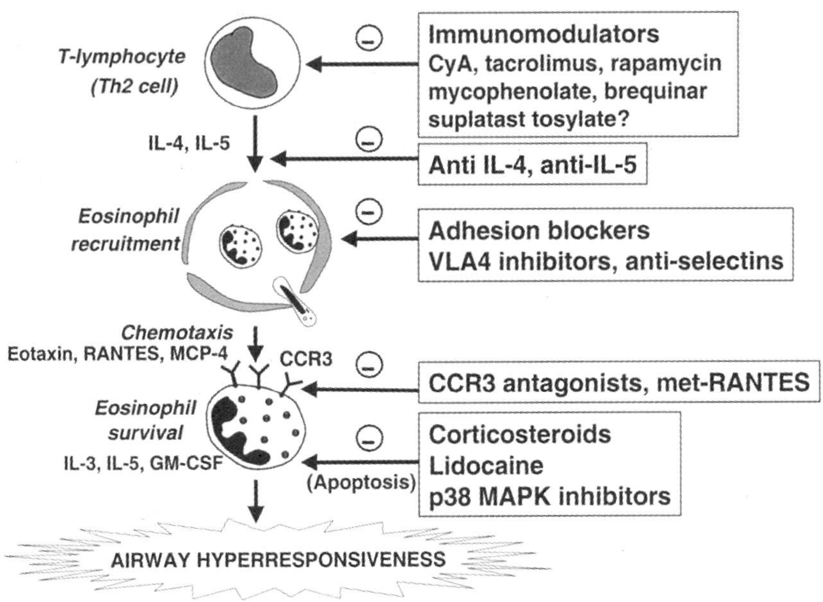

Figure 2 Inhibition of eosinophilic inflammation. Several strategies are possible to inhibit eosinophil inflammation in tissues, including immunomodulators, inhibitors of driving cytokines (IL-4 and IL-5), inhibition of critical adhesion molecules (VLA4, selectins, ICAM-1), blockade of chemokine receptors on eosinophils (CCR3), and induction of apoptosis.

cacy is limited, and side effects, particularly nephrotoxicity, limit routine clinical use (102). The possibility of using inhaled cyclosporin A is now being explored, because in animal studies the inhaled drug is effective in inhibiting the inflammatory response in experimental asthma (103). Immunomodulators, such as tacrolimus (FK506) and rapamycin, appear to be more potent and may be less toxic (see Chap. 13). Novel immunomodulators that inhibit purine or pyrimidine pathways, such as mycofenolate mofetil, leflunomide, and brequinar sodium, may be less toxic and therefore of greater potential value in long-term therapy (104). One problem with nonspecific immunomodulators is that they inhibit both Th1 and Th2 cells and therefore do not restore the imbalance between these Th1 and Th2 cells in atopy. They also inhibit suppressor T cells (Tc1 cells) that may modulate the inflammatory response. Selective inhibition of Th2 cells may be more effective and better tolerated, and there is now a search for such drugs.

$CD4^+$ T cells have been implicated in asthma, and a chimeric antibody directed against $CD4^+$ (keliximab) that reduces circulating $CD4^+$ cells appears to have some beneficial effect in asthma (105), although long-term safety of such a treatment might be a problem. Furthermore, there is increasing evidence that $CD8^+$ cells (Tc2 cells), through release of IL-5 and other cytokines, might also be involved in atopic diseases, particularly in response to infections with viruses (106).

B. Th2-Selective Inhibitors

More selective Th2-selective drugs may be safer for the treatment of asthma in the future. There has been a search for selective inhibitors of Th2 cells by identifying features that differentiate Th1 and Th2 cells. The transcription factor GATA-3 appears to be of particular importance in murine and human Th2 cells (107,108) and may be a target for selective immunomodulatory drugs. However, an argument against strategies to control atopic disease by targeting Th2 cells is that chronic stimulation (by exposure to allergen) results in cells that are relatively resistant to immune suppression (109). An inhibitor of Th2-cytokine release, suplatast tosilate (110), is reported to provide clinical benefit in asthma (111).

IX. Antiallergy Drugs

Most patients with asthma are atopic and commonly suffer from other allergic diseases, such as rhinitis and eczema. Drugs that target the underlying allergic inflammatory process may therefore be of particular benefit in asthma, and they are more selective than nonspecific anti-inflammatory drugs such as corticosteroids. Several drugs in development target the allergic inflammatory process (Fig. 3).

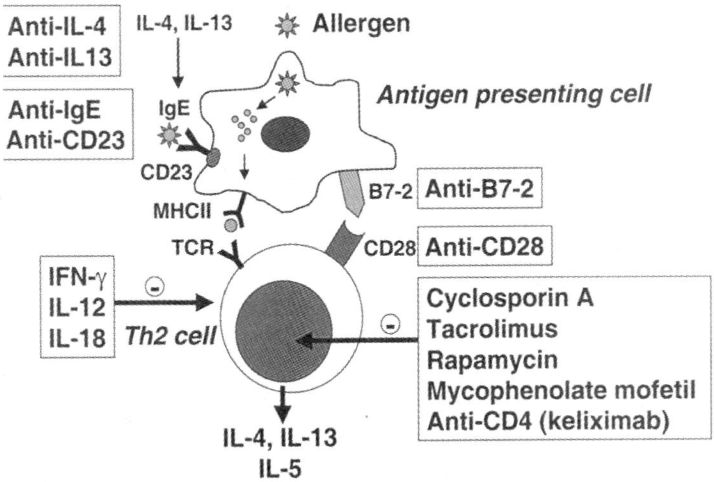

Figure 3 Inhibition of antigen-presenting cells (APCs) and Th2 lymphocytes. Therapies are based on inhibition of costimulatory molecules (B7-2, CD28), inhibition of IgE-driven APCs, and nonselective immunomodulators or cytokines that tip the balance away from Th1 cells toward Th2 cells (IFN-γ, IL-12, IL-18).

A. Cromones

Cromones (cromolyn sodium and nedocromil sodium) are the most specific antiallergy drugs so far discovered. However, they are only weakly effective, partly because of a short duration of action. Cromones appear to have a specific action on allergic inflammation, yet their molecular mechanism of action remains obscure. Although it was initially believed that the primary mode of action of cromones involves inhibiting mast cell mediator release, they affect several other inflammatory cells and sensory nerves. There is increasing evidence that cromones may act on certain types of chloride channels that are expressed in mast cells and sensory nerves (112). Cromolyn phosphorylates a specific cytoskeletal protein, moesin, in mast cells, indicating a possible mechanism that may inhibit degranulation (113). Both cromolyn and nedocromil sodium must be given topically, and all attempts to develop orally active drugs of this type have been unsuccessful, possibly suggesting that topical administration is critical to their efficacy.

B. Furosemide

The potent diuretic furosemide mimics many of the effects of cromones, in inhibiting indirect bronchoconstrictor challenges (allergen, exercise, cold air, adenosine, metabisulfite) but not direct bronchoconstriction (histamine, methacholine, prostaglandins) when given by inhalation (114,115). The mechanism of action of furosemide is not shared by the more potent loop diuretic bumetanide, indicating that some other mechanism than the inhibition of the $Na^+/K^+/Cl^-$ cotransporter must be involved. This is most likely to involve inhibition of the same chloride channel that is inhibited by cromones. Furosemide itself does not appear to be very effective when given regularly by metered dose inhaler in asthma (116), but it is possible that more potent and longer lasting chloride channel blockers might be developed in the future.

C. Costimulation Inhibitors

Costimulatory molecules may play a critical role in augmenting the interaction between antigen-presenting cells and $CD4^+$ T lymphocytes. The interaction between B7 and CD28 may determine whether a Th2-type cell response develops, and there is some evidence that B7-2 (CD86) skews toward a Th2 response. Blocking antibodies to B7-2 inhibit the development of specific IgE, pulmonary eosinophilia, and AHR in mice, whereas antibodies to B7-1 (CD80) are ineffective (117). A molecule on activated T cells, CTL4, appears to act as an endogenous inhibitor of T-cell activation, and a soluble fusion protein construct CTLA4-Ig is effective in blocking AHR in a murine model of asthma (118). Anti-CD28, anti-B7-2, and CTLA4-Ig all block the proliferative response of T cells to allergen (119), indicating that these are potential targets for novel therapies that might be effective in atopic diseases.

D. Anti-IgE

Strategies to block IgE are an obvious approach to the more specific treatment of atopic diseases and are discussed in Chapter 3. Clinical studies with a humanized murine monoclonal antibody (omalizumab) that binds to high affinity IgE-receptors (FcεRI) without activating the receptor show reduction in early and late responses to inhaled allergen and eosinophil counts in induced sputum. Recent studies in patients with moderate and severe asthma demonstrated significant steroid-sparing effects. In patients with severe asthma who require oral steroids there was a significant reduction in oral steroid requirements, and several patients were able to completely withdraw from oral steroids in comparison with a placebo (120). This represents an important advance in therapy (121). Although injections of antibody may not be feasible for the long-term treatment of mild asthma, they could be a realistic therapy for patients with severe asthma, particularly when there is severe concomitant rhinitis or eczema. It is of interest that corticosteroids do not suppress IgE and may even increase it, so this therapy may be directed toward an element of asthma that is currently not targeted by corticosteroids (122).

Allergen may also signal through a low-affinity IgE receptor (FcεR2,

CD23) that is expressed on B lymphocytes, macrophages, and eosinophils. An anti-CD23 Fab fragment blocks allergen-induced airway inflammation in mice, suggesting that this might be a therapeutic approach to inhibit allergic responses (123). Antibodies to CD23 are now in clinical development as a treatment for asthma.

X. Preventive Strategies

Atopy appears to be due to immune deviation from Th1 to Th2 cells, which may arise because of a failure to inhibit the normal Th2 preponderance at birth. This may be due to an absence of the environmental factors, such as bacterial infections and endotoxins, that stimulate the Th1 response.

A. Immunotherapy

Subcutaneous injection of small amounts of purified allergen has been used for many years in the treatment of allergy. It is effective in the treatment of insect venom anaphylaxis and hayfever and may induce prolonged remission (124) but is less effective in asthma. The molecular mechanism of desensitization is still uncertain. Cloning of several common allergen genes has now made it possible to prepare recombinant allergens for injection, although this purity may detract from their allergenicity, as most natural allergens contain several proteins. Intramuscular injection of rats with plasmid DNA expressing house dust mite allergen results in its long-term expression and prevents the development of IgE responses to inhaled allergen (125). This suggests that allergen gene immunization might be a useful specific therapeutic strategy in the future.

B. Peptide Immunotherapy

Small peptide fragments of allergen (epitopes) are able to block allergen-induced T-cell responses without inducing anaphylaxis (126). T-cell-derived peptides from cat allergen (*fel* d 1) are able to block allergen responses to cat dander (127) but may induce an isolated late response to allergen by direct T-cell activation (128). This appears to precede a prolonged period of unresponsiveness to allergen (anergy) (129). The problem with this approach is that it is specific for a particular allergen, and it is likely that for most patients several allergens can drive the inflammatory response.

C. Vaccination

A relative lack of infections may be a factor predisposing to the development of atopy in genetically predisposed individuals, leading to the concept that vaccination may induce protective Th1 responses to prevent sensitization and thus prevent the development of atopic diseases. BCG inoculation in mice 14 days before allergen sensitization reduced the formation of specific IgE in response to allergen and the eosinophilic response and AHR responses to allergen, with an increase in production of IFN-γ (130). This led to clinical trials of BCG to prevent the development of atopy. Similar results have been obtained in mice with a single injection of heat-killed *Mycobacterium vaccae*, another potent inducer of Th1 responses (131), and with *Listeria*. *Lactobacillus acidophilus* in yogurt, another potential means of tipping back the balance from Th2 to Th1 cells, weakly increases IFN-γ formation in adult asthmatic patients (132).

Immunostimulatory DNA sequences from bacteria, such as unmethylated cytosine-guanosine dinucleotide-containing oligonucleotides (CpG ODNs), are also potent inducers of Th1 cytokines. In mice, administration of CpG ODN increases the ratio of Th1 to Th2 cells, decreases formation of specific IgE, and reduces the eosinophilic response to allergen, an effect that lasts for over 6 weeks (133). These promising animal studies encourage the expectation that vaccination may prevent or cure atopic diseases in the future (134,135).

XI. Gene Therapy and the Impact of Molecular Genetics

Because asthma is polygenic, it is unlikely that gene therapy will be of value in long-term therapy. However, an understanding of the genes involved in atopic diseases and in disease severity may help to identify new molecular targets and also to predict the response to different forms of therapy (pharmacogenetics) (136). Transfer of anti-inflammatory genes may provide specific anti-inflammatory or inhibitory proteins in a convenient manner, and gene transfer by the use of viral vectors has been shown to be feasible in animals (137,138). Anti-inflammatory proteins relevant to asthma include IL-10, IL-12, and IκB. Antisense oligonucleotides may switch off specific genes, but there are considerable problems in getting these molecules into cells. An inhaled antisense oligonucleotide directed against the adenosine A_1 receptor has been shown to reduce AHR in a rabbit model of asthma, demonstrating the potential of this approach in treating asthma (139,140). Suitable target genes may be Th2 cytokines or their receptors. Considering the practical problems encountered in gene therapy, this approach is unlikely in the foreseeable future other than for proof-of-concept studies.

A. Role of Molecular Genetics

Sequencing of the human genome is likely to have an important impact on the future development of asthma therapy (141). All known drugs for human diseases target fewer than 500 molecules. As there are predicted to be over 200,000 human proteins coded by 30,000 genes, this gives scope to developing many new and more specific drugs that target known or novel genes that are associated with asthma.

Single nucleotide polymorphisms (SNPs) occur in most genes and account for the variability in gene expression between individuals. It is the combination of SNPs on different genes that produces genetic susceptibility to complex diseases such as asthma, and these SNPs are now being identified (142). Once we understand the relevant SNP maps it should be possible to predict the clinical progress of asthmatic patients and to identify patients who will develop severe or progressive disease. SNP maps may also be used to predict how a patient will respond to a particular drug and whether there is a risk of side effects. Although we diagnose asthma on the basis of a clinical pattern, it is likely that there are many variants and that these show different responses to treatments. For example, only a small number of asthmatic patients benefit from antileukotrienes, but at the moment we are unable to identify these individuals. In the future, it may be possible to precisely predict which patients may have differences in the synthesis of and response to leukotrienes (143). Similarly, patients with severe asthma who have a reduced responsiveness to corticosteroids may have differences in the genes that regulate corticosteroid responsiveness.

Being able to discriminate between asthmatic patients may also make clinical trials much more efficient, because only patients selected to have a good response without side effects will be selected, so that smaller numbers will be needed, which will accelerate the development of new asthma drugs.

References

1. Busse WW, Lemanske RF. Asthma. N Engl J Med 2001; 344:350–362.
2. Barnes PJ, Chung KF, Page CP. Inflammatory mediators of asthma: An update. Pharmacol Rev 1998; 50:515–596.
3. Pauwels RA, Lofdahl C-G, Postma DS, Tattersfield AE, O'Byrne PM, Barnes PJ, Ullman A. Effect of inhaled formoterol and budesonide on exacerbations of asthma. N Engl J Med 1997; 337:1412–1418.
4. Shrewsbury S, Pyke S, Britton M. Meta-analysis of increased dose of inhaled steroid or addition of salmeterol in symptomatic asthma (MIASMA). Br Med J 2000; 320:1368–1373.
5. Barnes PJ, Pauwels RA. Theophylline in asthma: Time for reappraisal? Eur Resp J 1994; 7:579–591.
6. Barnes PJ. New treatments for asthma. Eur J Intern Med 2000; 11:9–20.
7. Barnes PJ. Inhaled glucocorticoids for asthma. N Engl J Med 1995; 332:868–875.
8. Barnes PJ. Current issues for establishing inhaled corticosteroids as the anti-inflammatory agents of choice in asthma. J Allergy Clin Immunol 1998; 101:S427–S433.
9. Barnes PJ, Pedersen S, Busse WW. Efficacy and safety of inhaled corticosteroids: An update. Am J Respir Crit Care Med 1998; 157:S1–S53.

10. Tasche MJ, Uijen JH, Bernsen RM, de Jongste JC, van Der W. Inhaled disodium cromoglycate (DSCG) as maintenance therapy in children with asthma: A systematic review. Thorax 2000; 55:913–920.
11. Drazen JM, Israel E, O'Byrne PM. Treatment of asthma with drugs modifying the leukotriene pathway. N Engl J Med 1999; 340:197–206.
12. Busse W, Nelson H, Wolfe J, Kalberg C, Yancey SW, Rickard KA. Comparison of inhaled salmeterol and oral zafirlukast in patients with asthma. J Allergy Clin Immunol 1999; 103:1075–1080.
13. Bleecker ER, Welch MJ, Weinstein SF, Kalberg C, Johnson M, Edwards L, Rickard KA. Low-dose inhaled fluticasone propionate versus oral zafirlukast in the treatment of persistent asthma. J Allergy Clin Immunol 2000; 105:1123–1129.
14. Kim KT, Ginchansky EJ, Friedman BF, Srebro S, Pepsin PJ, Edwards L, Stanford RH, Rickard K. Fluticasone propionate versus zafirlukast: Effect in patients previously receiving inhaled corticosteroid therapy. Ann Allergy Asthma Immunol 2000; 85:398–406.
15. Nelson HS, Busse WW, Kerwin E, Church N, Emmett A, Rickard K, Knobil K. Fluticasone propionate/salmeterol combination provides more effective asthma control than low-dose inhaled corticosteroid plus montelukast. J Allergy Clin Immunol 2000; 106:1088–1095.
16. Robinson DS, Campbell DA, Barnes PJ. Addition of an anti-leukotriene to therapy in chronic severe asthma in a clinic setting: A double-blind, randomised, placebo-controlled study. Lancet 2001; 357:2007–2011.
17. Kidney JC, Dominguez M, Rose M, Aikman S, Chung KF, Barnes PJ. Immune modulation by theophylline: The effect of withdrawal of chronic treatment in asthma. Am J Respir Crit Care Med 1995; 151:1907–1914.
18. Ito K, Lim S, Adcock IM, Caramori G, Keller A, Barnes PJ. Effect of low dose theophylline on histone deacetylase activity in patients with mild asthma. Am J Resp Crit Care Med 2000; 161:A614.
19. Evans DJ, Taylor DA, Zetterstrom O, Chung KF, O'Connor BJ, Barnes PJ. A comparison of low-dose inhaled budesonide plus theophylline and high-dose inhaled budesonide for moderate asthma. N Engl J Med 1997; 337:1412–1418.
20. Ukena D, Harnest U, Sakalauskas R, Magyar P, Vetter N, Steffen H, Leichtl S, Rathgeb F, Keller A, Steinijans VW. Comparison of addition of theophylline to inhaled steroid with doubling of the dose of inhaled steroid in asthma. Eur Respir J 1997; 10:2754–2760.
21. Lim S, Jatakanon A, Gordon D, Macdonald C, Chung KF, Barnes PJ. Comparison of high dose inhaled steroids, low dose inhaled steroids plus low dose theophylline, and low dose inhaled steroids alone in chronic asthma in general practice. Thorax 2000; 55:837–841.
22. Hill SJ, Tattersfield AE. Corticosteroid sparing agents in asthma. Thorax 1995; 50: 577–582.
23. Frew AJ, Plummeridge MJ. Alternative agents in asthma. J Allergy Clin Immunol 2001; 108:3–10.
24. Palmqvist M, Arvidsson P, Beckman O, Peterson S, Lotvall J. Onset of bronchodilation of budesonide/formoterol vs. salmeterol/fluticasone in single inhalers. Pulm Pharmacol Ther 2001; 14:29–34.

25. Cochrane GM, Horne R, Chanez P. Compliance in asthma. Respir Med 1999; 93: 763–769.
26. Leynaert B, Neukirch F, Demoly P, Bousquet J. Epidemiologic evidence for asthma and rhinitis comorbidity. J Allergy Clin Immunol 2000; 106:S201–S205.
27. Barnes PJ, Woolcock AJ. Difficult asthma. Eur Respir J 1998; 12:1209–1218.
28. Szefler SJ, Leung DY. Glucocorticoid-resistant asthma: Pathogenesis and clinical implications for management. Eur Respir J 1997; 10:1640–1647.
29. Barnes PJ. Therapeutic strategies for allergic diseases. Nature 1999; 402:B31–B38.
30. Barnes PJ. New directions in allergic disease: Mechanism-based anti-inflammatory therapies. J Allergy Clin Immunol 2000; 106:5–16.
31. Barnes PJ. Efficacy of inhaled corticosteroids in asthma. J Allergy Clin Immunol 1998; 102:531–538.
32. Taylor DA, Jensen MW, Kanabar V, Englestatter R, Steinjans VW, Barnes PJ, O'Connor BJ. A dose-dependent effect of the novel inhaled corticosteroid ciclesonide on airway responsiveness to adenosine-5′-monophosphate in asthmatic patients. Am J Respir Crit Care Med 1999; 160:237–243.
33. Barnes PJ. Antiinflammatory actions of glucocorticoids: Molecular mechanisms. Clin Sci 1998; 94:557–572.
34. Ito K, Barnes PJ, Adcock IM. Glucocorticoid receptor recruitment of histone deacetylase 2 inhibits IL-1β-induced histone H4 acetylation on lysines 8 and 12. Mol Cell Biol 2000; 20:6891–6903.
35. Reichardt HM, Kaestner KH, Tuckermann J, Kretz O, Wessely O, Bock R, Gass P, Schmid W, Herrlich P, Angel P, Schutz G. DNA binding of the glucocorticoid receptor is not essential for survival [see comments]. Cell 1998; 93:531–541.
36. Vayssiere BM, Dupont S, Choquart A, Petit F, Garcia T, Marchandeau C, Gronemeyer H, Resche-Rigon M. Synthetic glucocorticoids that dissociate transactivation and AP-1 transrepression exhibit antiinflammatory activity in vivo. Mol Endocrinol 1997; 11:1245–1255.
37. Belvisi MG, Wicks SL, Battram CH, Bottoms SE, Redford JE, Woodman P, Brown TJ, Webber SE, Foster ML. Therapeutic benefit of a dissociated glucocorticoid and the relevance of in vitro separation of transrepression from transactivation activity. J Immunol 2001; 166:1975–1982.
38. Chung KF. Platelet-activating factor in inflammation and pulmonary disorders. Clin Sci 1992; 83:127–138.
39. Feldman M, Taylor P, Paleolog E, Brennan FM, Maini RN. Anti-TNFα therapy is useful in rheumatoid arthritis and Crohn's disease: Analysis of the mechanism of action predicts utility in other diseases. Transplant Proc 1998; 30:4126–4127.
40. Roquet A, Dahlen B, Kumlin M, Ihre E, Anstren G, Binks S, Dahlen SE. Combined antagonism of leukotrienes and histamine produces predominant inhibition of allergen-induced early and late phase airway obstruction in asthmatics. Am J Respir Crit Care Med 1997; 155:1856–1863.
41. Chung KF, Barnes PJ. Cytokines in asthma. Thorax 1999; 54:825–857.
42. Barncs, PJ. Cytokinc modulators as novel therapies for asthma. Ann Rev Pharmacol Toxicol 2002; 42:81–98.
43. Greenfeder S, Umland SP, Cuss FM, Chapman RW, Egan RW. The role of interleukin-5 in allergic eosinophilic disease. Respir Res 2001; 2:71–79.

44. Leckie MJ, ten Brincke A, Khan J, Diamant Z, O'Connor BJ, Walls CM, Mathur M, Cowley H, Chung KF, Djukanovic RJ, Hansel TT, Holgate ST, Sterk PJ, Barnes PJ. Effects of an interleukin-5 blocking monoclonal antibody on eosinophils, airway hyperresponsiveness and the late asthmatic response. Lancet 2000; 356:2144–2148.
45. Kips JC, O'Connor BJ, Langley SJ, Woodcock A, Kerstjens HAM, Postma DS, Danzig M, Cuss F, Pauwels RA. Results of a phase I trial with SCH55700, a humanized anti-IL-5 antibody in severe persistent asthma. Am J Resp Crit Care Med 2000; 161:A505.
46. Steinke JW, Borish L. Interleukin-4: Its role in the pathogenesis of asthma, and targeting it for asthma treatment with interleukin-4 receptor antagonists. Respir Res 2001; 2:66–70.
47. Borish LC, Nelson HS, Corren J, Bensch G, Busse WW, Whitmore JB, Agosti JM. Efficacy of soluble IL-4 receptor for the treatment of adults with asthma. J Allergy Clin Immunol 2001; 107:963–970.
48. Wills-Karp M, Luyimbazi J, Xu X, Schofield B, Neben TY, Karp CL, Donaldson DD. Interleukin-13: Central mediator of allergic asthma. Science 1998; 282:2258–2261.
49. Shimbara A, Christodoulopoulos P, Soussi-Gounni A, Olivenstein R, Nakamura Y, Levitt RC, Nicolaides NC, Holroyd KJ, Tsicopoulos A, Lafitte JJ, Wallaert B, Hamid QA. IL-9 and its receptor in allergic and nonallergic lung disease: Increased expression in asthma. J Allergy Clin Immunol 2000; 105:108–115.
50. Zhou Y, McLane M, Levitt RC. Interleukin-9 as a therapeutic target for asthma. Respir Res 2001; 2:80–84.
51. Thomas PS. Tumour necrosis factor-α: The role of this multifunctional cytokine in asthma. Immunol Cell Biol 2001; 79:132–140.
52. Markham A, Lamb HM. Infliximab: A review of its use in the management of rheumatoid arthritis. Drugs 2000; 59:1341–1359.
53. Rossi D, Zlotnik A. The biology of chemokines and their receptors. Annu Rev Immunol 2000; 18:217–242.
54. Proudfoot AE, Power CA, Wells TN. The strategy of blocking the chemokine system to combat disease. Immunol Rev 2000; 177:246–256.
55. Lloyd CM, Delaney T, Nguyen T, Tian J, Martinez A, Coyle AJ, Gutierrez-Ramos JC. CC chemokine receptor (CCR)3/eotaxin is followed by CCR4/monocyte-derived chemokine in mediating pulmonary T helper lymphocyte type 2 recruitment after serial antigen challenge in vivo. J Exp Med 2000; 191:265–274.
56. Jatakanon A, Uasaf C, Maziak W, Lim S, Chung KF, Barnes PJ. Neutrophilic inflammation in severe persistent asthma. Am J Respir Crit Care Med 1999; 160:1532–1539.
57. White JR, Lee JM, Young PR, Hertzberg RP, Jurewicz AJ, Chaikin MA, Widdowson K, Foley JJ, Martin LD, Griswold DE, Sarau HM. Identification of a potent, selective non-peptide CXCR2 antagonist that inhibits interleukin-8-induced neutrophil migration. J Biol Chem 1998; 273:10095–10098.
58. Barnes PJ, Lim S. Inhibitory cytokines in asthma. Mol Medicine Today 1998; 4:452–458.

59. Selig W, Tocker J. Effect of interleukin-1 receptor antagonist on antigen-induced pulmonary responses in guinea-pigs. Eur J Pharmacol 1992; 213:331–336.
60. Rosenwasser LJ. Biologic activities of IL-1 and its role in human disease. J Allergy Clin Immunol 1998; 102:344–350.
61. Barnes PJ. IL-10: A key regulator of allergic disease. Clin Exp Allergy 2001; 31: 667–669.
62. John M, Lim S, Seybold J, Robichaud A, O'Connor B, Barnes PJ, Chung KF. Inhaled corticosteroids increase IL-10 but reduce MIP-1α, GM-CSF and IFN-g release from alveolar macrophages in asthma. Am J Respir Crit Care Med 1998; 157:256–262.
63. Zuany-Amorim C, Haile S, Leduc D, Dumarey C, Huerre M, Vargaftig BB, Pretolani M. Interleukin-10 inhibits antigen-induced cellular recruitment into the airways of sensitized mice. J Clin Invest 1995; 95:2644–2651.
64. Akdis CA, Blesken T, Akdis M, Wuthrich B, Blaser K. Role of interleukin 10 in specific immunotherapy. J Clin Invest 1998; 102:98–106.
65. Fedorak RN, Gangl A, Elson CO, Rutgeerts P, Schreiber S, Wild G, Hanauer SB, Kilian A, Cohard M, LeBeaut A, Feagan B. Recombinant human interleukin 10 in the treatment of patients with mild to moderately active Crohn's disease. Gastroenterology 2000; 119:1473–1482.
66. Seldon PM, Barnes PJ, Giembycz MA. Interleukin-10 does not mediate the inhibitory effect of PDE4 inhibitors and other cAMP-elevating drugs on lipopolysaccharide-induced tumor necrosis factor-α generation from human peripheral blood monocytes. Cell Biochem Biophys 1998; 28:179–201.
67. Lack G, Bradley KL, Hamelmann E, Renz H, Loader J, Leung DY, Larsen G, Gelfand EW. Nebulized IFN-γ inhibits the development of secondary allergic responses in mice. J Immunol 1996; 157:1432–1439.
68. Boguniewicz M, Martin RJ, Martin D, Gibson U, Celniker A. The effects of nebulized recombinant interferon-γ in asthmatic airways. J Allergy Clin Immunol 1995; 95:133–135.
69. Benjaponpitak S, Oro A, Maguire P, Marinkovich V, DeKruyff RH, Umetsu DT. The kinetics of change in cytokine production by CD4 T cells during conventional allergen immunotherapy. J Allergy Clin Immunol 1999; 103:468–475.
70. Durham SR, Ying S, Varney VA, Jacobson MR, Sudderick RM, Mackay IS, Kay AB, Hamid QA. Grass pollen immunotherapy inhibits allergen-induced infiltration of CD4+ T lymphocytes and eosinophils in the nasal mucosa and increases the number of cells expressing messenger RNA for interferon-gamma. J Allergy Clin Immunol 1996; 97:1356–1365.
71. Gratzl S, Palca A, Schmitz M, Simon HU. Treatment with IFN-α in corticosteroid-unresponsive asthma. J Allergy Clin Immunol 2000; 105:1035–1036.
72. Gately MK, Renzetti LM, Magram J, Stern AS, Adorini L, Gubler U, Presky DH. The interleukin-12/interleukin-12-receptor system: Role in normal and pathologic immune responses. Annu Rev Immunol 1998; 16:495–521.
73. Gavett SH, O'Hearn DJ, Li X, Huang SK, Finkelman FD, Wills-Karp M. Interleukin 12 inhibits antigen-induced airway hyperresponsiveness, inflammation and Th2 cytokine expression in mice. J Exp Med 1995; 182:1527–1536.

74. Leonard JP, Sherman ML, Fisher GL, Buchanan LJ, Larsen G, Atkins MB, Sosman JA, Dutcher JP, Vogelzang NJ, Ryan JL. Effects of single-dose interleukin-12 exposure on interleukin-12-associated toxicity and interferon-gamma production. Blood 1997; 90:2541–2548.
75. Bryan S, O'Connor BJ, Matti S, Leckie MJ, Kanabar V, Khan J, Warrington S, Renzetti L, Rames A, Bock JA, Boyce M, Hansel TT, Holgate ST, Sterk PJ, Barnes PJ. Effects of recombinant human interleukin-12 on eosinophils, airway hyperreactivity and the late asthmatic response. Lancet 2000; 356:2149–2153.
76. Kim TS, DeKruyff RH, Rupper R, Maecker HT, Levy S, Umetsu DT. An ovalbumin-IL-12 fusion protein is more effective than ovalbumin plus free recombinant IL-12 in inducing a T helper cell type 1-dominated immune response and inhibiting antigen-specific IgE production. J Immunol 1997; 158:4137–4144.
77. Dinarello CA. Interleukin-18, a proinflammatory cytokine. Eur Cytokine Netw 2000; 11:483–486.
78. Walter DM, Wong CP, DeKruyff RH, Berry GJ, Levy S, Umetsu DT. Il-18 gene transfer by adenovirus prevents the development of and reverses established allergen-induced airway hyperreactivity. J Immunol 2001; 166:6392–6398.
79. Torphy TJ. Phosphodiesterase isoenzymes. Am J Respir Crit Care Med 1998; 157: 351–370.
80. Chan SC, Hanifin JM. Differential inhibitor effects on phosphodiesterase isoforms in atopic and normal leukocytes. J Lab Clin Med 1993; 121:44–51.
81. Muller T, Engels P, Fozard J. Subtypes of the type 4 cAMP phosphodiesterase: Structure, regulation and selective inhibition. Trends Pharmacol Sci 1996; 17:294–298.
82. Seybold J, Newton R, Wright L, Finney PA, Suttorp N, Barnes PJ, Adcock IM, Giembycz MA. Induction of phosphodiesterases 3B, 4A4, 4D1, 4D2, and 4D3 in Jurkat T-cells and in human peripheral blood T-lymphocytes by 8-bromo-cAMP and G_s-coupled receptor agonists. Potential role in β_2-adrenoreceptor desensitization. J Biol Chem 1998; 273:20575–20588.
83. Li L, Yee C, Beavo JA. CD3- and CD28-dependent induction of PDE7 required for T cell activation. Science 1999; 283:848–851.
84. Barnes PJ, Karin M. Nuclear factor-κB: A pivotal transcription factor in chronic inflammatory diseases. N Engl J Med 1997; 336:1066–1071.
85. Barnes PJ, Adcock IM. Transcription factors and asthma. Eur Respir J 1998; 12: 221–234.
86. Delhase M, Li N, Karin M. Kinase regulation in inflammatory response. Nature 2000; 406:367–368.
87. Nasuhara Y, Adcock IM, Catley M, Barnes PJ, Newton R. Differential IKK activation and IκBα degradation by interleukin-1β and tumor necrosis factor-α in human U937 monocytic cells: Evidence for additional regulatory steps in κB-dependent transcription. J Biol Chem 1999; 274:19965–19972.
88. Rao A, Luo C, Hogan PG. Transcription factors of the NFAT family: Regulation and function. Annu Rev Immunol 1997; 15:707–747.
89. Karin M. Mitogen-activated protein kinase cascades as regulators of stress responses. Ann NY Acad Sci 1998; 851:139–146.
90. Lee JC, Kumar S, Griswold DE, Underwood DC, Votta BJ, Adams JL. Inhibition

of p38 MAP kinase as a therapeutic strategy. Immunopharmacology 2000; 47:185–201.
91. Schafer PH, Wadsworth SA, Wang L, Siekierka JJ. p38α mitogen-activated protein kinase is activated by CD28-mediated signaling and is required for IL-4 production by human CD4+CD45RO+T cells and Th2 effector cells. J Immunol 1999; 162: 7110–7119.
92. Kankaanranta H, Giembycz MA, Barnes PJ, Lindsay DA. SB203580, an inhibitor of p38 mitogen-activated protein kinase, enhances constitutive apoptosis of cytokine-deprived human eosinophils. J Pharmacol Exp Ther 1999; 290:621–628.
93. Costello PS, Turner M, Walters AE, Cunningham CN, Bauer PH, Downward J, Tybulewicz VL. Critical role for the tyrosine kinase Syk in signalling through the high affinity IgE receptor of mast cells. Oncogene 1996; 13:2595–2605.
94. Yousefi S, Hoessli DC, Blaser K, Mills GB, Simon HU. Requirement of Lyn and Syk tyrosine kinases for the prevention of apoptosis by cytokines in human eosinophils. J Exp Med 1996; 183:1407–1414.
95. Amoui M, Draber P, Draberova L. Src family-selective tyrosine kinase inhibitor, PP1, inhibits both FcεRI- and Thy-1-mediated activation of rat basophilic leukemia cells. Eur J Immunol 1997; 27:1881–1886.
96. Lynch OT, Giembycz MA, Barnes PJ, Hellewell PG, Lindsay MA. 'Outside-in' signalling mechanisms underlying CD11b/CD18- mediated NADPH oxidase activation in human adherent blood eosinophils. Br J Pharmacol 1999; 128:1149–1158.
97. Lynch OT, Giembycz MA, Daniels I, Barnes PJ, Lindsay MA. Pleiotropic role of lyn kinase in leukotriene B_4-induced eosinophil activation. Blood 2000; 95:3541–3547.
98. Pilewski JM, Albelda SM. Cell adhesion molecules in asthma: Homing activation and airway remodelling. Am J Respir Cell Mol Biol 1995; 12:1–3.
99. Yuan Q, Strauch KL, Lobb RR, Hemler ME. Intracellular single-chain antibody inhibits integrin VLA-4 maturation and function. Biochem J 1996; 318:591–596.
100. Lin Kc, Ateeq HS, Hsiung SH, Chong LT, Zimmerman CN, Castro A, Lee WC, Hammond CE, Kalkunte S, Chen LL, Pepinsky RB, Leone DR, Sprague AG, Abraham WM, Gill A, Lobb RR, Adams SP. Selective, tight-binding inhibitors of integrin α4β1 that inhibit allergic airway responses. J Med Chem 1999; 42:920–934.
101. Alexander AG, Barnes NC, Kay AB. Trial of cyclosporin in corticosteroid-dependent chronic severe asthma. Lancet 1992; 339:324–328.
102. Evans DJ, Cullinan P, Geddes DM. Cyclosporin as an oral corticosteroid sparing agent in stable asthma. Cochrane Database Syst Rev 2001; 2:CD002993.
103. Underwood SL, McMillan S, Reeves R, Hunt J, Brealey CJ, Webber S, Foster M, Sargent CA. Effects of cyclosporin A administered into the airways against antigen-induced airway inflammation and hyperreactivity in the rat. Eur J Pharmacol 2001; 420:165–173.
104. Thompson AG, Starzl TC. New immunosuppressive drugs: Mechanistic insights and potential therapeutic advances. Immunol Rev 1993; 136:71–98.
105. Kon OM, Sihra BS, Compton CH, Leonard TB, Kay AB, Barnes NC. Randomised dose-ranging placebo-controlled study of chimeric antibody to CD4 (keliximab) in chronic severe asthma. Lancet 1998; 352:1109–1113.
106. Schwarze J, Cieslewicz G, Joetham A, Ikemura T, Hamelmann E, Gelfand EW.

CD8 T cells are essential in the development of respiratory syncytial virus-induced lung eosinophilia and airway hyperresponsiveness. J Immunol 1999; 162:4207–4211.

107. Zhang Z, Zimonjic DB, Popescu NC, Wang N, Gerhard DS, Stone EM, Arbour NC, De Vries HG, Scheffer H, Gerritsen J, Colle'e JM, Ten Kate LP, Mukherjee AB. Human uteroglobin gene: Structure, subchromosomal localization, and polymorphism. DNA Cell Biol 1997; 16:73–83.
108. Caramori G, Lim S, Ciaccia A, Fabbri LM, Barnes PJ, Adcock IM. GATA transcription factor expression in T cells, monocytes and bronchial biopsies of normal and asthmatic subjects. Am J Respir Crit Care Med 1999; 157:A908.
109. Murphy E, Shibuya K, Hosken N, Openshaw P, Maino V, Davis K, Murphy K, O'Garra A. Reversibility of T helper 1 and 2 populations is lost after long-term stimulation. J Exp Med 1996; 183:901–913.
110. Oda N, Minoguchi K, Yokoe T, Hashimoto T, Wada K, Miyamoto M, Tanaka A, Kohno Y, Adachi M. Effect of suplatast tosilate (IPD-1151T) on cytokine production by allergen-specific human Th1 and Th2 cell lines. Life Sci 1999; 65:763–770.
111. Tamaoki J, Kondo M, Sakai N, Aoshiba K, Tagaya E, Nakata J, Isono K, Nagai A. Effect of suplatast tosilate, a Th2 cytokine inhibitor, on steroid-dependent asthma: A double-blind randomised study. Lancet 2000; 356:273–278.
112. Heinke S, Szucs G, Norris A, Droogmans G, Nilius B. Inhibition of volume-activated chloride currents in endothelial cells by chromones. Br J Pharmacol 1995; 115:1393–1398.
113. Wang L, Correia I, Basu S, Theoharides TC. Ca^{2+} and phorbol ester effect on the mast cell phosphoprotein induced by cromolyn. Eur J Pharmacol 1999; 371:241–249.
114. Bianco S, Pieroni MG, Refini RM, Robuschi M, Vaghi A, Sestini P. Inhaled loop diuretics as potential new anti-asthmatic drugs. Eur Resp J 1993; 6:130–134.
115. Barnes PJ. Diuretics and asthma. Thorax 1993; 48:195–197.
116. Yates DH, O'Connor BJ, Yilmaz G, Aikman S, Chen-Worsdell M, Barnes PJ, Chung KF. Effect of acute and chronic inhaled furosemide on bronchial hyperresponsiveness in mild asthma. Am J Respir Crit Care Med 1995; 152:892–896.
117. Haczku A, Takeda K, Redai I, Hamelmann E, Cieslewicz G, Joetham A, Loader J, Lee JJ, Irvin C, Gelfand EW. Anti-CD86 (B7.2) treatment abolishes allergic airway hyperresponsiveness in mice. Am J Respir Crit Care Med 1999; 159:1638–1643.
118. Van Oosterhout AJ, Hofstra CL, Shields R, Chan B, van Ark I, Jardieu PM, Nijkamp FP. Murine CTLA4-IgG treatment inhibits airway eosinophilia and hyperresponsiveness and attenuates IgE upregulation in a murine model of allergic asthma. Am J Respir Cell Mol Biol 1997; 17:386–392.
119. van Neerven RJ, Van de Pol MM, van der Zee JS, Stiekema FE, De Boer M, Kapsenberg ML. Requirement of CD28-CD86 costimulation for allergen-specific T cell proliferation and cytokine expression. Clin Exp Allergy 1998; 28:808–816.
120. Milgrom H, Fick RB Jr, Su JQ, Reimann J, Bush RK, Watrous ML, Metzger WJ. Treatment of allergic asthma with monoclonal anti-IgE antibody. N Engl J Med 1999; 341:1966–1973.

121. Barnes PJ. Anti-IgE therapy in asthma: Rationale and therapeutic potential. Int Arch Allergy Immunol 2000; 123:196–204.
122. Barnes PJ. Corticosteroids, IgE, and atopy. J Clin Invest 2001; 107:265–266.
123. Dasic G, Juillard P, Graber P, Herren S, Angell T, Knowles R, Bonnefoy JY, Kosco-Vilbois MH, Chvatchko Y. Critical role of CD23 in allergen-induced bronchoconstriction in a murine model of allergic asthma. Eur J Immunol 1999; 29: 2957–2967.
124. Durham SR, Walker SM, Varga EM, Jacobson MR, O'Brien F, Noble W, Till SJ, Hamid QA, Nouri-Aria KT. Long-term clinical efficacy of grass-pollen immunotherapy. N Engl J Med 1999; 341:468–475.
125. Hsu CH, Chua KY, Tao MH, Lai YL, Wu HD, Huang SK, Hsieh KH. Immunoprophylaxis of allergen-induced immunoglobulin E synthesis and airway hyperresponsiveness in vivo by genetic immunization. Nat Med 1996; 2:540–544.
126. Yssel H, Fasler S, Lamb J, de Vries JE. Induction of non-responsiveness in human allergen specific type 2 helper cells. Curr Opin Immunol 1994; 6:847–852.
127. Norman PS, Ohman JL Jr, Long AA, Creticos PS, Gefter MA, Shaked Z, Wood RA, Eggleston PA, Hafner KB, Rao P, Lichtenstein LM, Jones NH, Nicodemus CF. Treatment of cat allergy with T-cell reactive peptides. Am J Respir Crit Care Med 1996; 154:1623–1628.
128. Haselden BM, Barry Kay A, Larche M. Immunoglobulin E-independent major histocompatibility complex-restricted T cell peptide epitope-induced late asthmatic reactions. J Exp Med 1999; 189:1885–1894.
129. Oldfield WL, Kay AB, Larche M. Allergen-derived T cell peptide-induced late asthmatic reactions precede the induction of antigen-specific hyporesponsiveness in atopic allergic asthmatic subjects. J Immunol 2001; 167:1734–1739.
130. Herz U, Gerhold K, Gruber C, Braun A, Wahn U, Renz H, Paul K. BCG infection suppresses allergic sensitization and development of increased airway reactivity in an animal model. J Allergy Clin Immunol 1998; 102:867–874.
131. Wang CC, Rook GA. Inhibition of an established allergic response to ovalbumin in BALB/c mice by killed Mycobacterium vaccae. Immunology 1998; 93:307–313.
132. Wheeler MA, Smith SD, Garcia Cardena G, Nathan CF, Weiss RM, Sessa WC. Bacterial infection induces nitric oxide synthase in human neutrophils. J Clin Invest 1997; 99:110–116.
133. Sur S, Wild JS, Choudhury BK, Sur N, Alam R, Klinman DM. Long term prevention of allergic lung inflammation in a mouse model of asthma by CpG oligodeoxynucleotides. J Immunol 1999; 162:6284–6293.
134. Krieg AM, Kline JN. Immune effects and therapeutic applications of CpG motifs in bacterial DNA. Immunopharmacology 2000; 48:303–305.
135. Horner AA, Van Uden JH, Zubeldia JM, Broide D, Raz E. DNA-based immunotherapeutics for the treatment of allergic disease. Immunol Rev 2001; 179:102–118.
136. Hall IP. Pharmacogenetics of asthma. Eur Respir J 2000; 15:449–451.
137. Xing Z, Ohkawara Y, Jordana M, Grahern FL, Gauldie J. Transfer of granulocyte-macrophage colony-stimulating factor gene to rat induces eosinophilia, monocytosis and fibrotic lesions. J Clin Invest 1996; 97:1102–1110.

138. Demoly P, Mathieu M, Curiel DT, Godard P, Bousquet J, Michel FB. Gene therapy strategies for asthma. Gene Ther 1997; 4:507–516.
139. Nyce JW, Metzger WJ. DNA antisense therapy for asthma in an animal model. Nature 1997; 385:721–725.
140. Metzger WJ, Nyce JW. Oligonucleotide therapy of allergic asthma. J Allergy Clin Immunol 1999; 104:260–266.
141. Lander ES, Linton LM, Birren B, Nusbaum C, Zody MC, Baldwin J, Devon K, Dewar K, Doyle M, FitzHugh W, Funke R, Gage D, Harris K, Heaford A, Howland J, Kann L, Lehoczky J, LeVine R, McEwan P, McKernan K, et al. Initial sequencing and analysis of the human genome. Nature 2001; 409:860–921.
142. Palmer LJ, Cookson WO. Genomic approaches to understanding asthma. Genome Res 2000; 10:1280–1287.
143. Drazen JM, Yandava CN, Dube L, Szczerback N, Hippensteel R, Pillari A, Israel E, Schork N, Silverman ES, Katz DA, Drajesk J. Pharmacogenetic association between ALOX5 promoter genotype and the response to anti-asthma treatment. Nat Genet 1999; 22:168–170.

AUTHOR INDEX

Italic numbers give the page on which the complete reference is cited.

A

B

C

D

E

F

I

K

M

N

O

P

Q

R

X

Y

Z

SUBJECT INDEX

B

D

E

H

I

J

K

N

O

P

T

V

W

Z